Biomarkers in Health and Medicine

Biomarkers in Health and Medicine

Edited by Ralph Bowen

hayle medical
New York

Hayle Medical,
750 Third Avenue, 9th Floor,
New York, NY 10017, USA

Visit us on the World Wide Web at:
www.haylemedical.com

ISBN: 978-1-63241-525-7

Printed in China.

Cataloging-in-Publication Data

Biomarkers in health and medicine / edited by Ralph Bowen.
p. cm.
Includes bibliographical references and index.
ISBN 978-1-63241-525-7
1. Biochemical markers. 2. Health. 3. Medicine. I. Bowen, Ralph.

R853.B54 B56 2018
572.8--dc23

Table of Contents

Preface

Biomarkers are the biological indicators of any biological state. They are usually used in detecting, screening, diagnosis and treatment of varied diseases. Biomarkers are also used to evaluate the therapeutic effect of specific pharmaceutical drugs. This book unfolds the innovative aspects of biomarkers which will be crucial for the progress of this field in the future. For someone with an interest and eye for detail, this book covers the most significant topics in the field of biomarkers.

After months of intensive research and writing, this book is the end result of all who devoted their time and efforts in the initiation and progress of this book. It will surely be a source of reference in enhancing the required knowledge of the new developments in the area. During the course of developing this book, certain measures such as accuracy, authenticity and research focused analytical studies were given preference in order to produce a comprehensive book in the area of study.

This book would not have been possible without the efforts of the authors and the publisher. I extend my sincere thanks to them. Secondly, I express my gratitude to my family and well-wishers. And most importantly, I thank my students for constantly expressing their willingness and curiosity in enhancing their knowledge in the field, which encourages me to take up further research projects for the advancement of the area.

Editor

1

Exposure to Organochlorine Pollutants and Type 2 Diabetes

Mengling Tang[1], Kun Chen[2], Fangxing Yang[1], Weiping Liu[1]*

1 MOE Key Laboratory of Environmental Remediation and Ecosystem Health, College of Environmental and Resource Sciences, Zhejiang University, Hangzhou, China, **2** Department of Epidemiology & Health Statistics, School of Public Health, Zhejiang University, Hangzhou, China

Abstract

Objective: Though exposure to organochlorine pollutants (OCPs) is considered a risk factor for type 2 diabetes (T2DM), epidemiological evidence for the association remains controversial. A systematic review and meta-analysis was applied to quantitatively evaluate the association between exposure to OCPs and incidence of T2DM and pool the inconsistent evidence.

Design and Methods: Publications in English were searched in MEDLINE and WEB OF SCIENCE databases and related reference lists up to August 2013. Quantitative estimates and information regarding study characteristics were extracted from 23 original studies. Quality assessments of external validity, bias, exposure measurement and confounding were performed, and subgroup analyses were conducted to examine the heterogeneity sources.

Results: We retrieved 23 eligible articles to conduct this meta-analysis. OR (odds ratio) or RR (risk ratio) estimates in each subgroup were discussed, and the strong associations were observed in PCB-153 (OR, 1.52; 95% CI, 1.19–1.94), PCBs (OR, 2.14; 95% CI, 1.53–2.99), and *p,p'*-DDE (OR, 1.33; 95% CI, 1.15–1.54) based on a random-effects model.

Conclusions: This meta-analysis provides quantitative evidence supporting the conclusion that exposure to organochlorine pollutants is associated with an increased risk of incidence of T2DM.

Editor: Noel Christopher Barengo, University of Tolima, Colombia

Funding: This study was supported by the National Natural Science Foundations of China (21177112, 21320102007). The funders had no role in study design, data collection and analysis, decision to publish, or preparation of the manuscript.

Competing Interests: The authors have declared that no competing interests exist.

* Email: wliu@zju.edu.cn

Introduction

Organochlorine pollutants (OCPs), represented by DDT (Dichlorodiphenyltrichloroethane) and PCBs (Polychlorinated biphenyls), are environmental contaminates of global concern because of their potential for bio-accumulate and bio-magnify in ecosystems and hazardous effects on human health. Though DDT and PCBs were forbidden in most countries in the 1970s [1] and 1980s [2], and the concentrations of these chemicals in the environment, organisms and human tissues were decreasing over the past 30 years, they can still be detected due to their characteristics of persistency, semi-volatility, lipid solubility, bioaccumulation and biomagnification [1]. In Ghana, DDE (Dichlorodiphenyldichloroethylene) was detected at the highest levels among DDT isomers at 44.8 and 7.1 ng/g in breast milk and serum, respectively [3]. In China, PCBs were detected at 0.9 ng/g in lipid in the placentas of women who had pregnancies affected by neural tube defects and at levels of 0.87 ng/g in lipid controls [4].

Type 2 diabetes mellitus (T2DM), formerly called adult-onset diabetes, is a noninsulin-dependent diabetes that accounts for 90–95% of all diabetes cases [5]. As a result of a metabolic disorder of glucose, T2DM has become a major global epidemic in recent years, and its prevalence will likely double over the next 20 years [6]. World Health Organization (WHO) projects that diabetes will be the 7th leading cause of death in 2030. The prevalence of T2DM may be affected by the interaction of conventional risk factors and a combination of genetic susceptibility [7], metabolic syndromes such as obesity [8] and hypertension [9], age, race, and poor diet. In addition, the accumulation of environmental pollutants in the human body has been suggested to have a significant contribution to the disease [10].

Within different populations, the positive associations were observed in the epidemiological studies about T2DM risk exposure to OCPs [11,12]. The associations may be attributed to certain mechanisms of the active ingredients of OCPs, such as γ-aminobutyric acid, which affect the neurotransmitter or ion channel systems involved in regulating pancreatic function and then influence glucose homeostasis [13]. Toxic effects through direct binding and activation of the aryl hydrocarbon receptor (AhR) pathway [14] and mediation through AhR-independent oxidative stress and mitochondrial dysfunction [15] have also been reported as biological mechanisms. Furthermore, toxic effects on estrogen receptor, peroxisome proliferator-activated receptor γ (PPARγ), and progesterone receptor were considered other mechanisms. However, the pathogenesis of exposure to OCPs is currently obscure.

To our knowledge, there have been many epidemiological studies regarding the association between exposure to OCPs and the prevalence of T2DM. However, the results showed contradictory. In order to fully evaluate and characterize the association and fill the vacancy of epidemiological evidence in the comprehensive summary, we performed a sub-group meta-analysis of the results of T2DM risk from exposure to OCPs. We systematically analyzed all studies on T2DM risk from exposure to OCPs up to August 2013.

Methods

Study Identification

We reported the meta-analysis according to the Preferred Reporting Items for Systematic Reviews and Meta-analyses (PRISMA) [16] (Checklist S1). Publications about epidemiological evidence of T2DM risk from exposure to OCPs were identified by a search on MEDLINE (National Library of Medicine, Bethesda, MD) and WEB OF SCIENCE databases. A preliminary total of 116 related studies published up to August 2013 were selected using various combinations of the following keywords: "diabetes", "DDE", "DDT", "PCB", and "organochlorine" with no restriction of publication type and date. The reference lists of the relevant publications identified were checked for additional studies and the recent articles in relevant journals were also scanned to identify other potential studies. The whole search was limited to studies published in English in the open literature in peer-reviewed journals.

Criteria for Inclusion

The systematic review and identification of eligible studies was performed. The titles and abstracts were screened to determine their relevance to the diabetes effects of humans when exposed to OCPs. The full text of potentially relevant studies was then examined and the eligibility criteria were applied to select the included studies.

A publication was considered eligible for review if it fulfilled the following six inclusion criteria. (1) It must be an original epidemiologic study using a case-control, cross-sectional, or prospective study design and other types of reviews, meta-analysis, case-reports, comments, letters, editorials, abstracts were excluded. (2) Papers should be written in the English language. (3) OCP exposure levels had to be measured in actual tissue samples (serum or serum lipid), not by environmental data or other indirect ways. (4) It unequivocally reported measures of association, including odds ratios (OR) and relative risk (RR) and confidence intervals (CIs) for diabetes risk and also considered papers that did not report these measures directly, but were able to extrapolate the relevant values. (5) Studies should use biomarkers of OCPs within our selected ones including PCB-153, PCBs, and *p,p'*-DDE, while others OCPs, for instance, using PCB-126 as the biomarker, were not included. (6) In addition, T2DM was confirmed by self-report or hospital diagnosis, and diseases related to T2DM as insulin resistence were excluded. Finally, 23 epidemiological studies were extracted for further systematic analysis.

Data Extraction

The authors examined the articles and independently extracted and tabulated the information. A standard data abstraction form was created to record the following information for each suitable article: first author name, year of publication, geographic region of the studies, epidemiologic design, subject selection, exposure pathways, type of OCP, biologic specimens, number of cases and controls, and a risk index calculated with the categories of the exposure and referent, corresponding 95% CI for T2DM. The risk indexes, adjusted for different confounding such as sex, BMI, cigarette smoking, and the ones stratified by age and sex were all extracted. The results of this abstraction were compared between the authors and consensus was obtained before the meta-analysis.

Stratification of the data were performed focusing on several variables that could influence the results, including exposure levels (background or high concentration exposure), study design (case-control, perspective, or cross-sectional study), population selection (general population or women), and biologic specimen (serum or serum lipid).

Quality Assessment

In order to assess evidence, all included studies underwent an independent quality assessment modified from the versions of the 1998 Downs and Black [17] and Wigle et al. checklists [18]. We discussed the individual items on the checklist to clarify their interpretation before conducting the quality assessment. The same to the version made by the latter group, we also added exposure measurement as the internal validity assessment to the checklist of quality assessment. However, some items that were either related only to reporting or were not applicable were removed from the checklist. No attempt was made to blind the reviewers of the authorship or publication status of the original studies. The evaluated factors including the representativeness of the selected participants, bias, and confounding were given a mark to assess the article quality. Finally, a total of 13 items and 16 scores were listed (Table S1). The results with higher scores were considered to be of superior quality. Differences in quality assessment were resolved by consensus.

Data Analysis

The heterogeneity across individual studies was quantified by the Q-test and I^2-test: when the result of the Q-test showed evidence of the heterogeneity ($p<0.1$), we used the random-effect analysis; otherwise, the I^2-test, which interpreted I^2 values of 25%, 50%, 75% as low, moderate, and high degrees of heterogeneity respectively, was used to assess heterogeneity. This is because the Q-test has low statistical power with few studies [19] and the fixed-effect analysis was conducted when $I^2<25\%$. $p<0.10$ or $I^2>25\%$ was considered significant heterogeneity which questions the validity of pooled estimates. The I^2 describes the percentage of total variation across studies due to heterogeneity rather than chance [20]. When heterogeneity exists, subgroup analyses were conducted to investigate potential sources of heterogeneity.

The risk estimates of OR or RR were combined for the evaluation of the dose-response relation between OCP exposure and T2DM prevalence. We assumed similarity between the OR and RR. When combined these binary variables, we aimed to choose the ones calculated between the highest exposed group and the references and the ones with the most adjusted variables. We attempted to combine adjusted OR or RR from primary studies, but if not possible, we pooled raw outcome data to yield unadjusted OR. In addition, we combined the risk estimates which were calculated by OCPs concentrations tested in serum lipid, otherwise we choose the values tested directly in serum. We considered all the OR stratified by ages and by BMI in each study. To conduct meta-analyses, we defined the least group as 4 articles with risk estimates [21], which corresponded to a minimum of 100 cases of T2DM.

We performed meta-analyses using Review Manager (RevMan) version 5.0 (Nordic Cochrane Centre, Cochrane Collaboration, Copenhagen, Denmark) to evaluate the overall risk of T2DM caused by exposure to OCPs. For the risk estimates presented as a binary variable, such as OR and RR, the inverse of variance for fixed-effects models using the Mantel-Haenszel [22] method which assumes that results across studies differ only by sampling error. The DerSimonian and Laird method [23] for random-effects models were used to combine the overall binaries and their corresponding 95% CI. The results of meta-analysis including all subgroup analysis were illustrated by forest plots.

Publication bias due to study size was investigated by visual inspection of funnel plots which showed the natural logarithm of the estimate of RR (lnRR) versus the inverse of standard error (1/SE). Funnel plot asymmetry can be illustrated by factors as the non-publication of small studies with negative results, differences in study quality and study heterogeneity.

To determine whether some of the decisions we made had a major impact on the results of the review, sensitivity analyses were conducted by (1) removing studies with the highest and lowest percentage weight in all included studies, (2) deleting studies with highest and lowest quality scores, (3) excluding studies reporting the lowest or highest estimator of binary variables.

Results

Study Characteristics

The searching process and selection studies was performed in Figure 1 and the characteristics of the 23 included studies [12,24,25,26,27,28,29,30,31,32,33,34,35,36,37,38,39,40,41,42,43-,44,45] are summarized in Table 1. Among the 32 related epidemiological studies, 2 were excluded because of their examination of other diseases related to T2DM [46,47]; 4 were removed because of the absence of dichotomous variables, OR or RR, and the CI [48,49,50,51]; 2 were excluded because the biomarkers were *p,p'*-DDT, PCB-126 [52] and PCB-170 [10], and not the ones (*p,p'*-DDE, PCBs, PCB-153) we selected for this study; and 1 was excluded because of the combination of both type 1 and type 2 diabetes [53].

From the 23 remaining studies, 1 were case-control studies [54], 18 were cross-sectional studies [24,25,26,27,28,29,30,31,32,33,35,36,37,38,39,40,41,42,44], and only 4 study was a prospective study [12,34,43,45]. 10 studies were conducted in the United States [12,25,26,32,34,38,40,41,45], 4 in Sweden [30,36,39,42], and the rest were conducted in Japan [27], the Faroe Islands [28], Korea [31], Slovakia [33], Canada [35], Belgium [43], Taiwan, China [37], Spain [24,44], and Finland [29].

13 studies used PCB-153 [24,26,27,29,30,34,35,36,38,39,41,42,45], 11 studies used PCBs [12,24,25,26,28,33,35,37,38,44,45] and 18 studies used *p,p'*-DDE as a biomarker [24,28,29,30,31,32,33,35,36,38,39,40,41,42,44,45]. Among these studies, different models were established to assess the OR or RR, and the related CI was adjusted by confounders such as age, body mass index (BMI), sex, or other factors. 2 studies estimated body burden levels of OCPs in both wet weight values (serum sample) and lipid-standardized values (serum lipid sample) [35,38]. In addition, 2 studies estimated the OR or RR of both men and women [25,37], and 1 study discussed the groups under and over the age of 55 years and also the total group separately [25]. The risk estimates from Wu et al. were obtained from two independent study [45].

In most studies, the study population was selected by background exposure to OCPs [24,27,29,30,31,32,34,36,38,40,41,43,44,45]. However, aquatic product exposure [12,28,35,39,42], heavy pollution area exposure [25,26,33], and specific diet exposure, such as rice-bran oil exposure [37], were also estimated in some studies. As a susceptible population, women were selected [36,39,45] in 3 studies. 6 studies collected serum as biologic specimens [12,24,25,30,36,37], while 12 chose serum lipids [26,28,29,32,33,34,39,41,42,43,44,45]. 5 studies detected the pollutants in both serum and serum lipid specimens [27,31,35,38,40].

Quality Assessment

The quality factor scores for the 23 studies are listed (Table S2). From the results of the quality assessment, all the included epidemiological studies accorded with most of the quality criteria we listed, but the items of participation rate, blind laboratory testing, data dredging, specific exposure measurement, and adequate adjustment for confounding were different among the original studies. The total quality scores were in the range from 9 to 14 with a possible maximum score of 16, reflecting the existing of study design limitations. More recent studies tended to have higher quality scores. Among these studies, only 4 studies had the external validity that participation rate for cases and controls reaches 70% [34,36,40,43]. Only 3 studies reported having made an attempt to blind those measuring the main outcomes of the OCPs exposure [29,31,37]. Most of the included studies got the scores of other 11 items.

Main Analysis

23 studies, contributing a total of 73 OR or RR estimators met the inclusion criteria and were taken into consideration. When combining the main data of all studies, the exposure to all 3 biomarkers showed positive associations with the prevalence of T2DM. The combined OR estimate of PCB-153 was 1.52 (95% CI, 1.19–1.94), for PCBs was 2.14 (95% CI, 1.53–2.99), and for *p,p'*-DDE was 1.33 (95% CI, 1.15–1.54) based on a random-effects model. Forest plots of the 3 organochlorine biomarkers, which show the weight of each study and the combined OR estimates, are provided in Figure 2. Considering the high evidence of heterogeneity for PCB-153 ($I^2 = 64\%$), PCBs ($I^2 = 59\%$) and *p,p'*-DDE ($I^2 = 56\%$), subgroup meta-analyses were conducted for the OR combining and further analyses of sources of heterogeneity. The results for the meta-analyses of 3 organochlorine biomarkers (PCB-153, PCBs, and *p,p'*-DDE) and their subgroups were analyzed and are summarized in Table 2.

Subgroup and Sensitivity Analyses

From the characteristics summary of the epidemiological studies, exposure levels (background or high concentration exposure), study design (case-control or cross-sectional study), population selection (general population or women), and biologic specimen (serum or serum lipid) were chosen as the stratifications for subgroup analyses to find the sources of heterogeneity.

For PCB-153, the exposure subgroup analyses may not be a heterogeneity source from the increased results of I^2 test. When the studies were stratified by the study design, heterogeneity and inconsistency among the epidemiological studies were eliminated in the perspective subgroup ($I^2 = 0\%$). When the studies were divided by the sex of the population, the consistency was observed among the women subgroup ($I^2 = 0\%$) and the heterogeneity between studies remained high for general population group ($I^2 = 71\%$). Finally, when the studies were stratified by biologic specimen, the high inconsistencies in both the serum ($I^2 = 74\%$) and serum lipid subgroup ($I^2 = 67\%$) also existed.

For PCBs, the background exposure subgroup ($I^2 = 30\%$) the subgroup of serum specimen exposure ($I^2 = 8\%$) resulted in a statistically decreasing heterogeneities from the total studies ($I^2 = 64\%$). The subgroup analysis of the case-control subgroup ($I^2 = 55\%$, n = 2 only), general population ($I^2 = 59\%$) and women

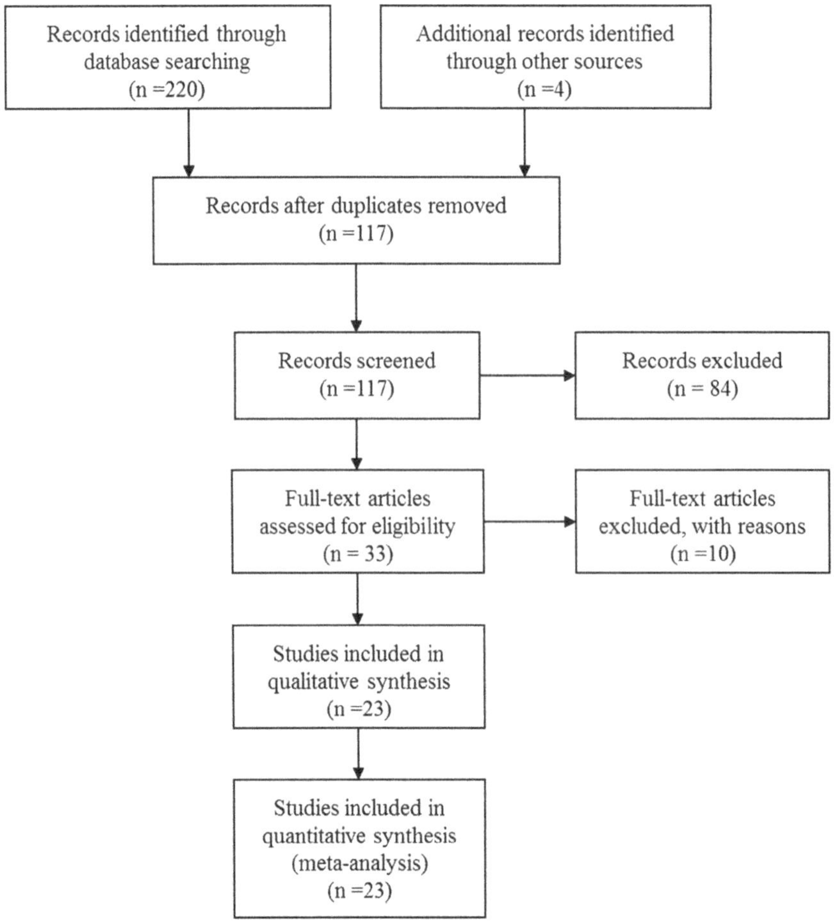

Figure 1. The study search and selection process.

population ($I^2 = 74\%$) gave the result that they still had relatively high heterogeneity.

The subgroup of background exposure from *p,p'*-DDE showed decreased heterogeneity ($I^2 = 25\%$) compared with total studies ($I^2 = 56\%$), and a risk factor was found from the combined OR (OR, 1.49; 95% CI, 1.18–1.88). Decreased heterogeneity was also found in the perspective group ($I^2 = 0\%$) and women subgroup ($I^2 = 0\%$) with a combined OR of 1.16 (95% CI, 0.87–1.55) and 1.27 (95% CI, 1.10–1.46). The heterogeneities in subgroups classified by biologic specimen were still in relatively high levels.

In general, findings from each sensitivity analysis did not substantially alter the results of the overall pooled estimate OR using the random effects model in direction and magnitude. Exclusion of the studies with the highest and lowest percentage weight, the highest and lowest quality scores, and the lowest or highest estimator of OR performed consistently with the pooled estimator OR for all indicators, including PCB-153, PCBs, and *p,p'*-DDE (data not shown).

Publication Bias

A funnel plot of standard error (SE) versus ln(OR) for the meta-analyses of the relationships between OCPs and T2DM, in which the number of studies was more than 10, are presented in Figure 3. Visual inspection of the funnel plot suggests that risk estimates stemmed mostly from large, precise studies, which are distributed in the superior part of the figure; however, possible publication bias was found from the evidence of asymmetry of some subgroup meta-analyses. Additionally, exclusion of studies published with non-English and other factors such as differences in study quality or heterogeneity, sample size, and study design may be other reasons for the asymmetries of the funnel plots.

Discussion

While a large number of studies about the association between OCPs exposure and the prevalence of T2DM were published, only few cohort studies are available. Among these studies, inconsistency was found among most of these epidemiological studies in different populations and different sources of exposure. However, our combined estimates of meta-analyses demonstrated a modest but statistically significant increase in the odds of T2DM with exposure to OCPs. For instance, a 52% increase of T2DM resulted from an exposure to PCB-153. In addition, all subgroup analyses stratified by exposure levels, design of the studies, study subjects and biologic specimen resulted in positive correlations. The consistency in the magnitude of increased risk indicates that this is unlikely to be a chance finding and these increased risks support the suggestion that exposure to OCPs may be a potential causal factor for prevalence of T2DM.

To determine the sources of heterogeneity of the studies and obtain the pooled estimates of PCBs, PCB-153, and *p,p'*-DDE in subgroups, subgroup analysis was conducted by stratified exposure levels, study designs, study subjects and biologic specimens.

Table 1. Study characteristics.

Reference	Country	Study design	age	Exposure pathway	biomarker	Biologic specimen	Cases/controls	OR or RR (95%CI)
Arrebola2013	Spain	Cross-sectional	16-	Background	*p,p'*-DDE	Serum lipid	34/352	1.69(0.54–5.22)[a]
Wu2012	USA	Prospective	30–55	Nurses	PCB-153	Serum lipid	10/214	2.19(0.72–6.68)[a]
			30–55	Nurses	PCB-153	Serum lipid	6/135	0.76(0.22–2.60)[a]
			30–55	Nurses	PCBs	Serum lipid	9/215	1.30(0.43–3.93)[a]
			30–55	Nurses	PCBs	Serum lipid	7/134	0.79(0.23–2.71)[a]
			30–55	Nurses	*p,p'*-DDE	Serum lipid	9/215	1.32(0.41–4.27)[a]
			30–55	Nurses	*p,p'*-DDE	Serum lipid	10/131	1.79(0.54–5.86)[a]
Persky2012	USA	Cross-sectional	35-	Electrical utilities company men	PCB-153	Serum lipid	7/56	3.1(1.2–7.8)[a]
			35-	Electrical utilities company men	PCBs	Serum lipid	7/56	3.0(1.3–7.2)[a]
Gasull2012	Spain	Cross-sectional	18–74	Background	PCB-153	Serum	77/192	1.6(1.2–2.4)[a]
			18–74	Background	PCBs	Serum	77/193	1.7(1.1–2.6)[a]
			18–74	Background	*p,p'*-DDE	Serum	73/207	1.1(0.7–1.7)[a]
Silverstone2012	USA	Cross-sectional	18-	PCBs plant area	PCBs	Serum	78/157	2.78(1.00–7.73)
			18–55	PCBs plant area	PCBs	Serum	27/111	4.78(1.11–20.6)
			55-	PCBs plant area	PCBs	Serum	51/47	4.19(0.26–68.12)
Lee 2011	Sweden	Prospective	70	background	PCB-153	Serum	12/277	1.7(0.5–6.2)
			70	background	*p,p'*-DDE	Serum	16/271	2.1(0.7–6.3)
Airaksinen2011	Finland	Cross-sectional	70	background	PCB-153	Serum lipid	69/398	1.64(0.92–2.93)[b]
			70	background	PCB-153	Serum lipid	10/121	1.03(0.25–4.18)[b]
			70	background	PCB-153	Serum lipid	23/184	1.97(0.75–5.23)[b]
			70	background	PCB-153	Serum lipid	36/93	2.3(0.87–6.11)[b]
			70	background	*p,p'*-DDE	Serum lipid	62/398	1.75(0.96–3.19)[b]
			70	background	*p,p'*-DDE	Serum lipid	7/120	0.88(0.18–4.35)[b]
			70	background	*p,p'*-DDE	Serum lipid	18/175	1.91(0.69–5.27)[b]
			70	background	*p,p'*-DDE	Serum lipid	37/103	1.82(0.71–4.65)[b]
Tanaka 2011	Japan	Cross-sectional	40–64	background	PCB-153	Serum	32/85	0.95(0.90–1.00)[a]
			40–64	background	PCB-153	Serum lipid	32/85	0.73(0.51–1.07)
Grandjean2011	Faroe Islands	Cross-sectional	70–74	Aquatic product	PCBs	Serum lipid	168/544	1.11(0.91–1.35)[a]
			70–74	Aquatic product	*p,p'*-DDE	Serum lipid	168/544	1.01(0.87–1.16)[a]
Son2010	Korea	Cross-sectional	40-	Background	*p,p'*-DDE	Serum	27/26	26.6(2.0–349.1)
			40-	Background	*p,p'*-DDE	Serum lipid	28/26	12.7(1.9–83.7)
Everett2010	USA	Cross-sectional	20-	Background	*p,p'*-DDE	Serum lipid	334/2715	1.08(0.58–2.03)[a]
Ukropec2010	Slovakia	Cross-sectional	21–75	Heavy pollution	PCBs	Serum lipid	120/699	1.86(1.09–3.17)

Table 1. Cont.

Reference	Country	Study design	age	Exposure pathway	biomarker	Biologic specimen	Cases/controls	OR or RR (95%CI)
			21–75	Heavy pollution	*p,p'*-DDE	Serum lipid	125/694	1.94(1.11–3.78)
Lee2010	USA	Perspective	18–30	Background	PCB-153	Serum lipid	39/45	0.8(0.2–2.6)[a]
			18–30	Background	*p,p'*-DDE	Serum lipid	47/45	0.7(0.2–1.9)[a]
Philibert2009	Canada	Cross-sectional	15–86	Aquatic product	PCB-153	Serum	25/101	4.91(1.27–19.01)
			15–86	Aquatic product	PCB-153	Serum lipid	25/101	6.46(2.07–36.63)
			15–86	Aquatic product	PCBs	Serum	25/101	4.91(1.27–19.01)
			15–86	Aquatic product	PCBs	Serum lipid	25/101	5.51(1.26–24.07)
			15–86	Aquatic product	*p,p'*-DDE	Serum	25/101	6.11(1.37–27.3)
			15–86	Aquatic product	*p,p'*-DDE	Serum lipid	25/101	3.56(0.97–13.08)
Rignell-Hydbom2009	Sweden	Prospective	50–59	Background women	PCB-153	Serum	371/371	0.99(0.71–1.4)[c]
			50–59	Background women	PCB-153	Serum	208/208	0.91(0.59–1.4)[c]
			50–59	Background women	PCB-153	Serum	163/163	1.1(0.66–1.9)[c]
			50–59	Background women	PCB-153	Serum	107/107	1.4(0.72–2.6)[c]
			50–59	Background women	PCB-153	Serum	74/74	1.4(0.67–3.1)[c]
			50–59	Background women	PCB-153	Serum	39/39	1.6(0.61–4.0)[c]
			50–59	Background women	*p,p'*-DDE	Serum	371/371	1.1(0.76–1.5)[c]
			50–59	Background women	*p,p'*-DDE	Serum	208/208	0.9(0.57–1.4)[c]
			50–59	Background women	*p,p'*-DDE	Serum	163/163	1.3(0.78–2.2)[c]
			50–59	Background women	*p,p'*-DDE	Serum	107/107	1.5(0.8–2.8)[c]
			50–59	Background women	*p,p'*-DDE	Serum	74/74	2.5(0.97–6.4)[c]
			50–59	Background women	*p,p'*-DDE	Serum	39/39	5.5(1.2–25)[c]
Turyk2009	USA	Prospective	25–76	Aquatic product	*p,p'*-DDE	Serum	24/285	7.1(1.6–31.9)
			25–76	Aquatic product	PCBs	Serum	21/293	1.8(0.6–5.0)
Wang2008	Taiwan, China	Cross-sectional	30-	Rice-bran oil men	PCBs	Serum	155/152	1.7(0.7–4.6)[a]
			30-	Rice-bran oil women	PCBs	Serum	233/218	5.5(2.3–13.4)[a]
Codru2007	USA	Cross-sectional	30-	Background	PCBs	Serum		2.8 (0.7–10.8)[a]
			30-	Background	PCBs	Serum lipid		2.6 (0.8–8.1)[a]
			30-	Background	PCB-153	Serum		3.0 (0.7–12.8)[a]
			30-	Background	PCB-153	Serum lipid		1.4 (0.4–4.8)[a]
			30-	Background	*p,p'*-DDE	Serum		2.6 (0.8–8.8)[a]
			30-	Background	*p,p'*-DDE	Serum lipid		2.4 (0.7–8.3)[a]
Rignell-Hydbom2007	Sweden	Cross-sectional	29–59	Aquatic product women	PCB-153	Serum lipid	15/528	1.4(0.8–2.5)[a]
			29–59	Aquatic product women	*p,p'*-DDE	Serum lipid	15/528	1.3(1.1–1.5)[a]

Table 1. Cont.

Reference	Country	Study design	age	Exposure pathway	biomarker	Biologic specimen	Cases/controls	OR or RR (95%CI)
Cox2007	USA	Cross-sectional	20–74	Background	*p,p'*-DDE	Serum	45/768	2.63(1.2–5.8)[a]
			20–74	Background	*p,p'*-DDE	Serum lipid	35/560	1.5(0.8–2.9)[a]
Lee2006	USA	Cross-sectional	12-	Background	PCB-153	Serum lipid	52/598	6.8(3.0–15.5)
			12-	Background	*p,p'*-DDE	Serum lipid	69/704	4.3(1.8–10.2)
Rylander2005	Sweden	Cross-sectional	49–84	Aquatic product	PCB-153	Serum lipid	22/358	1.16(1.03–1.32)
			49–84	Aquatic product	*p,p'*-DDE	Serum lipid	22/358	1.05(1.01–1.09)
Fierens2003	Belgium	Case-control	50.3–59.4	Background	PCBs	Serum lipid	9/248	7.6(1.58–36.3)

[a]Different models adjusted by confounding, such as sex, age, BMI, total cholesterol and triglycerides, and various compounds.
[b]stratified by BMI.
[c]stratified by the years diagnosed after the baseline investigation.

Specific exposure, such as seafood consumption and living in a high exposure area, did not show an increased risk of T2DM compared with background exposure studies. This result may be attributed to the limited studies of specific exposure and the discrepant results of exposure concentration in serum levels such as 70 to 70000 ng/g and 44.33 to 8863 ng/g PCBs found in a serum lipid in two aquatic food consumption studies [28,35], and 148 to 101413 ng/g PCBs found in a study on serum lipid in a heavily polluted area [33]. Additionally, the heterogeneity analysis indicated that background exposure was a group with smaller heterogeneity and specific exposure with higher heterogeneity for the significant differences of the exposure. With regard to study design and subjects, from the consistent I^2 test results of the subgroup analyses and the limited studies of the perspective study subgroup and women's subgroup, it may not be an obvious heterogeneity source of the meta-analyses for all organochlorine biomarkers in this study. The biologic specimen was considered a heterogeneity source for the decreasing I^2 test results from the serum subgroup.

Some studies preferred express OCP concentrations per weight of lipid rather than on a whole weight for the lipophilic character of the pollutants. Total lipid was defined using different formulas as total lipids (mg/dL) = 2.27×total cholesterol (mg/dL)+triglycerides (mg/dL)+62.3 [31,38] and total lipids = 1.13+1.13×(cholesterol+ triglycerides) [39]. Various definitions of total lipids may be one of the reasons that serum lipid is an obviously heterogeneity source. The gravimetric analysis of cholesterol and triglycerides with different detected method is another labile factor [55]. While, OCPs is lipophilic and likely to concentrate in serum lipid, so many studies used the concentrations based on serum lipid to present the residual levels in humans.

Furthermore, the different exposure contrast used in each study population may also be a larger source of heterogeneity. For instance, some studies [24,33] evaluated the increase in the odds comparing the 80th and the 20th percentiles of OCP concentrations, some studies used the quartiles for the comparison [25,34], while Airaksinen et al. calculated OR on the basis of percentile intervals <10th, 10th to <50th, 50th to <90th, and ≥90th. The diverse categories may cause the great heterogeneity among studies [29].

The original studies may be subject to limitations mainly related to the quality of potential sources of bias, exposure assessment, confounding, and the validity of the enrolled data. The bias in internal validity is most likely attributed to the misclassification of diabetes outcomes that only rely on self-reporting the prevalence of T2DM, the use of oral antidiabetic drugs or insulin, or that patients were on a specific diet [25,30,31,34,37,38,42,43] but lack of an accurate fasting glucose. Publication bias was also among the potential limitations from the evidence of asymmetry of the funnel plot. Some of the studies included in the meta-analysis were based on the same data, meaning that data for some subjects were included twice. For instance, some subjects from NHANES 1999–2004 was used both in the study of Everett et al. [32] and Lee et al. [41] and in both two studies, *p,p'*-DDE concentrations in serum were used as the indicator of the OCPs exposure. This may be a reason of the publication bias. However, this was not enough to negate the overall conclusion of an increased risk based on limited evidence for the deficit in small negative studies with effect sizes smaller than those from larger studies and in non-English published original studies.

It has been argued that exposure measurement is a typical effect factor for the quality of environmental epidemiology studies [56]. Though most studies gave a sufficient exposure gradient in the T2DM risk assessment (a dose-dependent manner across quantiles

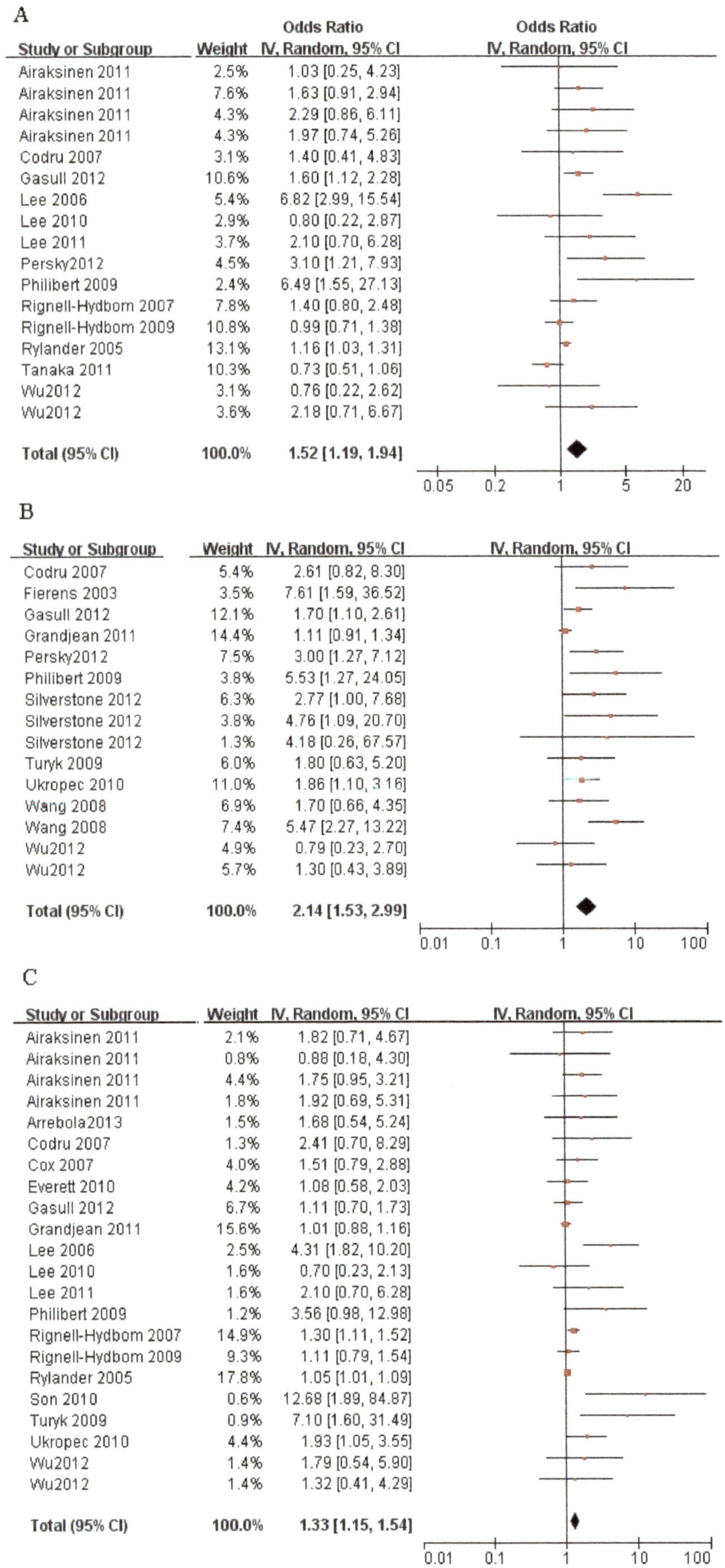
A
Odds Ratio
Odds Ratio
Study or Subgroup Weight IV, Random, 95% CI
IV, Random, 95% CI
Airaksinen 2011 2.5% 1.03 [0.25, 4.23]
Airaksinen 2011 7.6% 1.63 [0.91, 2.94]
Airaksinen 2011 4.3% 2.29 [0.86, 6.11]
Airaksinen 2011 4.3% 1.97 [0.74, 5.26]
Codru 2007 3.1% 1.40 [0.41, 4.83]
Gasull 2012 10.6% 1.60 [1.12, 2.28]
Lee 2006 5.4% 6.82 [2.99, 15.54]
Lee 2010 2.9% 0.80 [0.22, 2.87]
Lee 2011 3.7% 2.10 [0.70, 6.28]
Persky2012 4.5% 3.10 [1.21, 7.93]
Philibert 2009 2.4% 6.49 [1.55, 27.13]
Rignell-Hydbom 2007 7.8% 1.40 [0.80, 2.48]
Rignell-Hydbom 2009 10.8% 0.99 [0.71, 1.38]
Rylander 2005 13.1% 1.16 [1.03, 1.31]
Tanaka 2011 10.3% 0.73 [0.51, 1.06]
Wu2012 3.1% 0.76 [0.22, 2.62]
Wu2012 3.6% 2.18 [0.71, 6.67]
Total (95% CI) 100.0% 1.52 [1.19, 1.94]
0.05
0.2
1
5
20
B
Study or Subgroup Weight IV, Random, 95% CI
IV, Random, 95% CI
Codru 2007 5.4% 2.61 [0.82, 8.30]
Fierens 2003 3.5% 7.61 [1.59, 36.52]
Gasull 2012 12.1% 1.70 [1.10, 2.61]
Grandjean 2011 14.4% 1.11 [0.91, 1.34]
Persky2012 7.5% 3.00 [1.27, 7.12]
Philibert 2009 3.8% 5.53 [1.27, 24.05]
Silverstone 2012 6.3% 2.77 [1.00, 7.68]
Silverstone 2012 3.8% 4.76 [1.09, 20.70]
Silverstone 2012 1.3% 4.18 [0.26, 67.57]
Turyk 2009 6.0% 1.80 [0.63, 5.20]
Ukropec 2010 11.0% 1.86 [1.10, 3.16]
Wang 2008 6.9% 1.70 [0.66, 4.35]
Wang 2008 7.4% 5.47 [2.27, 13.22]
Wu2012 4.9% 0.79 [0.23, 2.70]
Wu2012 5.7% 1.30 [0.43, 3.89]
Total (95% CI) 100.0% 2.14 [1.53, 2.99]
0.01
0.1
1
10
100
C
Study or Subgroup Weight IV, Random, 95% CI
IV, Random, 95% CI
Airaksinen 2011 2.1% 1.82 [0.71, 4.67]
Airaksinen 2011 0.8% 0.88 [0.18, 4.30]
Airaksinen 2011 4.4% 1.75 [0.95, 3.21]
Airaksinen 2011 1.8% 1.92 [0.69, 5.31]
Arrebola2013 1.5% 1.68 [0.54, 5.24]
Codru 2007 1.3% 2.41 [0.70, 8.29]
Cox 2007 4.0% 1.51 [0.79, 2.88]
Everett 2010 4.2% 1.08 [0.58, 2.03]
Gasull 2012 6.7% 1.11 [0.70, 1.73]
Grandjean 2011 15.6% 1.01 [0.88, 1.16]
Lee 2006 2.5% 4.31 [1.82, 10.20]
Lee 2010 1.6% 0.70 [0.23, 2.13]
Lee 2011 1.6% 2.10 [0.70, 6.28]
Philibert 2009 1.2% 3.56 [0.98, 12.98]
Rignell-Hydbom 2007 14.9% 1.30 [1.11, 1.52]
Rignell-Hydbom 2009 9.3% 1.11 [0.79, 1.54]
Rylander 2005 17.8% 1.05 [1.01, 1.09]
Son 2010 0.6% 12.68 [1.89, 84.87]
Turyk 2009 0.9% 7.10 [1.60, 31.49]
Ukropec 2010 4.4% 1.93 [1.05, 3.55]
Wu2012 1.4% 1.79 [0.54, 5.90]
Wu2012 1.4% 1.32 [0.41, 4.29]
Total (95% CI) 100.0% 1.33 [1.15, 1.54]
0.01
0.1
1
10
100

Figure 2. Subgroup analysis forest plots of the studies on T2DM risk from exposure to all three biomarkers. *(A)* Result of exposure to PCB-153. *(B)* Result of exposure to PCBs. *(C)* Result of exposure to *p,p'*-DDE.

of the exposure levels), multiple quantile categories, such as tertile [31,44,45], quartile [24], quintile [25], percentile intervals [29] were used for the OR estimate via setting the lowest quantile or percentile intervals as the reference. Another limitation is the unspecific exposure measurements. In the present meta-analysis, we selected representative PCB-153, PCBs, and *p,p'*-DDE as the biomarkers. For PCBs, 209 congeners existed in the environment, and the selection of the representatives PCBs varied among studies. For instance, 15 PCB congeners were selected in a study on high level exposure [33], while another study conducted in a

Table 2. Subgroup analysis of the included epidemiological studies.

Subgroup	NO. of studies	Weight	Summary OR (95%CI)	Q test (p)	I^2
PCB-153					
Background exposure	10	76.6%	1.57(1.13–2.19)	0.0004	65%
Specific exposure	3	23.4%	-	0.05	66%
Total	13	100%	1.52(1.19–1.94)	0.0002	64%
Perspective study	4	23.5%	1.05(0.78–1.40)	0.60	0%
Cross-sectional study	9	76.5%	1.69(1.24–2.31)	<0.0001	72%
Total	13	100%	1.50(1.18–1.92)	0.0002	63%
General population	10	74.7%	1.69(1.23–2.33)	<0.0001	71%
Women	3	25.3%	1.11(0.85–1.46)	0.41	0%
Total	13	100%	1.52(1.19–1.94)	0.0002	64%
Serum	6	38.8%	1.36(0.95–1.95)	0.002	74%
Serum lipid	10	61.2%	1.62(1.18–2.24)	0.0002	67%
Total	13	100%	1.44(1.18–1.76)	<0.00001	74%
PCBs					
Background exposure	4	31.6%	1.74(1.22–2.48)[a]	0.22	30%
Specific exposure	7	68.4%	2.39(1.52–3.77)	0.001	67%
Total	11	100%	2.14(1.53–2.99)	0.002	59%
Case-control study	2	10.9%	2.83(1.18–6.81)[a]	0.14	55%
Cross-sectional study	8	89.1%	2.28(1.55–3.34)	0.001	66%
Total	10	100%	2.36(1.64–3.41)	0.0008	64%
General population	9	80.4%	2.18(1.50–3.16)	0.006	59%
Women	2	19.6%	1.88(0.56–6.26)	0.02	74%
Total	11	100%	2.19(1.54–3.13)	0.001	62%
Serum	6	48.3%	2.31(1.71–3.11)[a]	0.36	8%
Serum lipid	7	51.7%	1.91(1.20–3.04)	0.009	62%
Total	11	100%	2.24(1.62–3.10)	0.001	58%
p,p'-DDE					
Background exposure	12	45.2%	1.39(1.16–1.67)[a]	0.18	25%
Specific exposure	6	54.8%	1.20(1.01–1.43)	0.001	75%
Total	18	100%	1.33(1.15–1.54)	0.0007	56%
Perspective study	4	14.7%	1.16(0.87–1.55)[a]	0.64	0%
Cross-sectional study	13	85.3%	1.33(1.13–1.56)	0.0006	62%
Total	17	100%	1.29(1.12–1.48)	0.003	52%
General population	15	72.9%	1.41(1.17–1.71)	0.0008	59%
Women	3	27.1%	1.27(1.10–1.46)[a]	0.79	0%
Total	18	100%	1.33(1.15–1.54)	0.0007	56%
Serum	8	24.4%	2.22(1.32–3.73)	0.005	66%
Serum lipid	14	75.6%	1.34(1.14–1.57)	0.001	58%
Total	18	100%	1.45(1.24–1.70)	<0.0001	62%

[a]Based on fixed model, others based on random model.

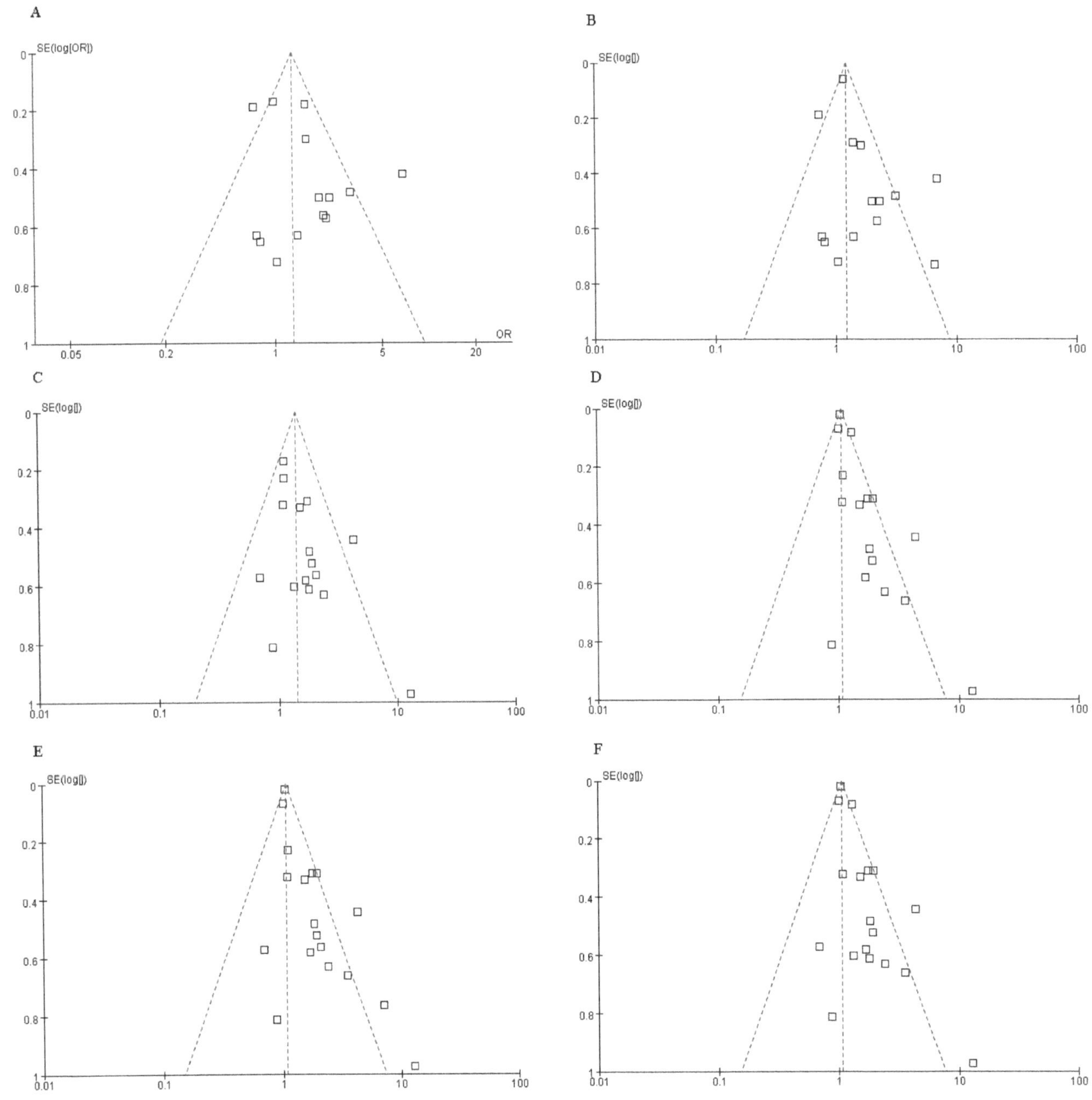

Figure 3. A funnel plot of SE versus ln(OR) for the meta-analyses. (*A*) Funnel plot for the meta-analysis on T2DM from background exposure to PCB-153. (*B*) Funnel plot for the subgroup analysis of serum lipid on T2DM from exposure to PCB-153. (*C*) Funnel plot for the subgroup analysis on T2DM from background exposure to *p,p'*-DDE. (*D*) Funnel plot for the subgroup analysis of the cross-sectional study on T2DM from exposure to *p,p'*-DDE. (*E*) Funnel plot for the subgroup analysis of the general population on T2DM from exposure to *p,p'*-DDE. (*F*) Funnel plot for the subgroup analysis of serum lipid on T2DM from exposure to *p,p'*-DDE.

fish consumption group selected only 8 PCB congeners as representatives of PCBs [35].

Confounding is also a potentially limited factor. Relevant confounders were selected from different adjusted models including basic demographics such as age, sex, and BMI and other major covariates, such as serum lipids, serum triglycerides, total cholesterol, fish consumption, smoking and alcohol. Models that were adjusted differently, including crude estimates, models with basic demographic variables, and models with all major confounders, led to discrepancies in the estimated OR. In the present meta-analyses, we selected the models with the most confounders which may give more accurate effects values to create pooled OR estimates. For instance, in a marine food consumption study, the model with basic demographic and all of the major confounders, was set and adjusted to evaluate the OR estimates [28].

Other than bias, exposure measurement, and confounding, the effect of the validity of the enrolled data is important. When outcome of interest was rare, such as the prevalence of cancer or birth defect, one can generally ignore the distinctions among the various measures of relative risk [57]. According to statistical data from the Ministry of Health of The People's Republic of China, the prevalence of T2DM were about 5 times the prevalence of cancer. In this study, we combined the binary variables of OR and RR. Considering the high prevalence of T2DM, the data processing may impact the consequence of the meta-analysis.

From the systematic screening of the relevant studies about the prevalence of T2DM exposure to OCPs, we found several other systematic reviews [58,59,60]. However, this study was the first meta-analysis to our knowledge to evaluate the pooled effect values. A previous systematic review assessed the risk for developing T2DM from exposure to organochlorine pesticides [58] but only analyzed the results at the qualitative and quantitative levels. Although the positive relationships were the same as our results, many limitations and uncertainties were proposed in that review. Exposure to OCPs cannot be concluded as being the only contributor to the prevalence of T2DM, and many factors other than exposure to OCPs may be causative for T2DM, such as obesity, race, gender, age, genetic susceptibility, dietary habits and lifestyle. From another review that discussed the impacts of OCPs on metabolic health [60], no associations between OCPs exposures and stages of glucose intolerance or markers of insulin resistance were observed [61]. This specific result is not in our meta-analysis because of the misclassification of T2DM outcomes, which may cause bias in our study. Additionally, a cross-sectional study conducted in Swedish [51] found that none of the PCB congeners selected were significantly associated with diabetes in age, BMI, weight change and region adjusted analyses. However, because of the lack of OR or RR estimates, we removed this study in our meta-analysis. Another cross-sectional study of 380 Swedish fishermen and their wives found significantly increased risk from exposure to PCB-153 congener in men but not in women [42]. For the subjects were either women or all overall population, it was not included. In the review of the relationship of PCBs with T2DM and hypertension, the author attributed these two results to hypothesis generating [59].

Overall, the findings from the present meta-analysis provide quantitative evidence consistent with the hypothesis that exposure to OCPs is a contributing risk factor for the prevalence of T2DM. From the heterogeneity analysis, the specific exposure and biologic specimen of serum lipid may be the heterogeneity sources for the large disparities of the concentration of this class of environmental pollutants. Based on our sensitivity analysis, sources of bias, exposure assessment, and confounding are unlikely to significantly affect the results. In regards to the possible observed publication bias, more studies with small samples and adverse results should be included in future research. Apart from the conventional etiologies that include genetic susceptibility, metabolic disorder and obesity, the finding of the meta-analysis indicates that environmental factors, especially exposure to OCPs, may also be a risk factor of T2DM.

Supporting Information

Table S1 Modified Downs and Black checklist for the quality assessment of epidemiological studies.

Table S2 Quality assessment of the included epidemiological studies.

Checklist S1 PRISMA (Preferred Reporting Items for Systematic Reviews and Meta-Analyses) 2009 Checklist.

Acknowledgments

We would like to thank the authors of the original studies included in this meta-analysis.

Author Contributions

Conceived and designed the experiments: MT KC WL. Performed the experiments: MT FY. Analyzed the data: MT KC WL. Wrote the paper: MT WL.

References

1. Govarts E, Nieuwenhuijsen M, Schoeters G, Ballester F, Bloemen K, et al. (2012) Birth Weight and Prenatal Exposure to Polychlorinated Biphenyls (PCBs) and Dichlorodiphenyldichloroethylene (DDE): A Meta-analysis within 12 European Birth Cohorts. Environ Health Perspect 120: 162–170.
2. Lopez-Cervantes M, Torres-Sanchez L, Tobias A, Lopez-Carrillo L (2004) Dichlorodiphenyldichloroethane burden and breast cancer risk: A meta-analysis of the epidemiologic evidence. Environ Health Perspect 112: 207–214.
3. Ntow WJ, Tagoe LM, Drechsel P, Kelderman P, Gijzen HJ, et al. (2008) Accumulation of persistent organochlorine contaminants in milk and serum of farmers from Ghana. Environ Res 106: 17–26.
4. Ren AG, Qiu XH, Jin L, Ma J, Li ZW, et al. (2011) Association of selected persistent organic pollutants in the placenta with the risk of neural tube defects. Proc Natl Acad Sci U S A 108: 12770–12775.
5. Navas-Acien A, Silbergeld EK, Streeter RA, Clark JM, Burke TA, et al. (2006) Arsenic exposure and type 2 diabetes: A systematic review of the experimental and epidemiologic evidence. Environ Health Perspect 114: 641–648.
6. Chiasson JL, Josse RG, Gomis R, Hanefeld M, Karasik A, et al. (2002) Acarbose for prevention of type 2 diabetes mellitus: the STOP-NIDDM randomised trial. Lancet 359: 2072–2077.
7. Sladek R, Rocheleau G, Rung J, Dina C, Shen L, et al. (2007) A genome-wide association study identifies novel risk loci for type 2 diabetes. Nature 445: 881–885.
8. Kahn SE, Hull RL, Utzschneider KM (2006) Mechanisms linking obesity to insulin resistance and type 2 diabetes. Nature 444: 840–846.
9. Gress TW, Nieto FJ, Shahar E, Wofford MR, Brancati FL (2000) Hypertension and antihypertensive therapy as risk factors for type 2 diabetes mellitus. Atherosclerosis risk in communities study. N Engl J Med 342: 905–912.
10. Patel CJ, Bhattacharya J, Butte AJ (2010) An environment-wide association study (EWAS) on type 2 diabetes mellitus. PLoS One 5: e10746.
11. Everett CJ, Frithsen IL, Diaz VA, Koopman RJ, Simpson WM, et al. (2007) Association of a polychlorinated dibenzo-p-dioxin, a polychlorinated biphenyl, and DDT with diabetes in the 1999–2002 National Health and Nutrition Examination Survey. Environ Res 103: 413–418.
12. Turyk M, Anderson H, Knobeloch L, Imm P, Persky V (2009) Organochlorine exposure and incidence of diabetes in a cohort of Great Lakes sport fish consumers. Environ Health Perspect 117: 1076–1082.
13. Thayer KA, Heindel JJ, Bucher JR, Gallo MA (2012) Role of environmental chemicals in diabetes and obesity: a national toxicology program workshop review. Environ Health Perspect 120: 779–789.
14. Remillard RB, Bunce NJ (2002) Linking dioxins to diabetes: epidemiology and biologic plausibility. Environ Health Perspect 110: 853–858.
15. Wallace DC (2005) A mitochondrial paradigm of metabolic and degenerative diseases, aging, and cancer: a dawn for evolutionary medicine. Annu Rev Genet 39: 359–407.
16. Liberati A, Altman DG, Tetzlaff J, Mulrow C, Gøtzsche PC, et al. (2009) The PRISMA statement for reporting systematic reviews and meta-analyses of studies that evaluate health care interventions: explanation and elaboration. PLoS Med 6(7): e1000100.
17. Downs SH, Black N (1998) The feasibility of creating a checklist for the assessment of the methodological quality both of randomised and non-randomised studies of health care interventions. J Epidemiol Community Health 52: 377–384.
18. Wigle DT, Turner MC, Krewski D (2009) A systematic review and meta-analysis of childhood leukemia and parental occupational pesticide exposure. Environ Health Perspect 117: 1505–1513.
19. Hardy RJ, Thompson SG (1998) Detecting and describing heterogeneity in meta-analysis. Stat Med 17: 841–856.
20. Higgins J, Thompson SG, Deeks JJ, Altman DG (2003) Measuring inconsistency in meta-analyses. Br Med J 327: 557–560.
21. Vrijheid M, Martinez D, Manzanares S, Dadvand P, Schembari A, et al. (2011) Ambient air pollution and risk of congenital anomalies: a systematic review and meta-analysis. Environ Health Perspect 119: 598–606.

22. Mantel N, Haenszel W (1959) Statistical aspects of the analysis of data from retrospective studies of disease. J Natl Cancer Inst 22: 719–748.
23. Dersimonian R, Laird N (1986) Meta-analysis in clinical-trials. Controlled Clin Trials 7: 177–188.
24. Gasull M, Pumarega J, Tellez-Plaza M, Castell C, Tresserras R, et al. (2012) Blood concentrations of persistent organic pollutants and prediabetes and diabetes in the general population of catalonia. Environ Sci Technol 46: 7799–7810.
25. Silverstone AE, Rosenbaum PF, Weinstock RS, Bartell SM, Foushee HR, et al. (2012) Polychlorinated biphenyl (PCB) exposure and diabetes: results from the Anniston Community Health Survey. Environ Health Perspect 120: 727–732.
26. Persky V, Piorkowski J, Turyk M, Freels S, Chatterton RJ, et al. (2012) Polychlorinated biphenyl exposure, diabetes and endogenous hormones: a cross-sectional study in men previously employed at a capacitor manufacturing plant. Environ Health 11: 57.
27. Tanaka T, Morita A, Kato M, Hirai T, Mizoue T, et al. (2011) Congener-specific polychlorinated biphenyls and the prevalence of diabetes in the Saku Control Obesity Program. Endocr J 58:589–596.
28. Grandjean P, Henriksen JE, Choi AL, Petersen MS, Dalgard C, et al. (2011) Marine food pollutants as a risk factor for hypoinsulinemia and type 2 diabetes. Epidemiology 22: 410–417.
29. Airaksinen R, Rantakokko P, Eriksson JG, Blomstedt P, Kajantie E, et al. (2011) Association between type 2 diabetes and exposure to persistent organic pollutants. Diabetes Care 34: 1972–1979.
30. Lee DH, Lind PM, Jacobs DJ, Salihovic S, van Bavel B, et al. (2011) Polychlorinated biphenyls and organochlorine pesticides in plasma predict development of type 2 diabetes in the elderly: the prospective investigation of the vasculature in Uppsala Seniors (PIVUS) study. Diabetes Care 34: 1778–1784.
31. Son HK, Kim SA, Kang JH, Chang YS, Park SK, et al. (2010) Strong associations between low-dose organochlorine pesticides and type 2 diabetes in Korea. Environ Int 36: 410–414.
32. Everett CJ, Matheson EM (2010) Biomarkers of pesticide exposure and diabetes in the 1999–2004 national health and nutrition examination survey. Environ Int 36: 398–401.
33. Ukropec J, Radikova Z, Huckova M, Koska J, Kocan A, et al. (2010) High prevalence of prediabetes and diabetes in a population exposed to high levels of an organochlorine cocktail. Diabetologia 53: 899–906.
34. Lee DH, Steffes MW, Sjodin A, Jones RS, Needham LL, et al. (2010) Low dose of some persistent organic pollutants predicts type 2 diabetes: a nested case-control study. Environ Health Perspect 118: 1235–1242.
35. Philibert A, Schwartz H, Mergler D (2009) An exploratory study of diabetes in a First Nation community with respect to serum concentrations of *p,p'*-DDE and PCBs and fish consumption. Int J Environ Res Public Health 6: 3179–3189.
36. Rignell-Hydbom A, Lidfeldt J, Kiviranta H, Rantakokko P, Samsioe G, et al. (2009) Exposure to *p,p'*-DDE: a risk factor for type 2 diabetes. PLoS One 4: e7503.
37. Wang SL, Tsai PC, Yang CY, Guo YL (2008) Increased risk of diabetes and polychlorinated biphenyls and dioxins - A 24-year follow-up study of the Yucheng cohort. Diabetes Care 31: 1574–1579.
38. Codru N, Schymura MJ, Negoita S, Rej R, Carpenter DO (2007) Diabetes in relation to serum levels of polychlorinated biphenyls and chlorinated pesticides in adult Native Americans. Environ Health Perspect 115: 1442–1447.
39. Rignell-Hydbom A, Rylander L, Hagmar L (2007) Exposure to persistent organochlorine pollutants and type 2 diabetes mellitus. Hum Exp Toxicol 26: 447–452.
40. Cox S, Niskar AS, Narayan KM, Marcus M (2007) Prevalence of self-reported diabetes and exposure to organochlorine pesticides among Mexican Americans: Hispanic health and nutrition examination survey, 1982–1984. Environ Health Perspect 115: 1747–1752.
41. Lee DH, Lee IK, Song K, Steffes M, Toscano W, et al. (2006) A strong dose-response relation between serum concentrations of persistent organic pollutants and diabetes - Results from the National Health and Examination Survey 1999–2002. Diabetes Care 29: 1638–1644.
42. Rylander L, Rignell-Hydbom A, Hagmar L (2005) A cross-sectional study of the association between persistent organochlorine pollutants and diabetes. Environ Health 4: 28.
43. Fierens S, Mairesse H, Heilier JF, De Burbure C, Focant JF, et al. (2003) Dioxin/polychlorinated biphenyl body burden, diabetes and endometriosis: findings in a population-based study in Belgium. Biomarkers 8: 529–534.
44. Arrebola JP, Pumarega J, Gasull M, Fernandez MF, Martin-Olmedo P, et al. (2013) Adipose tissue concentrations of persistent organic pollutants and prevalence of type 2 diabetes in adults from Southern Spain. Environ Res 122: 31–37.
45. Wu HY, Bertrand KA, Choi AL, Hu FB, Laden F, et al. (2013) Persistent organic pollutants and type 2 diabetes: a prospective analysis in the nurses' health study and meta-analysis. Environ Health Perspect 121: 153–161.
46. Lee DH, Jacobs DJ, Steffes M (2008) Association of organochlorine pesticides with peripheral neuropathy in patients with diabetes or impaired fasting glucose. Diabetes 57: 3108–3111.
47. Lee DH, Lee IK, Jin SH, Steffes M, Jacobs DJ (2007) Association between serum concentrations of persistent organic pollutants and insulin resistance among nondiabetic adults: results from the National Health and Nutrition Examination Survey 1999–2002. Diabetes Care 30: 622–628.
48. Turyk M, Anderson HA, Knobeloch L, Imm P, Persky VW (2009) Prevalence of diabetes and body burdens of polychlorinated biphenyls, polybrominated diphenyl ethers, and *p,p'*-diphenyldichloroethene in Great Lakes sport fish consumers. Chemosphere 75: 674–679.
49. Montgomery MP, Kamel F, Saldana TM, Alavanja MC, Sandler DP (2008) Incident diabetes and pesticide exposure among licensed pesticide applicators: Agricultural Health Study, 1993–2003. Am J Epidemiol 167: 1235–1246.
50. Vasiliu O, Cameron L, Gardiner J, Deguire P, Karmaus W (2006) Polybrominated biphenyls, polychlorinated biphenyls, body weight, and incidence of adult-onset diabetes mellitus. Epidemiology 17: 352–359.
51. Glynn AW, Granath F, Aune M, Atuma S, Darnerud PO, et al. (2003) Organochlorines in Swedish women: determinants of serum concentrations. Environ Health Perspect 111: 349–355.
52. Everett CJ, Frithsen IL, Diaz VA, Koopman RJ, Simpson WJ, et al. (2007) Association of a polychlorinated dibenzo-p-dioxin, a polychlorinated biphenyl, and DDT with diabetes in the 1999–2002 National Health and Nutrition Examination Survey. Environ Res 103: 413–418.
53. Longnecker MP, Klebanoff MA, Brock JW, Zhou H (2001) Polychlorinated biphenyl serum levels in pregnant subjects with diabetes. Diabetes Care 24: 1099–1101.
54. Fierens S, Mairesse H, Heilier JF, De Burbure C, Focant JF, et al. (2003) Dioxin/polychlorinated biphenyl body burden, diabetes and endometriosis: findings in a population-based study in Belgium. Biomarkers 8: 529–534.
55. Bernert JT, Turner WE, Patterson DG, Needham LL (2007) Calculation of serum "total lipid" concentrations for the adjustment of persistent organo-halogen toxicant measurements in human samples. Chemosphere 68: 824–831.
56. Turner MC, Wigle DT, Krewski D (2010) Residential pesticides and childhood leukemia: a systematic review and meta-analysis. Environ Health Perspect 118: 33–41.
57. Greenland S (1987) Quantitative methods in the review of epidemiologic literature. Epidemiol Rev 9: 1–30.
58. Henley P, Hill J, Moretti ME, Jahedmotlagh Z, Schoeman K, et al. (2012) Relationships between exposure to polyhalogenated aromatic hydrocarbons and organochlorine pesticides and the risk for developing type 2 diabetes: a systematic review and a meta-analysis of exposures to 2,3,7,8-tetrachlorodibenzo-p-dioxin (TCDD). Toxicol Environ Chem 94: 814–845.
59. Everett CJ, Frithsen I, Player M (2011) Relationship of polychlorinated biphenyls with type 2 diabetes and hypertension. J Environ Monit 13: 241–251.
60. Langer P (2010) The impacts of organochlorines and other persistent pollutants on thyroid and metabolic health. Fron Neuroendocrinol 31: 497–518.
61. Jorgensen ME, Borch-Johnsen K, Bjerregaard P (2008) A cross-sectional study of the association between persistent organic pollutants and glucose intolerance among Greenland Inuit. Diabetologia 51: 1416–1422.

Determination of Morphological, Biometric and Biochemical Susceptibilities in Healthy Eurasier Dogs with Suspected Inherited Glaucoma

Thomas Boillot[1]ⓢ, Serge G. Rosolen[2,3,4,5]*ⓢ, Thomas Dulaurent[6]ⓢ, Frédéric Goulle[7], Philippe Thomas[8], Pierre-François Isard[6], Thierry Azoulay[9], Stéphanie Lafarge-Beurlet[10], Mike Woods[11], Sylvie Lavillegrand[5], Ivana Ivkovic[2,3,4], Nathalie Neveux[12,13], José-Alain Sahel[2,3,4,14,15,16], Serge Picaud[2,3,4,14], Nicolas Froger[2,3,4]*

1 Clinique Vétérinaire Vetea, Saintes, France, **2** INSERM, U968, Institut de la Vision, Paris, France, **3** Sorbonne Universités, UPMC Univ Paris 06, UMR_S 968, Institut de la Vision, Paris, France, **4** CNRS, UMR 7210, Institut de la Vision, Paris, France, **5** Clinique Veterinaire Voltaire, Asnières sur Seine, France, **6** Centre Hospitalier Veterinaire Saint-Martin, Saint-Martin de Bellevue, France, **7** Clinique Veterinaire Aquivet, Eysines, France, **8** Clinique Veterinaire Saint-Pierre, Saint-Chamond, France, **9** Clinique Veterinaire des Halles, Strasbourg, France, **10** Vébio, Arcueil, France, **11** Pimrose Hill Veterinary Clinic, Dun Laoghaire, Co. Dublin, Ireland, **12** Department of Nutrition, Faculty of Pharmacy, Paris Descartes University, Paris, France, **13** Clinical Chemistry, Hôtel-Dieu-Cochin Hospitals, AP-HP, Paris, France, **14** Fondation Ophtalmologique Adolphe de Rothschild, Paris, France, **15** Centre hospitalier d'ophtalmologie des Quize-Vingts, Paris, France, **16** University College London, London, United Kingdom

Abstract

In both humans and dogs, the primary risk factor for glaucoma is high intraocular pressure (IOP), which may be caused by iridocorneal angle (ICA) abnormalities. Oxidative stress has also been implicated in retinal ganglion cell damage associated with glaucoma. A suspected inherited form of glaucoma was recently identified in Eurasier dogs (EDs), a breed for which pedigrees are readily available. Because of difficulties in assessing ICA morphology in dogs with advanced glaucoma, we selected a cohort of apparently healthy dogsfor the investigation of ICA morphological status, IOP and plasma concentrations of oxidative stress biomarkers. We aimed to establish correlations between these factors, to identify predictive markers of glaucoma in this dog breed. A cohort of 28 subjects, volunteered for inclusion by their owners, was selected by veterinary surgeons. These dogs were assigned to four groups: young males, young females (1–3 years old), adult males and adult females (4–8 years old). Ocular examination included ophthalmoscopy, tonometry, gonioscopy, biometry and ultrasound biomicroscopy (UBM), and the evaluation of oxidative stress biomarkers consisting of measurements of plasma glutathione peroxidase (GP) activity and taurine and metabolic precursor (methionine and cysteine) concentrations in plasma. The prevalence of pectinate ligament abnormalities was significantly higher in adult EDs than in young dogs. Moreover, in adult females, high IOP was significantly correlated with a short axial globe length, and a particularly large distance between Schwalbe's line and the anterior lens capsule. GP activity levels were significantly lower in EDs than in a randomized control group of dogs, and plasma taurine concentrations were higher. Hence, ICA abnormalities were associated with weaker antioxidant defenses in EDs, potentially counteracted by higher plasma taurine concentrations. This study suggests that EDs may constitute an appropriate canine model for the development of glaucoma. This cohort will be used as a sentinel for longitudinal monitoring.

Editor: Thomas Claudepierre, Université de Lorraine, France

Funding: This work was supported by Institut National de la Santé et de la Recherche Médicale (INSERM), Pierre et Marie Curie University (UPMC), Centre National de la Recherche Scientifique (CNRS), the Fondation pour la Recherche Médicale and from the Fondation Rolland Bailly, Agence Nationale pour la Recherche (ANR: GLAUCOME, VISIOWEST), the Fédération des Aveugles de France, IRRP, the city of Paris, the Regional Council of Ile-de-France, and the French State program "Investissements d'Avenir" managed by the Agence Nationale de la Recherche [LIFESENSES: ANR-10-LABX-65]. Nicolas Froger received postdoctoral fellowships from the Fondation pour la Recherche Médicale and from the Fondation Rolland Bailly. The funders had no role in study design, data collection and analysis, decision to publish, or preparation of the manuscript.

Competing Interests: Thomas Boillot, Serge G. Rosolen, Frederic Goulle, Philippe Thomas, and Thierry Azoulay are employed by Clinique Vétérinaire, Stéphanie Lafarge-Beurlet by Vébio, and Mike Woods by Pimrose Hill Veterinary Clinic. There are no patents, products in development or marketed products to declare.

* Email: nicolas.froger@inserm.fr (NF); sg.rosolen@orange.fr (SR)

ⓢ These authors contributed equally to this work.

Introduction

Glaucoma, the second most common cause of blindness worldwide [1], is a group of ophthalmic diseases characterized by the loss of retinal ganglion cells (RGCs) whose function is to transfer visual information to the brain through the optic nerve. High intraocular pressure (IOP) is considered a major risk factor for glaucomatous neuropathies [2]. IOP level is partly regulated by the rate of aqueous humor (AH) formation, which normally equals the rate of outflow. Abnormalities in AH turnover have been implicated in most types of hypertensive glaucoma [3]. However, a progressive loss of vision can occur in patients with normal tension as well as when their IOP is controlled with drugs [4,5], and oxidative stress is now well known to play a critical role in RGC degeneration [6]. This role has been suggested by (i) the decrease in systemic glutathione levels in patients with primary open-angle glaucoma [7] and (ii) the association of this form of glaucoma with a polymorphism of the glutathione S-transferase gene [8]. The importance of combating oxidative stress to ensure RGC survival was confirmed by the prevention of RGC degeneration by taurine, a major antioxidant [9].

The dog, an animal of intermediate size with an ocular anatomy and physiology similar to that of humans and living in the same environment as humans, may constitute a suitable model for the investigation of susceptibilities to glaucoma because spontaneous glaucomas are observed in certain dog breeds [10,11,12,13,14]. As in humans, the primary risk factor for glaucoma in dogs seems to be high IOP [15], also regulated by AH turnover [15,16,17]. AH drainage mechanisms involve the iridocorneal angle (ICA) and the anterior opening of the ciliary cleft (CC), which are spanned by the comb-like pectinate ligament. The passage of AH between the intraligamentary spaces leads to its entry into the uveal and then the corneoscleral trabecular meshwork before being collected by the angular aqueous plexus, the intrascleral plexus, and the vortex venous drainage system [15]. Drainage via this conventional route accounts for 85% of AH outflow in dogs [18]. Pectinate ligament abnormalities (PLA), involving a lack of resorption of the mesenchymatous tissue filling the anterior part of the ciliary cleft during embryonic development, have often been reported in association with primary narrow and closed-angle glaucoma [10,19]. Primary glaucomas are further classified as having an open or narrow ICA on the basis of either gonioscopic examination [20] or imaging by ultrasound biomicroscopy (UBM) [21,22].

The underlying genetic susceptibilities potentially contributing to the development and progression of primary glaucoma have never been clearly identified. Glaucoma is genetically heterogeneous, and many genes have been reported to be linked to primary open-angle glaucoma in both humans and dogs [23,24,25,26]. In several dog breeds, including the Chow Chow [27], the Samoyed [28], and the Keeshound [29], primary glaucoma is considered to be hereditary with a prevalence of 4.7% and 1.6%, in Chow Chow and Samoyed dogs, respectively [30]. These two breeds were used to generate Eurasier dogs (EDs): a breed obtained in the early 1960s by Julius Whipfel in Germany and characterized by a small population size and intense inbreeding.

In a preliminary study, we observed high rates of blindness in EDs from France, associated with the clinical signs of glaucoma (e.g. mydriasis, episcleral congestion and diffuse corneal edema) and high IOP [31]. We therefore established a cohort of apparently healthy EDs to determine whether these dogs displayed any morphological and biochemical features conferring a predisposition to glaucoma. Our ultimate objective was to determine whether the ED could be considered a genuine animal model of glaucoma for subsequent therapeutic and genetic investigations.

Materials and Methods

Dogs were included in the study by veterinary surgeons from the European *Réseau Européen d'Ophtalmologie Vétérinaire et de Vision Animale* (REOVVA) network.

The specific protocols were approved by the joint ethics committee of the Vision Institute, the Pierre et Marie Curie University and REOVVA. All animals were examined with the consent of their owners.

Animal cohorts

Three cohorts of dogs were recruited by the REOVVA network:

1) The first cohort (cohort 1) was used in the preliminary study investigating the blindness associated with high IOP that occurs in EDs.
2) Imaging was not possible in the animals of the first cohort due to severe corneal edema and mydriasis. We therefore established a second cohort (cohort 2) of apparently healthy EDs.
3) The third cohort (cohort 3) of randomized healthy dogs of various breeds was established for a comparison of biochemical parameters with those of the second cohort.

Glaucomatous dogs (cohort 1). Cohort 1 was identified by clinical examination. All animals were presented by their owners for an abnormal appearance of the eyes and vision problems. Ophthalmic examinations were performed and included indirect ophthalmoscopy, slit-lamp examination and IOP measurements. This cohort included 18 dogs (11 males and 7 females from 14 generations; age: 6.7± 1.0 years old; mean±SEM).

Apparently healthy EDs (cohort 2). We ensured that this cohort included a representative distribution of EDs by including dogs from 8 generations of a family of 830 individuals. The family tree was constructed with GenoPro software according to data obtained for pedigrees from the website "Chiens de France" (cross-linked sources). Dogs were selected from various lineages and were volunteered for participation by their owners. The dogs were obtained from different breeders and owners from across the country, but the rate of interbreeding was nevertheless as high as 60% in some individuals. The selected dogs were healthy and had no apparent macroscopic clinical signs of glaucoma (e.g., mydriasis, episcleral congestion, diffuse corneal edema). The normal range of IOP has not been determined for this breed, so we did not use IOP as an inclusion criterion. Cohort 2 included 28 dogs (age: 4.0±0.6 years old; means±SEM) divided into homogeneous groups on the basis of age and sex: 7 young males (age: 1–3 years old; weight: 20–30 kg), 9 young females (age: 1–3 years old; weight: 16–26 kg), 6 adult males (age: 4–8 years old; weight: 24–31 kg), and 6 adult females (age: 4–8 years old; weight: 20–26 kg).

Control dogs (cohort 3). An additional cohort of healthy dogs was used as a control for biochemical comparisons with EDs. This cohort was randomized for sex, age, weight and breed. It included 39 dogs (15 males; 24 females; age: 3.10±1.7 years old; weight: 20.5±2.2 kg; means±SEM) from 25 different breeds other than the ED such that the values could not be biased by a breed with specific features. The breeds included in this control cohort were not known to be prone to either primary ocular or any other diseases. For example, we did not include the Basset Hound, the American Cocker Spaniel or the Welsh Terrier, three breeds known to develop primary glaucoma, in this cohort. Blood samples were collected primarily for reasons unrelated to this study.

Clinical examinations and tonometry (cohorts 1, 2)

Complete ocular examinations were performed on all animals, including slit-lamp examination, indirect ophthalmoscopy (with 20D and 30D lenses), and tonometry. We harmonized procedures and decreased individual variation by systematically performing ophthalmoscopy with devices equipped with small-pupil systems to prevent pupil dilation [32]. This was considered important because it is not possible to evaluate the pectinate ligament precisely once the pupil has become dilated. The optic nerve head was evaluated by indirect ophthalmoscopy with a Volk Macula Plus 5.5X for enlargement. IOP was always determined at the same time of day, between noon and 3 p.m., to minimize the effects of circadian variations [33,34], with a rebound tonometer (Tono-Vet, Tiolat, Espoo, Finland). The IOP values recorded for each eye were the mean of three successive tonometer readings on the central cornea.

Gonioscopy (cohort 2)

Before bilateral gonioscopy, the cornea was anesthetized by the topical application of proxymetacaine (Proparacaine 0.5%, Bausch & Lomb, Chauvin Pharmaceuticals Ltd., Aubenas, France). Direct gonioscopy was performed with a 17 mm Koeppe goniolens (Ocular Instruments, Bellevue, WA, USA) filled with hydroxyethylcellulose fluid (Gelaser, Alcon, Rueil Malmaison, France) before being placed in contact with the cornea, ensuring that there were no air bubbles or nictitating membrane entrapment. Examinations were performed on conscious animals whenever possible, but anesthesia was used if necessary (induction: 2 µg/kg medethomidine, 5 mg/kg ketamine intramuscularly, followed by the inhalation of 1.5 to 3% isoflurane gas in a mixture of 30% air and 70% oxygen). General anesthesia likely influences the ICA morphology, but there is no reference in dog because gonioscopy is a qualitative examination.

The anesthetized animals were placed in a lateral recumbent position with the head positioned so as to ensure that the plane of the iris was parallel to the table. The ICA was viewed with a hand-held slit-lamp biomicroscope (Kowa SL-2, SL-14 or SL-15). The entire ICA and the opening of the CC were systematically examined for the presence of PLAs. Goniophotography was performed according to a standardized procedure (DSLR camera +100 mm macro lens + Koeppe lens 17 mm + Gelaser + Finoff transilluminator) for each eye and each quadrant. In cases of PLA detection, the abnormality was quantified by assigning a percentage of the 360° after systematically viewing the entire circumference of the ICA, and a grade was attributed according to the ICA percentage. All quantifications were carried out by the same investigator (Thomas Dulaurent) who received the data without any additional information about age, sex, breed or animal status. The grading used corresponds to that recommended by the French Eye Panellists/Maladies Héréditaires Oculaires Canines (AFEP/MHOC)] Association eye scheme.

Ultrasonography (cohort 2)

B-mode ultrasonography (10 MHz probe, OTI, EDC Vet, Carvin, France) was performed on each animal and on each eye to measure the axial globe length (AGL) from the corneal epithelial surface to the inner retinal surface. Only one image per eye was selected by veterinarians and used for measurements. Images were sent to the same investigator (Thomas Dulaurent) to minimize the individual coefficient of variation in the analysis.

Ultrasound biomicroscopy (UBM) (cohort 2)

For each animal, and for each eye, a 48 MHz (Accutome, UBM-Plus, Malvern PA, USA) monotransducer with geometric focalization and line scanning was used for this study. As previously described, anesthetized animals were positioned in a recumbent position with the head stabilized with a hollow cushion [22]. A series of video sequences was recorded and sent to the same investigator (Thomas Dulaurent) in each case, and he selected one image among 20 images, which optimally demonstrated the maximal distance between the corneal endothelium in the region of the vertex and the most anterior portion of the length capsule. For analyses, the transducer was positioned in the central region of the anterior chamber to measure the anterior chamber length (ACL), determined as the distance between the corneal endothelium in the region of the corneal vertex and the anterior pole of the lens. For ICA parameter measurements, outflow pathways were evaluated in the dorsal quadrant. The transducer was placed perpendicularly to the corneoscleral limbus, in the 12 o'clock position, and scanning was then carried out from the 10 to 2 o'clock positions.

Collection of blood samples (cohorts 2, 3)

For determinations of biomarkers of inflammation and oxidative stress, we collected blood samples (5 ml) from the cephalic veins of fasted, awake animals. Half the blood sample was used for the extraction of plasma which was then immediately frozen at -20°C.

Determination of biomarkers of inflammation and oxidative stress (cohorts 2 & 3)

Inflammatory biomarkers, including albumin, C-reactive (CRP) and haptoglobin, were determined in the plasma by spectrophotometry with diagnostic kits (previously validated in dogs) and controls from Thermofisher, and a KONELAB 60 (Thermofisher) clinical chemistry analyzer. These biomarkers were selected as representative of the different phases of the inflammatory response [35,36]. CRP is a biomarker of the very early phase (several hours) whereas haptoglobin increases at a slower rate (few days) but remains high for longer amounts of time. By contrast, albumin synthesis decreases during inflammation.

Glutathione peroxidase (GP) activity in the plasma was assessed by spectrophotometry with a diagnostic kit and controls from Randox Laboratories and a KONELAB 60 (Thermofisher) clinical chemistry analyzer. Finally, plasma concentrations of taurine, methionine and cysteine were determined by ion exchange chromatography, as previously described [37].

Statistical analysis (cohort 2, 3)

For each ED subgroup, qualitative data are expressed as the proportion (%) of examined eyes considered to be abnormal. These proportions were compared in chi-squared (χ^2) tests to identify significant differences in the distribution of these events between subgroups. Quantitative data are presented as means ± SD. We used the non-parametric Mann & Witney test to compare mean values between two groups. For simultaneous comparisons of more than two groups, we carried out the non-parametric Kruskal-Wallis comparison of variance, followed, if significant, by a Dunn's post-hoc test to compare the means of the groups considered. Differences were considered significant if $p<0.05$.

We used the non-parametric Spearman's rank correlation test to detect non-linear correlations between parameters. The correlation was considered significant if $p\leq0.05$. Linear correlation analyses were also carried out and were considered significant if $r^2>0.52$.

Results

Clinical examination and tonometry (Cohort 1, 2)

Cohort 1. Diagnosed by an initial exam, EDs from cohort 1 displayed clinical signs of glaucoma including diffuse corneal edema, episcleral congestion, and mydriasis. These dogs included ten (4 males and 6 females) with an IOP>35 mmHg who were already blind, and eight (7 males and 1 females) with an IOP of between 25 and 35 mmHg who were not blind. When compared with the IOP value in normal dogs (19.0 mmHg with a range of 11

(5%) and 29 (95%) mmHg [38]), this cohort had elevated levels and many individuals exceeded the limit>35 mmHg defined as abnormal by Gelatt et al. [15]. Due to the severe corneal edema and mydriasis, neither gonioscopy nor UBM could be performed in these dogs to assess ICA morphology.

Cohort 2. Because we undertook the first study in healthy EDs it was important to mention all ocular abnormalities and IOP levels. On clinical examination, none of the animals examined presented clinical signs of glaucoma (e.g. mydriasis, episcleral congestion, diffuse corneal edema), but 25.0% of the eyes were found to display ocular abnormalities other than those specifically related to glaucoma and identifiable with the AFEP/MHOC scheme (see below).

The prevalence of these abnormalities was higher (i) in females than in males and (ii) in adults than in young dogs (**Table 1**). The prevalence of clinical eye abnormalities was significantly higher in adult females (33.3%) than in young females ($p<0.05$; χ^2 test; **Table 1**).

Mean IOP values for each group were towards the upper limit of the normal range for dogs with a similar morphology [39,40,41]. No significant differences in IOP levels were found between the ED subgroups (p = 0.16, Kruskall-Wallis ANOVA, **Table 1**). However, a surprising decrease of IOP (−13%) was found in adult EDs when compared to young EDs (**Table 1**). An even larger decrease was observed in the analyses restricted to females (−15%; **Table 1**). Regarding the glaucoma prevalence in EDs (see cohort 1 above), healthy dogs with IOP of 25–35 mmHg are not considered clinically glaucomatous because normal IOP ranges are unknown in EDs.

Gonioscopy (Cohort 2)

When the ICA was viewed with a hand-held slit-lamp biomicroscope (**see Fig. 1a**), the entire ICA and opening of the ciliary cleft were systematically scrutinized for the presence of PLA (**Fig.1b-d**). Such abnormalities were rated as being at different stages of progression: stage 1 (fibrae latae) corresponded to abnormally broad and thickened pectinate ligament fibers; stage 2 (lamina) corresponded to the appearance of solid sheets of pectinate ligament tissue; stage 3 (occlusion) was characterized by the persistence of an embryonic sheet of ICA tissue and an absence of intraligamentary spaces.

For PLA quantification, the grades were as follow: grade 0 corresponded to an absence of PLA (**Fig. 1a**); grade 1 corresponded to a mild (stage 1 and/or stage 2; **Fig. 1b**) PLA affecting less than 25% of the ICA; grade 2 corresponded to a moderate PLA (stage 1 and/or stage 2) involving between 25% and 75% of the ICA circumference (stage 2; **Fig. 1c**); grade 3 corresponded to severe PLA (stage 1 and/or stage 2 affecting more than 75% of the ICA and/or the presence of an occlusion), regardless of the percentage of the circumference affected (stage 3; **Fig. 1d**). PLA scoring was performed by an independent investigator on anonymous pictures to ensure the attribution of an unbiased grade.

The prevalence of PLA was higher in females (53.3%) than in males (38.4%) in an analysis of all grades together ($p<0.05$, χ^2 test; **Fig. 1e**). However, males were more frequently affected by the minor forms of PLA (grade 1: 60.0%), whereas females displayed more severe forms of PLA (grades 2 & 3: 56.3%; **Table 2**).

Interestingly, the frequency of PLA increased with age; as such abnormalities were found in 79.2% of adult EDs and only in 21.8% in young EDs ($p<0.001$, χ^2 test; **Fig. 1e**). Minor forms of PLA (grade 1) were more prominent in adult EDs (45.8%), whereas the more severe forms (grades 2 & 3) were observed mostly in young EDs (15.7%; **Table 2**). In addition, PLA was

Table 1. Ocular abnormalities and tonometry in the cohort of healthy Eurasier dogs (cohort 2).

Clinical Observations and tonometry	Male dogs (*N*=13)	Female dogs (*N*=15)	Young dogs (*N*=16)	Adult dogs (*N*=12)	Young males (*N*=7)	Young females (*N*=9)	Adult males (*N*=6)	Adult females (*N*=6)
Eyelid abnormalities	2	3	5	-	2	3	-	-
Corneal dystrophies	-	2	-	2	-	-	-	2
Lens opacities	3	1	1	3	-	1	3	-
Micropapilla	1	-	1	-	1	-	-	-
Choroidal hypoplasia	-	2	-	2	-	-	-	2
Total abnormalities (%)	6 (23.1%) (n = 26)	8 (26.7%) (n = 30)	7 (21.9%) (n = 32)	7 (29.2%) (n = 24)	3 (21.4%) (n = 14)	4 (22.3%) (n = 18)	3 (25.0%) (n = 12)	4 (33.3%) (n = 12)
IOP (mm Hg)	17.7±4.5 (*n*=26)	15.7±3.4 (*n*=29)	17.8±4.2 (*n*=31)	15.5±3.5 (*n*=24)	18.8±5.2 (*n*=14)	16.9±2.9 (*n*=17)	16.5±3.1 (*n*=12)	14.4±3.6 (*n*=12)

Abnormalities were observed on clinical examinations other than gonioscopy examination. Data represent the numbers for each category of abnormalities observed in each subgroup of EDs and the total numbers of abnormalities (with a percentage) are presented in the last line.
Tonometric data are expressed as means ± standard deviation (SD).
n refers to the number of eyes examined in each group whereas *N* is the number of dogs in each group.
IOP: intraocular pressure.

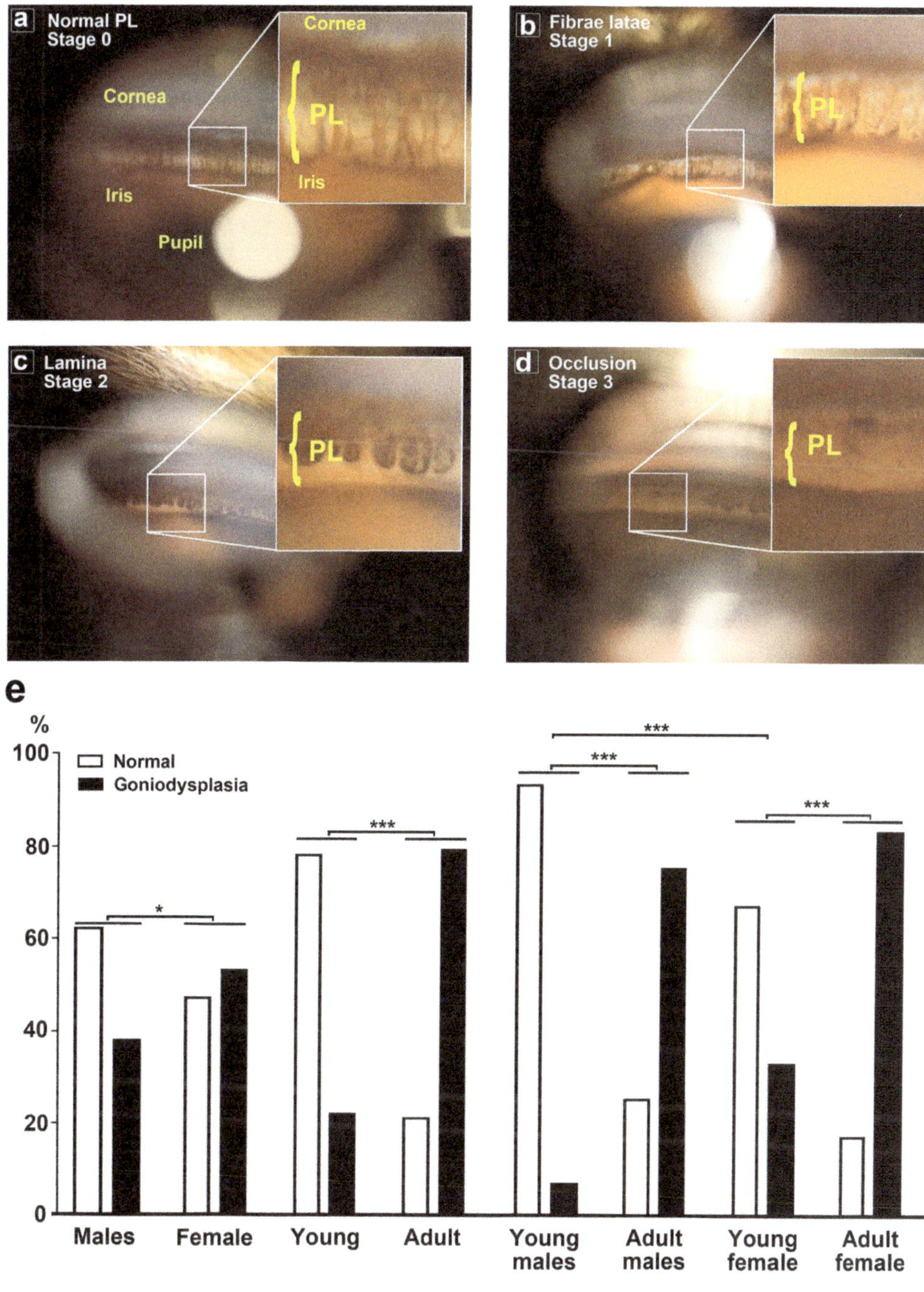

Figure 1. Pectinate ligament abnormalities (PLA) evaluated by gonioscopic examination in Eurasier dogs. (a) Normal pectinate ligament (PL) visible when rarefaction of the initial fibrilar sheet was almost complete, by 2 to 4 weeks after birth, leaving strands of intertwining collagen, progressively encased by attenuate trabecular cells, confluent with the anterior surface of the iris (stage 0). (b-d) The entire ICA and opening of the CC were systematically examined for the presence of a PLA, defined as abnormally broad and thickened pectinate ligament fibers (stage 1) (**b**) or solid sheets (stage 2) (**c**) of PL tissue, with or without "holes" (stage 3) (**d**). (e) Percentage of PLA (including grade 1, 2 and 3; black bars) with respect to normal pectinate ligament (white bars) in each category of the ED cohort. $^*p<0.05$ and $^{***}p<0.001$ indicate significant differences in the prevalence of PLA between the indicated groups (χ^2 test).

more prevalent in young females (33.4%) than in young males (7.2%; $p<0.001$, χ^2 test; **Fig. 1e**), and young females displayed predominantly severe forms (27.8% for grades 2 & 3). By contrast, in adult EDs, PLA affected both sexes equally (75% for males and 83.4% for females; **Fig. 1e**), but the forms detected were essentially minor (50% grade 1 for females and 41.7% for males; **Table 2**).

Biometry and UBM examinations (Cohort 2)

Biometric examinations were carried out to measure (i) AGL, defined as the distance between the corneal epithelial surface and the inner retinal surface (**figure 2**), and (ii) ACL, defined as the distance between the corneal endothelium at the corneal vertex and the anterior pole of the lens. Analyses of biometric results revealed significant differences in AGL between the different ED

Table 2. Morphological appearance of the pectinate ligament in the cohort of healthy Eurasier dogs (cohort 2).

PL aspects (%)	Male dogs ($N=13$)	Female dogs ($N=15$)	Young dogs ($N=16$)	Adult dogs ($N=12$)	Young males ($N=7$)	Young females ($N=9$)	Adult males ($N=6$)	Adult females ($N=6$)
Grade 0 (normal)	16	14	25	5	13	12	3	2
Grade 1	6	7	2	11	1	1	5	6
Grade 2	1	3	1	3	0	1	1	2
Grade 3	3	6	4	5	0	4	3	2

The PL was observed by gonioscopy. In cases of pectinate ligament abnormalities, quantification was performed by assigning a percentage of the 360° after systematically viewing the entire circumference of the ICA, and a grade was attributed according to the percentage of the ICA affected (AFEP/MHOC). Grade 0 corresponds to an absence of goniodysplasia (see figure 1a), grade 1 corresponds to mild goniodysplasia (stage 1 in figure 1b), grade 2 corresponds to moderate goniodysplasia (stage 2 in figure 1c), and grade 3 corresponds to severe goniodysplasia (stage 3 in figure 1d). PLA grades are provided separately for the two eyes because PLA did not progress uniformly in the two eyes.

Data are expressed as the number of eyes affected by the various grades of goniodysplasia for each group of EDs. *N* is the number of dogs in each group.

subgroups considered ($p<0.01$; Kruskall-Wallis ANOVA; **table 3**). In particular, AGL was found to be significantly lower in female EDs than in male EDs ($p<0.05$, Dunn's post-hoc test; **table 3**). This decrease in females was found to be more significant when compared to adult males ($p<0.001$, Dunn's post-hoc test; **table 3**). In males, AGL of adults was significantly higher ($p<0.01$, Dunn's post-hoc test) than that of young dogs **(Table 3)**. By contrast, no significant difference in ACL was found between any of the subgroups considered (**Table 3**).

The "en face" CC opening can only be visualized by gonioscopy, whereas the entire cleft can be imaged by ultrasound biomicroscopy (UBM) **(Fig. 3 a-b)**, allowing the measurement of its width and length. Three parameters were evaluated for each eye, as described in **figure 3**: (i) the width of the entrance of the CC (CCW), determined as the distance between the corneoscleral limbus and the iris root **(Fig. 3c,d)**, (ii) the length of the CC (CCL), determined as the distance between the pectinate ligament (or the most anterior visible portion of the uveal trabecular meshwork) and the anterior portion of the ciliary body **(Fig. 3e-f)** and, finally, (iii) the distance between Schwalbe's line (the peripheral termination of Descemet's membrane, i.e., the borderline between the cornea and sclera) and the anterior capsule of the lens (DSAC) (**Fig. 3g-h**). This last distance is considered a suitable parameter for the comparison of UBM measurements between dogs with different body sizes/weights [42].

No significant difference in the mean values of CCW, CCL and DSAC was found between the subgroups of EDs (**Table 3**). Thus, UBM measurements indicated that the anatomy of the CC was unaffected by age or sex in the cohort of EDs studied (cohort 2).

Correlation between IOP biometry and UBM parameters (Cohort 2)

We investigated the possible effect of changes in biometric and UBM parameters on changes in IOP; and vice versa, by carrying out statistical tests to evaluate the correlation between IOP and

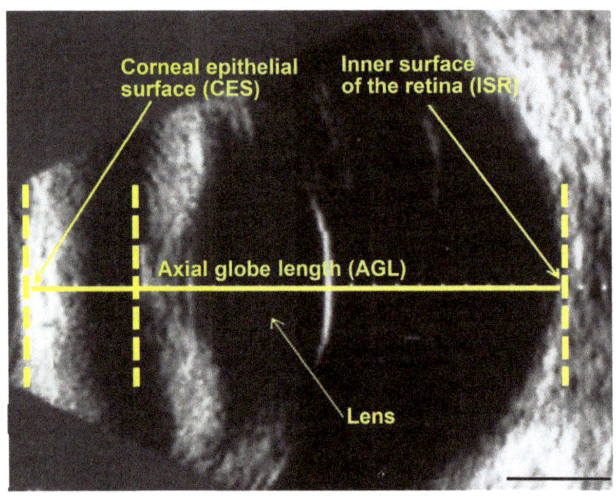

Figure 2. Biometry of the dog eyeball. Representative image from a normal dog obtained by B-mode ultrasound: a standard 10 MHz transducer was placed directly on the cornea after the instillation of topical anesthetic into the eye. A vertical axial scan was performed, making it possible to measure axial globe length (AGL) — the length from the corneal epithelial surface (CES) to the inner surface of the retina (ISR). The normal lens is translucent and only the posterior lens capsule is visible, as a highly reflective concave line. The anterior chamber and the vitreous are clear and anechoic and appear as homogeneous black areas. The scale bar represents 1 mm.

Table 3. Biometry and UBM measurements for the cohort of healthy Eurasier dogs (cohort 2).

Biometric measurements	Male dogs (N = 13)	Female dogs (N = 15)	Young dogs (N = 16)	Adult dogs (N = 15)	Young males (N = 7)	Young females (N = 9)	Adult males (N = 6)	Adult females (N = 6)
AGL (mm)	19.9±0.6 (n = 26)	19.5±0.6* (n = 26)	19.6±0.5 (n = 28)	19.9±0.7 (n = 24)	19.6±0.6 (n = 14)	19.5±0.5 (n = 14)	20.3±0.5°°° ¶¶ (n = 12)	19.5±0.8## (n = 12)
ACL (mm)	3.7±0.2 (n = 26)	3.8±0.4 (n = 26)	3.8±0.2 (n = 28)	3.8±0.4 (n = 24)	3.7±0.3 (n = 14)	3.8±0.3 (n = 14)	3.7±0.2 (n = 12)	3.9±0.5 (n = 12)
CCL (mm)	2.6±0.6 (n = 25)	2.5±0.6 (n = 28)	2.5±0.5 (n = 31)	2.6±0.7 (n = 22)	2.5±0.5 (n = 14)	2.4±0.5 (n = 17)	2.6±0.8 (n = 11)	2.6±0.7 (n = 11)
CCW (mm)	0.27±0.09 (n = 25)	0.25±0.09 (n = 28)	0.24±0.09 (n = 31)	0.28±0.08 (n = 22)	0.23±0.10 (n = 14)	0.25±0.09 (n = 17)	0.30±0.06 (n = 11)	0.26±0.09 (n = 11)
DSAC (mm)	2.8±0.2 (n = 20)	2.8±0.3 (n = 27)	2.9±0.3 (n = 26)	2.8±0.2 (n = 21)	2.9±0.2 (n = 10)	2.9±0.3 (n = 16)	2.8±0.2 (n = 10)	2.8±0.2 (n = 11)

Data are expressed as means ± standard deviation (SD) and n is the number of eyes examined in each group whereas N is the number of dogs in each group. We did not include all the eyes, because some of the images could not be exploited.
AGL: axial globe length; ACL: anterior chamber length; CCW: ciliary cleft width; CCL: ciliary cleft length; DSAC: distance from Schwalbe's line to the anterior capsule of the lens.
*$p<0.05$ versus the male group; °°°$p<0.001$ versus females; ##$p<0.01$ versus the adult males and ¶¶$p<0.01$ versus the young male group (Kruskal-Wallis ANOVA followed by a Dunn's post-hoc test).

quantitative parameters assessing ICA morphology (biometric and UBM parameters, respectively).

A plot of the IOP levels of all EDs against biometric parameters (AGL, ACL) revealed a significant inverse correlation between IOP and AGL (**Fig. 4a**), suggesting that a decrease in AGL may lead to an increase in IOP ($p = 0.05$; Spearman's test). Similar correlations were found for analyses limited to the male ED subgroup (**Fig. 4b**) and the adult female ED subgroup (**Fig 4c**).

In an analysis that included all EDs, no significant correlation was found between IOP and the UBM parameter: DSAC ($p = 0.17$; Spearman's test; **Fig 4d**). However, we found a significant positive correlation between these parameters for the adult subgroup (**Fig. 4e**) and for adult females (**Fig. 4f**). This observation indicates that decreases in IOP may be associated with decreases in DSAC, or vice versa.

Biochemical investigations (Cohort 2, 3)

Concentrations of various biomarkers of inflammation (albumin, CRP, haptoglobin) and oxidative stress (GP activity, taurine and its precursors: methionine and cysteine) were measured in the plasma of healthy EDs (cohort 2) and compared to those measured in the control dogs (cohort 3).

No significant differences in concentrations of inflammatory biomarkers were found between these two cohorts of dogs. Similarly, no differences in the levels of these biomarkers were found between the various ED subgroups (**Table 4**). These results suggest that levels of inflammatory biomarkers in EDs are identical to those in the general dog population.

GP activity was significantly lower in healthy EDs than in the control dogs (**Fig. 5a**). This enzymatic activity was also significantly lower in each of the subgroups of EDs than in the control dogs ($p<0.001$, Kruskal-Wallis ANOVA followed by a Dunn's post-hoc test; see **Fig. 5e**). GP activity was stronger in young than in adults EDs, but this difference was not statistically significant (**Fig. 5e**).

Surprisingly, plasma taurine concentrations were higher in EDs than in the control dogs ($p<0.001$, Mann & Whitney test; **Fig. 5b**). By contrast, the plasma concentrations of methionine and cysteine were similar in the EDs and the control dogs (**Fig. 5c-d**). Each subgroup of EDs displayed a significantly higher plasma taurine concentration than the control dogs, except for the adult male subgroup (**Fig. 5f**). This suggests that such increase in plasma taurine concentration was not dependent on age or sex in healthy EDs, but instead is typical of the breed. However, the lower plasma taurine concentration observed in the adult male EDs was linearly correlated ($p = 0.05$ and $r^2 = 0.68$) with the lower level of GP activity, suggesting an increased vulnerability to oxidative stress with age in male EDs.

Discussion

Primary glaucoma has been reported to occur at a high prevalence in various dog breeds which is consistent with the existence of hereditary forms [27] [28] [29] [30]. We recently published the first report of high rates of spontaneous glaucoma affecting both sexes of adult EDs in France [31], as shown by severe visual problems and clinical signs of glaucoma on clinical examination, together with high IOP.

In a cohort of healthy EDs without a diagnosis of glaucoma, we found that IOP values were towards the upper end of the mean values obtained for dogs with Tonovet [39,40,43], but that these values tend to decrease with age. Because no reference describing IOP ranges in EDs is available, we have no explanation for the decline of IOP with age, although a similar phenomenon was

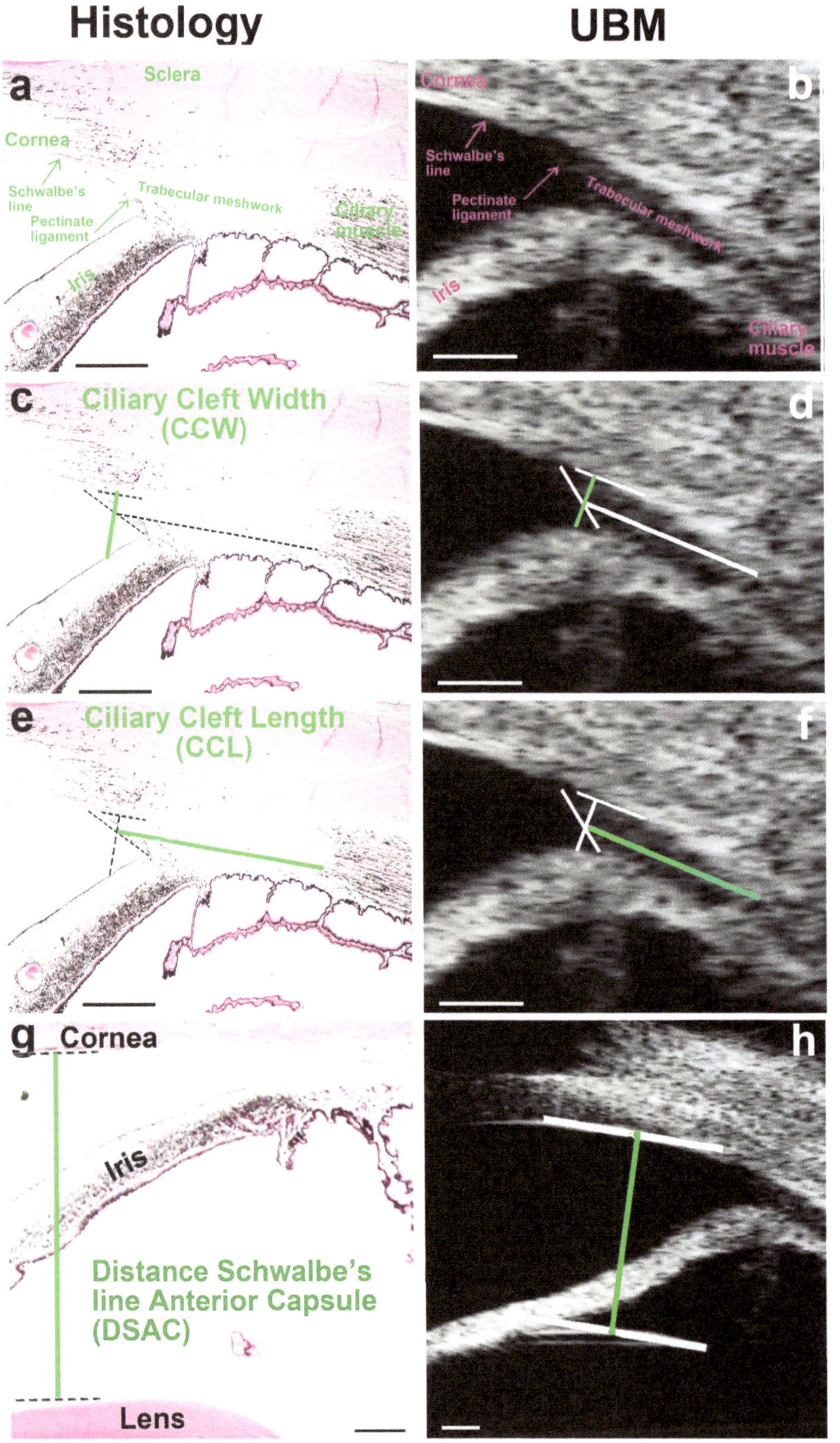

Figure 3. Iridocorneal angle (ICA) in dogs: images from ICA sections versus ultrasound biomicroscopy. (a-b) Normal histological sections of the ICA (stained with hematoxilin/eosin) are shown on the left, with the corresponding UBM images on the right. ICA structures in (a) are compared with those obtained by UBM (b). The pectinate ligament corresponds to the anterior delineation of the ciliary cleft. The trabecular meshwork, which fills the ciliary cleft (CC), is clearly visible. (c-d) The width of the entrance of the ciliary cleft (CCW) was measured by determining the distance between the corneoscleral limbus and the iris root as follows. A line outlining the pectinate ligament was traced. Another line, outlining the inner wall of the sclera in the anterior portion of the CC, was then traced. The CCW corresponds to a line perpendicular to the inner wall of the sclera and crossing the pectinate ligament halfway along its length. (e-f) The length of the CC (CCL) was determined as the distance from the pectinate ligament (or the most anterior visible portion of the uveal trabecular meshwork) to the anterior portion of the ciliary body as follows. A line was

traced outlining the pectinate ligament. The CCL corresponds to a line parallel to the long axis of the CC, crossing the pectinate ligament halfway along its length at the anterior and reaching the ciliary muscle at the posterior. (g-h) Determination of the distance between Schwalbe's line (the peripheral termination of Descemet's membrane, i.e. the borderline between the cornea and sclera) and the anterior capsule of the lens (DSAC). The scale bar corresponds to 1 mm for all images. The ICA sections were obtained from the same dog as the UBM images.

already described in other breeds [38]. Clinical investigation revealed the presence of ocular abnormalities in all ED subgroups, regardless of age or sex. PLA accounted for 50% of all abnormalities and was more frequent (~80%) in adult EDs, suggesting that changes in ICA morphology may be correlated with aging in this dog breed, particularly in females. This observation was already described in another breed (Flat coated retriever), but remains under debate, and it cannot exclude an

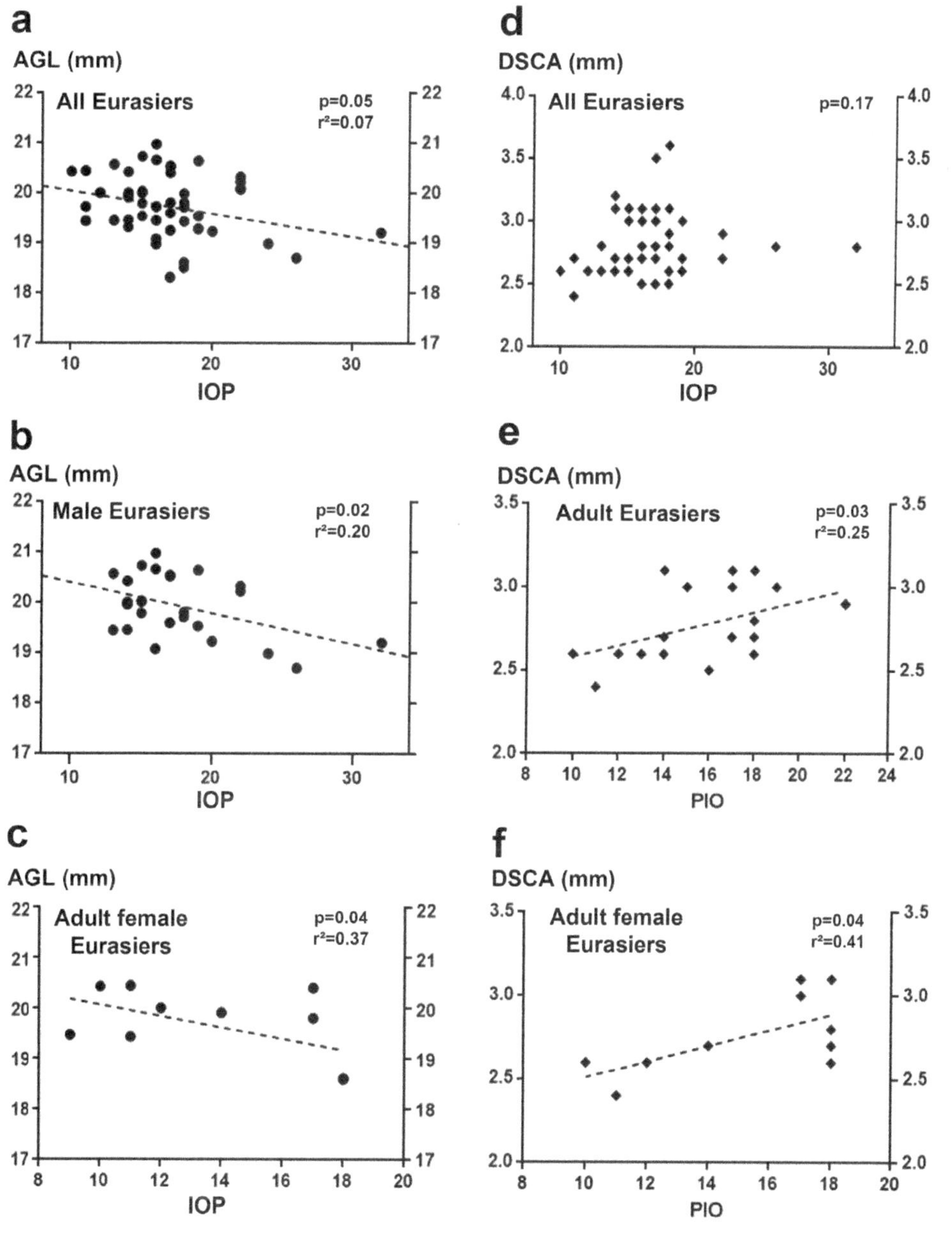

Figure 4. Correlation between intraocular pressure (IOP) and axial globe length biometric parameters in the various subgroups of the ED cohort. (a-c) Correlation between IOP and axial globe length (AGL) in all EDs from the cohort: increasing IOP was significantly associated with decreasing AGL ($p = 0.05$, Spearman's test; a). Similar significant correlations were also found for adult EDs ($p = 0.03$; b) and for female adult EDs ($p = 0.05$; c). The linear regression analysis (hatched lines) demonstrated the non-linear status of the correlations, because $r^2 < 0.5$ in all cases (a-c). (d-f) Correlation between IOP and distance between Schwalbe's line and the anterior capsule of the lens (DSAC): increasing IOP was significantly associated with increasing DSAC in male EDs ($p = 0.03$; e) and adult female EDs ($p = 0.05$; f), whereas no significant correlation between these parameters was found when all EDs were considered together ($p = 0.17$; d). Linear regression analysis (hatched lines) indicated that the significant correlations observed were not linear ($r^2 < 0.52$ in all cases; d-f).

Table 4. Biochemical markers of inflammation determined in plasma from the cohort of healthy Eurasier dogs (cohort 2).

Biochemical markers	Male dogs (*N*=13)	Female dogs (*N*=15)	Young dogs (*N*=16)	Adult dogs (*N*=12)	Young males (*N*=7)	Young females (*N*=9)	Adult males (*N*=6)	Adult females (*N*=6)
Albumin (g/l)	30.0±2.0	29.6±2.3	29.5±2.4	30.2±1.7	30.3±2.3	28.8±2.4	29.7±1.7	30.7±1.8
CRP (mg/l)	6.3±1.7	6.8±1.6	6.5±1.7	6.7±1.6	5.9±1.1	7.0±2.1	6.8±2.3	6.5±0.5
Haptoglobin (g/l)	0.7±0.4	0.2±0.2	0.4±0.4	0.6±0.4	0.6±0.4	0.2±0.2	0.8±0.3	0.3±0.3

Data are expressed as means ± standard deviation (SD) for each group. *N* is the number of dogs in each group.
CRP: C-reactive protein.

effect of the breed selection [44]. The relationship between glaucoma and PLA has never been clearly established in dogs, although it was suspected by some studies in various breeds [11,20,44,45]. In addition, « dysplasia » is a controversial notion amongst veterinary ophthalmologists because theoretically a normal dysplasia cannot change with time. Surprisingly, young dogs displayed more severe forms of PLA than adult dogs, suggesting the possibility of changes in the appearance of the pectinate ligament over time in dogs, consistent with a recent study in another dog breed (Flat-Coated Retriever) [46]. The high prevalence of minor forms of PLA (grade 1) in adults in our study may be accounted for by the progression of asymptomatic forms (grade 0) to minor forms (grade 1), but this hypothesis requires confirmation in a longitudinal follow-up study of this cohort. The higher prevalence of PLA in female EDs suggests that females are more prone to the development of primary glaucoma [15], as previously reported in other breeds [47] and even in humans, with women being more frequently affected than men [1]. This finding is also consistent with the reported two-fold higher risk of primary angle closure glaucoma in females than in males [48,49].

Very few studies including biometric UBM analyses for ICA phenotyping have been performed in dogs, and no such studies have been performed on EDs. Our data therefore provide the reference values for this breed. We found that AGL (i) increased with age, particularly in males, and (ii) was higher in males than in females, probably due to the higher size/weight ratio in males (27.3±3.7 kg in males versus 21.8±2.7 kg in females; $p<0.001$), as described in Samoyeds [28]. Regarding the higher value of AGL in adult males, similar result was described in normal eyes Samoyed [50], without any rationale to explain such a phenomenon. The other parameters studied (ACL, CCL and CCW) displayed no significant change with aging. We found an inverse correlation between IOP and AGL, particularly for the adult female subgroup (high IOP and low AGL). This suggests that the smaller AGL in female EDs may render them more susceptible to the development of a high IOP. A more surprising positive correlation was found between DSAC and IOP in adult females. With age, the lens increases in volume [43,51,52] and may move backwards, towards the posterior chamber of eye. The anterior capsule of the lens is thicker and more rigid in dogs [53] than in humans [54], potentially resulting in equatorial and posterior lens deformation, keeping the ACL constant but decreasing the DSAC. High IOP has been identified as a major risk factor for the initiation and development of glaucoma, but the correlation of IOP with biometric parameters (AGL and DSCA) suggests that changes in these parameters could serve as alternative biomarkers and/or risk factors for the development of glaucoma. Furthermore, these correlations were more marked in adult female EDs, a subgroup particularly affected by PLA. Accordingly, these dogs present ICA abnormalities which are relevant to the development of glaucoma.

Oxidative stress has been identified as a major mechanism underlying the development of glaucoma and RGC degeneration [6]. The importance of this role was highlighted by the decrease in systemic glutathione concentrations observed in patients with primary open glaucoma [7] and the association of this form of glaucoma with a polymorphism of the glutathione S-transferase M1 gene [8]. The activity of GP, a crucial enzyme for the glutathione cycle [55], was very low in EDs. Taurine, another important retinal antioxidant [56], has also recently been reported to play a major role in RGC survival [9]. Surprisingly, we found that plasma taurine levels were higher in EDs than in the control dogs, whereas methionine and cysteine concentrations were similar in these two groups. Taurine is endogenously involved in

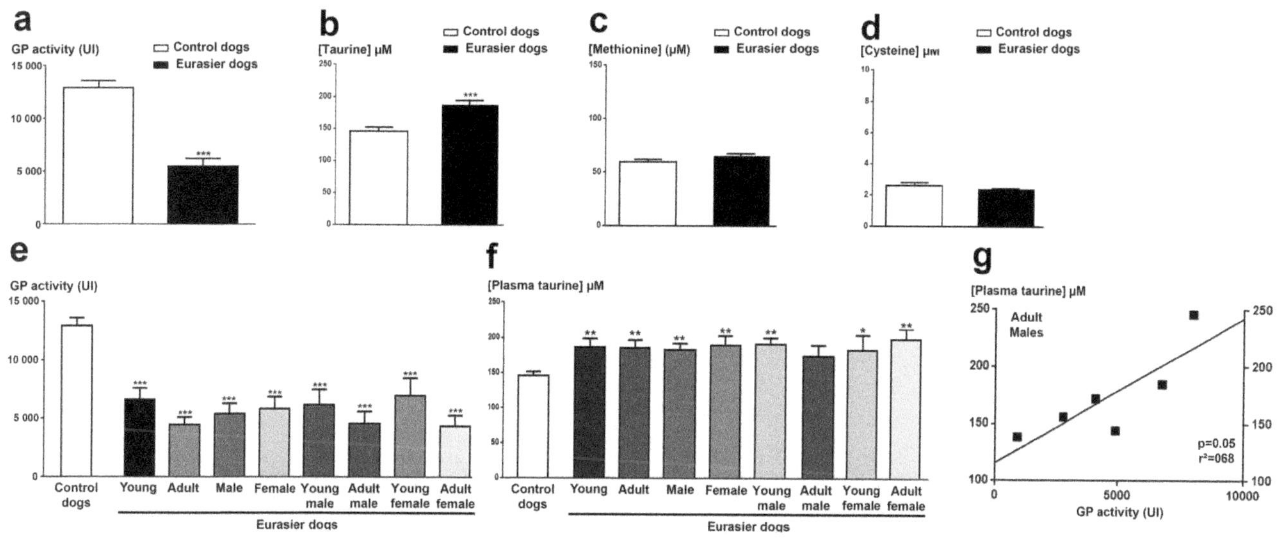

Figure 5. Determinations of biomarkers of oxidative stress in the plasma of Eurasier dogs. (a) Plasma glutathione peroxidase (GP) activity in all EDs (black bar), compared with a cohort of randomized control dogs (white bar). (b) Measurement of plasma taurine concentrations in EDs (black bar), compared with control dogs (white bar). (c-d) Determination of the concentrations of the taurine's precursors, methionine and cysteine, in plasma from EDs (black bar) and control dogs (white bar). (e): Measurement of plasma GP activity in the various subgroups of the ED cohort. (f): Measurement of plasma taurine concentration in the various subgroups of EDs. (g) Correlation between GP activity and plasma taurine concentration in the adult male subgroup of EDs, demonstrating a significant association of low levels of GP activity with a low plasma taurine concentration ($p<0.05$; Spearman's correlation test). This correlation was shown to be linear ($r^2>0.52$). $^{***}p<0.001$ versus the control dogs (Mann Whitney test for a, b,c and Kruskal-Wallis ANOVA followed by the Dunn's post-hoc test for d, e, f).

the process of ROS detoxification in mitochondria [57]. The plasma taurine concentrations may be higher due to an increase in taurine transporter activity responsible for the plasma taurine concentrations. Given the powerful antioxidant action of taurine, these high plasma taurine levels may compensate for the lower level of GP activity. However, the linear correlation between GP activity and plasma taurine concentration suggests that this compensatory effect of taurine may change with age, which possibly would render EDs more susceptible to oxidative stress as adults.

EDs may therefore constitute a genuine canine model for glaucoma. Unlike human patients, the ED breed of dogs is characterized by a very high percentage of inbreeding, which should facilitate the search for the genetic origins of the ICA and glutathione phenotypes. However, it is necessary to study a larger number of dogs to assess the genetic transmission of these phenotypes. The cohort studied here is now being monitored longitudinally with the genotyping of putative candidate genes. In addition, therapeutic treatments, such as beta-blockers and/or carbonic anhydrase inhibitors and/or prostaglandins, will be proposed to animals showing an apparition of glaucomatous symptoms.

We aim to investigate the correlation between ICA modifications and glaucoma development and to identify the cause of susceptibility to glaucoma. This work is based on the notion that there are biomarkers of glaucoma common to humans and dogs, consistent with involvement of the same causal genes in the two species [58]. This study thus provides an illustration of the "one disease, one medicine" concept [59], to the mutual benefit of humans and dogs [60].

Acknowledgments

We thank the members of the *Reseau Europeen d'Ophtalmologie Veterinaire et de Vision Animale* (REOVVA) who participated in the recruitment of animals, the owners of the dogs, and the Conseil Supérieur de l'Ordre des Vétérinaires.

Author Contributions

Conceived and designed the experiments: SR TB TD NF SP. Performed the experiments: SR TB TD FG PT PFI TA SLB II NN NF SL. Analyzed the data: SR NF TB TD NN SLB. Contributed reagents/materials/analysis tools: SR TB TD SLB NN NF. Wrote the paper: NF SR SP TB TD MW JAS.

References

1. Quigley HA, Broman AT (2006) The number of people with glaucoma worldwide in 2010 and 2020. Br J Ophthalmol 90: 262–267.
2. Quigley HA, Dunkelberger GR, Green WR (1989) Retinal ganglion cell atrophy correlated with automated perimetry in human eyes with glaucoma. Am J Ophthalmol 107: 453–464.
3. Goel M, Picciani RG, Lee RK, Bhattacharya SK (2010) Aqueous humor dynamics: a review. Open Ophthalmol J 4: 52–59.
4. Burgoyne CF, Downs JC (2008) Premise and prediction-how optic nerve head biomechanics underlies the susceptibility and clinical behavior of the aged optic nerve head. J Glaucoma 17: 318–328.
5. Burgoyne CF, Downs JC, Bellezza AJ, Suh JK, Hart RT (2005) The optic nerve head as a biomechanical structure: a new paradigm for understanding the role of IOP-related stress and strain in the pathophysiology of glaucomatous optic nerve head damage. Prog Retin Eye Res 24: 39–73.
6. Andersen JK (2004) Oxidative stress in neurodegeneration: cause or consequence? Nat Med 10 Suppl: S18–25.
7. Gherghel D, Griffiths HR, Hilton EJ, Cunliffe IA, Hosking SL (2005) Systemic reduction in glutathione levels occurs in patients with primary open-angle glaucoma. Invest Ophthalmol Vis Sci 46: 877–883.
8. Yildirim O, Ates NA, Tamer L, Oz O, Yilmaz A, et al. (2005) May glutathione S-transferase M1 positive genotype afford protection against primary open-angle glaucoma? Graefes Arch Clin Exp Ophthalmol 243: 327–333.
9. Froger N, Cadetti L, Lorach H, Martins J, Bemelmans AP, et al. (2012) Taurine Provides Neuroprotection against Retinal Ganglion Cell Degeneration. PLoS One 7: e42017.

10. Bedford PG (1977) A gonioscopic study of the iridocorneal angle in the English and American breeds of Cocker Spaniel and the Basset Hound. J Small Anim Pract 18: 631–642.
11. Bjerkas E, Ekesten B, Farstad W (2002) Pectinate ligament dysplasia and narrowing of the iridocorneal angle associated with glaucoma in the English Springer Spaniel. Vet Ophthalmol 5: 49–54.
12. Cottrell BD, Barnett KC (1988) Primary glaucoma in the Welsh springer spaniel. Journal of Small Animal Practice 29: 185–190.
13. Read RA, Wood JL, Lakhani KH (1998) Pectinate ligament dysplasia (PLD) and glaucoma in Flat Coated Retrievers. I. Objectives, technique and results of a PLD survey. Vet Ophthalmol 1: 85–90.
14. Strom AR, Hassig M, Iburg TM, Spiess BM (2011) Epidemiology of canine glaucoma presented to University of Zurich from 1995 to 2009. Part 1: Congenital and primary glaucoma (4 and 123 cases). Vet Ophthalmol 14: 121–126.
15. Gelatt KN, Brooks DE, Källberg ME (2007) The canine glaucomas. In: Gelatt KN, editor. Veterinary Ophthalmology 4th edn. Iowa: Blackwell Publishing. pp. 753–811.
16. Bedford PG, Grierson I (1986) Aqueous drainage in the dog. Res Vet Sci 41: 172–186.
17. Samuelson DA, Gelatt KN (1984) Aqueous outflow in the beagle. I. Postnatal morphologic development of the iridocorneal angle: pectinate ligament and uveal trabecular meshwork. Curr Eye Res 3: 783–794.
18. Gum GG, Gelatt KN, Esson D (2007) Physiology of the eye. In: Gelatt KN, editor. Veterinary Ophthalmology 4th edn. Iowa: Blackwell Publishing. pp. 149–182.
19. Ekesten B (1993) Correlations of intraocular distences to the iridocorneal angle in Samoyeds with special reference to angle-closure glaucoma. Progress in Veterinary and Comparative Ophthalmology 3: 67–73.
20. Ekesten B, Narfstrom K (1991) Correlation of morphologic features of the iridocorneal angle to intraocular pressure in Samoyeds. Am J Vet Res 52: 1875–1878.
21. Crumley W, Gionfriddo JR, Radecki SV (2009) Relationship of the iridocorneal angle, as measured using ultrasound biomicroscopy, with post-operative increases in intraocular pressure post-phacoemulsification in dogs. Vet Ophthalmol 12: 22–27.
22. Dulaurent T, Goulle F, Dulaurent A, Mentek M, Peiffer RL, et al. (2012) Effect of mydriasis induced by topical instillations of 0.5% tropicamide on the anterior segment in normotensive dogs using ultrasound biomicroscopy. Vet Ophthalmol 15 Suppl 1: 8–13.
23. Kanemaki N, Tchedre KT, Imayasu M, Kawarai S, Sakaguchi M, et al. (2013) Dogs and humans share a common susceptibility gene SRBD1 for glaucoma risk. PLoS One 8: e74372.
24. Kato K, Kamida A, Sasaki N, Shastry BS (2009) Evaluation of the CYP1B1 gene as a candidate gene in beagles with primary open-angle glaucoma (POAG). Mol Vis 15: 2470–2474.
25. Kumar A, Basavaraj MG, Gupta SK, Qamar I, Ali AM, et al. (2007) Role of CYP1B1, MYOC, OPTN, and OPTC genes in adult-onset primary open-angle glaucoma: predominance of CYP1B1 mutations in Indian patients. Mol Vis 13: 667–676.
26. Yang M, Guo X, Liu X, Shen H, Jia X, et al. (2009) Investigation of CYP1B1 mutations in Chinese patients with primary congenital glaucoma. Mol Vis 15: 432–437.
27. Corcoran KA, Koch SA, Peiffer RLJ (1994) Primary glaucoma in the chow chow. Veterinary & Comparative Ophthalmology 4: 197.
28. Ekesten B, Torrang I (1995) Heritability of the depth of the opening of the ciliary cleft in Samoyeds. Am J Vet Res 56: 1138–1143.
29. Gelatt KN, Brooks DE, Källberg ME (1999) The canine glaucomas. In: Gelatt KN, editor. Veterinary Ophthalmology 3thr edn. Baltimore: Lippincott & Wilkins. pp. 701–754.
30. Gelatt KN, MacKay EO (2004) Prevalence of the breed-related glaucomas in pure-bred dogs in North America. Vet Ophthalmol 7: 97–111.
31. Boillot T, Boderiou Y, Maller D, Rosolen SG (2012) Bilateral glaucoma affecting a population of adult Eurasier dogs in France: a possible inherited disease?. ESVO proceedings 2012 Veterinary Ophthalmology 1–5: DOI:10.1111/vop.12010.
32. Taylor NR, Zele AJ, Vingrys AJ, Stanley RG (2007) Variation in intraocular pressure following application of tropicamide in three different dog breeds. Vet Ophthalmol 10 Suppl 1: 8–11.
33. Giannetto C, Piccione G, Giudice E (2009) Daytime profile of the intraocular pressure and tear production in normal dog. Vet Ophthalmol 12: 302–305.
34. Piccione G, Giannetto C, Fazio F, Giudice E (2010) Influence of different artificial lighting regimes on intraocular pressure circadian profile in the dog (Canis familiaris). Exp Anim 59: 215–223.
35. Ceron JJ, Eckersall PD, Martynez-Subiela S (2005) Acute phase proteins in dogs and cats: current knowledge and future perspectives. Vet Clin Pathol 34: 85–99.
36. Eckersall PD, Bell R (2010) Acute phase proteins: Biomarkers of infection and inflammation in veterinary medicine. Vet J 185: 23–27.
37. Rosolen SG, Neveux N, Sahel JA, Picaud S, Froger N (2013) Evaluation of the taurine concentrations in dog plasma and aqueous humour: a pilot study. Advances in Experimental Medicine and Biology 775: 145–154.
38. Gelatt KN, MacKay EO (1998) Distribution of intraocular pressure in dogs. Vet Ophthalmol 1: 109–114.
39. Gorig C, Coenen RT, Stades FC, Djajadiningrat-Laanen SC, Boeve MH (2006) Comparison of the use of new handheld tonometers and established applanation tonometers in dogs. Am J Vet Res 67: 134–144.
40. Leiva M, Naranjo C, Pena MT (2006) Comparison of the rebound tonometer (ICare) to the applanation tonometer (Tonopen XL) in normotensive dogs. Vet Ophthalmol 9: 17–21.
41. von Spiessen L, Karck J, Rohn K, Meyer-Lindenberg A (2013) Clinical comparison of the TonoVet rebound tonometer and the Tono-Pen Vet applanation tonometer in dogs and cats with ocular disease: glaucoma or corneal pathology. Vet Ophthalmol.
42. Kawata M, Hasegawa T (2013) Evaluation of the distance between Schwalbe's line and the anterior lens capsule as a parameter for the correction of ultrasound biomicroscopic values of the canine iridocorneal angle. Vet Ophthalmol 16: 169–174.
43. Williams DL (2004) Lens morphometry determined by B-mode ultrasonography of the normal and cataractous canine lens. Vet Ophthalmol 7: 91–95.
44. Kato K, Sasaki N, Matsunaga S, Mochizuki M, Nishimura R, et al. (2006) Possible association of glaucoma with pectinate ligament dysplasia and narrowing of the iridocorneal angle in Shiba Inu dogs in Japan. Vet Ophthalmol 9: 71–75.
45. van der Linde-Sipman JS (1987) Dysplasia of the pectinate ligament and primary glaucoma in the Bouvier des Flandres dog. Vet Pathol 24: 201–206.
46. Pearl R, Gould D, Spiess B (2013) Progression of pectinate ligament dysplasia over time in two populations of Flat-Coated Retrievers. Vet Ophthalmol.
47. Tsai S, Bentley E, Miller PE, Gomes FE, Vangyi C, et al. (2012) Gender differences in iridocorneal angle morphology: a potential explanation for the female predisposition to primary angle closure glaucoma in dogs. Vet Ophthalmol 15 Suppl 1: 60–63.
48. Slater MR, Erb HN (1986) Effects of risk factors and prophylactic treatment on primary glaucoma in the dog. J Am Vet Med Assoc 188: 1028–1030.
49. Vajaranant TS, Nayak S, Wilensky JT, Joslin CE (2010) Gender and glaucoma: what we know and what we need to know. Curr Opin Ophthalmol 21: 91–99.
50. Ekesten B, Torrang I (1995) Age-related changes in ocular distances in normal eyes of Samoyeds. Am J Vet Res 56: 127–133.
51. Hoffer KJ (1993) Axial dimension of the human cataractous lens. Arch Ophthalmol 111: 914–918.
52. Perkins ES (1988) Lens thickness in early cataract. Br J Ophthalmol 72: 348–353.
53. Samuelson DA (2007) Ophthalmic anatomy. In: Gelatt KN, editor. Veterinary Ophthalmology 4th edn. Iowa: Blackwell Publishing. pp. 37–148.
54. Piatigorsky J (1981) Lens differentiation in vertebrates. A review of cellular and molecular features. Differentiation 19: 134–153.
55. Brigelius-Flohe R, Maiorino M (2013) Glutathione peroxidases. Biochim Biophys Acta 1830: 3289–3303.
56. Schaffer SW, Azuma J, Mozaffari M (2009) Role of antioxidant activity of taurine in diabetes. Can J Physiol Pharmacol 87: 91–99.
57. Froger N, Moutsimilli L, Cadetti L, Jammoul F, Wang QP, et al. (2014) Taurine: The comeback of a neutraceutical in the prevention of retinal degenerations. Prog Retin Eye Res 41C: 44–63.
58. Pennisi E (2007) Genetics. The geneticist's best friend. Science 317: 1668–1671.
59. Zinsstag J, Schelling E, Wyss K, Mahamat MB (2005) Potential of cooperation between human and animal health to strengthen health systems. Lancet 366: 2142–2145.
60. Enserink M (2007) Medicine. Initiative aims to merge animal and human health science to benefit both. Science 316: 1553.

Measurement of Glycosylated Alpha-Fetoprotein Improves Diagnostic Power over the Native Form in Hepatocellular Carcinoma

Hyunsoo Kim[1]⁹, Kyunggon Kim[2]⁹, Jonghwa Jin[2], Jiyoung Park[1], Su Jong Yu[3], Jung-Hwan Yoon[3], Youngsoo Kim[1,2]*

1 Department of Biomedical Sciences, Seoul National University College of Medicine, Seoul, Republic of Korea, **2** Department of Biomedical Engineering, Seoul National University College of Medicine, Seoul, Republic of Korea, **3** Department of Internal Medicine, Seoul National University College of Medicine, Seoul, Republic of Korea

Abstract

Serum alpha-fetoprotein (AFP) has long been used as a diagnostic marker for hepatocellular carcinoma (HCC), albeit controversially. Although it remains widely used in clinics, the value of AFP in HCC diagnosis has recently been challenged due to its significant rates of false positive and false negative findings. To improve the efficacy of AFP as HCC diagnostic marker, we developed a method of measuring total and glycosylated AFP by multiple reaction monitoring (MRM)-MS. In this study, we verified the total amount of AFP (nonglycopeptide levels) and the degree of glycosylated AFP (deglycopeptide levels) in 60 normal (41 men and 19 women; mean age 53 years; range 32–74 years), 35 LC (23 men and 12 women; mean age 56 years; range 43–78 years; HBV-related), and 60 HCC subjects (42 men and 18 women; mean age 58 years; range 38–76 years; HBV-related; 30 stage I, 15 stage II, and 10 stage III). By MRM-MS analysis, the nonglycopeptide had 56.7% sensitivity, 68.3% specificity, and an AUC of 0.687 [cutoff value: ≥0.02 (light/heavy ratio)], comparing the normal and HCC group, whereas the deglycopeptide had 93.3% sensitivity, 68.3% specificity, and an AUC of 0.859 [cutoff value: ≥0.02 (light/heavy ratio)]. In comparing the stage I HCC subgroup with the LC group, the nonglycopeptide had a sensitivity of 66.7%, specificity of 80.0%, and an AUC of 0.712 [cutoff value: ≥0.02 (light/heavy ratio)], whereas the deglycopeptide had a sensitivity of 96.7%, specificity of 80.0%, and an AUC of 0.918 [cutoff value: ≥0.02 (light/heavy ratio)]. These data demonstrate that the discriminatory power of the deglycopeptide is greater than that of the nonglycopeptide. We conclude that deglycopeptide can distinguish cancer status between normal subjects and HCC patients better than nonglycopeptide.

Editor: Lian-Yue Yang, Xiangya Hospital of Central South University, China

Funding: This work was supported by a National Research Foundation of Korea grant (No. 2011-0030740) and the Proteogenomic Research Program, funded by the Korea government [MISP]. This work was also supported by the Industrial Strategic Technology Development Program (#10045352), funded by the Ministry of Knowledge Economy (MKE, Korea). The funders had no role in study design, data collection and analysis, decision to publish, or preparation of the manuscript.

Competing Interests: The authors have declared that no competing interests exist.

* Email: biolab@snu.ac.kr

⁹ These authors contributed equally to this work.

Introduction

Glycosylation is one of the most important and common post-translational modifications (PTMs) of proteins that are secreted into serum. Glycosylation influences many functional aspects of proteins, including their structure and functions [1]. The expression and degree of glycosylation is significantly altered by various diseases, such as cancer, and thus, glycoproteins are associated with abnormal phenomena in patients with cancer [2–4]. To this end, quantitative measurements of glycoproteins might be useful in discovering biomarkers for cancer.

The carbohydrates on glycosylated protein biomarkers undergo modifications in cancer. For example, the carbohydrate moieties of AFP are altered in cancer, and such changes are considered to be more useful markers of HCC [5]. Studies from the past several decades have demonstrated that total AFP is a collection of heterogeneous glycoproteins that can be fractionated by affinity electrophoresis into 3 glycoforms–AFP-L1, AFP-L2, and AFP-L3–based on their reactivity with the lectin Lens culinaris agglutinin (LCA). AFP-L3 binds strongly to LCA through an α1-6 bond between its additional fucose and the reducing terminus of N-acetylglucosamine, in contrast to AFP-L1 [6–8].

AFP levels are sometimes elevated in patients with chronic hepatitis and cirrhosis who have no evidence of HCC [9]. AFP has a reported sensitivity of 39% to 65% and a specificity of 65% to 94%; approximately one-third of early-stage HCC patients with small tumors (<3 cm) have normal AFP levels [10,11]. Thus, clinicians are dissatisfied with AFP as a marker due to its high false-positive and false-negative rates [12].

Multiple reaction monitoring (MRM)-based quantification using triple quadrupole mass spectrometry (MS) is especially useful for measuring glycosylated biomarkers. MRM-MS, a multiplexed, targeted proteomic platform, is a rapid and cost-effective approach for measuring protein biomarkers for preclinical verification [13]. Nonglycopeptides (unmodified native peptides) and glycopeptides (glycosylated peptides) of glycoprotein markers are valuable biomarkers for the diagnosis and prediction of diseases, because their expression levels and degree of glycosylation reflect quantitative differences of disease states, as in cancer.

In this study, we measured total AFP and glycosylated AFP by MRM-MS. Total AFP was represented by common nonglycopeptides among all forms of AFP, and glycosylated AFP comprised the portion of deglycosylated peptides after treatment of glycosylated peptides with PNGase F. Measurement of the deglycopeptide fraction from the glycosylated AFP yielded better AUC values than the nonglycopeptides of total AFP. Consequently, on measuring AFP concentrations in serum from HCC patients versus normal healthy controls and early-stage HCC versus liver cirrhosis by MRM-MS, AFP deglycopeptides had greater power in distinguishing, compared with nonglycopeptides.

Notably, total AFP and glycosylated AFP were measured effectively by MRM-MS in the form of nonglycopeptides and deglycopeptides, respectively, improving our diagnosis of HCC versus normal and early-stage HCC versus LC serum. In addition, MRM-MS is a platform that improves the measurement of total AFP and glycosylated AFP in glycoprotein biomarker assays, which is more advantageous compared with conventional methods, such as antibody-based measurements by lectin affinity electrophoresis and liquid-phase binding assays.

Materials and Methods

Materials

Standard glycoprotein (origin: yeast) was purchased from Sigma-Aldrich (St. Louis, MO). Trypsin was obtained from Promega (Madison, WI). Peptide-N-glycosidase F (PNGase F) was purchased from New England Biolabs (NEB, Beverly, MA). HPLC-grade water and acetonitrile were obtained from Thermo Fisher Scientific (Bremen, Germany). Serum depletion was performed for the 6 most abundant proteins using a multiple affinity removal system (MARS), consisting of an LC column (Agilent, 5185–5984); buffer A for sample loading, washes, and equilibration (Agilent, 5185–5987); and buffer B for elution (Agilent, 5185–5988). Stable isotope-labeled peptides [isotopically labeled (^{13}C and ^{15}N) amino acids] were obtained from JPT (Berlin, Germany).

Clinical sample information

The institutional review board (IRB) of Seoul National University Hospital (approval No. H-1103-056-355) approved the study protocol, and written informed consent was obtained from each patient or legally authorized representative. The clinical characteristics of the patients are shown in Table 1.

The clinical sample set comprised healthy controls (n = 60), patients with liver cirrhosis (n = 35), and patients with hepatocellular carcinoma (n = 60). The healthy control group (normal group) comprised sixty healthy volunteers who visited the Healthcare Center of Seoul National University Hospital. All control subjects were confirmed, based on normal liver function test results, including serum alanine and aspartate aminotransferases, and were negative for hepatitis B virus surface antigen and anti-hepatitis C virus. Liver ultrasonography was performed to screen for fatty liver disease, and all healthy controls had normal findings.

The liver cirrhosis group (LC group) included 35 patients with compensated HBV cirrhosis and no HCC. The cirrhosis group had at least 1 year of follow-up from the time that serum was obtained for these studies. Patients were diagnosed with cirrhosis, based on established clinical, laboratory, and imaging criteria with ultrasound examination.

Sixty patients before HCC treatment who were infected with hepatitis B virus (HBV) were also enrolled, from whom serum samples were collected and defined as the HCC group. The diagnosis of HCC was made per the American Association for the Study of Liver Diseases by a hepatologist with more than 20 years of experience [14]. To reduce causal heterogeneity, HCC patients who had other types of chronic liver disease, except chronic hepatitis B, such as chronic hepatitis C and alcoholic hepatitis, were excluded.

HCC stage was classified per the tumor-node-metastasis (TNM) staging system (7th edition, 2010, the American Joint Committee on Cancer staging system). TNM staging of the 55 cases demonstrated stage I in 30 cases, stage II in 15 cases, stage III in 10 cases, and stage IV in 0 cases. Insufficient information was available to assign stage in 5 HCC cases.

All subjects (n = 155) were recruited during the study period from September 2005 to August 2012 and collected by the Liver Research Institute, Seoul National University College of Medicine. Blood samples were centrifuged immediately at 3000 rpm for 10 min at 4°C to fractionate the serum. The resulting supernatant was aliquoted (100 μL) and stored at −80°C until analysis.

Sample size calculations

We calculate the sample size that was needed for clinical MRM verification with reference to previous studies using AUC (area under the curve) [15]. The sample size was calculated, based on an AUC with a type I error rate α of 0.05 and type II error rate β of 0.10 (90% power). To anticipate similar AUC values as in previous studies, we needed a sample size of 29 each in the normal and HCC groups, each totaling 58, and 24 each in the HCC and recovery groups, totaling 48. A minimum sample size of 29 per group was necessary for the MRM assays to determine a significant difference between groups (Table S1).

Standard glycoprotein preparation

Standard glycoprotein (INV1) was prepared to 100 μg/μL. Standard glycoprotein samples were denatured with 6 M urea, 100 mM Tris, pH 8.0, and 20 mM dithiothreitol (DTT) at 37°C for 60 min and alkylated with 50 mM iodoacetamide (IAA) at room temperature in the dark for 30 min. The urea was diluted 15-fold with 100 mM Tris, pH 8.0. One INV1 sample was deglycosylated with 2 μL of PNGase F (500,000 units/mL) at 37°C for 12 h and incubated and digested in a solution of 1:50 trypsin (w/w) at 37°C for 16 h. The other INV1 sample was incubated in 2 μL 100 mM Tris, pH 8.0 (untreated PNGase F) at 37°C for 12 h and digested as described above. The 2 INV1 digests were dried on a speed vacuum, diluted in mobile phase A, and spiked with stable isotope-labeled standard (SIS) peptide, as needed.

Clinical serum sample preparation

The 6 most abundant proteins in human serum (albumin, transferrin, IgG, IgA, haptoglobin, and α1-antitrypsin) were depleted on an HPLC system (Shimadzu Co., Kyoto, Japan) that was equipped with a multiple affinity removal system LC column (Agilent Technologies, Santa Clara, CA). Crude human serum samples were diluted by a factor of 5 with buffer A and passed through 0.22-μm filters by centrifugation (12,000 g, room temperature, 2–3 min). Diluted crude serum was injected at 0.25 mL/min, and flowthrough fractions were collected and stored at −80°C. Depleted serum samples were concentrated by

Table 1. Characteristics of clinical subjects for MRM-MS analysis.

	Normal group	LC group	HCC group
Total patient number	60	35	60
Gender (Male/Female)	41/19	23/12	42/18
Age (Mean, Range)	53 (32–74)	56 (43–78)	58 (38–76)
Etiology of liver disease		HBV, 35 (100%)	HBV, 60 (100%)
AFP value (mean, range)			
<20 ng/ml	60	35	26
20–400 ng/ml	0	0	18
>400 ng/ml	0	0	16
Albumin (g/dL)	4.3±0.18	4.2±0.3	3.6±0.5
Bilirubin (mg/dL)	1.3±0.4	1.4±0.7	1.3±0.8
AST (IU/L)	22.5±6.0	32.3±24.3	89.1±142.3
ALT (IU/L)	20.2±8.3	37.6±35.0	97.1±249.9
ALP (IU/L)	41.7±19.2	78.4±20.6	123.5±77.6
HBV DNA levels (IU/mL)[a]			
Not detected		11	1
Detected (<10^3/units)		9	3
Detected (≥10^3/units)		6	25
Antiviral therapy[b]			
Yes (%)		23 (65.7%)	17 (28.3%)
No (%)		12 (34.3%)	43 (71.7%)
Treatment type			
Surgical resection			1
RFA			3
PEIT			22
TACE			30
TACE & PEIT			4
Tumor size (cm)[c]			
<2			21
2~5			16
>5			3
Tumor stage[d]			
I			30
II			15
III			10
IV			0
Target lesion response			
CR			38
PR			19
SD			3
PD			0

Abbreviations
TACE: Transcatheter arterial chemoembolization.
PEIT: Percutaneous ethanol injection therapy.
RFA: Radiofrequency ablation.
AFP: Alpha-fetoprotein.
ALT: Alanine aminotransferase; AST: Aspartate aminotransferase; ALP: Alkaline phosphatase.
CR: Complete Response; PR: Partial Response; SD: Stable disease; PD: Progressive disease.
Albumin, Bilirubin, AST, ALT, ALP, and HBV DNA levels data are presented as mean ± SD.
[a]HBV DNA levels were provided for 26 among a total of 35 liver cirrhosis patients, and 29 among the 60 HCC patients.
[b]Antiviral therapy was treatment with Entecavir, Tenofovir, Zeffix, Hepsera and Revovir.
[c]Tumor size was provided for 40 among a total of 60 HCC patients.
[d]According to American Joint Committee on Cancer (AJCC) staging system (7th edition, 2010).

centrifugal filtration using a 3000-Da molecular weight cutoff (MWCO) (Millipore, Bedford, MA). Concentrated serum protein was quantified by bicinchoninic acid (BCA) assay.

Aliquots of serum samples (100 μg) were denatured and digested as described above. Tryptic digestion was stopped with formic acid (FA) at a final concentration of 1% and desalted on OASIS HLB 1-cc (30 mg) extraction cartridges (Waters Corp., Milford, MA). The cartridges were equilibrated sequentially with 3 mL acetonitrile (ACN) and 5 mL water/0.1% FA prior to loading of the tryptic digestions. The cartridges were washed with 3 mL water/ 0.1% FA and eluted with 1 mL of 60% ACN/0.1% FA. The eluted samples were frozen and lyophilized on a speed vacuum. Before MRM-MS analysis, the samples were reconstituted in mobile phase A to 1 μg/μL.

MRM-MS transition (Q1/Q3) selection

Skyline software was used to generate a list of all possible b-, y-series fragment ions for 2^+ precursor ion charge states, spanning the m/z range from 300 to 1400. In brief, full-length protein sequences were imported into Skyline in FASTA format and designed into peptides, each with a list of product ions for monitoring by MRM-MS. In selecting transitions through Skyline, the peptide filter condition was as follows: maximum length of peptide of 24, including at least 6 amino acids.

Peptides with repeat arginines (Arg, R) or lysines (Lys, K) were discarded. If methionine (Met, M) was included in the peptide, it was discarded to avoid the risk of modification. If proline (Pro, P) was next to arginine (Arg, R) or lysine (Lys, K), the peptide was discarded. If a peptide contained histidine (His, H), it was discarded to avoid the risk of charge alterations. Peptides that satisfied these conditions were used as Q1 transitions. Next, we selected a maximum of 10 Q3 transitions from the fragmentation ions that were derived from the Q1 transitions in descending order.

For glycopeptides, theoretical transition values were selected, based on the original FASTA sequences after changing asparagine (Asn, N) in the NxS/T motif into aspartic acid (Asp, D), using Skyline. In addition, to verify that the measured peptides originated from the endogenous peptide that was tested, a stable isotope-labeled standard (SIS) peptide was used. The sequence of the SIS peptide is identical to that of the measured peptide but has ^{13}C and ^{15}N in the C-terminal arginine (Arg, R) and lysine (Lys, K). This result is described in Table S2.

Quantification by multiple reaction monitoring

An Agilent 1260 Infinity HPLC system was used to inject 5 μL of digestion samples directly into a reversed phase analytical column (150 mm×0.5 mm i.d., Agilent Zorbax SB-C18, 3.5-μm particle size) that was maintained at 40°C. Mobile phase A consisted of water/0.1% FA, and mobile phase B comprised ACN/0.1% FA. The peptides were separated and eluted at 20 μL/min on a linear gradient of mobile phase B from 3% to 40% B in 45 min. The gradient was ramped to 70% B for 5 min and 3% B for 10 min to equilibrate the column for the next run. The total LC run time was 60 min.

The MRM-MS data were analyzed using ESI on an Agilent 6490 triple quadrupole (QQQ) mass spectrometer (Agilent Technologies, Santa Clara, CA) that was equipped with an iFunnel Technology source and controlled by MassHunter Workstation software (Agilent, B.06.00). The MRM-MS analysis was conducted in the positive ion mode with the ion spray capillary voltage and nozzle voltage set to 2500 and 2000 V, respectively. The drying gas temperature was set to 250°C at 15 L/min, and the sheath gas temperature was 350°C at 12 L/min. The nebulizer was set to 30 psi, the fragmentor voltage was 380 V, and the cell accelerator voltage was 5 V. For the MRM-MS acquisition, delta EMV was set to 200 V. Quadrupoles 1 and 3 were maintained at unit (0.7 FWHM) resolution.

Collision energy optimization

The initial collision energy (CE) linear equation was derived from our optimized experiments, prior to the Skyline CE optimization step, using 600 stable isotope-labeled standard (SIS) peptides that were measured (data not shown). In the CE optimization module in Skyline, "Step count" was set to 5 on either side of the equation-predicted value, and "Step size" was set to 2V. The b and y ions for 2^+ precursor ion charge states were used, and in total, 11 collision energy voltage values were considered for each fragment ion. The maximum number of concurrent measurements was set to 132. The data were acquired and imported into Skyline for peak area integration, which was reviewed manually and finalized by a single investigator.

Study design for blocking and randomization

Blocking and randomization can prevent the negative impacts of nonbiologic effects on molecular biomarker discovery [16]. In our experiments, nonbiologic effects could have been introduced during the sample preparation (order of MARS depletion and order of tryptic digestion) and MRM-MS analysis (order of injection). Three step where the experimenter's subjectivity could have led to bias of sample groups was negated by blocked randomization method.

We applied the blocked randomization design when assigning the sample group to remove confounding nonbiologic effects. There were equal numbers of cases (HCC group) and controls (normal group) in every block, with random block size. We then assigned each group of order to a random permutation of the samples in the corresponding group (Table S3). Blocked randomization was performed using Excel (2013, Microsoft) and Random Allocation (version 1.00, University of Medical Sciences).

Statistical analysis of MRM-MS data

To analyze the MRM-MS data, raw MRM-MS data files were processed in Skyline. To increase the accuracy of the peak area integration, we manually confirmed and corrected the wrong automatic assignments for each targeted peak area. In our peak integration step, we used the Savitzky-Golay smoothing algorithm. Differences were analyzed by *T*-test between the normal versus HCC group and the LC versus stage I HCC subgroup. To evaluate the discriminatory power of the serum biomarkers between groups, we analyzed the receiver operator characteristic (ROC) curves and generated interactive plots. ROC curves were compared using DeLong's method [17]. All statistical analyses were performed using MedCalc (Mariakerke, Belgium, version 12.2.1).

Results

Overall scheme

We performed a combined measurement in a single run of the total AFP concentration and glycosylated AFP fraction after PNGase F treatment. There are 3 glycosylated forms of AFP–AFP-L1, L2, and L3–based on its reactivity to Lens culinaris agglutinin (LCA) by affinity electrophoresis (Figure S1A). The concentration of total AFP and the N-linked glycosylated AFP fraction (AFP-L1, L2 and L3) that can be cleaved by PNGase F (Figure S1B) could be measured by MRM-MS in the same MRM run.

To develop an MRM-MS method for measuring glycoprotein concentration, such as AFP, we measured a standard glycoprotein of INV1 to determine whether MRM-MS was suitable for measuring glycoprotein concentrations and applied MRM-MS to measure AFP concentrations (Figure 1). The total AFP concentration was measured, based on nonglycopeptides, whereas the glycosyated AFP fraction was represented by the corresponding deglycopeptide that was generated by PNGase F treatment. Consequently, the discriminatory power was examined for total AFP and glycosylated AFP in serum samples from normal healthy controls versus HCC patients and liver cirrhosis versus early-stage HCC patients.

Establishment of MRM-MS measurement using standard glycoprotein

We first determine whether MRM-MS is suitable for measuring glycoproteins using standard glycoproteins, such as yeast INV1. Four peptides were examined in developing and assessing the MRM-MS method (Figure S2A and Table S2): 2 peptides (IEIYSSDDLK and VVDFGK) were nonglycopeptides, and 2 were glycopeptides (NPVLAA*N*STQFR and FAT*N*TTLTK).

In examining their ability to be detected, all nonglycopeptides and deglycopeptides (SIS standard: Asn to Asp) coeluted with the corresponding SIS heavy peptides, whereas glycopeptides did not coelute with its SIS heavy peptide form (SIS standard: Asn with no

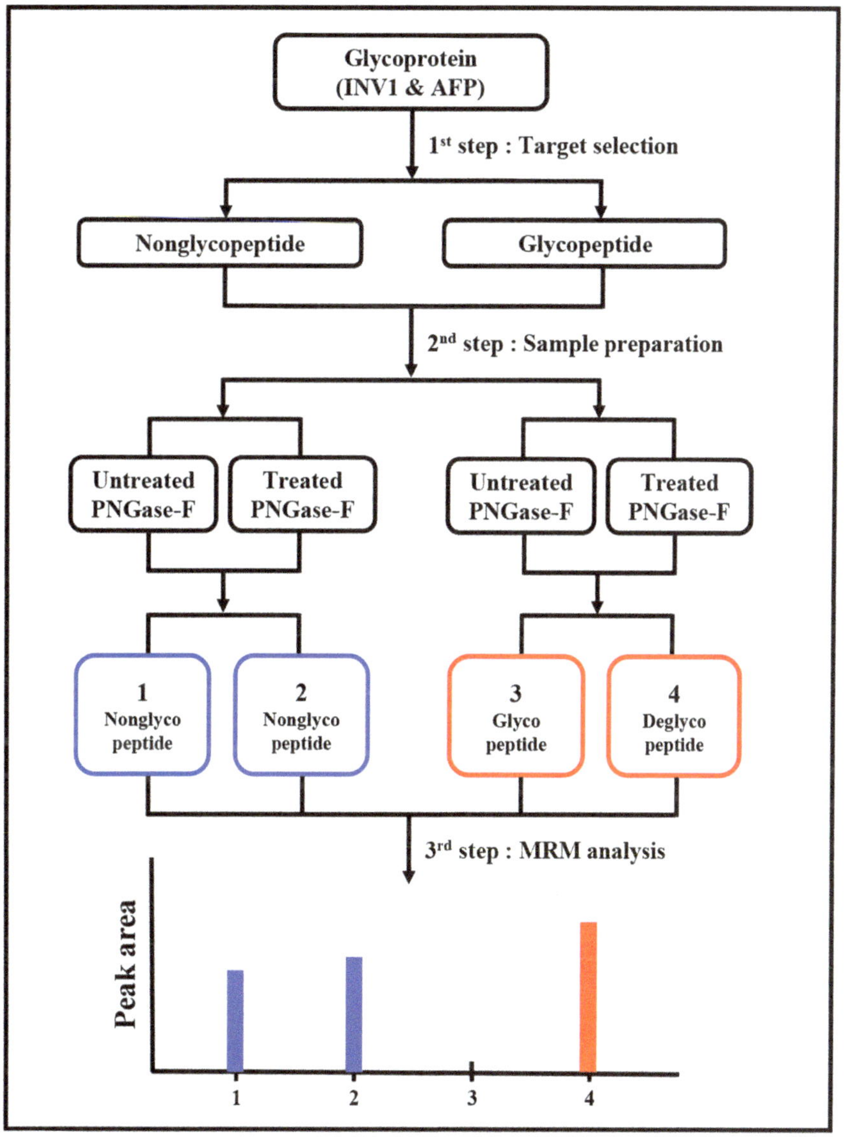

Figure 1. Development of MRM-MS method for measuring glycoproteins. To develop the MRM-MS method for measuring nonglycopeptides, glycopeptides, and deglycopeptides, we determined whether our MRM-MS approach was suitable for measuring glycoproteins using a standard glycoprotein, such as yeast invertase 1 (INV1), and applied the MRM-MS method to measure the alpha-fetoprotein (AFP) in human serum samples.

glycan). Because the SIS heavy peptides were synthesized only using Asn with no glycan, the SIS heavy peptide that represents the glycopeptide comprises only amino acid residues; thus, the existence of a glycopeptide is measured alternatively in the form as in the MRM-MS (eg, glycosylated Asn is measured as Asn or Asp). We measured the 4 peptides using the corresponding SIS heavy peptides, as detailed in Figure S3A–H. Because we could not use glycosylated SIS heavy peptides for the 2 glycopeptides, we measured the SIS heavy peptides NPVLAADSTQFR and FATDTTLTK indirectly as substitutes for the glycopeptides NPVLAANSTQFR and FATNTTLTK (Figure S3E & S3G).

Two nonglycopeptides (IEIYSSDDLK; Figure S3A & S3B, and VVDFGK; Figure S3C & S3D) were detected in the PNGase F-untreated (S3A, S3C) and PNGase F-treated (S3B, S3D) samples; the 2 nonglycopeptides had slightly greater intensity with PNGase F treatment (Figure S4). It is possible that PNGase F removes the glycan of a peptide, which may effect the absence of steric hindrance due to the glycan, allowing trypsin approach to a target peptide more easily. Consequently this accessibility might increase digestion and affect the peak intensity of MS/MS spectra [18].

The 2 glycopeptides (NPVLAANSTQFR and FATNTTLTK) were detected only with PNGage F treatment as peaks of the corresponding deglycopeptides (NPVLAADSTQFR; Figure S3F, and FATDTTLTK; Figure S3H). In the PNGase F-untreated, no extracted ion chromatogram (XIC) was detected for the endogenous glycopeptide forms, whereas SIS heavy peptides were detected with unglycosylated Asn (NPVLAANSTQFR; Figure S3E, and FATNTTLTK; Figure S3G). In the MRM-MS analysis, glycopeptides could not be detected, because they were measured, based on the original sequence–ie, NPVLAANSTQFR and FATNTTLTK, respectively. Conversely, the corresponding deglycosylated sequences for PNGage F-treated glycopeptides–NPVLAADSTQFR and FATDTTLTK–were detected as MRM peaks for the glycosylated peptides of NPVLAANSTQFR and FATNTTLTK, respectively.

To develop the quantitative method, we evaluated the linearity of nonglycopeptides, glycopeptides, and deglycopeptides that originated from INV1 by analyzing the standard curves of serial dilutions for known concentrations of SIS heavy peptides. To generate calibration curves for the 3 types of peptides, SIS heavy peptides were serially diluted (0, 4, 13, 40, 120, and 370 fmol), with the light peptides as internal standards. Digested light yeast peptide (370 nmol) was added to each diluted sample. Each experiment was repeated in triplicate to generate coefficients of variation (%CV) and calibration curve values (R^2).

The calibration curves demonstrated linearity over more than 2 orders of magnitude for the concentration ranges and strong linear correlation (R^2>0.99) in all 3 peptide forms (Figure S5A–D). By MRM-MS analysis using the standard peptides, we developed the MRM-MS method for measuring glycoprotein concentrations. Notably, the PNGase F-untreated endogenous light glycopeptides (NPVLAANSTQFR and FATNTTLTK, filled downward arrows) did not generate peaks from MRM, as shown in Figure S5C–D.

Preliminary MRM-MS using pooled serum samples

Prior to MRM-MS of AFP using individual samples, we first selected predictable transitions using Skyline, in which the N-linked glycopeptide included the NxS/T motif, whereas the nonglycopeptide did not. Table 2 shows 3 AFP peptides that were used in the MRM-MS; the sequences of the nonglycopeptide, glycopeptide, and deglycopeptide of AFP were GYQELLEK, VNFTEIQK, and VDFTEIQK, respectively. For MRM-MS of the 3 AFP peptides, we determined their detectability in the preliminary MRM-MS run.

Nonglycopeptides (GYQELLEK) and deglycopeptide (VDFTEIQK) of AFP coeluted with the endogenous light and SIS heavy peptides at the same retention time. In brief, the nonglycopeptide (GYQELLEK) was coeluted in the PNGase F-untreated (Figure S6A) and PNGase F-treated (Figure S6B) conditions. However, the glycopeptide was not detected (Figure S6C) when the PNGase F-untreated glycosylated peptide was analyzed by the glycopeptide form with the no-glycan form (VNFTEIQK). The PNGage F-treated glycosylated peptide coeluted (Figure S6D) with the deglycopeptide form (VDFTEIQK).

Serum AFP concentrations rise in HCC patients versus normal subjects [19–22]; thus, we examined this difference between the normal healthy and HCC group using MRM-MS measurements. 20 normal samples and 20 HCC samples were pooled separately and analyzed by MRM-MS using the nonglycopeptide (GYQELLEK). The MS/MS intensity for the nonglycopeptide increased in the normal versus HCC group (Figure 2).

With regard to measuring glycopeptide concentrations, because the glycosylated glycopeptide form (VNFTEIQK) could not be detected directly using MRM-MS, we analyzed the deglycopeptide form (VDFTEIQK), which was generated by treating VNFTEIQK with PNGase F. The normalized peak area for the nonglycopeptide and deglycopeptide increased in HCC patients versus the normal group (Figure 2). Particularly, the peak area ratio of HCC to the normal group was 6.5 and 66.5 for the nonglycopeptide and deglycopeptide, respectively, indicating that total AFP concentration is a useful index for liver cancer diagnostics and that measuring the fraction of glycosylated AFP that has been treated by PNGase F is a more important element in HCC diagnosis.

Linearity of calibration curve for SIS AFP peptide

In the quantitative MRM-MS analysis, we determined the linearity of the nonglycopeptide (GYQELLEK) and deglycopeptide (VDFTEIQK) with regard to AFP, which was performed by generating a standard curve for the nonglycopeptide and deglycopeptide, composed of serial dilutions for known concentrations of SIS heavy peptides. SIS heavy peptides were serially diluted (9 concentrations: 0.0, 0.8, 1.6, 3.1, 6.3, 12.5, 25.0, 50.0, and 100.0 fmol) with the endogenous light peptide as an internal standard (pooled serum: 5 μg), added to each serially diluted sample. Each experiment was repeated in triplicate to generate coefficients of variation (%CV) and calibration curve values (R^2). The calibration curves were linear over more than 2 orders of magnitude in concentration, wherein the nonglycopeptide (GYQELLEK) and deglycopeptide (VDFTEIQ) showed strong linearity (R^2>0.99) (Figure 3).

MRM-MS measurements of AFP peptides using individual serum samples

To measure the nonglycopeptide (GYQELLEK) and deglycopeptide (VDFTEIQK) of AFP using MRM-MS in individual normal and HCC serum samples, we determined the optimal spiking concentrations for SIS heavy peptides that minimized the measurement errors for the peak area ratio between endogenous light peptide and SIS heavy peptide. By MRM analysis using pooled samples, which comprised endogenous light (pooled serum: 5 μg) and serially diluted SIS heavy peptides (0–200 fmol), we determined the optimal range of SIS heavy peptide for spiking (peak area ratio of light peptide to heavy peptide = 1). The concentrations of SIS heavy peptides for the nonglycopeptide (GYQELLEK) and deglycopeptide (VDFTEIQK) that were used to spike were 10.3 and 7.3 fmol, respectively.

Table 2. AFP peptides and their parameters for MRM-MS.

Peptide type	Peptide sequence	Q1 (m/z)	Q1 ion charge	Q3 (m/z)	Q3 ion charge	Q3 ion type	Retention time (min)	Isotope	Fragmentor (volt)	Initial CE (volt)	Optimized CE (volt)
Nonglycopeptide	GYQELLEK	490.3	2	759.4	1	y6	23.6	light	380	17.3	11.3
				631.4	1	y5	23.6	light	380	17.3	13.3
				502.3	1	y4	23.6	light	380	17.3	15.3
				389.2	1	y3	23.6	light	380	17.3	17.3
				276.2	1	y2	23.6	light	380	17.3	21.3
				221.1	1	b2	23.6	light	380	17.3	11.3
				349.2	1	b3	23.6	light	380	17.3	9.3
				591.3	1	b5	23.6	light	380	17.3	11.3
				704.4	1	b6	23.6	light	380	17.3	7.3
				833.4	1	b7	23.6	light	380	17.3	9.3
	GYQELLEK	494.3	2	767.4	1	y6	23.6	heavy	380	17.3	11.3
				639.4	1	y5	23.6	heavy	380	17.3	13.3
				510.3	1	y4	23.6	heavy	380	17.3	15.3
				397.3	1	y3	23.6	heavy	380	17.3	17.3
				284.2	1	y2	23.6	heavy	380	17.3	21.3
				221.1	1	b2	23.6	heavy	380	17.3	11.3
				349.2	1	b3	23.6	heavy	380	17.3	9.3
				591.3	1	b5	23.6	heavy	380	17.3	11.3
				704.4	1	b6	23.6	heavy	380	17.3	7.3
				833.4	1	b7	23.6	heavy	380	17.3	9.3
Glycopeptide[a]	V*N*FTEIQK	489.8	2	879.5	1	y7	22.0	light	380	17.3	13.3
				765.4	1	y6	22.0	light	380	17.3	13.3
				618.3	1	y5	22.0	light	380	17.3	15.3
				517.3	1	y4	22.0	light	380	17.3	11.3
				388.3	1	y3	22.0	light	380	17.3	21.3
				275.2	1	y2	22.0	light	380	17.3	21.3
				361.2	1	b3	22.0	light	380	17.3	9.3
				462.2	1	b4	22.0	light	380	17.3	9.3
				591.3	1	b5	22.0	light	380	17.3	11.3
				704.4	1	b6	22.0	light	380	17.3	9.3
				832.4	1	b7	22.0	light	380	17.3	7.3
	V*N*FTEIQK	493.8	2	887.5	1	y7	22.0	heavy	380	17.3	13.3
				773.4	1	y6	22.0	heavy	380	17.3	13.3
				626.4	1	y5	22.0	heavy	380	17.3	15.3
				525.3	1	y4	22.0	heavy	380	17.3	11.3
				396.3	1	y3	22.0	heavy	380	17.3	21.3

Table 2. Cont.

Peptide type	Peptide sequence	Q1 (m/z)	Q1 ion charge	Q3 (m/z)	Q3 ion charge	Q3 ion type	Retention time (min)	Isotope	Fragmentor (volt)	Initial CE (volt)	Optimized CE (volt)
				283.2	1	y2	22.0	heavy	380	17.3	21.3
				361.2	1	b3	22.0	heavy	380	17.3	9.3
				462.2	1	b4	22.0	heavy	380	17.3	9.3
				591.3	1	b5	22.0	heavy	380	17.3	11.3
				704.4	1	b6	22.0	heavy	380	17.3	9.3
				832.4	1	b7	22.0	heavy	380	17.3	7.3
Deglycopeptide	VDFTEIQK	490.3	2	880.4	1	y7	22.7	light	380	17.3	13.3
				765.4	1	y6	22.7	light	380	17.3	13.3
				618.3	1	y5	22.7	light	380	17.3	15.3
				517.3	1	y4	22.7	light	380	17.3	11.3
				388.3	1	y3	22.7	light	380	17.3	21.3
				275.2	1	y2	22.7	light	380	17.3	21.3
				362.2	1	b3	22.7	light	380	17.3	9.3
				463.2	1	b4	22.7	light	380	17.3	9.3
				592.3	1	b5	22.7	light	380	17.3	11.3
				705.3	1	b6	22.7	light	380	17.3	9.3
				833.4	1	b7	22.7	light	380	17.3	7.3
	VDFTEIQK	494.3	2	888.5	1	y7	22.7	heavy	380	17.3	13.3
				773.4	1	y6	22.7	heavy	380	17.3	13.3
				626.4	1	y5	22.7	heavy	380	17.3	15.3
				525.3	1	y4	22.7	heavy	380	17.3	11.3
				396.3	1	y3	22.7	heavy	380	17.3	21.3
				283.2	1	y2	22.7	heavy	380	17.3	21.3
				362.2	1	b3	22.7	heavy	380	17.3	9.3
				463.2	1	b4	22.7	heavy	380	17.3	9.3
				592.3	1	b5	22.7	heavy	380	17.3	11.3
				705.3	1	b6	22.7	heavy	380	17.3	9.3
				833.4	1	b7	22.7	heavy	380	17.3	7.3

[a]The molecular mass of glycopeptide is estimated based on Asn with no glycan moiety.

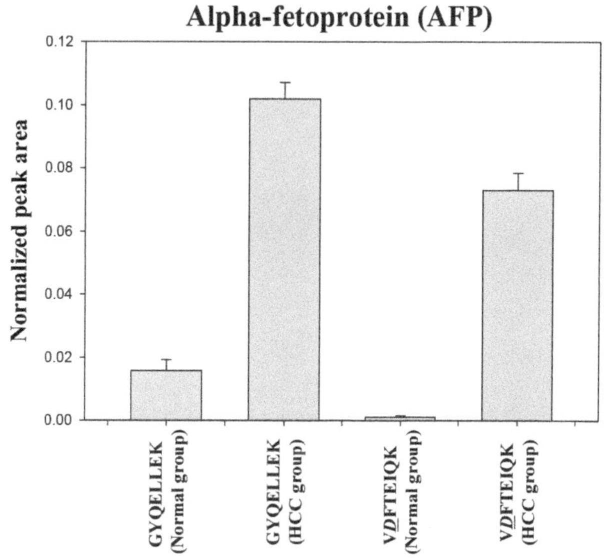

	Nonglycopeptide (GYQELLEK)		Deglycopeptide (V*D*FTEIQK)	
	Normal group	HCC group	Normal group	HCC group
1 set	0.0183	0.1064	0.0016	0.0675
2 set	0.0118	0.0963	0.0010	0.0782
3 set	0.0173	0.1032	0.0008	0.0734
Average	0.0158	0.1020	0.0011	0.0731
STDEV	0.0035	0.0051	0.0004	0.0054
CV (%)	22.3	5.0	38.5	7.3
Fold-change (HCC / Normal)		**6.5**		**66.1**

Figure 2. Preliminary MRM-MS analysis using pooled serum samples. Normal samples (n = 20) and HCC samples (n = 20) were pooled separately and analyzed by MRM-MS using the nonglycopeptide (GYQELLEK) and deglycopeptide (V*D*FTEIQK).

Individual serum samples were analyzed using the MRM-MS measurements with the spiked SIS heavy peptide mixture of nonglycopeptide (GYQELLEK) and deglycopeptide (V*D*FT EIQK) as the internal standard. Based on the MRM measurements using 155 individual serum samples, we measured the concentrations of the nonglycopeptide (GYQELLEK) and deglycopeptide (V*D*FTEIQK) of AFP in the normal (n = 60), LC group (n = 35) and HCC group (n = 60). The MRM measurements were imported into Skyline, and the peak areas of each transition were calculated, after normalization by the peak area of the spiked SIS heavy peptide (Figure S7). Next, the relative quantities of each transition were compared between the nonglycopeptide (GYQELLEK) and deglycopeptide (V*D*FTEIQK) in the normal versus HCC group and the LC versus stage I HCC subgroup.

To determine the efficacy of serum biomarkers in distinguishing HCC versus normal controls and the stage I HCC subgroup versus LC group, we drew receiver operator characteristic (ROC) curves and interactive plots, and the MRM-MS data on the nonglycopeptide (GYQELLEK) and deglycopeptide (V*D*F TEIQK) from both groups were analyzed. (Figure 4).

HCC group was compared to normal control group, the nonglycopeptide had a sensitivity of 56.7%, specificity of 68.3%, AUC of 0.687 [cutoff value: ≥0.02 (light/heavy ratio)] whereas the deglycopeptide had sensitivity of 93.3%, specificity of 68.3%, AUC of 0.859 [cutoff value: ≥0.02 (light/heavy ratio)] (Figure 4A).

In comparing the stage I HCC subgroup with the LC group, the nonglycopeptide had a sensitivity of 66.7%, specificity of 80.0%, and AUC of 0.712 [cutoff value: ≥0.02 (light/heavy ratio)], whereas the deglycopeptide had a sensitivity of 96.7%, specificity of 80.0%, and AUC of 0.918 [cutoff value: ≥0.02 (light/heavy ratio)] (Figure 4B). Thus, the discriminatory power of the deglycopeptide was greater versus the nonglycopeptide.

Pairwise differences in AUC values between nonglycopeptide and deglycopeptide estimations were analyzed by DeLong test [17]–the difference in AUC values was significant (normal vs HCC: *P*-value = 0.0010; LC vs stage I HCC: *P*-value = 0.0042) (Table S4).

Notably, considering that the nonglycopeptide (GYQELLEK) is measuring total AFP, it would be more advantageous to measure the deglycopeptide (V*D*FTEIQK) or take a combined measurement of nonglycopeptide (GYQELLEK) and deglycopeptide (V*D*FTEIQK), which could improve the diagnostic power in HCC.

Discussion

Most protein biomarkers are based on the premise that native proteins are differentially expressed in normal versus disease states. Recent studies have also demonstrated that protein biomarkers can discriminate such states according to the degree of glycosylation of native proteins [23–28].

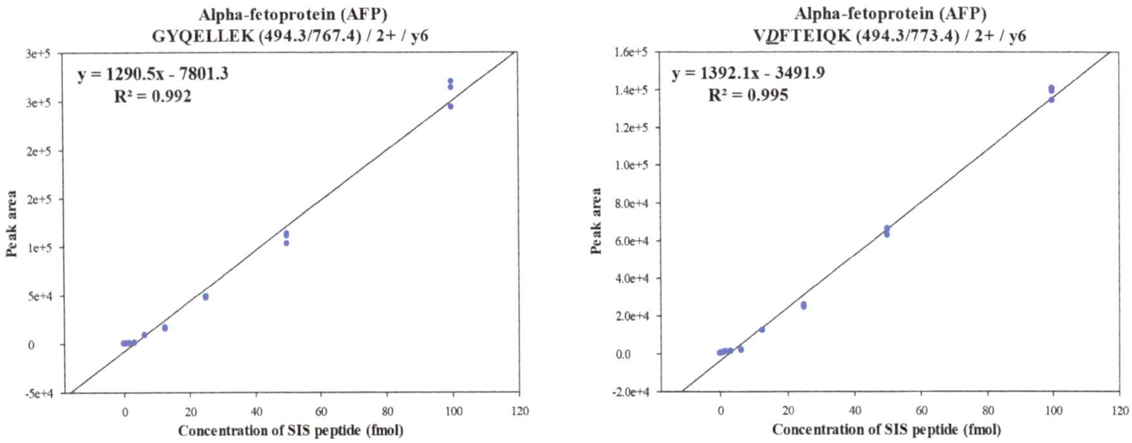

GYQELLEK (494.3/767.4) / 2+ / y6

Conc. (fmol)	Blank	0.0	0.8	1.6	3.1	6.3	12.5	25.0	50.0	100.0
Mean Area	7.33	70.67	441.00	524.33	1064.33	8809.33	16086.33	48325.33	109508.67	259150.09
STDEV	2.31	48.60	9.64	28.45	121.23	277.69	809.40	1110.34	5383.50	13769.43
CV (%)	31.49	68.78	2.19	5.43	11.39	3.15	5.03	2.30	4.92	5.31

VDFTEIQK (494.3/773.4) / 2+ / y6

Conc. (fmol)	Blank	0.0	0.8	1.6	3.1	6.3	12.5	25.0	50.0	100.0
Mean Area	7.00	307.00	640.00	1109.33	1296.67	1900.33	12319.33	25216.00	64973.00	138138.00
STDEV	5.57	14.11	61.59	83.20	12.90	194.20	76.85	669.63	1838.58	3336.99
CV (%)	79.54	4.60	9.62	7.50	0.99	10.22	0.62	2.66	2.83	2.42

Figure 3. Generation of calibration curve for nonglycopeptide (GYQELLEK) and deglycopeptide (VDFTEIQK) of AFP. To generate a calibration curve for the nonglycopeptide and deglycopeptide, SIS heavy peptides were serially diluted (9 concentration points: 0.0, 0.8, 1.6, 3.1, 6.3, 12.5, 25.0, 50.0, and 100.0 fmol) with the endogenous light peptide as an internal standard (pooled serum: 5 μg), added to each serially diluted sample. Each experiment was performed in triplicate to generate coefficients of variation (%CV) and calibration curve values (R^2).

In this study, we performed MRM measurements for 2 types of peptides (nonglycopeptide and deglycopeptide) that target a glycoprotein and serum AFP, wherein the amount of nonglycopeptide represents the total glycoprotein concentration and the deglycopeptide represents the glycosylated fraction of the glycoprotein. Based on our hypothesis, we compared the total AFP

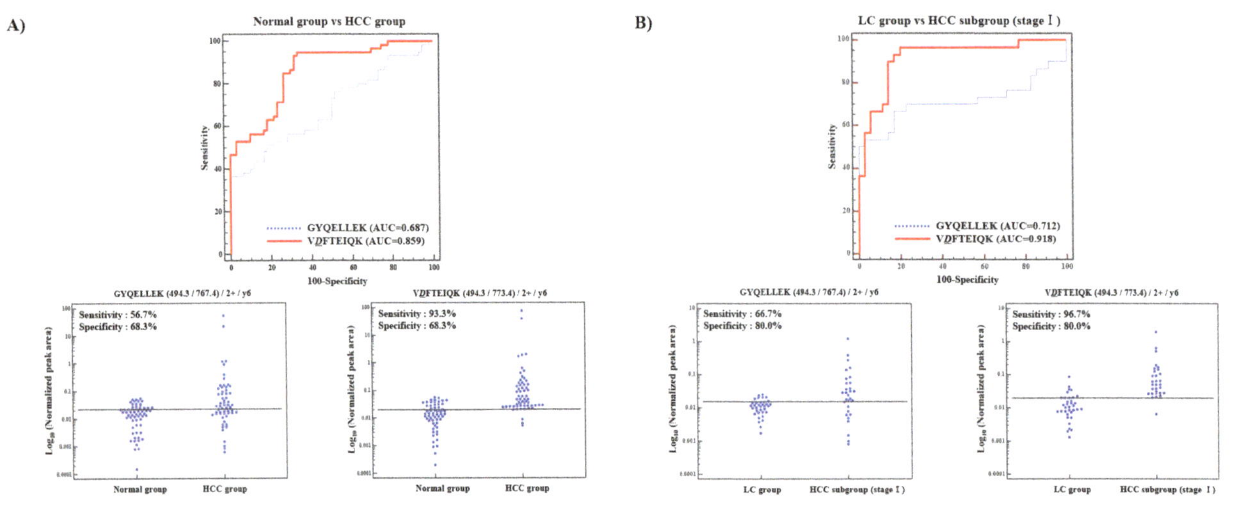

Figure 4. Receiver operating characteristic (ROC) curves and interactive plots for the nonglycopeptide (GYQELLEK) and deglycopeptide (VDFTEIQK) of AFP, respectively. The normalized peak areas of transitions were compared between normal and HCC group. In the interactive plots, sensitivity was calculated based on a specificity of 68.3%, which was calculated per an AFP cutoff value of 20 ng/mL (56.7% sensitivity), representing significant prognostic impact for HCC (A) LC was compared to Stage I HCC subgroup, in the interactive plots, sensitivity was calculated based on a specificity of 80.0% which was calculated with optimal deglycopeptide level (B).

concentration (represented as nonglycopeptide: GYQELLEK) with the glycosylated AFP fraction (represented as deglycopeptide: VDFTEIQK) between the normal, LC, and HCC groups.

To quantitatively analyze the total AFP and glycosylated AFP, respectively, we established an MRM-MS method for measuring the nonglycopeptide and deglycopeptide that corresponded to the glycosylated glycopeptide in serum samples. In developing this method, we first assessed whether the MRM-MS approach was suitable for measuring glycoprotein levels. We observed that MRM-MS measured the nonglycopeptide and deglycopeptide as alternatives to total AFP concentration and the glycosylated AFP fraction that was cleaved by PNGase F, respectively. Then, we performed MRM measurements for the endogenous light peptides and the SIS heavy peptides that coeluted with them as internal standards.

The nonglycopeptide was detected in the PNGase F-untreated and PNGase F-treated conditions, whereas the glycosylated glycopeptide was seen only after PNGase F treatment in the deglycopeptide form, because the original amino acid sequence with glycan could not be detected by MRM-MS. Specifically, although the PNGase F-treated deglycosylated state could be measured based on the deglycopeptide sequence (Asn changed to Asp), no glycopeptide could be detected by MRM in the glycosylated state (PNGase F-untreated). Thus, this sequence-based approach to the MRM measurements is useful in measuring the glycoprotein concentrations.

AFP is a significant marker for the clinical diagnosis and evaluation of suspected HCC patients. As a diagnostic tool for HCC, AFP level is determined by immunoenzymatic chemiluminescence; the cutoff of serum AFP levels for significant prognostic impact for HCC is 20 ng/mL (AFP-negative: <20 ng/mL and AFP-positive: ≥20 ng/mL) [22].

However, some reports have demonstrated that AFP level (cutoff value: ≥20 ng/mL) is a poor diagnostic tool in HCC, with a sensitivity of 54%. For example, 46%, 36%, and 18% of 1158 HCC patients had normal (<20 ng/mL), elevated (20–400 ng/mL), and diagnostic AFP levels (>400 ng/mL), respectively [29,30]. We noted the similar trend in AFP level in our HCC patients–as shown in Table 1, 43%, 30%, and 27% of 60 HCC patients had normal (<20 ng/mL), elevated (20–400 ng/mL), and diagnostic levels of AFP (>400 ng/mL), respectively (yielding a sensitivity of 56.7%). This result suggests that solely using total AFP level is not an effective method for distinguishing HCC from healthy subjects.

There are other biomarkers besides AFP that can be used to screen for HCC, such as DCP, also known as prothrombin induced by vitamin K absence II (PIVKA II). DCP is an abnormal product of liver carboxylation during thrombogen formation. The serum level of DCP in patients with HCC is significantly higher than in healthy adults and patients with nonmalignant hepatopathy (chronic hepatitis and cirrhosis) [31,32].

DCP can be used as a prognostic indicator for patients with small HCC tumors. High serum levels of DCP are also associated with a greater risk of HCC recurrence and worse overall survival in patients with an HCC tumor under 3 cm [33,34]. DCP can be used to evaluate the prognosis of patients with small HCC tumors but remains insufficient in the primary screening of HCC patients [35].

Recently, AFP-L3 (%) has been used as an additional indicator of total AFP in the diagnosis of HCC, demonstrating superior performance compared with measuring total AFP alone [36–41]. Similarly, we developed a MRM-based measurement approach using a deglycopeptide of AFP as an alternative to the glycosylated AFP fraction (AFP-L1, L2 and L3). By MRM-MS, the nonglycopeptide had a sensitivity of 56.7%, specificity of 68.3%, and AUC of 0.687 in distinguishing normal and HCC subjects versus 93.3%, 68.3%, and 0.859, respectively with the deglycopeptide. Also, the nonglycopeptide had a sensitivity of 66.7%, specificity of 80.0%, and AUC of 0.712 in distinguishing LC and the stage I HCC subgroup versus 96.7%, 80.0%, and 0.918, respectively, with the deglycopeptide. Thus, the discriminatory power of the deglycopeptide was better than that of the nonglycopeptide (Figure 4). To compare the nonglycopeptide and deglycopeptide of AFP accurately, we fixed their specificity in calculating the sensitivity.

In total, 30 HCC patients were primarily TNM stage I–ie, the early stage of HCC–suggesting that these findings can be applied to clinical settings in discriminating early-stage HCC from LC. Thus, deglycopeptide levels can differentiate small tumors from cirrhotic liver, which is significant, because other markers can not distinguish between early-stage HCC and LC. Our data indicate that upregulated deglycopeptide levels in early-stage HCC patients function in tumorigenesis and can be used as a marker for the early detection of a cirrhotic liver that progresses to HCC.

Our MRM-MS-based method has benefits in verifying glycoprotein biomarkers in human samples, because it does not require any complex or irreproducible glycoprotein enrichment steps. Further, determining the amount and extent of glycosylation in glycoproteins is difficult through conventional methods. Specifically, the differences in expression and degree of glycosylation of AFP have not been compared using antibody-based assays, such as western blot and ELISA (enzyme-linked immunosorbent assay).

Ultimately, 2 types of peptide markers–a nonglycopeptide and deglycopeptide–were used to distinguish HCC from normal controls and early-stage HCC from the LC group. Further verification of their value in larger samples should facilitate the development of better biomarkers for HCC.

Supporting Information

Figure S1

Figure S2

Figure S3

Figure S4

Figure S5

Figure S6

Figure S7

Table S1

Table S2

Table S3

Table S4

Author Contributions

Conceived and designed the experiments: J-HY YK. Performed the experiments: HK KK. Analyzed the data: JJ SJY JP. Contributed reagents/materials/analysis tools: J-HY YK. Contributed to the writing of the manuscript: HK KK. Modified the manuscript: J-HY YK.

References

1. Bertozzi CR, Sasisekharan R (2009) Glycomics. In: Varki A, Cummings RD, Esko JD, Freeze HH, Stanley P, et al., editors. Essentials of Glycobiology. Cold Spring Harbor NY: The Consortium of Glycobiology Editors, La Jolla, California.
2. Durand G, Seta N (2000) Protein glycosylation and diseases: blood and urinary oligosaccharides as markers for diagnosis and therapeutic monitoring. Clin Chem 46: 795–805.
3. Spiro RG (2002) Protein glycosylation: nature, distribution, enzymatic formation, and disease implications of glycopeptide bonds. Glycobiology 12: 43R-56R.
4. Anderson NL, Anderson NG (2002) The human plasma proteome: history, character, and diagnostic prospects. Mol Cell Proteomics 1: 845–867.
5. Miyoshi E, Noda K, Yamaguchi Y, Inoue S, Ikeda Y, et al. (1999) The alpha1-6-fucosyltransferase gene and its biological significance. Biochim Biophys Acta 1473: 9–20.
6. Kamoto T, Satomura S, Yoshiki T, Okada Y, Henmi F, et al. (2002) Lectin-reactive alpha-fetoprotein (AFP-L3%) curability and prediction of clinical course after treatment of non-seminomatous germ cell tumors. Jpn J Clin Oncol 32: 472–476.
7. Li D, Mallory T, Satomura S (2001) AFP-L3: a new generation of tumor marker for hepatocellular carcinoma. Clin Chim Acta 313: 15–19.
8. Khien VV, Mao HV, Chinh TT, Ha PT, Bang MH, et al. (2001) Clinical evaluation of lentil lectin-reactive alpha-fetoprotein-L3 in histology-proven hepatocellular carcinoma. Int J Biol Markers 16: 105–111.
9. Chu CW, Hwang SJ, Luo JC, Lai CR, Tsay SH, et al. (2001) Clinical, virologic, and pathologic significance of elevated serum alpha-fetoprotein levels in patients with chronic hepatitis C. J Clin Gastroenterol 32: 240–244.
10. Wang B, Chen D, Chen Y, Hu Z, Cao M, et al. (2012) Metabonomic profiles discriminate hepatocellular carcinoma from liver cirrhosis by ultraperformance liquid chromatography-mass spectrometry. J Proteome Res 11: 1217–1227.
11. Daniele B, Bencivenga A, Megna AS, Tinessa V (2004) Alpha-fetoprotein and ultrasonography screening for hepatocellular carcinoma. Gastroenterology 127: S108–112.
12. Colli A, Fraquelli M, Casazza G, Massironi S, Colucci A, et al. (2006) Accuracy of ultrasonography, spiral CT, magnetic resonance, and alpha-fetoprotein in diagnosing hepatocellular carcinoma: a systematic review. Am J Gastroenterol 101: 513–523.
13. Boja E, Rivers R, Kinsinger C, Mesri M, Hiltke T, et al. (2010) Restructuring proteomics through verification. Biomark Med 4: 799–803.
14. Bruix J, Sherman M (2011) Management of hepatocellular carcinoma: an update. Hepatology 53: 1020–1022.
15. Kim H, Kim K, Yu SJ, Jang ES, Yu J, et al. (2013) Development of biomarkers for screening hepatocellular carcinoma using global data mining and multiple reaction monitoring. PLoS One 8: e63468.
16. Qin LX, Zhou Q, Bogomolniy F, Villafania L, Olvera N, et al. (2014) Blocking and randomization to improve molecular biomarker discovery. Clin Cancer Res 20: 3371–3378.
17. DeLong ER, DeLong DM, Clarke-Pearson DL (1988) Comparing the areas under two or more correlated receiver operating characteristic curves: a nonparametric approach. Biometrics 44: 837–845.
18. Lee JY, Kim JY, Park GW, Cheon MH, Kwon KH, et al. (2011) Targeted mass spectrometric approach for biomarker discovery and validation with nonglycosylated tryptic peptides from N-linked glycoproteins in human plasma. Mol Cell Proteomics 10: M111 009290.
19. Malaguarnera G, Giordano M, Paladina I, Berretta M, Cappellani A, et al. (2010) Serum markers of hepatocellular carcinoma. Dig Dis Sci 55: 2744–2755.
20. Witjes CD, van Aalten SM, Steyerberg EW, Borsboom GJ, de Man RA, et al. (2013) Recently introduced biomarkers for screening of hepatocellular carcinoma: a systematic review and meta-analysis. Hepatol Int 7: 59–64.
21. Lai Q, Melandro F, Pinheiro RS, Donfrancesco A, Fadel BA, et al. (2012) Alpha-fetoprotein and novel tumor biomarkers as predictors of hepatocellular carcinoma recurrence after surgery: a brilliant star raises again. Int J Hepatol 2012: 893103.
22. Zhou L, Rui JA, Wang SB, Chen SG, Qu Q (2012) The significance of serum AFP cut-off values, 20 and 400 ng/mL in curatively resected patients with hepatocellular carcinoma and cirrhosis might be of difference. Hepatogastroenterology 59: 840–843.
23. Alavi A, Axford JS (2008) Glyco-biomarkers: potential determinants of cellular physiology and pathology. Dis Markers 25: 193–205.
24. Peracaula R, Barrabes S, Sarrats A, Rudd PM, de Llorens R (2008) Altered glycosylation in tumours focused to cancer diagnosis. Dis Markers 25: 207–218.
25. An HJ, Kronewitter SR, de Leoz ML, Lebrilla CB (2009) Glycomics and disease markers. Curr Opin Chem Biol 13: 601–607.
26. Drake PM, Cho W, Li B, Prakobphol A, Johansen E, et al. (2010) Sweetening the pot: adding glycosylation to the biomarker discovery equation. Clin Chem 56: 223–236.
27. Hua S, An HJ (2012) Glycoscience aids in biomarker discovery. BMB Rep 45: 323–330.
28. Reis CA, Osorio H, Silva L, Gomes C, David L (2010) Alterations in glycosylation as biomarkers for cancer detection. J Clin Pathol 63: 322–329.
29. Farinati F, Marino D, De Giorgio M, Baldan A, Cantarini M, et al. (2006) Diagnostic and prognostic role of alpha-fetoprotein in hepatocellular carcinoma: both or neither? Am J Gastroenterol 101: 524–532.
30. Kulik LM (2007) Advancements in hepatocellular carcinoma. Curr Opin Gastroenterol 23: 268–274.
31. Cui R, Wang B, Ding H, Shen H, Li Y, et al. (2002) Usefulness of determining a protein induced by vitamin K absence in detection of hepatocellular carcinoma. Chin Med J (Engl) 115: 42–45.
32. Marrero JA, Su GL, Wei W, Emick D, Conjeevaram HS, et al. (2003) Des-gamma carboxyprothrombin can differentiate hepatocellular carcinoma from nonmalignant chronic liver disease in american patients. Hepatology 37: 1114–1121.
33. Khan KN, Yatsuhashi H, Yamasaki K, Yamasaki M, Inoue O, et al. (2000) Prospective analysis of risk factors for early intrahepatic recurrence of hepatocellular carcinoma following ethanol injection. J Hepatol 32: 269–278.
34. Nagaoka S, Yatsuhashi H, Hamada H, Yano K, Matsumoto T, et al. (2003) The des-gamma-carboxy prothrombin index is a new prognostic indicator for hepatocellular carcinoma. Cancer 98: 2671–2677.
35. Koike Y, Shiratori Y, Sato S, Obi S, Teratani T, et al. (2001) Des-gamma-carboxy prothrombin as a useful predisposing factor for the development of portal venous invasion in patients with hepatocellular carcinoma: a prospective analysis of 227 patients. Cancer 91: 561–569.
36. Taketa K, Endo Y, Sekiya C, Tanikawa K, Koji T, et al. (1993) A collaborative study for the evaluation of lectin-reactive alpha-fetoproteins in early detection of hepatocellular carcinoma. Cancer Res 53: 5419–5423.
37. Aoyagi Y, Suzuki Y, Isemura M, Nomoto M, Sekine C, et al. (1988) The fucosylation index of alpha-fetoprotein and its usefulness in the early diagnosis of hepatocellular carcinoma. Cancer 61: 769–774.
38. Aoyagi Y, Saitoh A, Suzuki Y, Igarashi K, Oguro M, et al. (1993) Fucosylation index of alpha-fetoprotein, a possible aid in the early recognition of hepatocellular carcinoma in patients with cirrhosis. Hepatology 17: 50–52.
39. Oda K, Ido A, Tamai T, Matsushita M, Kumagai K, et al. (2011) Highly sensitive lens culinaris agglutinin-reactive alpha-fetoprotein is useful for early detection of hepatocellular carcinoma in patients with chronic liver disease. Oncol Rep 26: 1227–1233.
40. Yamashiki N, Seki T, Wakabayashi M, Nakagawa T, Imamura M, et al. (1999) Usefulness of Lens culinaris agglutinin A-reactive fraction of alpha-fetoprotein (AFP-L3) as a marker of distant metastasis from hepatocellular carcinoma. Oncol Rep 6: 1229–1232.
41. Hayashi K, Kumada T, Nakano S, Takeda I, Sugiyama K, et al. (1999) Usefulness of measurement of Lens culinaris agglutinin-reactive fraction of alpha-fetoprotein as a marker of prognosis and recurrence of small hepatocellular carcinoma. Am J Gastroenterol 94: 3028–3033.

4

Circulating MicroRNAs as Easy-to-Measure Aging Biomarkers in Older Breast Cancer Patients: Correlation with Chronological Age but Not with Fitness/Frailty Status

Sigrid Hatse[1]*, Barbara Brouwers[1], Bruna Dalmasso[1,2], Annouschka Laenen[3], Cindy Kenis[1,4], Patrick Schöffski[1], Hans Wildiers[1]

1 Laboratory of Experimental Oncology (LEO), Department of Oncology, KU Leuven, and Department of General Medical Oncology, University Hospitals Leuven, Leuven Cancer Institute, Leuven, Belgium, **2** Department of Internal Medicine, Istituto di Ricerca a Carattere Clinico e Scientifico (IRCCS), Azienda Ospedaliera Universitaria (AOU) San Martino Istituto Nazionale Tumori (IST), Genoa, Italy, **3** Interuniversity Centre for Biostatistics and Statistical Bioinformatics, Leuven, Belgium, **4** Department of Geriatric Medicine, University Hospitals Leuven, Leuven, Belgium

Abstract

Circulating microRNAs (miRNAs) hold great promise as easily accessible biomarkers for diverse (patho)physiological processes, including aging. We have compared miRNA expression profiles in cell-free blood from older versus young breast cancer patients, in order to identify "aging miRNAs" that can be used in the future to monitor the impact of chemotherapy on the patient's biological age. First, we assessed 175 miRNAs that may possibly be present in serum/plasma in an exploratory screening in 10 young and 10 older patients. The top-15 ranking miRNAs showing differential expression between young and older subjects were further investigated in an independent cohort consisting of another 10 young and 20 older subjects. Plasma levels of miR-20a-3p, miR-30b-5p, miR106b, miR191 and miR-301a were confirmed to show significant age-related decreases (all $p \leq 0.004$). The remaining miRNAs included in the validation study (miR-21, miR-210, miR-320b, miR-378, miR-423-5p, let-7d, miR-140-5p, miR-200c, miR-374a, miR376a) all showed similar trends as observed in the exploratory screening but these differences did not reach statistical significance. Interestingly, the age-associated miRNAs did not show differential expression between fit/healthy and non-fit/frail subjects within the older breast cancer cohort of the validation study and thus merit further investigation as true aging markers that not merely reflect frailty.

Editor: Consuelo Borras, University of Valencia, Spain

Funding: HW is a recipient of the 'Fonds voor Wetenschappelijk Onderzoek – Vlaanderen (FWO).' BB is a recipient of the 'Vlaamse Liga tegen Kanker (VLK).' The funders had no role in study design, data collection and analysis, decision to publish, or preparation of the manuscript.

Competing Interests: The authors have declared that no competing interests exist.

* Email: sigrid.hatse@med.kuleuven.be

Introduction

Given the increasing proportion of older people in the general population, oncologists nowadays encounter the great challenge of proper cancer management in older patients. A major problem is the heterogeneous health condition among older cancer patients, making it difficult to rely on standard treatment guidelines established for distinct cancer types and, hence, demanding a more individualized approach. Secondly, long-term impact of chemotherapy on the patient's global health condition may be more pronounced and, at the same time, less predictable in older individuals.

Body aging is a complex phenomenon involving several, partly overlapping, molecular mechanisms. Among others, these include the accumulation of oxidative stress [1] and DNA damage [2], the shortening of telomeres [3,4]and neuroendocrine and immunologic changes [5,6].

It is generally assumed that chemotherapy may accelerate the aging process through interference at the level of one or several of these aging driving forces [7]. For example, free radical intermediates are generated during the metabolism anthracyclines, alkylating agents directly cause DNA damage, while topoisomerase inhibitors, such as epirubicin, inhibit DNA repair enzymes. Also, chemotherapy may accelerate leukocyte telomere attrition, due to telomerase inhibition [8] and/or repeated cycles of intense hematological repopulation [9–11]. Moreover, chemoradiotherapy may have more severe effects on the replicative capacity of blood cells in older as compared to younger patients [12]. Finally, neuroendocrine and immune functions can also be affected by chemotherapeutic agents and by corticosteroids that are often incorporated in chemotherapeutic regimens [7].

At the cellular level, aging is intimately linked with tumorigenesis through the mechanism of cellular senescence [13], a cancer-protective stress response that causes irreversible growth arrest in order to prevent further proliferation of damaged, potentially harmful cells. While being a potent anti-tumor mechanism early in life, cellular senescence is at the same time responsible for tissue aging at older age, through accumulation of non-proliferative cells [13], finally resulting in tissue dysfunction and age-related diseases. Standard chemotherapy and radiotherapy might function in part by inducing senescence within the tumor mass [14,15], but might concurrently cause increased senescence induction in healthy, proliferating tissues as well.

Taken together, chemotherapeutic treatment may potentially lead to accelerated aging and/or premature onset of frailty in older cancer patients [7]. Therefore, the patient's biological aging profile is of particular relevance in geriatric oncology and may aid in oncological decision making and individual treatment optimization. Several aging biomarkers have already been described, most particularly mean leukocyte telomere length and $p16^{INK4a}$ mRNA expression in T lymphocytes [16–18]. However, none of these so far made its way into routine clinical practice and the search for robust and easy-to-measure aging biomarkers is still ongoing.

MicroRNA's (miRNAs) are short (20–24 nt), non-coding and highly stable RNA's that are involved in post-transcriptional regulation of gene expression. They are known as fine-tuning mediators of a wide variety of normal physiological pathways, developmental processes and pathological conditions; it is thus plausible that they also play a role in cellular senescenceand tissue/ body aging [19,20]. Several miRNAs involved in DNA damage response, cellular senescence and cell death (such as let-7, miR-34 and miR-43), were indeed identified in the widely used *C. elegans* aging model and turned out to be highly conserved among species [21]. In aging mice, miR-34a was shown to be upregulated, concomitantly with a decreased mRNA expression of its primary target gene SIRT1, in brain tissue but also in peripheral blood mononuclear cells and plasma [22]. Therefore, it was suggested that circulatory miR-34a may hold great promise as an accessible biomarker for brain aging.

Circulating miRNAs actually are attractive candidate biomarkers for clinical use, because of their easy accessibility and outstanding stability in serum/plasma [23]. Here, we describe the potential use of microRNA signatures expressed in serum/ plasma for the assessment of biological age in breast cancer patients. We compared a panel of 175 different microRNAs, known to be among the most relevant in serum/plasma, between older and young breast cancer patients and validated the findings of this initial exploratory screening in an independent breast cancer cohort. At least 5 circulating microRNAs emerged from this study that are worth to be further explored as potential aging biomarkers in larger cohorts of young *versus* old fit *versus* old frail individuals, both within and beyond a cancer background.

Results

The experimental design of our study is shown in Fig. 1. In the first stage, the expression profiles of 175 miRNAs were analyzed in serum samples of 10 young (mean age 34.5 years) and 10 older (mean age 82.8 years) breast cancer patients. Distinct breast cancer subtypes were equally represented in both groups (see Table 1). From this initial screening experiment, the 15 top-ranking miRNAs (showing the highest significance for differential expression between both groups) were selected, together with 4 candidate reference miRNAs (showing stable expression among all samples). In the second stage, the selected potential aging miRNAs and candidate reference miRNAs were re-evaluated by individual RT-qPCR in plasma samples from a new, independent study cohort consisting of 10 young (mean age 41 years) and 20 older (mean age 78 years) breast cancer patients, all diagnosed with lymph node negative, luminal A (grade 1–2, ER-positive, PR-positive, HER2-negative) tumors (see Table 2). Geriatric assessment in the older cohort was performed as described by Kenis *et al.* [24].

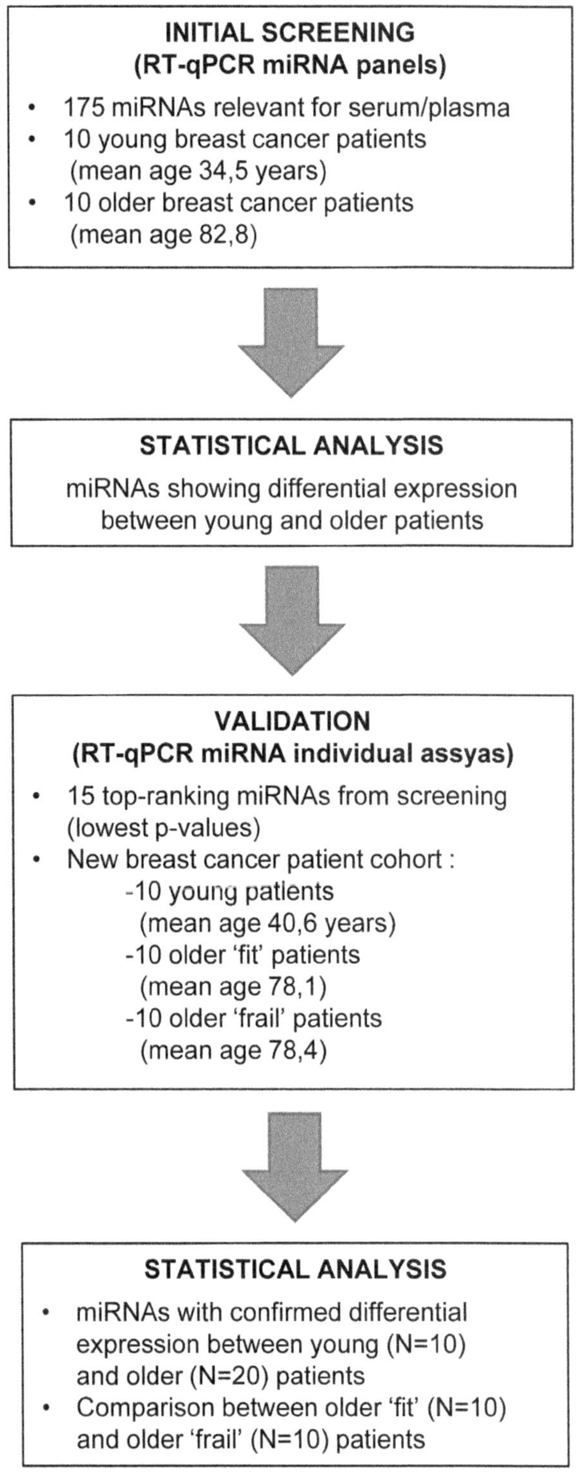

Figure 1. Experimental study design.

Table 1. Patient and tumor characteristics of the pilot study cohort.

	Young group	Older group
	N = 10	N = 10
Age at diagnosis		
Mean (years)	34,5	82,8
Range (years)	28–38	80–89
Breast cancer subtype		
Luminal A-like phenotype	7	7
Luminal B-like phenotype	1	1
Triple negative-like phenotype	2	2
Tumor grade		
I	2	2
II	7	5
III	1	3
Histological subtype		
Invasive ductal carcinoma	9	7
Invasive lobular carcinoma	1	1
Other	0	2
Estrogen receptor status		
Positive	8	8
Negative	2	2
Progesteron receptor status		
Positive	7	8
Negative	3	2
HER-2 receptor status		
Positive	0	0
Negative	10	10
Pathological staging (pT)		
pT1a	1	0
pT1b	0	1
pT1c	4	1
pT2	4	8
x	1	0
Nodal status		
pN0	10	10

Exploratory screening for differentially expressed miRNAs in older versus young breast cancer patients

Profiles of circulating miRNAs were analyzed in the 10 young and 10 older breast cancer patients of the exploratory cohort using the Exiqon miRNA serum/plasma focus panels, including 175 different miRNAs (refer to File S2 for a complete list of included miRNAs). Plate-to-plate variations in qPCR efficiency were small: the standard deviation of Cp values obtained for the individual interplate calibrator wells was 0.33 cycles, and no outliers (deviation of 4 times the standard deviation or more) were detected. Comparable RNA extraction and reverse transcription efficiency across all samples of the cohort was ascertained by the UniSp6 spike-in control : standard deviation of the UniSp6 PCR Cp values (after interplate calibration) was 0.55 cycles (mean Cp was 25,99) and no outliers were detected, indicating that no inhibitors of reverse transcription and/or PCR reactions were present. The average signal of all miRNAs was comparable in both age categories : the global mean Cp of the young patient group was 33.80±2.01, compared to 33.90±1.67 for the old group. Thus, there were no significant age-related changes in total miRNA content of the serum samples.

After global mean normalisation (i.e. normalisation to the average signal of all miRNAs included in the panel) [25], statistical analysis of the results revealed 37 miRNAs with significantly different ($p<0.05$) expression in serum samples from the older compared to the young patient group. The first 50 miRNAs of the t-test p-value ranking are listed in Table 3. Interestingly, older and young patients clustered in two relatively distinct groups in a principal component analysis incorporating these top 50-ranking miRNAs (Fig. 2A), whereas patients were randomly scattered when PCA analysis was performed with the bottom 50-ranking miRNAs (Fig. 2B). The dendrogram in Fig. 3 also clearly demonstrates a high degree of clustering of the patients from both age groups. This indicates that there are indeed important

Table 2. Patient and tumor characteristics of the validation study cohort.

	Young group (N = 10)	Older 'fit' group (N = 10)	Older 'non-fit' group (N = 10)
Age at diagnosis			
Mean (years)	41	78	78
Range (years)	37–43	71–83	73–91
Frailty status (Balducci)			
Frail	N/A	0	9
Vulnerable	N/A	4	1
Fit	N/A	6	0
Frailty status (LOFS[a])			
0–2 (severely frail)	N/A [b]	0	1
3–4 (frail)	N/A	0	1
5–6 (vulnerable)	N/A	0	8
7–8 (slightly vulnerable)	N/A	0	0
9–10 (fit)	N/A	10	0
Breast cancer subtype			
Luminal A-like	10	10	10[c]
Tumor grade			
I	4	2	2
II	6	8	8
III	0	0	1[c]
Histological subtype			
Invasive ductal carcinoma	8	6	5
Invasive lobular carcinoma	2	3	2
Other	0	1	3
Estrogen receptor status			
Positive	10	10	10
Negative	0	0	0
Progesteron receptor status			
Positive	10	10	10
Negative	0	0	0
HER-2 receptor status			
Positive	0	0	0
Negative	10	10	10
Pathological staging (pT)			
pT1a	0	0	0
pT1b	4	1	2
pT1c	2	3	1
pT2	4	5	7
pT3	0	1	0
Nodal staging (pN)			
pN0	10	10	10

[a]Leuven Oncology Frailty Score : refer to File S1 for more details.
[b]N/A : not applicable.
[c]One patient had a mixed luminal A (grade II)/luminal B (grade III) tumor.

age-related differences in circulating miRNA profiles. Some miRNAs showed an age-related increase in abundance, while others were found to be down-regulated in older, as compared to young, patients. When considering the 15 miRNAs exhibiting the most pronounced age-related changes (lowest p-values), increased abundance in serum of older *versus* young patients was noted for miR-21, miR-210, miR-320b, miR-378 and miR-423-5p (Fig. 4). Conversely, circulating levels of let-7d, miR-20a-3p, miR-301a, miR-374a, miR-376a, miR-191, miR-200c, miR-30b-5p, miR-

Table 3. Exploratory serum/plasma miRNA panel screening of circulating miRNAs in older (N = 10) *versus* young (N = 10) breast cancer patients.

miRNA[a]	Age-related change[b]	Fold change	t-test P value
hsa-miR-320b	up	2.10	0.0003
hsa-miR-301a	down	3.34	0.0012
hsa-miR-210	up	2.48	0.0024
hsa-miR-21	up	2.32	0.0025
hsa-miR-376a	down	3.24	0.0036
hsa-miR-378	up	2.87	0.0037
hsa-miR-374a	down	2.13	0.0038
hsa-miR-423-5p	up	1.66	0.0044
hsa-miR-20a-3p	down	8.64	0.0049
hsa-let-7d	down	2.33	0.0052
hsa-miR-191	down	1.49	0.0061
hsa-miR-200c	down	4.88	0.0063
hsa-miR-30b-5p	down	1.78	0.0063
hsa-miR-140-5p	down	2.00	0.0064
hsa-miR-106b-5p	down	2.17	0.0097
hsa-miR-382	down	2.66	0.0109
hsa-miR-495	down	2.81	0.0132
hsa-miR-199a-3p	down	1.80	0.0141
hsa-miR-146a	up	1.83	0.0203
hsa-miR-15b*	down	2.31	0.0213
hsa-miR-320a	up	5.17	0.0218
hsa-miR-551b	down	7.10	0.0227
hsa-miR-766	up	2.24	0.0244
hsa-miR-409-3p	down	4.82	0.0261
hsa-miR-543	down	3.75	0.0308
hsa-miR-10b	up	2.06	0.0328
hsa-miR-34a	up	2.36	0.0367
hsa-miR-331-3p	down	2.37	0.0368
hsa-miR-423-5p	up	5.41	0.0383
hsa-miR-222	up	2.43	0.0410
hsa-miR-199a-5p	down	2.13	0.0436
hsa-miR-33a	up	2.09	0.0451
hsa-miR-92a	up	2.06	0.0470
hsa-miR-324-5p	down	1.51	0.0471
hsa-miR-130a	down	1.44	0.0474
hsa-miR-151-5p	down	1.39	0.0484
hsa-miR-486-5p	up	2.50	0.0489
hsa-miR-150	up	2.16	0.0511
hsa-miR-126	up	2.38	0.0568
hsa-miR-342-3p	up	1.94	0.0703
hsa-miR-15a	up	1.60	0.0759
hsa-miR-30e	up	1.29	0.0823
hsa-miR-424	up	3.15	0.0825
hsa-miR-660	up	1.53	0.0899
hsa-miR-10a	up	1.69	0.0924
hsa-miR-885-5p	down	2.44	0.0943
hsa-miR-30c	down	1.53	0.0948
hsa-miR-324-3p	up	2.07	0.0963
hsa-miR-152	up	1.58	0.1003

Table 3. Cont.

miRNA[a]	Age-related change[b]	Fold change	t-test P value
hsa-miR-326	down	1.83	0.1055

[a]This table only shows the top-50 ranking miRNAs for differential expression according to t-test. A list of all miRNAs included in the entire panel is shown in File S2.
[b]up : higher plasma levels found in older compared to young subjects; down : lower plasma levels found in older compared to young subjects.

140b-5p and miR-106b were decreased in older compared to young patients (Fig. 4).

Identification of candidate reference miRNAs via miRNA serum/plasma panel screening

A second purpose of the initial screening experiment was the identification of stably expressed miRNAs that could serve as valuable references for normalisation in future validation experiments. As subsequent experiments will probably only include a limited number of selected miRNAs, global mean normalisation, requiring at least 50 genes, will not be possible anymore. To this end, the 10 miRNAs most resembling the behaviour of the global mean, i.e. the miRNAs having least variation after global mean normalisation, were selected as candidate reference miRNAs (Table 4). From these selected candidates, miR-191 was excluded since it ranged within the top 15 of age-related differential expression in the panel screening (see Table 3). The remaining 9 miRNAs, i.e. let-7i, miR-484, miR-29a, miR-29c, miR-140-3p, miR-30e, miR-30d, miR-29b and miR-590-5p, were further evaluated by the use of Normfinder [26] and GeNorm [27], two popular algorithms to select the most stably expressed reference genes from a set of tested candidate genes in a given sample panel. Normfinder, which basically calculates for each candidate reference gene the standard deviation from the global average expression (and thus mirrors the variance after global mean normalisation), yielded the following stability order: let-7i>miR-140-3p> miR-29c>miR-29a>miR-484> miR-30e>miR-29b> miR-30d>miR-590-5p. The respective stability values ranged between 0.27 for let-7i and 0.56 for miR-590-5p, with superior stability indicated by the lowest value (Table 4). Normfinder analysis also indicated that 4 is a reasonable number of normalisation genes: accumulated standard deviation values were 0.27, 0.21, 0.18, 0.16, 0.16, 0.15, 0.15, 0.14 and 014 when the number of normalizing genes was increased from just 1 to 9. Thus, the inclusion of a fourth reference gene still afforded a substantial reduction of variation retained in the dataset, while additional reference genes only contributed a minor further improvement. GeNorm analysis, which is based on a different mathematical approach, resulted in a slightly different stability ranking: miR-29a = miR-29c>miR-140-3p>let-7i>miR-29b>miR-484> miR-30e>miR-30d>miR-590-5p. The corresponding M-values (gene stability measure) increased from 0.31 for let-7i to 0.59 for miR-590-5p, again with the most stably expressed genes having the lowest M-values (Table 4). Taken together, both algorithms pointed at let-7i, miR-29a, miR-29c and miR-140-3p as the common best reference miRNAs for normalisation, which all had GeNorm and Normfinder stability values below the 0.50 cut-off for suitable reference genes [26,27]. However, we decided not to retain let-7i since it was previously reported to be involved in genome-wide miRNA signatures of human longevity [28] and might thus be somehow age-related, which would not be desirable for the current study. Based on the above-described results, we instead selected miR-484 as the fourth reference gene.

Validation of age-associated miRNAs

To further examine potential aging miRNAs, we focussed on the 15 miRNAs that emerged from the pilot study as those showing the most significantly different expression levels in young *versus* older individuals. For this validation study, a new independent breast cancer patient cohort was selected that basically consisted of a young group (<45 years, N = 10) and an older group (>70 years, N = 20). The latter comprised a subgroup (N = 10) of 'fit' older breast cancer patients and a second subgroup (N = 10) of 'frail' patients. These two subcategories were included to investigate whether the observed age-associated differences in plasma miRNA levels were truly related to the aging process itself (i.e. pure "aging biomarkers"), or were caused by age-related pathologies and functional decline (i.e. "frailty biomarkers").

Individual PCR assays were carried out for each of the selected candidate aging miRNAs (i.e. miR-320b, miR-301a, miR-210, miR-21, miR-376a, miR-378, miR-374a, miR-423-5p, miR-20a-3p, let-7d, miR-191, miR-200c, miR-30b-5p, miR-140-5p and miR-106b), along with the 4 selected normalisation miRNAs (i.e. miR-29a, miR-29c, miR-140-3p and miR-484). In addition, miR-451 and miR-23a-3p were also included for hemolysis control (see Materials and Methods section). Comparable RNA extraction and reverse transcription efficiency across all 30 samples of the validation cohort was ascertained by the UniSp6 spike-in control: standard deviation of the UniSp6 PCR Cp values (after interplate calibration) was ≤0.37 cycles (mean Cp value was 20.48 cycles).

Analysis of the data first confirmed miR-29a, miR-29c, miR-140-3p and miR-484 as reliable normalisation references, all GeNorm M-values being lower than 0.5 (data not shown). However, miR-23a-3p was additionally identified as an excellent reference miRNA. This is not surprising; miR-23a-3p is incorporated in the hemolysis control test because of its stable expression in serum/plasma samples and is often used as a suitable reference miRNA for normalisation. Hence, we decided to add it to our reference miRNA panel, which thus finally consisted of 5 miRNAs.

When comparing older (N = 20) with young (N = 10) patients, significantly *decreased* miRNA plasma levels were confirmed for miR-20a-3p, miR-301a, miR-374a, miR-30b-5p, miR-106b-5p and miR-191, whereas let-7d, miR-140-5p, miR-200c and miR-376a did not reach statistical significance at the 5% significance level (Table 5). When applying Bonferroni correction for multiple testing, p-values for miR-20a-3p, miR-30b-5p, miR-106b-5p, miR-191 and miR301a were still below the corrected significance threshold of 0.00341 (Table 5).

Increased expression in older compared to young subjects was only confirmed for miR-378 (p = 0.0077) and was close to the 5% significance threshold for miR-320b (p = 0.0585) and miR-423-5p (p = 0.0566), while miR-21 and miR-210 were not close to statistical significance in the validation experiment. However, none of these miRNAs showing apparently *increased* expression in older subjects remained significant after Bonferroni correction for multiple testing (Table 5). An overview of upregulated and

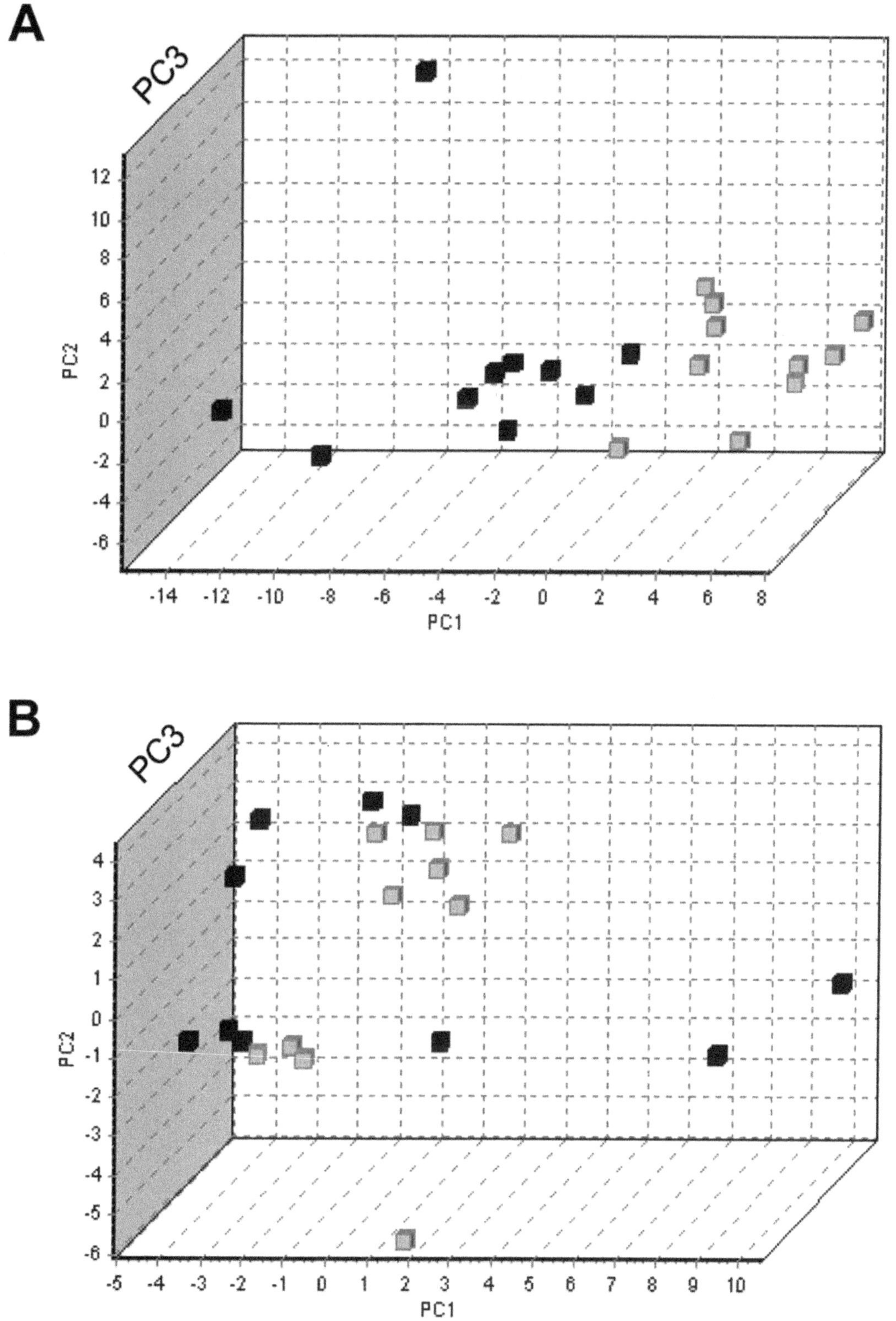

Figure 2. Principal component analysis (PCA) of the panel screening results. (**A**) PCA analysis of the top-50 ranking (lowest P-values in t-test) miRNAs of the panel screening; (**B**) PCA analysis of the bottom-50 ranking miRNAs (highest P-values in t-test). Black symbols represent young patients; grey symbols represent older, frail patients. PC1, PC2 and PC3 on X, Y and Z-axis represent the 3 principal components generated by this statistical algorithm.

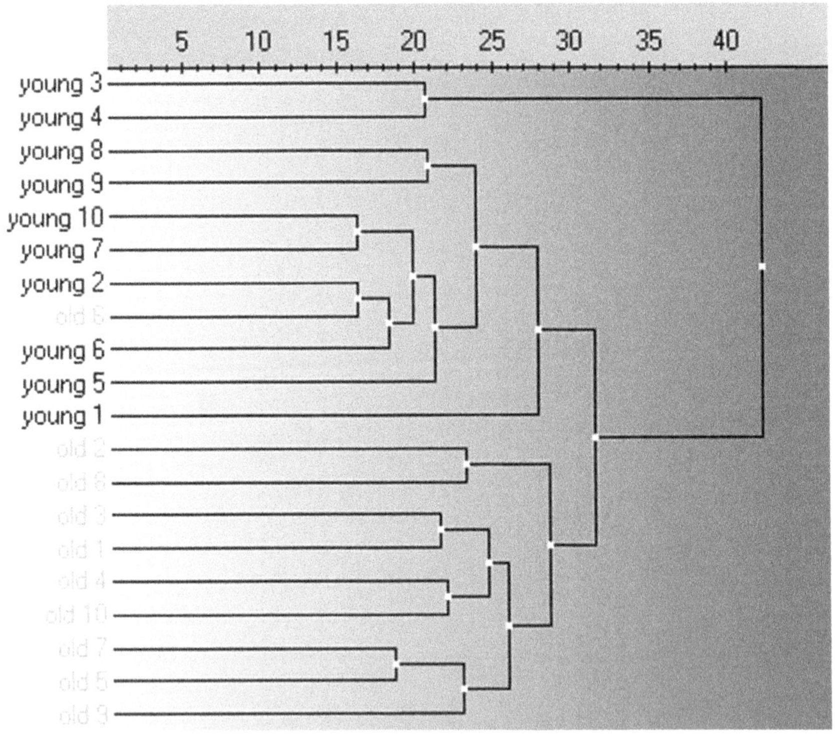

Figure 3. Dendrogram showing hierarchical clustering of patients according to the exploratory miRNA screening panel results. Young patients are shown in black, older patients are shown in grey. The clustering was performed on all 20 patients of the exploratory cohort and on the entire miRNA screening panel, applying complete linkage as the clustering method and Euclidean distance as the distance measure.

downregulated miRNAs in the exploratory screening and the validation study is shown in Fig. 5.

Interestingly, no significant differences were revealed in a subanalysis comparing the 'fit' and 'non-fit' subgroups of the older cohort for any of the microRNAs included in this validation study (all $p>0.1$) (Table 5). These results indicate that the observed differences in plasma miRNA levels between young and older breast cancer patients reflect a pure aging effect and do not result from age-associated changes in the patient's global health status.

Discussion

MicroRNA's circulating in plasma are particularly interesting as easily accessible biomarkers for aging and age-related diseases. However, relatively little data are presently available on age-related changes in miRNA expression that can directly be monitored in human plasma. A previous study in humans has compared the miRNA expression profile in peripheral blood mononuclear cells from older versus young individuals and revealed significant age-associated down-regulation of miR-24,

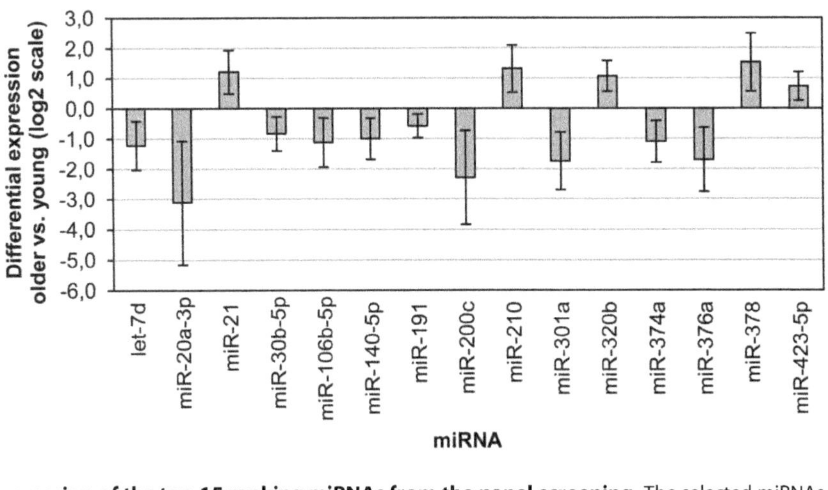

Figure 4. Differential expression of the top-15 ranking miRNAs from the panel screening. The selected miRNAs are displayed in numerical order. Bars represent the difference in expression in older compared to young patients on a 2-logarithmic scale, with indication of the 95% confidence interval (based on t-test).

Table 4. Candidate reference miRNAs identified by exploratory serum/plasma miRNA panel screening.

miRNA	Variance[a]	Normfinder	GeNorm
	after GMN	SD[b]	M-value[c]
hsa-let-7i	0.09	0.27	0.40
hsa-miR-484	0.10	0.44	0.49
hsa-miR-29a	0.18	0.36	0.31
hsa-miR-29c	0.20	0.34	0.31
hsa-miR-140-3p	0.22	0.32	0.35
hsa-miR-30e	0.23	0.46	0.53
hsa-miR-30d	0.24	0.51	0.56
hsa-miR-191	0.25	–	–
hsa-miR-29b	0.26	0.50	0.45
hsa-miR-590-5p	0.28	0.57	0.59

[a]Variance after global mean normalisation (GMN) : reflects the deviation of a specific miRNA from the behavior of the global mean (i.e. average signal of all miRNAs included).
[b]Standard deviation returned by NormFinder algorithm.
[c]Expression stability measure (M) returned by GeNorm algorithm (the lower, the more stable the expression).

miR-103, miR-107, miR-128, miR-130a, miR-155, miR-221, miR-496 and miR-1538 [29], but Hunter et al. reported marked differences in miRNA expression between the peripheral blood mononuclear cells and plasma fractions of human blood [30]. In order to identify plasma microRNAs implicated in the aging process, we have compared circulating microRNA's between young and older subjects, by applying a comprehensive RT-qPCR platform for focused microRNA profiling on serum/plasma, using samples from the large blood bank of breast cancer patients that has been established at our institution. We have chosen to perform this search for aging miRNAs in a female breast cancer population, on the plasma samples readily available from our biorepositories, in view of our eventual aim to investigate the

Table 5. Validation of differentially expressed miRNAs in older (N = 10) *versus* young (N = 20) breast cancer patients and comparison between older 'fit' (N = 10) and older 'frail' (N = 10) subjects.

miRNA	Older vs. young		Older 'fit' vs. 'frail'
	P-value[a]	Fold change[b]	P-value[a]
Decreased expression			
hsa-let-7d	*0.1083*	1.59	0.7861
hsa-miR-20a-3p	**0.0004***	**2.48**	0.7405
hsa-miR-30b-5p	**<0.0001***	**2.47**	0.8428
hsa-miR-106b-5p	**0.0001***	**1.56**	0.8784
hsa-miR-140-5p	*0.8431*	1.06	*0.2413*
hsa-miR-191	**0.0010***	**2.23**	0.5611
hsa-miR-200c	*0.5235*	1.21	0.5097
hsa-miR-301a	**0.0024***	**2.34**	0.6111
hsa-miR-374a	**0.0109**	**2.36**	0.6765
hsa-miR-376a	*0.4679*	1.23	0.4195
Increased expression			
hsa-miR-21	0.4133	1.12	0.8749
hsa-miR-210	*0.1528*	1.29	*0.3447*
hsa-miR-320b	0.0585	1.25	0.6679
hsa-miR-378	**0.0077**	**1.71**	0.2817
hsa-miR-423-5p	0.0566	1.34	0.7050

[a]P-values are derived from parametric t-test (unpaired, 2-tail, C.I = 95%), unless data are not normally distributed (values indicated *in italic*). In such cases, P-value derived from Mann-Whitney test is displayed. **Bold values** indicate significant values according to the 5% significance threshold. Values indicated with an asterisk (*) remained significant after correction for multiple testing.
[b]Negative values indicate x-fold *decreased* expression, positive values indicate x-fold *increased* expression.

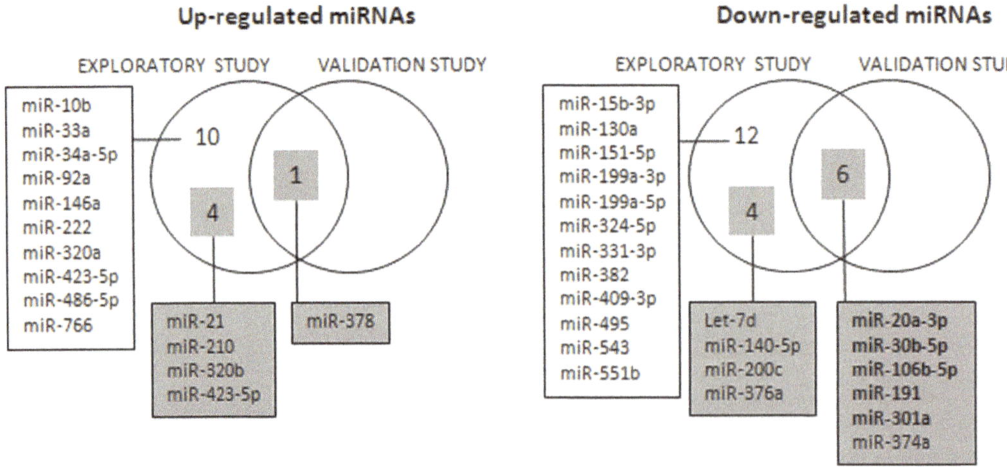

Figure 5. Venn diagram showing up-regulated and down-regulated miRNAs in the exploratory screening and the validation study. In the exploratory screening, there were in total 37 circulating miRNAs exhibiting age-related expression ($p<0.05$). Of those, only the top-15 miRNAs with the lowest p-values (shown in grey boxes) were further investigated in the validation study. Seven age-related miRNAs were confirmed in the validation study ($p<0.05$), of which 5 (all showing decreased expression) remained significant after correction for multiple testing; these are indicated in bold. Obviously, the right-hand zone (i.e. miRNAs showing altered expression in the validation study but not the exploratory screening) cannot contain any miRNAs, since the validation study only included those miRNAs that emerged from the exploratory study as the most significantly age-related ones.

impact of chemotherapeutic treatments on the biological age of older breast cancer patients.

For 5 miRNAs, i.e. miR-301a, miR-20a-3p, miR-106b-5p, miR-191 and miR-30b-5p, plasma expression levels were convincingly confirmed to significantly correlate with chronological age. Six other miRNAs that were selected from the intial screening (i.e. let-7d, miR-21, miR-140, miR200c, miR-210 and miR-376a) showed no significant differences between young and older patients in the validation experiment, two (i.e. miR-320b and miR-423-5p) were close to the 5% significance level and two (i.e. miR-374a and miR-378) actually reached statistical significance, but were not retained after correction for multiple testing. Nevertheless, each of the miRNAs included in the validation study consistently showed the same trend, regarding decreased or increased expression in older *versus* young subjects, as observed in the exploratory screening. It should be kept in mind that patient numbers were rather small in both the initial screening and the validation. This might explain why several miRNAs, emerging as candidate aging miRNAs from the exploratory experiment, did not reach statistical significance in the subsequent validation step. On the other hand, we neither can exclude the possibility that for these miRNAs, the 'differences' initially observed in the screening study did not reflect 'real' differential expression but were merely coincidental findings due to multiple testing. Another aspect that may explain inconsistencies between the screening and validation steps is the use of different specimens : because of sample availability issues, the validation study was done on plasma, while serum was used in the initial screening. Nevertheless, one can argue that if the same five miRNA were found to be differentially expressed between age categories in both serum and plasma, regardless of the preparation procedure, these can be considered as particularly strong biomarkers.

It is well possible that we 'missed' significant aging-related miRNAs, either because they are not included in the initial screening panel (which contains a selection of the 175 most commonly detected circulating miRNAs out of the ~300–400 miRNAs that have ever been annotated to serum/plasma), or because they were not among the top-15 ranking differentially expressed miRNAs in the pilot study and were thus not selected for further investigation, future studies will not exclusively be limited to the five aging miRNAs identified here. For instance, we have observed significantly increased expression of miR-34a in older compared to young subjects in our exploratory screening, which is in line with previous findings [22]. However, miR-34a was not included in our validation experiment because for the present study, we have chosen for an unbiased, straight-forward selection of the top 15 differentially expressed miRNAs to be included in the validation study. We are currently starting a miRNA profiling study including miR-34a in older breast cancer patients receiving chemotherapy.

Interestingly, of the 15 potential aging-related miRNAs selected from the initial screening, 8 miRNAs (i.e. let-7d, miR-106b-5p, miR-20a-3p, miR-21, miR-301a, miR-320b, miR-374a and miR-423-5p) were previously reported to be associated with healthy longevity in a recent study by El Sharawy et al. on genome-wide miRNA signatures [28]. In line with our current findings, this study also revealed age-related down-regulation of let-7d, miR-106b-5p, miR-20a-3p, miR-301a and miR-374a, while miR-320b and miR-423-5p were shown to be upregulated with increasing age. The 7 other potential aging miRNAs that were selected from our initial screening, i.e. miR-140-5p, miR-200c, miR-210, miR-376a, miR-378, miR-191, miR-30b-5p, were not reported to show age-related changes in the longevity study, although the latter two miRNAs were definitely confirmed in our validation study. On the other hand, several miRNAs showing age-related differential expression in the longevity study were also included in our initial screening panel but did not show significant differences between young and older patients and were therefore not further investigated. However, the different context of both studies must be underscored : while the study by El Sharawy and coworkers refers to healthy aging and longevity, the age-related miRNAs reported here are found in a breast cancer background. Moreover, both studies were conducted on relatively small patient cohorts, each containing only ≤20 older patients. Thus, it is well possible that they both lacked sufficient statistical power to detect subtle differences between young and older patients. This, together with the use of different experimental methodology and statistical thresholds, may account for the partial discrepancies. Nonetheless, it is quite remarkable that such highly significant age-related changes in circulating miRNAs, as observed in our study for miR-301a, miR-20a-3p, miR-106b-5p, miR-191 and miR-30b-5p, can be evidenced with as little as 10 patients per age group, suggesting that these miRNAs can be considered as robust and reliable aging biomarkers.

Several of the top-ranking miRNAs for age-related differences between young and older breast cancer patients in our exploratory study have already been linked with cellular senescence in previous reports. A study using diverse human cellular as well as organismal aging models revealed miR-17, miR-19b, miR-20a and miR-106a as biomarkers of aging [31]. These miRNAs, which all belong to the oncogenic miR-17~92 cluster [32,33], prevent cellular senescence by down-regulating the cell cycle inhibitor p21/CDKN1A. Likewise, family members of the paralog miR-106b~25 cluster also promote cell cycle progression – and thus inhibit senescence – by directly targeting p21/CDKN1A [34]. Consistent with these findings, we observed a highly significant age-related decrease in plasma levels of miR-20a and miR-106b, which might thus correspond to an increased level of senescence. Notably, these two miRNAs have previously also been reported to be down-regulated in peripheral blood mononuclear cells from octogenarians *versus* young people, whereas centenarians exhibiting a healthy aging phenotype seemed capable of maintaining high levels of these senescence inhibitors [35]. We found no evidence, however, pointing to miR-17, miR-19b or miR-106a as circulating aging markers, although these miRNAs were also included in the serum/plasma screening panel used in our exploratory study. Neither did we find age-related changes in plasma expression of miR-24, which has been shown to suppress the expression of the senescence gene $p16^{INK4A}$ in human diploid fibroblasts [36]. As opposed to the senescence inhibiting miRNAs miR20a and miR-106b, 6 other miRNAs that were identified as candidate circulating aging miRNAs in our initial exploratory study (i.e. miR-21, miR-191, miR-200c, miR-210, miR-376a and let-7d) have been reported to *trigger* cellular senescence in specific cell types [20,37–40]; miR-21 has even been described as a new circulating marker of inflammaging [41]. Yet, only miR-191 was convincingly confirmed in our validation study; its significant age-associated down-regulation in serum/plasma is in agreement with earlier findings in mononuclear cells [35]. The remaining 7 candidate aging miRNAs miR-320b, miR-301a, miR-378, miR-374a, miR-423, miR-30b, miR-140 that emerged from our initial screening and of which two (i.e. miR-301a and miR-30b) were convincingly confirmed in the validation study, have previously not been linked with cellular senescence and are now for the first time directly associated with aging in humans. It should be mentioned, though, that one of the target genes of miR-320 family members is IGFBP5 (insulin-like growth factor binding protein 5), an important modulator of the aging-related insulin/IGF-1 signaling pathway. IGFBP5 and miR-320 are expressed in a wide variety of overlapping tissues (e.g. liver, brain, lung, kidney, heart, colon …) and are secreted into the circulation. Serum IGFBP5 concentrations have been reported to decline with age and to show a significant positive correlation with circulating levels of IGF-1 [42]. Thus, the age-associated increase in circulating miR-320b observed in our present study – albeit not statistically significant in the validation experiment – might possibly be linked with our previous finding that plasma IGF-1 levels are decreased in older compared to younger patients (our own data, manuscript in preparation). Therefore, miR-320b will still be considered as a potential miRNA of interest in our future aging biomarker studies.

For reasons outlined above, we are not studying aging miRNAs in a healthy population but in a breast cancer context. In order to minimize cancer-related confounding effects, we have selected highly homogeneous cohorts with regard to tumor characteristics. Nevertheless, it cannot be excluded that the organismal response to breast cancer disease might override otherwise regulated miRNAs. Small age-related changes in plasma miRNA expression might possibly be masked by substantial cancer-related under- or overexpression of particular miRNAs in older breast cancer patients. The processes of aging and carcinogenesis are indeed intimately linked, since cellular senescence constitutes an intrinsic tumor suppressor mechanism *in vivo* but, at the same time, is the major driving force in age-related tissue degeneration and – dysfunction [43]. It is thus conceivable that miRNAs implicated in aging are also modulated in human cancers and *vice versa*. Several miRNAs that emerged from our exploratory screening as candidate aging miRNAs have actually been reported as "oncomirs" or "tumor suppressor miRNAs". For instance, let-7d is considered a tumor suppressor microRNA, as it is strongly down-regulated in poorly differentiated lung and breast tumor cells [44]. Also, miR-376a is downregulated in several tumors and makes part of a miRNA cluster frequently silenced in malignant melanoma [45]. In contrast, miR-20a, miR-21, miR-378, miR-106b and miR-191 were found to exert oncogenic activity and are overexpressed in several types of cancer [20,31,34,46,47]. Moreover, high (tumor) expression of miR-210 has been associated with higher risk of recurrence in breast cancer [48]. Serum miR-200c was reported as a novel prognostic and metastasis-predictive biomarker in colorectal cancer [49], while miR-423-5p was found to be upregulated in serum from patients with gastric cancer [50]. Therefore, it should be kept in mind when interpreting our data that certain miRNAs exert their action at the interface between cancer and aging. To our knowledge, this is the first miRNA study comparing "fit" and "non-fit/frail" older individuals. We did not observe any significant differences between those two subgroups, at least not with regard to the miRNAs investigated in the validation study. This is somewhat surprising, since several of these miRNAs have also been implicated in age-related diseases. For instance, let-7d, miR-191 and miR-301a make part of a unique circulating 7-miRNA signature that can distinguish patients with Alzheimer's disease from normal controls [51], and miR-20a and miR-106b are both implicated in transcriptional inhibition of Alzheimer's amyloid precursor protein (APP) [52]. Also, miR-320 was shown to be upregulated in neurodegeneration in mice [53]. Furthermore, miR-21 expression has been reported to be higher in patients suffering from cardiovascular disease [41] and loss of miR-140 contributes to the development of age-related osteoarthritis-like changes in mice [54]. However, other miRNAs than those included in our validation study have been more consistently associated with age-related physical and mental decline: e.g. the miRNA most clearly associated with age-related neurodegeneration in the aging *Drosophila* brain is miR-34 [55]. Our data indicate that the observed age-related differential expression of the 5 validated aging miRNAs represents a direct effect of physiological aging and is not merely associated to the age-related frailty syndrome. Yet, the newly identified aging miRNAs should be further validated in larger cohorts of frail *verus* non-frail older persons that are not affected by cancer, in order to ultimately sustain this conclusion. A search for "frailty miRNAs" is another issue of clinical interest, which would, however, demand a different experimental set-up, such as exploratory screening and subsequent validation in healthy *versus* frail subjects of comparable age.

In conclusion, we have discovered five miRNAs (miR-301a, miR-20a-3p, miR-106b-5p, miR-191 and miR-30b-5p) that can be used as aging biomarkers in future research projects. Since we have chosen for a straight-forward selection of 15 miRNAs from the initial screening, certain potentially interesting miRNAs, most particularly miR-34a, were not further investigated in this study. These, together with several miRNAs that remained inconclusive because of borderline statistical significance (e.g. miR-320b, miR-374a, miR-378, miR-423), might yet merit further attention in future studies. The newly identified aging miRNAs will now be examined in a prospective study that has recently been conducted in our institution with the aim to investigate the impact of chemotherapy on the biological age of older breast cancer patients. While common acute adverse events of chemotherapy, such as neutropenia and mucosal degeneration, are well-known and may be tolerated/accepted by the patient, the long term impact of cytotoxic treatments (and perhaps other anti-cancer therapies such as hormonal drugs, monoclonal antibiodies and oral targeted agents) on healthy tissues is actually poorly documented. For instance, premature telomere shortening due to DNA-targeting chemotherapeutic drugs may impact on the long-term replicative potential of regenerative tissues like hair follicles, the hematopoietic and gastrointestinal system, and germline and skin cells [56]. To learn more about such delayed aging-related side effects in long-term survivors of cancer, a better insight into aging mechanisms and associated biomarkers is mandatory, along with detailed investigation of the impact of common chemotherapeutic regimens on these aging biomarkers.

Materials and Methods

Ethics statement

This study was performed in compliance with the Helsinki Declaration and national law. All patients included in the study gave written informed consent for future translational research. Blood sampling, collection of patient data and genetic analysis were approved by the ethics committee of our institution (Ethics Committee of the University Hospitals Leuven, study number S53608; Approval number : ML7994).

Patients

Since 2003, the Leuven Multidisciplinary Breast Center (University Hospitals Leuven) has systematically collected plasma and serum from all consenting (i.e. ±75%) breast cancer patients at the time of diagnosis, before initiation of any local or systemic therapy. All breast cancer patients are also included in a clinical database, containing extensive general and tumor-related information, as well as clinical follow-up. In addition, most older (70+) breast cancer patients diagnosed since 2009 are also included in one of the large-scale geriatric cancer projects running in our institution: geriatric assessment (GA) – integrating two geriatric screening tools G8 and Flemish version of the Triage Risk Screening Tool (fTRST), Activities of Daily Living (ADL), instrumental Activities of Daily Living (iADL), Geriatric Depression Scale, Mini Mental State Examination, and Mini Nutritional Assessment – is systematically performed prior to initiation of any chemotherapy, radiotherapy or surgery [24]. Furthermore, the Charlson Comorbidity Index (at the time of diagnosis) can easily be calculated retrospectively using the patient's electronic file.

Selection of the exploratory cohort

For an initial exploratory pilot experiment, eligible subjects were selected from the clinical breast cancer database based on the following inclusion criteria: (i) diagnosed with primary (i.e. non-relapse) early (i.e. non-locally advanced, non-metastatic) invasive breast cancer *without* lymph node involvement; (ii) received primary surgery and pathological confirmation in our institution; (iii) serum collected at the time of diagnosis (i.e. before initiation of any treatment); (iv) all pathological parameters available to identify histological subtype according to recent guidelines [57,58]. A study group of 10 young (<45 years) patients and 10 older (>70 years) patients (all female), the latter with GA performed at the time of diagnosis (i.e. before initiation of any treatment), was selected and both age groups were matched in order to contain an equal distribution of different breast cancer subtypes: 7 so-called luminal A, 1 luminal B, 2 triple negative [58]. Tumor characteristics are summarized in Table 1. Determination of tumor grading and estrogen receptor (ER), progesterone receptor (PR), and HER2/*neu* status was done according to standard procedures. ER and PR were considered positive if >1% of cells stained positive on immunohistochemistry. HER2 was considered positive if the fluorescent in situ hybridization (FISH) test, systematically performed in all immunohistochemistry (IHC) 2+ tumors, showed HER2 genomic amplification or, in the absence of FISH, if IHC was 3+.

Selection of the validation study cohort

For the subsequent validation experiment, an independent cohort of early breast cancer patients (all with primary invasive, node-negative luminal A tumors) was selected consisting of 10 young (<45 years) female patients and 20 older (>70 years) female patients, from whom 10 were 'fit' while 10 others were classified as 'non-fit'. Fitness/frailty status was estimated based on the results of the GA, which were condensed into (i) the generally used Balducci score [59] and (ii) the novel Leuven Oncogeriatric Frailty Score (LOFS), a final score from 0 (severly frail) to 10 (entirely fit), described in File S1. Patients of the older 'fit' group had LOFS = 9–10, whereas patients of the older 'non-fit' group had LOFS ≤5. Clinical characteristics of patients from the validation study cohort are summarized in Table 2.

Serum and plasma collection

Peripheral blood was routinely sampled in 4-mL BD Vacutainer SST II Advance tubes (for serum collection) and in 4-mL BD Vacutainer EDTA K2E tubes (for plasma collection). The blood samples were incubated at room temperature for 20 to 60 min. After centrifugation at 1600xg for 10 min at 4°C, the supernatant (serum/plasma) was isolated and stored in aliquots at −80°C. Because of sample availability issues, the validation study was done on plasma specimens, whereas the exploratory screening was done on serum.

MicroRNA isolation

After spinning down thawed serum/plasma to remove debris, the absorbance spectrum of the sample was recorded on a NanoDrop ND-1000 in order to detect hemolysis, which may cause severe perturbation of serum/plasma miRNA profiles due to cell-derived microRNA contamination. Samples showing a clear absorption peak at 415 nm (i.e. absorbance maximum of hemoglobin) were excluded from the experiment. Absence of hemolysis in the included samples was further verified after qPCR (see below). RNA was purified from non-hemolysed serum/plasma samples using the miRNeasy Mini kit (Qiagen) following the manufacturer's protocol with slight modifications in order to achieve optimal microRNA extraction from serum/plasma samples, which typically contain very low amounts of RNA. Briefly, to 200 µL of serum/plasma, 1 µg of carrier MS2 RNA (Roche) was added, together with 750 µL of QIAzol (Qiagen).

Subsequently, 1 µL of a synthetic RNA spike-in (UniSp6 at 10^8 copies/µL, Exiqon) was added to allow evaluation of the efficiency and uniformity of the entire RNA extraction/cDNA synthesis procedure. After 5 min of incubation, 200 µL chloroform was added. After incubation and centrifugation according to the normal procedure, the upper aqueous phase was isolated, 1.5 volumes of ethanol was added and the sample was loaded onto the spin column. The column was washed once with RWT buffer and three times with RPE buffer (both included in the kit). After air-drying of the column, the RNA sample was eluted with 50 µL of nuclease-free water and immediately frozen at −80°C until further analysis. In both the pilot and the validation experiment, duplicate RNA extractions were performed in parallel from each plasma sample.

cDNA synthesis

Because of the very low amounts of RNA in serum/plasma and, therefore, the use of an RNA carrier during the extraction procedure, standard spectrophotometric measurement of RNA yield and quality is not suitable for serum/plasma RNA extracts. Therefore, RNA input in the reverse transcription (RT) reaction was based on sample volume and not RNA quantity. Preliminary test experiments with several commonly used control miRNAs (i.e. miR-103, miR-191, miR-423-3p and miR-451) were carried out to determine the optimal amount of RNA template to be used in the RT reaction; these titration experiments showed that an RNA input of 4 µL mostly resulted in good RT efficiency and subsequent PCR amplification without significant interference by RT and/or PCR inhibitors, which are frequently present in RNA preparations from serum/plasma. Thus, cDNA was synthesized from each of both duplicate RNA extracts using 4 µL of RNA in a 20-µL reaction by use of the Universal cDNA synthesis kit II (Exiqon) according to the manufacturer's instructions. cDNA samples were stored frozen until PCR analysis was performed.

RT-qPCR-based miRNA assays

In the initial experiment, a broad exploratory miRNA screening was performed using the 96-well Serum/Plasma Focus microRNA PCR Panel (Exiqon) that comprises microRNA PCR assays for 175 different microRNAs that are commonly found in serum/plasma. Since individual samples are assessed on separate plates, the panel assay also includes triplicate wells of an interplate calibrator (UniSp3) to account for technical run-to-run differences in amplification signal. Data from different plates were normalized using the Cp-values of the interplate calibrator. For each serum sample, both duplicate cDNA samples were pooled before running the miRNA panel assay. Assays were carried out following the manufacturer's protocol. Briefly, pooled cDNA was diluted 50x in nuclease-free water and mixed with an equal volume of 2x SYBR Green master mix (Exiqon). Final reaction volume was 10 µL. Plates were run on a LightCycler 480 (LC480, Roche) instrument applying the following thermal cycling protocol : activation step (10 min at 95°C); 45 amplification cycles (10 s at 95°C, 1 min at 60°C, ramp rate 1,6°C/s); melting curve analysis.

In the subsequent validation study on plasma samples from a different, independent patient cohort, 21 selected miRNAs were assessed by the use of individual PCR assays (MicroRNA LNA PCR primer sets, Exiqon). These included the 15 top-ranking candidate aging miRNAs, showing the most pronounced age-related differences in the pilot screening experiment. In addition, 4 miRNAs that were identified as good reference candidates in the pilot experiment and 2 additonal quality control miRNAs were also included. For each plasma sample, duplicate RNA extracts were prepared and reverse transcribed and separate PCR assays were run on each of both duplicate cDNA samples. All PCR assays were done in triplicate microplate wells (96-well format). Reaction mixtures were prepared according to the provided assay protocol and contained 4 µL of 40-fold diluted cDNA (20-fold diluted for miR-20a-3p) in a final volume of 10 µL. For each miRNA, all samples were run together on the same plate to avoid bias introduced by plate-to-plate variations in qPCR efficiency. Plates were run on the LC480 instrument using the same thermal cycling protocol as described above for the panel assays.

Data analysis

RT-qPCR Cp values were determined by the LC480 instrument software using the second derivative method and were subsequently imported and further processed by GenEx Pro software (MultiID Analyses). The absence of hemolysis in the initial serum/plasma samples was verified by means of the miR-451/miR-23a-3p hemolysis test: ΔCp values between miR-23a-3p, known to be stably expressed in serum/plasma samples, and miR-451a, known to show highly increased expression in hemolysed samples, were below 5 for all samples.

Data of the initial screening experiment were normalized using the global mean of the entire miRNA panel [25]. Candidate reference miRNAs were then identified by variance analysis of the normalized dataset and were further examined using the specified algorithms GeNorm [27] and Normfinder [26], which are both incorporated in the GenEx Pro software package (MultiID Analyses). Five miRNAs with superior expression stability among all samples were used for data normalisation in the subsequent validation study.

Statistical tools incorporated in the GenEx software package were applied to assess differences in serum/plasma miRNA expression between the different patient groups. These included parametric t-test (unpaired, two-tailed) for normally distributed miRNA results and Mann-Whitney test (unpaired, two-tailed) for cases where the data were not normally distributed. Normality was assessed with the Kolmogorov-Smirnov test. In the exploratory study, principal component analysis and hierarchical clustering were additionally applied to reveal sample grouping patterns in the multivariate dataset. In the validation study, the age effect was first assessed by comparing the young patient group ($N = 10$) with the total older patient group ($N = 20$), combining both 'fit' ($N = 10$) and 'frail' ($N = 10$) subgroups. Subsequently, a comparison between 'fit' and 'frail' patients was done within the older cohort. Correction for multiple testing was done according to the Dunn-Bonferroni method.

Supporting Information

File S1 Leuven Oncogeriatric Frailty Score (LOFS). Description and illustration of the composition of the new, refined scoring system that was used to evaluate the fitness/frailty status of the patients.

File S2 List of all microRNAs included in the exploratory screening panel.

File S3 Data set of the exploratory screening study.

File S4 Data set of the validation study.

Acknowledgments

We thank Kathleen Corthouts for excellent technical assistance.

Author Contributions

Conceived and designed the experiments: SH BB CK HW. Performed the experiments: SH. Analyzed the data: SH BD AL PS HW. Contributed reagents/materials/analysis tools: SH BB CK AL. Contributed to the writing of the manuscript: SH BB BD AL CK PS HW.

References

1. Balaban RS, Nemoto S, Finkel T (2005) Mitochondria, oxidants, and aging. Cell 120: 483–495.
2. Lombard DB, Chua KF, Mostoslavsky R, Franco S, Gostissa M, et al. (2005) DNA repair, genome stability, and aging. Cell 120: 497–512.
3. Blasco MA (2007) Telomere length, stem cells and aging. Nat Chem Biol 3: 640–649.
4. Campisi J, Kim SH, Lim CS, Rubio M (2001) Cellular senescence, cancer and aging: the telomere connection. Exp Gerontol 36: 1619–1637.
5. Zhang G, Li J, Purkayastha S, Tang Y, Zhang H, et al. (2013) Hypothalamic programming of systemic ageing involving IKK-beta, NF-kappaB and GnRH. Nature 497: 211–216.
6. Alcedo J, Flatt T, Pasyukova EG (2013) Neuronal inputs and outputs of aging and longevity. Front Genet 4: 71.
7. Maccormick RE (2006) Possible acceleration of aging by adjuvant chemotherapy: a cause of early onset frailty? Med Hypotheses 67: 212–215.
8. Li P, Hou M, Lou F, Bjorkholm M, Xu D (2012) Telomere dysfunction induced by chemotherapeutic agents and radiation in normal human cells. Int J Biochem Cell Biol 44: 1531–1540.
9. Franco S, Ozkaynak MF, Sandoval C, Tugal O, Jayabose S, et al. (2003) Telomere dynamics in childhood leukemia and solid tumors: a follow-up study. Leukemia 17: 401–410.
10. Schroder CP, Wisman GB, de Jong S, van der Graaf WT, Ruiters MH, et al. (2001) Telomere length in breast cancer patients before and after chemotherapy with or without stem cell transplantation. Br J Cancer 84: 1348–1353.
11. Wynn RF, Cross MA, Hatton C, Will AM, Lashford LS, et al. (1998) Accelerated telomere shortening in young recipients of allogeneic bone-marrow transplants. Lancet 351: 178–181.
12. Unryn BM, Hao D, Gluck S, Riabowol KT (2006) Acceleration of telomere loss by chemotherapy is greater in older patients with locally advanced head and neck cancer. Clin Cancer Res 12: 6345–6350.
13. Serrano M, Blasco MA (2007) Cancer and ageing: convergent and divergent mechanisms. Nat Rev Mol Cell Biol 8: 715–722.
14. Roninson IB (2003) Tumor cell senescence in cancer treatment. Cancer Res 63: 2705–2715.
15. Chang BD, Swift ME, Shen M, Fang J, Broude EV, et al. (2002) Molecular determinants of terminal growth arrest induced in tumor cells by a chemotherapeutic agent. Proc Natl Acad Sci U S A 99: 389–394.
16. Liu Y, Sanoff HK, Cho H, Burd CE, Torrice C, et al. (2009) Expression of p16(INK4a) in peripheral blood T-cells is a biomarker of human aging. Aging Cell 8: 439–448.
17. Vandenberk B, Brouwers B, Hatse S, Wildiers H (2011) p16(INK4a): A central player in cellular senescence and a promising aging biomarker in elderly cancer patients. Journal of Geriatric Oncology 2: 259–269.
18. Pallis AG, Hatse S, Brouwers B, Pawelec G, Falandry C, et al. (2013) Evaluating the physiological reserves of older patients with cancer: The value of potential biomarkers of aging? Journal of Geriatric Oncology in press.
19. Grillari J, Grillari-Voglauer R (2010) Novel modulators of senescence, aging, and longevity: Small non-coding RNAs enter the stage. Exp Gerontol 45: 302–311.
20. Olivieri F, Rippo MR, Monsurro V, Salvioli S, Capri M, et al. (2013) MicroRNAs linking inflamm-aging, cellular senescence and cancer. Ageing Res Rev.
21. Inukai S, Slack F (2013) MicroRNAs and the genetic network in aging. J Mol Biol 425: 3601–3608.
22. Li X, Khanna A, Li N, Wang E (2011) Circulatory miR34a as an RNAbased, noninvasive biomarker for brain aging. Aging (Albany NY) 3: 985–1002.
23. Mitchell PS, Parkin RK, Kroh EM, Fritz BR, Wyman SK, et al. (2008) Circulating microRNAs as stable blood-based markers for cancer detection. Proc Natl Acad Sci U S A 105: 10513–10518.
24. Kenis C, Bron D, Libert Y, Decoster L, Van Puyvelde K, et al. (2013) Relevance of a systematic geriatric screening and assessment in older patients with cancer: results of a prospective multicentric study. Ann Oncol 24: 1306–1312.
25. Mestdagh P, Van Vlierberghe P, De Weer A, Muth D, Westermann F, et al. (2009) A novel and universal method for microRNA RT-qPCR data normalization. Genome Biol 10: R64.
26. Andersen CL, Jensen JL, Orntoft TF (2004) Normalization of real-time quantitative reverse transcription-PCR data: a model-based variance estimation approach to identify genes suited for normalization, applied to bladder and colon cancer data sets. Cancer Res 64: 5245–5250.
27. Vandesompele J, De Preter K, Pattyn F, Poppe B, Van Roy N, et al. (2002) Accurate normalization of real-time quantitative RT-PCR data by geometric averaging of multiple internal control genes. Genome Biol 3: RESEARCH0034.
28. ElSharawy A, Keller A, Flachsbart F, Wendschlag A, Jacobs G, et al. (2012) Genome-wide miRNA signatures of human longevity. Aging Cell 11: 607–616.
29. Noren Hooten N, Abdelmohsen K, Gorospe M, Ejiogu N, Zonderman AB, et al. (2010) microRNA expression patterns reveal differential expression of target genes with age. PLoS One 5: e10724.
30. Hunter MP, Ismail N, Zhang X, Aguda BD, Lee EJ, et al. (2008) Detection of microRNA expression in human peripheral blood microvesicles. PLoS One 3: e3694.
31. Hackl M, Brunner S, Fortschegger K, Schreiner C, Micutkova L, et al. (2010) miR-17, miR-19b, miR-20a, and miR-106a are down-regulated in human aging. Aging Cell 9: 291–296.
32. Grillari J, Hackl M, Grillari-Voglauer R (2010) miR-17-92 cluster: ups and downs in cancer and aging. Biogerontology 11: 501–506.
33. He L, Thomson JM, Hemann MT, Hernando-Monge E, Mu D, et al. (2005) A microRNA polycistron as a potential human oncogene. Nature 435: 828–833.
34. Ivanovska I, Ball AS, Diaz RL, Magnus JF, Kibukawa M, et al. (2008) MicroRNAs in the miR-106b family regulate p21/CDKN1A and promote cell cycle progression. Mol Cell Biol 28: 2167–2174.
35. Serna E, Gambini J, Borras C, Abdelaziz KM, Belenguer A, et al. (2012) Centenarians, but not octogenarians, up-regulate the expression of microRNAs. Sci Rep 2: 961.
36. Lal A, Kim HH, Abdelmohsen K, Kuwano Y, Pullmann R, Jr., et al. (2008) p16(INK4a) translation suppressed by miR-24. PLoS One 3: e1864.
37. Dellago H, Preschitz-Kammerhofer B, Terlecki-Zaniewicz L, Schreiner C, Fortschegger K, et al. (2013) High levels of oncomiR-21 contribute to the senescence-induced growth arrest in normal human cells and its knock-down increases the replicative lifespan. Aging Cell 12: 446–458.
38. Lena AM, Mancini M, Rivetti di Val Cervo P, Saintigny G, Mahe C, et al. (2012) MicroRNA-191 triggers keratinocytes senescence by SATB1 and CDK6 downregulation. Biochem Biophys Res Commun 423: 509–514.
39. Magenta A, Cencioni C, Fasanaro P, Zaccagnini G, Greco S, et al. (2011) miR-200c is upregulated by oxidative stress and induces endothelial cell apoptosis and senescence via ZEB1 inhibition. Cell Death Differ 18: 1628–1639.
40. Faraonio R, Salerno P, Passaro F, Sedia C, Iaccio A, et al. (2012) A set of miRNAs participates in the cellular senescence program in human diploid fibroblasts. Cell Death Differ 19: 713–721.
41. Olivieri F, Spazzafumo L, Santini G, Lazzarini R, Albertini MC, et al. (2012) Age-related differences in the expression of circulating microRNAs: miR-21 as a new circulating marker of inflammaging. Mech Ageing Dev 133: 675–685.
42. Mohan S, Farley JR, Baylink DJ (1995) Age-related changes in IGFBP-4 and IGFBP-5 levels in human serum and bone: implications for bone loss with aging. Prog Growth Factor Res 6: 465–473.
43. Finkel T, Serrano M, Blasco MA (2007) The common biology of cancer and ageing. Nature 448: 767–774.
44. Yu F, Yao H, Zhu P, Zhang X, Pan Q, et al. (2007) let-7 regulates self renewal and tumorigenicity of breast cancer cells. Cell 131: 1109–1123.
45. Zehavi L, Avraham R, Barzilai A, Bar-Ilan D, Navon R, et al. (2012) Silencing of a large microRNA cluster on human chromosome 14q32 in melanoma: biological effects of mir-376a and mir-376c on insulin growth factor 1 receptor. Mol Cancer 11: 44.
46. Lee DY, Deng Z, Wang CH, Yang BB (2007) MicroRNA-378 promotes cell survival, tumor growth, and angiogenesis by targeting SuFu and Fus-1 expression. Proc Natl Acad Sci U S A 104: 20350–20355.
47. Volinia S, Calin GA, Liu CG, Ambs S, Cimmino A, et al. (2006) A microRNA expression signature of human solid tumors defines cancer gene targets. Proc Natl Acad Sci U S A 103: 2257–2261.
48. Camps C, Buffa FM, Colella S, Moore J, Sotiriou C, et al. (2008) hsa-miR-210 Is induced by hypoxia and is an independent prognostic factor in breast cancer. Clin Cancer Res 14: 1340–1348.
49. Toiyama Y, Hur K, Tanaka K, Inoue Y, Kusunoki M, et al. (2013) Serum miR-200c Is a Novel Prognostic and Metastasis-Predictive Biomarker in Patients With Colorectal Cancer. Ann Surg.
50. Liu R, Zhang C, Hu Z, Li G, Wang C, et al. (2011) A five-microRNA signature identified from genome-wide serum microRNA expression profiling serves as a fingerprint for gastric cancer diagnosis. Eur J Cancer 47: 784–791.
51. Kumar P, Dezso Z, MacKenzie C, Oestreicher J, Agoulnik S, et al. (2013) Circulating miRNA biomarkers for Alzheimer's disease. PLoS One 8: e69807.
52. Hebert SS, Horre K, Nicolai L, Bergmans B, Papadopoulou AS, et al. (2009) MicroRNA regulation of Alzheimer's Amyloid precursor protein expression. Neurobiol Dis 33: 422–428.
53. Saba R, Goodman CD, Huzarewich RL, Robertson C, Booth SA (2008) A miRNA signature of prion induced neurodegeneration. PLoS One 3: e3652.
54. Miyaki S, Sato T, Inoue A, Otsuki S, Ito Y, et al. (2010) MicroRNA-140 plays dual roles in both cartilage development and homeostasis. Genes Dev 24: 1173–1185.

55. Aw S, Cohen SM (2012) Time is of the essence: microRNAs and age-associated neurodegeneration. Cell Res 22: 1218–1220.
56. Beeharry N, Broccoli D (2005) Telomere dynamics in response to chemotherapy. Curr Mol Med 5: 187–196.
57. Brouckaert O, Schoneveld A, Truyers C, Kellen E, Van Ongeval C, et al. (2013) Breast cancer phenotype, nodal status and palpability may be useful in the detection of overdiagnosed screening-detected breast cancers. Ann Oncol 24: 1847–1852.
58. Goldhirsch A, Winer EP, Coates AS, Gelber RD, Piccart-Gebhart M, et al. (2013) Personalizing the treatment of women with early breast cancer: highlights of the St Gallen International Expert Consensus on the Primary Therapy of Early Breast Cancer 2013. Ann Oncol 24: 2206–2223.
59. Balducci L, Extermann M (2000) Management of the frail person with advanced cancer. Crit Rev Oncol Hematol 33: 143–148.

5

Efficacy of Short-Term High-Dose Statin Pretreatment in Prevention of Contrast-Induced Acute Kidney Injury: Updated Study-Level Meta-Analysis of 13 Randomized Controlled Trials

Joo Myung Lee[1], Jonghanne Park[1]**, Ki-Hyun Jeon[1], Ji-hyun Jung[1], Sang Eun Lee[1], Jung-Kyu Han[1], Hack-Lyoung Kim[2], Han-Mo Yang[1], Kyung Woo Park[1], Hyun-Jae Kang[1], Bon-Kwon Koo[1], Sang-Ho Jo[3], Hyo-Soo Kim[1,4]***

1 Department of Internal Medicine and Cardiovascular Center, Seoul National University Hospital, Seoul, Korea, **2** Cardiovascular Center, Seoul National University, Boramae Medical Center, Seoul, Korea, **3** Division of Cardiology, Department of Internal Medicine, Hallym University Sacred Heart Hospital, Anyang-si, Gyeonggi-do, Korea, **4** Department of Molecular Medicine and Biopharmaceutical Sciences, Graduate School of Convergence Science and Technology, Seoul National University, Seoul, Korea

Abstract

Background: There have been conflicting results across the trials that evaluated prophylactic efficacy of short-term high-dose statin pre-treatment for prevention of contrast-induced acute kidney injury (CIAKI) in patients undergoing coronary angiography (CAG). The aim of the study was to perform an up-to-date meta-analysis regarding the efficacy of high-dose statin pre-treatment in preventing CIAKI.

Methods and Results: Randomized-controlled trials comparing high-dose statin versus low-dose statin or placebo pre-treatment for prevention of CIAKI in patients undergoing CAG were included. The primary endpoint was the incidence of CIAKI within 2–5days after CAG. The relative risk (RR) with 95% CI was the effect measure. This analysis included 13 RCTs with 5,825 total patients; about half of them (n = 2,889) were pre-treated with high-dose statin (at least 40 mg of atorvastatin) before CAG, and the remainders (n = 2,936) pretreated with low-dose statin or placebo. In random-effects model, high-dose statin pre-treatment significantly reduced the incidence of CIAKI (RR 0.45, 95% CI 0.35–0.57, $p<0.001$, $I^2 = 8.2\%$, NNT 16), compared with low-dose statin or placebo. The benefit of high-dose statin was consistent in both comparisons with low-dose statin (RR 0.47, 95% CI 0.34–0.65, $p<0.001$, $I^2 = 28.4\%$, NNT 19) or placebo (RR 0.34, 95% CI 0.21–0.58, $p<0.001$, $I^2 = 0.0\%$, NNT 16). In addition, high-dose statin showed significant reduction of CIAKI across various subgroups of chronic kidney disease, acute coronary syndrome, and old age (≥60years), regardless of osmolality of contrast or administration of N-acetylcystein.

Conclusions: High-dose statin pre-treatment significantly reduced overall incidence of CIAKI in patients undergoing CAG, and emerges as an effective prophylactic measure to prevent CIAKI.

Editor: Giuseppe Remuzzi, Mario Negri Institute for Pharmacological Research and Azienda Ospedaliera Ospedali Riuniti di Bergamo, Italy

Funding: This study was supported by grants from the Bio & Medical Technology Development Program of the National Research Foundation (NRF) funded by the Korean government (2010-0020258) and from the IRICT, Seoul National University Hospital (A062260), sponsored by the Ministry of Health and Welfare, Republic of Korea. The funders had no role in study design, data collection and analysis, decision to publish, or preparation of the manuscript.

Competing Interests: The authors have declared that no competing interests exist.

* Email: hyosoo@snu.ac.kr

These authors contributed equally to this work.

Introduction

Contrast-induced acute kidney injury (CIAKI) is a well-recognized complication of coronary angiography (CAG) with iodinated contrast medium and is the third leading cause of hospital-acquired acute renal failure. CIAKI has been known to be associated with prolonged hospitalization, increased costs, and increased short and long-term morbidity and mortality. [1] The incidence of CIAKI varies widely depending on the patient's underlying co-morbidities, definition criteria, and preventive strategies. But, certain subgroup of coronary heart disease patients, especially with acute coronary syndrome or chronic kidney disease, showed higher risk for the CIAKI. [2,3] Investigators have examined several strategies to prevent CIAKI, such as fenolopam, mannitol, theophylline, iloprost, furosemide, dopamine, hemofiltration, ascorbic acid, and N-acetylcystein (NAC). [4] However, none of the agents were proved to be effective in preventing CIAKI. [4,5] Currently, recommendations of the

European Society of Cardiology/European Association for Cardio-Thoracic Surgery (ESC/EACTS) or the ACCF/AHA/SCAI guideline are limited to the prophylactic intravenous hydration, use of iso- or low-osmolar contrast agents, and reduced dosages of contrast agents to prevent occurrence of CIAKI. [6,7] Since a few observational studies suggested that 3-hydroxyl-3-methylglutaryl coenzyme A reductase inhibitors (statins) may reduce CIAKI incidence, several RCTs have evaluated the potential benefit of statin in prevention of CIAKI. [8,9]Statin's postulated mechanism of kidney protection was through its pleotropic effects, i.e. antioxidant, anti-inflammatory, and anti-thrombotic actions. However, these previous RCTs and meta-analysis of high-dose statin pre-treatment showed disappointing results. [10–12] Recently, three RCTs with relatively large sample size (NAPLES II, PRATO-ACS, TRACK-D trial) have reported promising results favoring prophylactic efficacy of high-dose statin in prevention of CIAKI. [13–15] Considering insufficient evidences regarding efficacy of high-dose statin pre-treatment and prognostic importance of CIAKI, we therefore performed a systematic review and comprehensive meta-analysis of all published randomized control trials, in order to evaluate the efficacy of high-dose statin pre-treatment to reduce the incidence of CIAKI in various clinical situations including overall population, chronic kidney disease, or acute coronary syndrome.

Methods

Data Sources and Searches

Relevant published or unpublished studies were independently searched in PubMed, Cochrane Central Register of Controlled Trials, EMBASE, the United States National Institutes of Health registry of clinical trials (www.clinicaltrials.gov), and relevant websites (www.crtonline.org, www.clinicaltrialresults.com, www.tctmd.com, www.cardiosource.com, and www.pcronline.com) were also searched. Detailed search strategy was presented in the Method S1. The electronic search strategy was complemented by manual review of reference lists of included articles. References of recent reviews, editorials, and meta-analyses were also examined. No restrictions were imposed on language, study period, or sample size.

Study Selection

We included RCTs assessing preventive strategies for CIAKI that met following criteria. First, we selected studies which enrolled adult patients undergoing CAG with or without percutaneous coronary intervention (PCI). Second, the intervention was high-dose statin (defined as a daily dose of at least 40 mg of Atorvastatin or equivalent dose of available statins including Simvastatin, Pitavastatin, Fluvastatin, Lovastatin, Pravastatin, or Rosuvastatin), compared with low-dose statin (defined as a daily dose of less than 40 mg of Atorvastatin or equivalent dose of available statins), placebo or none of medication pre-treatment. In cases where a concomitant prophylactic measures were used (for example, NAC, sodium bicarbonate, or other preventive medications), both arms must have shared the same concomitant prophylactic measures, with only a difference in statin protocol. Finally, the incidences of post-procedural CIAKI were reported in both arms, regardless of its definition or the timing of data collection. We excluded RCTs conducted on pediatric patients (including neonates and preterm infants) and randomized crossover trials that assigned patients to both high-dose and low-dose or placebo arms.

Data Extraction and Quality Assessment

Data extraction and quality assessment was performed as previously described. [16] Summarized data as reported in the published manuscripts were used in the analysis. A standardized form was used to extract characteristics of trials, study design (including randomization sequence generation, allocation concealment, crossover between assigned groups, number of post-randomization withdrawals or follow-up loss), number of study patients, age, eligibility criteria of each trials, definition of CIAKI in each trials, baseline serum creatinine and estimated glomerular filtration rates (eGFR), mean change of serum creatinine after procedure, total cumulative dose of statin before procedure, protocols for statin treatment, hydration protocols, type or mean dosage of radio-contrast agents, the proportion of diabetes mellitus, hypertension, chronic kidney disease, timing of data collection, length of follow-up, adverse events data associated with statin treatment reported on an intention-to-treat basis. We primarily focused our analysis on the effect of prophylactic treatment with high-dose statin on the incidence of CIAKI, not on the surrogate markers of inflammation or oxidative stress. The quality of eligible RCTs was assessed using the Cochrane Collaboration's tool for assessing the risk of bias for RCTs (Table S1 in File S1). Because most previous meta-analyses have reported the methodological quality of each trial using the Jadad score, we also provided this score, as well as the Cochran Collaboration's tool, for each RCT. [17] Two investigators (JML and JP) independently performed screening of titles and abstracts, identified duplicates, reviewed full articles, and determined their eligibility. Disagreements were resolved by discussions. The last search was performed in February 2014.

Outcomes and Definitions

The primary outcome was the incidence of post-procedural CIAKI within 2–5 days after index procedure. Secondary outcomes included the incidence of post-procedural CIAKI, stratified according to the various subgroups for example, type of contrast agents (iso-osmolar or low-osmolar) used, mean age of the study patients, presence of underlying chronic kidney disease, patients with acute coronary syndrome, NAC usage, or placebo control. All of the patients and outcomes were analyzed according to the originally assigned group.

Data Synthesis and Analysis

Data synthesis and analsysis was performed as described in detail previously [16], The primary outcome was analyzed by both a random effects model and a fixed effects model. Relative risks (RR) with 95% confidence interval (CI) were presented as summary statistics. The pooled RR was calculated with the DerSimonian and Laird method for random effects model, as well as the Mantel–Haenszel method for fixed effects model. [18] To evaluate the effect of progressive chronological change in study design, such as study population, protocol of statin pre-treatment, hydration protocols or concomitant prophylactic medications including NAC or sodium bicarbonate, we evaluated the impact of publication date on the overall effect of pooled RRs for incidence of CIAKI by a cumulative meta-analysis. Stratified subgroup analyses were performed to assess treatment effects according to the control group (low-dose statin, placebo, or no medication), type of contrast agent, mean age of the patients, underlying chronic kidney disease, acute coronary syndrome, and usage of NAC along with tests for interaction derived from random effects meta-regression. Statistical heterogeneity was assessed by Cochran's Q via a $\chi 2$ test and was quantified with the I^2 test. [19] Publication bias was assessed by funnel plot asymmetry, along with Egger's and Begg's test. The κ statistic was used to assess agreement between investigators for study selection. Results were considered statistically significant at 2-sided $p<0.05$. Statistical analysis was performed with the use of STATA/SE 12.0 (Stata Corp LP, College Station, Texas, USA). The present study was performed in compliance with the Preferred Reporting Items for Systematic Reviews and Meta-Analyses (PRISMA) guidelines and the review protocol has not been registered (Checklist S1). [20]

Results

Search Results

We identified 465 citations from searches as previously described. Among these, 24 studies were retrieved for detailed evaluation, of which 13 RCTs met inclusion criteria (Figure 1). [11–15,21–28] These 13 RCTs included a total of 5,825 adult patients, 2,889 (49.6%) of which were allocated to the high-dose statin group and 2,936 (50.4%) of which were allocated to the control group (low-dose statin or placebo group). The characteristics of 11 excluded studies after full article review are summarized in the Method S2. The inter-observer agreement for study selection was high ($\kappa = 0.92$).

Trial Characteristics

The main characteristics of the individual studies are summarized in Table 1 and 2. All trials reported the incidence of CIAKI within 2-5days from index procedure using contrast agents. Four trials exclusively enrolled the patients with chronic kidney disease, which was defined as eGFR of less than 60 ml/min/1.73 m^2 in PROMISS, Toso et al, and NAPLES II trial, and eGFR of between 30–90 ml/min/1.73 m^2 in TRACK-D trial. [11–14] Only one trial (TRACK-D) exclusively enrolled type 2 diabetes mellitus patients, whereas the others enrolled the patients regardless of diabetes mellitus. [14] Among the 13 trials, 4 trials compared high-dose statin versus low-dose statin pre-treatment. [21,22,25,27] Majority of trials used Atorvastin, whereas 2 trials [11,21] used Simvastatin, and 2 trials [14,15] used Rosuvastatin. Total cumulative dose of statin in high-dose statin group ranged from 40 mg to 560 mg of Atorvastatin equivalent dose from 1 to 7 days before CAG. The detailed medication protocols in each included trials are summarized in Table 1. The definition of CIAKI slightly differed across trials. Ten trials [11,14,15,21, 22,24–28] used an increase in serum creatinine of $\geq$0.5mg/dL or $\geq$25% from baseline within 48–72 hours after radiocontrast exposure, whereas 2 trials [12,23] regarded an absolute increase in serum creatinine of $\geq$0.5 mg/dL within 5 days as their primary definition of CIAKI. One trial (NAPLES II) used an increase in serum cystatin C $\geq$10% from baseline, which was used in this analysis, although they reported the incidence of CIAKI on the base of the change in serum creatinine as secondary outcomes. [13] All trials evaluated patients with coronary artery disease undergoing CAG with or without percutaneous coronary intervention. Among the trials, 5 studies [15,21,26–28] exclusively enrolled the patients with acute coronary syndrome including unstable angina and non ST-segment elevation myocardial infarction, and 2 of these 5 studies [21,28] further included the patients with ST-segment elevation myocardial infarction. Four trials [12,13,15,24] used NAC (600 mg or 1200 mg twice daily) as additional preventive measure of CIAKI in both arms, and 1 trial

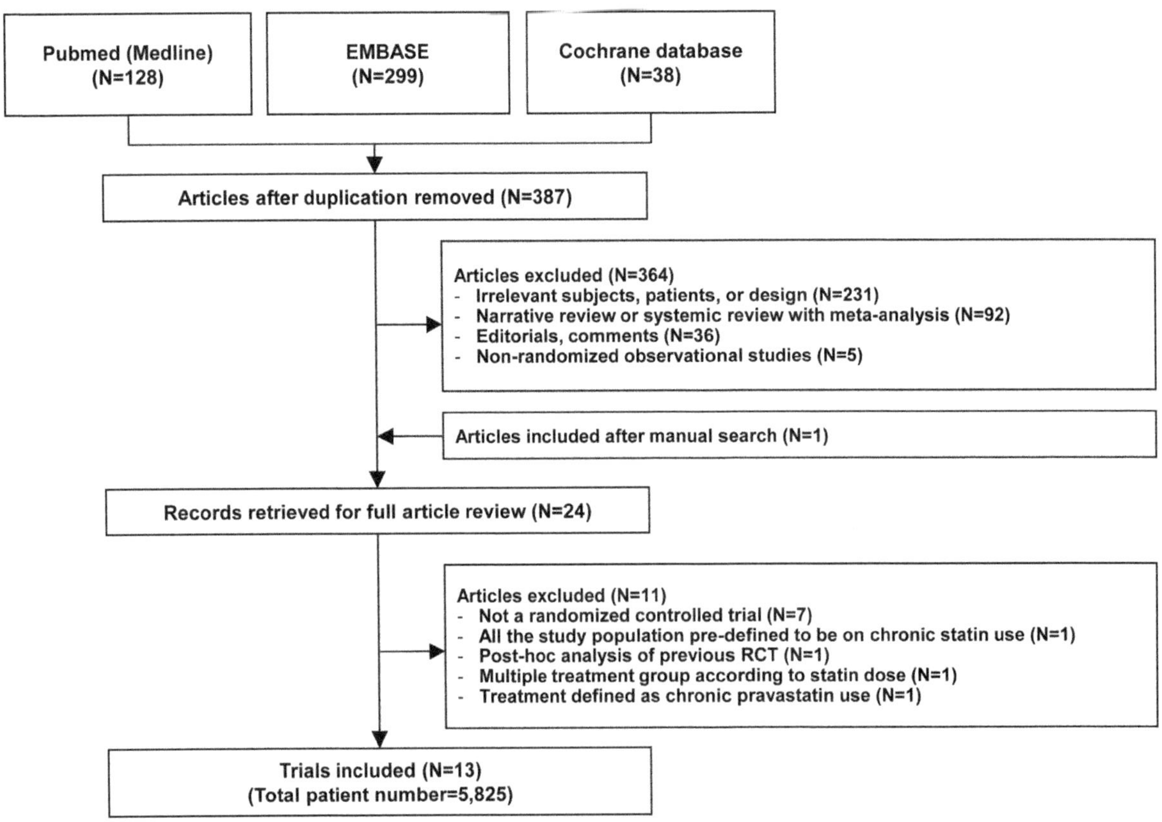

Figure 1. Flow diagram of trial selection. Abbreviations: RCT, randomized controlled trial.

Table 1. Characteristics of the study, trial characteristics and protocols.

Trial (Year)	Patients number		Inclusion criteria	Definition of CIN	Medication Protocols		Contrast agent	Contrast volumes (mean), ml		Hydration protocols
	Statin (N = 2889)	Control (N = 2936)			Statin	Control		Statin	Control	
PROMISS (2008)	118	118	CKD patients undergoing CAG or PCI, CrCl≤60 mL/min or SCr≥ 1.1 mg/dL	Increase of SCr≥ 0.5 mg/dL or ≥25% at 48 hours	Simvastatin 40 mg bid, 1 day pre-procedure and 1 day post-procedure	Placebo	Visipaque (iodixanol)	173.3	190.9	NS 1 mg/kg/h for 12 h before and 12 h after procedure
Toso et al. (2009)	152	152	CKD patients undergoing CAG or PCI, CrCl<60 mL/min	Increase of SCr≥ 0.5 mg/dl within 5 days.	Atorvastatin 80 mg/day 2 days pre-procedure and 2 days post-procedure, NAC 1200 mg bid from 1 day before to 1 day post-procedure	Placebo + NAC 1200 mg bid from 1day before to 1 day post-procedure	Visipaque (iodixanol)	151.0	164.0	NS 1 ml/kg/h for 12 h before and after the procedure
Xinwei et al. (2009)	113	115	ACS (UA/NSTEMI) including STEMI patients undergoing PCI	Increase of SCr≥ 0.5 mg/dL or ≥25% at 48 hours	Simvastatin 80 mg/ day from admission to the day before, 20 mg/day after procedure	Simvastatin, 20 mg/day from admission to the end	Visipaque (iodixanol) for CKD, Omnipaque (iohexol) for non-CKD	227.0	240.0	NS 1 ml/kg/h for 6 to 12 h before and 12 h after procedure
Zhou Xia et al. (2009)	50	50	Patients undergoing CAG or PCI	Increase of SCr≥ 0.5 mg/dL or ≥ 25% at 72 hours	Atorvastatin 80 mg/ day before for 1day,10 mg/day for 6days after procedure	Atorvastatin 10 mg/day for 7 days	Iopamidol 370 mg/ml	118.7	112.9	NS 1000 mL infusion, for 12 h before and 12 h after intervention
Acikel et al. (2010)	80	80	Patients undergoing elective CAG or PCI (excluding ACS), LDL≥ 70 mg/dl, eGFR≥60 ml/min/ 1.73 m^2	Increase of SCr≥ 0.5 mg/dL at 48 hours	Atorvastatin 40 mg/ day 3 days pre-procedure and 2 days post-procedure	None	Omnipaque(iohexol)	105.0	103.0	NS 1 ml/kg/h starting 4 h before and continuing until 24 h after procedure
Ozhan et al. (2010)	60	70	Patients undergoing CAG or PCI, eGFR≥70 ml/min/1.73 m^2 or SCr≤1.5 mg/dL	Increase of SCr≥ 0.5 mg/dL or ≥25% at 48 hours	Atorvastatin 80 mg 1 day pre-procedure and 2 days post-procedure, NAC 600 mg bid pre-procedure	No statin pre-procedure, NAC 600 mg bid pre-procedure	Iopamidol	97.0	93.0	NS 1000 ml infusion during 6 h after procedure
Hua et al. (2010)	76	97	Patients undergoing CAG or PCI	Increase of SCr≥ 0.5 mg/dL or ≥25% at 72 hours	Atorvastatin 80 mg/day pre-procedure	Atorvastatin 20 mg/day pre-procedure	Iopromide	173.0	177.0	NR
ARMYDA-CIN (2011)	120	121	ACS (UA/NSTEMI) Patients undergoing CAG or PCI (excluding high-risk NSTEMI requiring emergency PCI), SCr≤3 mg/dl	Increase of SCr≥ 0.5 mg/dL or ≥25% at 48 hours	Atorvastatin 80 mg (12 h before) → 40 mg (2 h before), 40 mg for 2days after procedure	Placebo before procedure → Atorvastatin 40 mg for 2days after procedure	Xenetix (iobitridol)	209.0	213.0	For patients CrCl < 60 ml/min, NS 1 ml/ kg/h for 12 h before and 24 h after intervention

Table 1. Cont.

Trial (Year)	Patients number		Inclusion criteria	Definition of CIN	Medication Protocols		Contrast agent	Contrast volumes (mean), ml		Hydration protocols
	Statin (N = 2889)	Control (N = 2936)			Statin	Control		Statin	Control	
Wei Li et al. (2012)	78	83	STEMI patients undergoing emergency PCI within 12 hours of symptom onset	Increase of SCr≥ 0.5 mg/dL or ≥25% at 72 hours	Atorvastatin 80 mg loading pre-procedure, long-term 40 mg/day after procedure	Placebo 801mg loading pre-procedure, long-term 40 mg/day after procedure	Ultravist 370 (iopromide)	100.0	103.6	NS 1 ml/kg/h before the procedure and for 12 h after the procedure
NAPLES II (2012)	202	208	CKD patients undergoing CAG or PCI, eGFR<60 ml/min/1.73 m^2	Increase of Serum Cystatin C concentration ≥10% at 24 hours	Atorvastatin 80 mg before procedure, NAC 1200 mg bid the day before and the day of procedure	No statin pre-procedure, NAC 1200 mg bid the day before and the day of procedure	Visipaque (iodixanol)	177.0	184.0	Sodium bicarbonate solution (154 mEq/L), initial bolus of 3 mL/kg/h for 1 h before procedure, 1 mL/kg/h during and for 6 h after the procedure
CAO et al. (2012)	90	90	Patients undergoing CAG or PCI	Increase of SCr≥ 0.5 mg/dL or ≥25% at 72 hours	Atorvastatin 40 mg/day from 3days before procedure, 20 mg/day after procedure	Atorvastatin 20 mg/day from 3days before procedure, 20 mg/day after procedure	NR	162.3	158.9	NR
PRATO-ACS (2014)	252	252	ACS (UA/NSTEMI) patients undergoing CAG or PCI (excluding STEMI and high-risk NSTEMI requiring emergency PCI), SCr≤ 3 mg/dl	Increase of SCr≥ 0.5 mg/dL or ≥25% at 72 hours	Rosuvastatin 40 mg loading → 20 mg/day before procedure, Rosuvastatin 20 mg/day continued after procedure, NAC 1200 mg bid the day before and the day of procedure	No statin pre-procedure, Atorvastatin 40 mg/day after procedure, NAC 1200 mg bid the day before and the day of pro cedure	Visipaque (iodixanol)	149.7	138.2	NS 1 ml/kg/h for 12 h both before and after the procedure. Hydration rate was reduced to 0.5 ml/kg/h in both arms for patients with LVEF <40%
TRACK-D (2014)	1498	1500	Stage 2 or 3 CKD and type II DM patients undergoing CAG or PCI, eGFR ≥30 ml/min/1.73 m^2 and < 90 ml/min/1.73 m^2 (excluded stage 0,1,4,5 CKD patients)	Increase of SCr≥ 0.5 mg/dL or ≥25% at 72 hours	Rosuvastatin 10 mg/day from 2 days before to 3 days after procedure → continued after procedure	No statin pre-procedure, Rosuvastatin 10 mg. day 3 days after procedure	Visipaque (iodixanol)	120.0	110.0	NS 1 ml/kg/h started 12 h before and continued for 24 h after procedure

Abbreviations: ACS, acute coronary syndrome; CAG, coronary angiography; CIN, contrast induced nephropathy; CKD, chronic kidney disease; CrCl, creatinine clearance; DM, diabetes mellitus; eGFR, estimated glomerular filtration rate; LDL, low-density lipoprotein; LVEF, left ventricular ejection fraction; NAC, N-acetylcystein; NR, not reported; NS, normal saline (isotonic saline, 0.9%); NSTEMI, non ST-segment elevation myocardial infarction; PCI, percutaneous coronary intervention; SCr, serum creatinine; STEMI, ST-segment elevation myocardial infarction; UA, unstable angina.

Table 2. Characteristics of the study, baseline characteristics.

	Mean age, year		Mean baseline SCr (mg/dL)		Mean baseline eGFR (ml/min)					
Trial (Year)	**Statin**	**Control**	**Statin**	**Control**	**Statin**	**Control**	**Male proportion**	**Diabetes Mellitus proportion**	**Hypertension proportion**	**Additional measures**
PROMISS (2008)	65	66	1.29	1.25	53.46	55.40	72.5%	25.9%	63.2%	None
Toso et al. (2009)	75	76	1.20	1.18	46.00	46.00	64.5%	21.1%	60.5%	NAC
Xinwei et al. (2009)	65	66	0.82	0.83	86.50	93.60	36.0%	20.6%	63.6%	None
Zhou Xia et al. (2009)	60	61	1.04	1.08	76.88	70.54	59.0%	20.0%	75.0%	None
Acikel et al. (2010)	59	61	0.84	0.85	97.70	97.00	63.8%	24.4%	58.1%	None
Ozhan et al. (2010)	54	55	0.88	0.88	92.00	89.00	59.2%	16.2%	22.3%	NAC
Hua et al. (2010)	65	65	1.34	1.40	68.20	66.70	67.1%	26.6%	74.6%	None
ARMYDA-CIN (2011)	65	66	1.04	1.04	79.80	77.00	77.6%	28.2%	75.1%	None
Wei Li et al. (2012)	66	65	0.93	0.93	NR	NR	75.8%	28.0%	80.7%	None
NAPLES II (2012)	70	70	1.32	1.29	42.00	43.00	54.4%	41.2%	86.3%	NAC, bicarbonate
CAO et al. (2012)	63	63	0.85	0.83	109.60	106.80	57.2%	21.7%	37.2%	None
PRATO-ACS (2014)	66	66	0.95	0.96	69.90	69.30	65.7%	21.2%	55.8%	NAC
TRACK-D (2014)	62	61	1.08	1.07	74.16	74.43	65.2%	100.0%	71.9%	None

Abbreviations: ACS, acute coronary syndrome; CAG, coronary angiography; CIN, contrast induced nephropathy; CKD, chronic kidney disease; CrCl, creatinine clearance; DM, diabetes mellitus; eGFR, estimated glomerular filtration rate; LDL, low-density lipoprotein; LVEF, left ventricular ejection fraction; NAC, N-acetylcystein; NR, not reported; NS, normal saline (isotonic saline, 0.9%); NSTEMI, non ST-segment elevation myocardial infarction; PCI, percutaneous coronary intervention; SCr, serum creatinine; STEMI, ST-segment elevation myocardial infarction; UA, unstable angina.

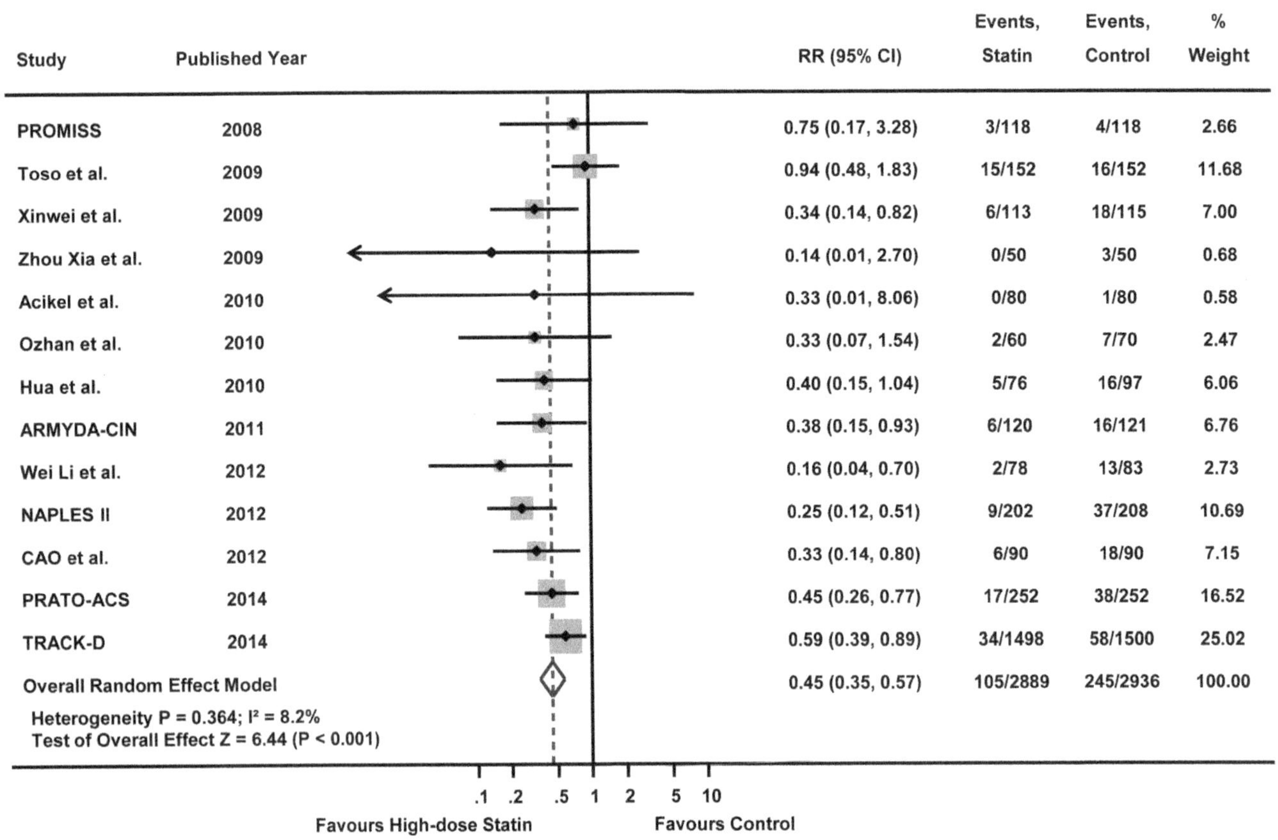

Figure 2. The effect of high-dose statin on the incidence of contrast-induced acute kidney injury by random effects model. Forest plot with relative risks for the incidence of contrast-induced acute kidney injury associated with high-dose statin pre-treatment, compared with control group (low-dose statin or placebo) for individual trials and the pooled population. Abbreviations: CI, confidence intervals; RR, relative risks.

[13] used sodium bicarbonate solution as primary hydration protocol.

Risk of Bias within Trials

Figure S1 in File S1 shows the risk of bias graph illustrating the proportion of studies with each of the judgments ('Yes', 'No', 'Unclear') for each entry in the Cochrane Collaboration's tool. A full description of the summary of risk of bias judgments of each study is available in Figure S2 and Table S1 in File S1. All of the included trials were RCTs and no substantial risk of bias was observed in random sequence generation. The included trials showed relatively high methodological quality. Among the 13 RCTs, 5 trials [11,12,15,26,28] had double-blinded design, whereas others were open-label or non-blinded trials. However, all trials used objective findings (serum creatinine or cystatin C) to define the primary endpoint (the incidence of CIAKI), the authors, therefore, judged that the outcomes were not likely to be influenced by lack of blinding.

Effect of Statin on the Incidence of Contrast-Induced Acute Kidney Injury

As shown in Figure 1, this meta-analysis included 13 RCTs [11–15,21–28], all of which provided the incidence of CIAKI. Figure 2 illustrates the RRs of individual study and pooled RR in regards to the incidence of CIAKI, the primary outcome. The overall incidence of CIAKI in the intention-to-treat population was 3.6% (105/2889) in high-dose statin group and 8.3% (245/2936) in control group, respectively. In pooled analysis using random effects model, patients receiving high-dose statin pre-treatment had 55% less risk of CIAKI compared with the control group (RR 0.45, 95% CI 0.35–0.57, $p<0.001$) (Figure 2). A fixed effects model yielded a similar result (RR 0.44, 95% CI 0.35–0.55, $p<0.001$) (Figure S3 in File S1). The number needed to treat (NNT) of high-dose statin was 16 in random effects model which means that treatment of 16 patients with high-dose statin will reduce 1 event of CIAKI. There was no significant heterogeneity in either the random effects or the fixed effects model ($I^2 = 8.2\%$, heterogeneity $p = 0.364$ for both random and fixed effects model). Since 4 trials compared high-dose versus low-dose statin group and 9 trials compared high-dose versus placebo or no treatment, we performed stratified analysis according to the type of treatment (Figure 3). High-dose statin significantly reduced the risk of CIAKI by 53% (RR 0.47, 95% CI 0.34–0.65, $p<0.001$, $I^2 = 28.4\%$, heterogeneity $p = 0.192$) or 66% (RR 0.34, 95% CI 0.21–0.58, $p< 0.001$, $I^2 = 0.0\%$, heterogeneity $p = 0.931$), when compared with placebo or low-dose statin group, respectively.

Visual estimation of the funnel plot indicated no apparent publication or small study effect bias with the support of the Egger's test ($p = 0.128$) and Begg's test ($p = 0.625$) (Figure S4 in File S1). No individual study unduly influenced the pooled estimate of high-dose statin for the incidence of CIAKI (Figure S5 in File S1). Cumulative meta-analysis, which sorts trials chronologically, showed no apparent progressive shift of pooled estimate of high-dose statin from a negative to a positive effect, despite of differences in practice patterns or patient populations from 2008 to 2014 (Figure S6 in File S1). Along with the

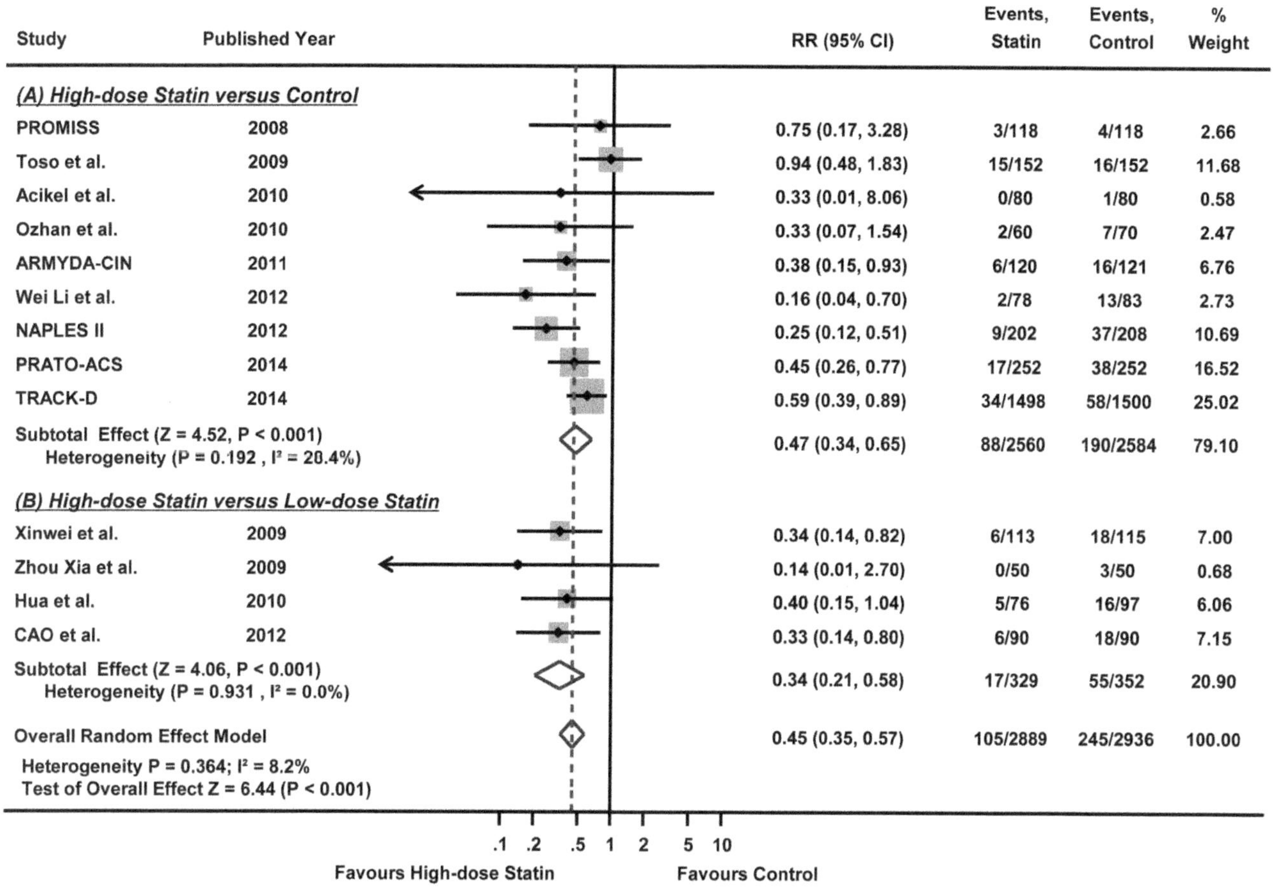

Figure 3. The effect of high-dose statin on the incidence of contrast-induced acute kidney injury, stratified according to the high-dose versus low-dose statin or high-dose versus placebo. Forest plot with relative risks for the incidence of contrast-induced acute kidney injury associated with (A) high-dose statin versus low-dose statin or (B) high-dose statin versus placebo for individual trials and the pooled population. Abbreviations: CI, confidence intervals; RR, relative risks.

significantly reduced incidence of CIAKI in high-dose statin group, mean change of post-procedural serum creatinine was also significantly lower in the high-dose statin group, compared with control group (SMD −0.37, 95% CI −0.59 to −0.15, p = 0.001) (Figure S7 in File S1).

Subgroup Analysis

The results of subgroup analysis are presented in Figure 4. The beneficial effect of high-dose statin pre-treatment was consistent across all the subgroups, except the subgroup of age less than 60 years old. The high-dose statin showed significantly less development of CIAKI in the patients with old age (≥60 years old), underlying chronic kidney disease, or acute coronary syndrome. When the high-risk subgroup was defined with the patients with chronic kidney disease or acute coronary syndrome, the high-dose statin showed also significant beneficial effect in reducing CIAKI in both high-risk and low-risk subgroup. In addition, the protective effect of high-dose statin was also significant regardless of the osmolality of the contrast agents (iso- or low-osmolar) or concomitant treatment of NAC. Lastly, high-dose statin significantly reduced the incidence of CIAKI compared with placebo or low-dose statin. The NNT of high-dose statin ranged from 12 to 26 (Figure 4). Detailed results of pooled analysis in each subgroup are summarized in the Figure S8-S12 in File S1.

Discussion

The results of this meta-analysis indicate that high-dose statin pre-treatment in patients undergoing CAG with or without PCI significantly reduced the incidence of CIAKI, compared with control (placebo or low-dose statin). The beneficial effect of high-dose statin was obvious in various subgroups of patients including underlying chronic kidney disease, acute coronary syndrome, or old age (≥60 years). The effect of high-dose statin was also clear regardless of type of contrast agent or concomitant treatment of NAC.

This study is the most up-to-date comprehensive meta-analysis with improved statistical power to address the effect of statin for CIAKI prevention in CAG. [10,29–33] The inconclusive results of previous meta-analyses regarding the efficacy of statin pre-treatment, might mainly originate from the limited sample size of included trials. [29–31] Some of these studies included both randomized and non-randomized clinical trials, which might have led to potential bias. [10,32] In the most recent meta-analysis by Li et al. [33], the authors showed significant benefit of statin pre-treatment in reducing the incidence of CIAKI. However, they argued that statin pre-treatment had no protective effect in the patients with underlying chronic kidney disease (RR 0.79, 95% CI 0.47–1.32, p = 0.37), however, the included studies in this subgroup analysis were only 3 studies with total sample size of

	No. of Trials	No. of Patients	Relative Risks (95% CI) for CIN	NNT	I^2 (heterogeneity P)	Interaction P
Statistical Model						
Fixed effects	13	5825	0.44 (0.35-0.55)	22	8.2% (0.364)	
Radom Effects	13	5825	0.45 (0.35-0.57)	16	8.2% (0.364)	
Type of Intervention						**0.356**
High-dose Statin versus Control	9	5144	0.47 (0.34-0.65)	19	28.4% (0.192)	
High-dose Statin versus Low-dose Statin	4	681	0.34 (0.21-0.58)	16	0.0% (0.931)	
Type of Contrast agent						**0.156**
Iso-osmolar, non-ionic contrast	5	4452	0.52 (0.34-0.79)	21	50.2% (0.090)	
Low-osmolar, non-ionic contrast	7	1193	0.33 (0.21-0.52)	14	0.0% (0.962)	
Mean Age of the Population						**0.718**
≥ 60 years old	11	5535	0.44 (0.34-0.58)	14	22.3% (0.231)	
< 60 years old	2	290	0.33 (0.08-1.33)	31	0.0% (1.000)	
Chronic Kidney Disease						**0.144**
Exclusively enrolled CKD patients	4	3948	0.55 (0.31-0.96)	26	60.5% (0.055)	
Others	9	1877	0.37 (0.27-0.51)	13	0.0% (0.973)	
Acute coronary syndrome						**0.265**
Exclusively enrolled ACS patients	5	1314	0.37 (0.26-0.53)	10	0.0% (0.776)	
Others	8	4511	0.50 (0.34-0.73)	24	24.2% (0.236)	
N-acetylcystein was administered						**0.710**
Yes	4	1348	0.46 (0.25-0.83)	13	59.9% (0.058)	
No	9	4477	0.45 (0.34-0.60)	18	0.0% (0.695)	
Placebo controlled or Not						**0.047**
Placebo controlled	5	3940	0.56 (0.36-0.88)	28	32.5% (0.205)	
No	8	1885	0.35 (0.26-0.49)	12	0.0% (0.953)	
Risk of CIAKI						
High-risk (CKD or ACS patient)	9	5262	0.45 (0.33- 0.61)	14	34.1% (0.145)	**0.583**
Low-risk (Others)	4	563	0.35 (0.16-0.75)	19	0.0% (0.932)	

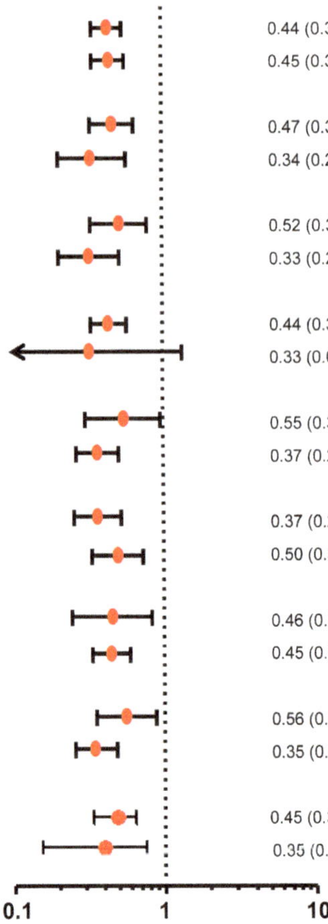

Figure 4. Subgroup analyses according to the study protocols. The forest plot shows relative risks (by random effects model) for the incidence of contrast-induced acute kidney injury associated with high-dose statin pre-treatment, compared with control group (low-dose statin or placebo), stratified according to (1) type of intervention, (2) type of contrast agent, (3) mean age of the patients, (4) underlying chronic kidney disease, (5) acute coronary syndrome, (6) N-acetylcystein as concomitant prophylactic measure, and (7) placebo controlled trial or not. Abbreviations: ACS, acute coronary syndrome; CI, confidence intervals; CKD, chronic kidney disease; RR, relative risks.

390 in high-dose statin versus 391 in control group. [33] In the present meta-analysis we evaluated over 5,800 patients from 13 RCTs, the benefit of high-dose statin was consistently observed in both overall population and various subgroups including patients with chronic kidney disease (RR 0.55, 95% CI 0.31–0.96, $p = 0.036$). The limited sample size of the pooled analysis and larger chance of type II error would explain the negative result of Li et al.

Previous studies have suggested that statin protects CIAKI through its pleotropic effect rather than its lipid lowering effect. The pleotropic effect includes enhancement of nitric oxide production, anti-inflammatory, and antioxidative effect. [34,35] These pleotropic effects could decrease renal cell injury after iodinated contrast exposure. In the NAPLES II trial, high-dose atorvastatin reduced contrast-induced JNK activation and p53 phosphorylation which is the key steps of oxidative stress induced intrinsic apoptosis. [13] Also, statin may modulate the kidney hypoperfusion after radio-contrast exposure by down-regulation of angiotensin receptors and by decrease of endothelin-1 synthesis. [36] Lastly, anti-inflammatory effect of statin may prevent renal cell damage through decrease of pro-inflammatory cytokines which induce tissue factor expression by macrophage and activate nuclear factor-kappa B [37].

Although high-dose statin showed clear beneficial effect in preventing CIAKI, the risk of high-dose statin should be considered. Among the 13 RCTs, only 2 trials reported adverse events related with high-dose statin treatment. [14,28] Wei Li et al. reported that the rates of hepatotoxicity (defined as>3 times of upper normal limits of alanine aminotransferase within 1 month of the procedure) were 3.85% in high-dose statin group and 1.20% in control group ($p = 0.57$). In TRACK-D trial, they described that the rates of muscle pain, liver function abnormality, gastrointestinal disorders, edema or rash were not statistically different between high-dose statin and control group without presentation of actual numbers of the complications. Since limited data of adverse events in the included trials, the hazard of high-dose statin pre-treatment could not be evaluated in this meta-analysis. Previous meta-analysis of 35 RCTs comparing statin versus placebo, which was not a meta-analysis for CIAKI, reported that the absolute risk differences (RD) of most frequent adverse drug reactions were as follows; transaminase elevation (RD 4.2%, 95% CI 1.5 to 6.9%), myalgia (RD 2.7%, 95% CI −3.2 to 8.7%), rhabdomyolysis (RD 0.4%, 95% CI −0.1 to 0.9%), and discontinuation due to any adverse drug reaction (RD −0.5%, 95% CI −4.3 to 3.3%). [38] According to this report, the number needed to harm of statin treatment regarding adverse drug reaction are from 24 (hepatotoxicity) to 250 (rhabdomyolysis, defined as creatinine kinase elevations ≥10 times upper normal limit). Considering substantially lower NNT of 16 in this meta-analysis for reducing CIAKI and the clinical importance of CIAKI, high-dose statin pre-treatment before CAG with or without PCI could be considered as an effective prophylactic measure to prevent CIAKI.

Limitations

Several important limitations of the study should not be ignored. First, this meta-analysis included clinically- and methodologically-diverse studies. Although we included only RCTs to the final analysis and assured statistically insignificant heterogeneity, there were some differences in the enrollment criteria (some studies exclusively enrolled patients with chronic kidney disease or diabetes mellitus), definition of the CIAKI, medication or hydration protocols. Also, basically this meta-analysis comprising 13 RCTs inherently shares the limitations of each trial. Second, variations in the type, dose, and duration of statin pretreatment among the included trials might have potential effects to our results, since all statins may not be equivalent to each other in their pleotropic and nephroprotective effects. Finally, as this study was a study-level meta-analysis, individual patient data were not included in the analysis, and therefore, we could not adjust for patient-level confounders.

Conclusion

High-dose statin pre-treatment significantly reduced the incidence of CIAKI in patients undergoing CAG. Considering prognostic importance of CIAKI and clear beneficial effect of statin in this meta-analysis, high-dose statin pre-treatment may be more actively employed as an effective prophylactic measure to prevent CIAKI.

Supporting Information

Checklist S1 PRISMA checklist.

File S1 Supporting information files. Method S1, Search Strategy on Medline, EMBASE and Cochran Central. Method S2, Characteristics of the Excluded Study. Table S1, The Cochrane Collaboration's tool for assessing risk of bias. Figure S1, Risk of bias assessment graph. Risk of bias of each included trial was assessed with the Cochrane Collaboration's tool. This 'risk of bias graph' illustrates the proportion of studies with each of the judgments for each entry in the tool. Green represents 'Yes (low risk of bias)'; yellow, 'Unclear'; red, 'No (high risk of bias)'. Figure S2, Risk of bias assessment summary. Risk of bias of each included trial was assessed with the Cochrane Collaboration's tool. This 'risk of bias summary' figure presents all of the judgments in a cross-tabulation of study by entry. Green represents 'Yes (low risk of bias)'; yellow, 'Unclear'; red, 'No (high risk of bias)'. Figure S3, The effect of High-dose statin on the incidence of contrast-induced nephropathy by fixed effects model. Forest plot with relative risks for the incidence of contrast-induced nephropathy associated with high-dose statin versus low-dose statin or placebo for individual trials and the pooled population. The squares and the horizontal lines indicate the relative risks (by fixed effects model) and the 95% confidence intervals (CI) for each trial included; the size of each square is proportional to the statistical weight of a trial in the frequentist meta-analysis; diamond indicates the effect estimate derived from meta-analysis, with the center indicating the point estimate and the left and the right ends the 95% CI. Abbreviations: CI, confidence intervals; RR, relative risks. Figure S4, The effect of High-dose statin on mean change of post-procedural serum creatinine. Forest plot with standardized mean difference (SMD) for the mean change of post-procedural serum creatinine from the baseline value associated with high-dose statin versus low-dose statin or placebo for individual trials and the pooled population. The squares and the horizontal lines indicate the SMD (by random effects model) and the 95% confidence intervals (CI) for each trial included; the size of each square is proportional to the statistical weight of a trial in the frequentist meta-analysis; diamond indicates the effect estimate derived from meta-analysis, with the center indicating the point estimate and the left and the right ends the 95% CI. Abbreviations: CI, confidence intervals; SD, standard deviation; SMD, standardized mean difference. Figure S5, Funnel plot for evaluation of publication and small study bias. Figure S6, Influence of individual studies Abbreviations: CI, confidence intervals; RR, relative risks. Figure S7, Cumulative Meta-analysis of high-dose statin on the incidence of contrast-induced nephropathy. The first row shows the effect of one study, the second row shows the cumulative pooled estimates based on the two studies, and so on. The squares and the horizontal lines indicate the cumulative relative risks (by random effects model) and the 95% confidence intervals (CI) for each trial included. Abbreviations: CI, confidence intervals; RR, relative risks. Figure S8, The effect of High-dose statin on the incidence of contrast-induced nephropathy, stratified according to the type of contrast. The squares and the horizontal lines indicate the relative risks (by random effects model) and the 95% confidence intervals (CI) for each trial included; the size of each square is proportional to the statistical weight of a trial in the meta-analysis; diamond indicates the effect estimate derived from meta-analysis, with the center indicating the point estimate and the left and the right ends the 95% CI. Abbreviations: CI, confidence intervals; RR, relative risks. Figure S9, The effect of High-dose statin on the incidence of contrast-induced nephropathy, stratified according to the mean age of the patients. The squares and the horizontal lines indicate the relative risks (by random effects model) and the 95% confidence intervals (CI) for each trial included; the size of each square is proportional to the statistical weight of a trial in the meta-analysis; diamond indicates the effect estimate derived from meta-analysis, with the center indicating the point estimate and the left and the right ends the 95% CI. Abbreviations: CI, confidence intervals; RR, relative risks. Figure S10, The effect of High-dose statin on the incidence of contrast-induced nephropathy, stratified according to the underlying chronic kidney disease. The squares and the horizontal lines indicate the relative risks (by random effects model) and the 95% confidence intervals (CI) for each trial included; the size of each square is proportional to the statistical weight of a trial in the meta-analysis; diamond indicates the effect estimate derived from meta-analysis, with the center indicating the point estimate and the left and the right ends the 95% CI. Abbreviations: CI, confidence intervals; CKD, chronic kidney disease; eGFR, estimated glomerular filtration rates; RR, relative risks. Figure S11, The effect of High-dose statin on the incidence of contrast-induced nephropathy, stratified according to the acute coronary syndrome. The squares and the horizontal lines indicate the relative risks (by random effects model) and the 95% confidence intervals (CI) for each trial included; the size of each square is proportional to the statistical weight of a trial in the meta-analysis; diamond indicates the effect estimate derived from meta-analysis, with the center indicating the point estimate and the left and the right ends the 95% CI. Abbreviations: CI, confidence intervals; RR, relative risks. Figure S12, The effect of High-dose statin on the incidence of contrast-induced nephropathy, stratified according to the concomitant treatment of N-acetylcystein. The squares and the horizontal lines indicate the relative risks (by random effects model) and the 95% confidence intervals (CI) for each trial included; the size of each square is proportional to the statistical weight of a trial in the meta-analysis; diamond indicates the effect estimate derived from meta-analysis, with the center indicating the point estimate and the left and the right ends the 95% CI. Abbreviations: CI, confidence intervals; RR, relative risks.

Author Contributions

Conceived and designed the experiments: JML JP HSK. Analyzed the data: JML JP KHJ JHJ SEL JKH HLK HMY KWP HJK BKK SHJ HSK. Contributed reagents/materials/analysis tools: JHJ SEL JKH HLK HMY KWP HJK BKK SHJ. Wrote the paper: JML JP.

References

1. McCullough PA (2008) Contrast-induced acute kidney injury. J Am Coll Cardiol 51: 1419–1428.
2. McCullough PA, Adam A, Becker CR, Davidson C, Lameire N, et al. (2006) Epidemiology and prognostic implications of contrast-induced nephropathy. Am J Cardiol 98: 5K–13K.
3. Klein LW, Sheldon MW, Brinker J, Mixon TA, Skelding K, et al. (2009) The use of radiographic contrast media during PCI: a focused review: a position statement of the Society of Cardiovascular Angiography and Interventions. Catheter Cardiovasc Interv 74: 728–746.
4. Kelly AM, Dwamena B, Cronin P, Bernstein SJ, Carlos RC (2008) Meta-analysis: effectiveness of drugs for preventing contrast-induced nephropathy. Ann Intern Med 148: 284–294.
5. Kitzler TM, Jaberi A, Sendlhofer G, Rehak P, Binder C, et al. (2012) Efficacy of vitamin E and N-acetylcysteine in the prevention of contrast induced kidney injury in patients with chronic kidney disease: a double blind, randomized controlled trial. Wien Klin Wochenschr 124: 312–319.
6. O'Gara PT, Kushner FG, Ascheim DD, Casey DE Jr, Chung MK, et al. (2013) 2013 ACCF/AHA guideline for the management of ST-elevation myocardial infarction: executive summary: a report of the American College of Cardiology Foundation/American Heart Association Task Force on Practice Guidelines: developed in collaboration with the American College of Emergency Physicians and Society for Cardiovascular Angiography and Interventions. Catheter Cardiovasc Interv 82: E1–27.
7. Task Force on Myocardial Revascularization of the European Society of C, the European Association for Cardio-Thoracic S, European Association for Percutaneous Cardiovascular I, Wijns W, Kolh P, et al. (2010) Guidelines on myocardial revascularization. Eur Heart J 31: 2501–2555.
8. Attallah N, Yassine L, Musial J, Yee J, Fisher K (2004) The potential role of statins in contrast nephropathy. Clin Nephrol 62: 273–278.
9. Khanal S, Attallah N, Smith DE, Kline-Rogers E, Share D, et al. (2005) Statin therapy reduces contrast-induced nephropathy: an analysis of contemporary percutaneous interventions. Am J Med 118: 843–849.
10. Pappy R, Stavrakis S, Hennebry TA, Abu-Fadel MS (2011) Effect of statin therapy on contrast-induced nephropathy after coronary angiography: a meta-analysis. Int J Cardiol 151: 348–353.
11. Jo SH, Koo BK, Park JS, Kang HJ, Cho YS, et al. (2008) Prevention of radiocontrast medium-induced nephropathy using short-term high-dose simvastatin in patients with renal insufficiency undergoing coronary angiography (PROMISS) trial—a randomized controlled study. Am Heart J 155: 499 e491–498.
12. Toso A, Maioli M, Leoncini M, Gallopin M, Tedeschi D, et al. (2010) Usefulness of atorvastatin (80 mg) in prevention of contrast-induced nephropathy in patients with chronic renal disease. Am J Cardiol 105: 288–292.
13. Quintavalle C, Fiore D, De Micco F, Visconti G, Focaccio A, et al. (2012) Impact of a high loading dose of atorvastatin on contrast-induced acute kidney injury. Circulation 126: 3008–3016.
14. Han Y, Zhu G, Han L, Hou F, Huang W, et al. (2014) Short-term rosuvastatin therapy for prevention of contrast-induced acute kidney injury in patients with diabetes and chronic kidney disease. J Am Coll Cardiol 63: 62–70.
15. Leoncini M, Toso A, Maioli M, Tropeano F, Villani S, et al. (2014) Early high-dose rosuvastatin for contrast-induced nephropathy prevention in acute coronary syndrome: Results from the PRATO-ACS Study (Protective Effect of Rosuvastatin and Antiplatelet Therapy On contrast-induced acute kidney injury and myocardial damage in patients with Acute Coronary Syndrome). J Am Coll Cardiol 63: 71–79.
16. Lee JM, Bae W, Lee YJ, Cho YJ (2014) The efficacy and safety of prone positional ventilation in acute respiratory distress syndrome: updated study-level meta-analysis of 11 randomized controlled trials. Crit Care Med 42: 1252–1262.
17. Jadad AR, Moore RA, Carroll D, Jenkinson C, Reynolds DJ, et al. (1996) Assessing the quality of reports of randomized clinical trials: is blinding necessary? Control Clin Trials 17: 1–12.
18. DerSimonian R, Laird N (1986) Meta-analysis in clinical trials. Control Clin Trials 7: 177–188.
19. Higgins JP, Thompson SG, Deeks JJ, Altman DG (2003) Measuring inconsistency in meta-analyses. BMJ 327: 557–560.
20. Moher D, Liberati A, Tetzlaff J, Altman DG (2009) Preferred reporting items for systematic reviews and meta-analyses: the PRISMA statement. Ann Intern Med 151: 264–269, W264.
21. Xinwei J, Xianghua F, Jing Z, Xinshun G, Ling X, et al. (2009) Comparison of usefulness of simvastatin 20 mg versus 80 mg in preventing contrast-induced nephropathy in patients with acute coronary syndrome undergoing percutaneous coronary intervention. Am J Cardiol 104: 519–524.
22. Zhou X, Jin YZ, Wang Q, Min R, Zhang XY (2009) [Efficacy of high dose atorvastatin on preventing contrast induced nephropathy in patients underwent coronary angiography]. Zhonghua Xin Xue Guan Bing Za Zhi 37: 394–396.
23. Acikel S, Muderrisoglu H, Yildirir A, Aydinalp A, Sade E, et al. (2010) Prevention of contrast-induced impairment of renal function by short-term or long-term statin therapy in patients undergoing elective coronary angiography. Blood Coagul Fibrinolysis 21: 750–757.
24. Ozhan H, Erden I, Ordu S, Aydin M, Caglar O, et al. (2010) Efficacy of short-term high-dose atorvastatin for prevention of contrast-induced nephropathy in patients undergoing coronary angiography. Angiology 61: 711–714.
25. X-p H, R-x W, Y Y, Zheng C, Bin C (2010) Prevention of contrast-induced nephropathy using high-dose atorvastatin in patients with coronary heart disease undergoing elective percutaneous coronary intervention] [in Chinese. Milit Med J South China 24: 448–451.
26. Patti G, Ricottini E, Nusca A, Colonna G, Pasceri V, et al. (2011) Short-term, high-dose Atorvastatin pretreatment to prevent contrast-induced nephropathy in patients with acute coronary syndromes undergoing percutaneous coronary intervention (from the ARMYDA-CIN [atorvastatin for reduction of myocardial damage during angioplasty—contrast-induced nephropathy] trial. Am J Cardiol 108: 1–7.
27. Cao S, Wang P, Cui K, Zhang L, Hou Y (2012) [Atorvastatin prevents contrast agent-induced renal injury in patients undergoing coronary angiography by inhibiting oxidative stress]. Nan Fang Yi Ke Da Xue Xue Bao 32: 1600–1602.
28. Li W, Fu X, Wang Y, Li X, Yang Z, et al. (2012) Beneficial effects of high-dose atorvastatin pretreatment on renal function in patients with acute ST-segment elevation myocardial infarction undergoing emergency percutaneous coronary intervention. Cardiology 122: 195–202.
29. Takagi H, Umemoto T (2011) A meta-analysis of randomized trials for effects of periprocedural atorvastatin on contrast-induced nephropathy. Int J Cardiol 153: 323–325.
30. Zhang BC, Li WM, Xu YW (2011) High-dose statin pretreatment for the prevention of contrast-induced nephropathy: a meta-analysis. Can J Cardiol 27: 851–858.
31. Zhang L, Zhang L, Lu Y, Wu B, Zhang S, et al. (2011) Efficacy of statin pretreatment for the prevention of contrast-induced nephropathy: a meta-analysis of randomised controlled trials. Int J Clin Pract 65: 624–630.
32. Zhang T, Shen LH, Hu LH, He B (2011) Statins for the prevention of contrast-induced nephropathy: a systematic review and meta-analysis. Am J Nephrol 33: 344–351.
33. Li Y, Liu Y, Fu L, Mei C, Dai B (2012) Efficacy of short-term high-dose statin in preventing contrast-induced nephropathy: a meta-analysis of seven randomized controlled trials. PLoS One 7: e34450.
34. John S, Schneider MP, Delles C, Jacobi J, Schmieder RE (2005) Lipid-independent effects of statins on endothelial function and bioavailability of nitric oxide in hypercholesterolemic patients. Am Heart J 149: 473.

35. Ridker PM, Rifai N, Clearfield M, Downs JR, Weis SE, et al. (2001) Measurement of C-reactive protein for the targeting of statin therapy in the primary prevention of acute coronary events. N Engl J Med 344: 1959–1965.
36. Ichiki T, Takeda K, Tokunou T, Iino N, Egashira K, et al. (2001) Downregulation of angiotensin II type 1 receptor by hydrophobic 3-hydroxy-3-methylglutaryl coenzyme A reductase inhibitors in vascular smooth muscle cells. Arterioscler Thromb Vasc Biol 21: 1896–1901.
37. Bonetti PO, Lerman LO, Napoli C, Lerman A (2003) Statin effects beyond lipid lowering—are they clinically relevant? Eur Heart J 24: 225–248.
38. Kashani A, Phillips CO, Foody JM, Wang Y, Mangalmurti S, et al. (2006) Risks associated with statin therapy: a systematic overview of randomized clinical trials. Circulation 114: 2788–2797.

Circulating AIM as an Indicator of Liver Damage and Hepatocellular Carcinoma in Humans

Tomoko Yamazaki[1], Mayumi Mori[1], Satoko Arai[1], Ryosuke Tateishi[2], Masanori Abe[3], Mihoko Ban[4], Akemi Nishijima[1], Maki Maeda[4], Takeharu Asano[5], Toshihiro Kai[1¤], Kiyohiro Izumino[4], Jun Takahashi[4], Kayo Aoyama[1], Sei Harada[6], Toru Takebayashi[6], Toshiaki Gunji[7], Shin Ohnishi[8], Shinji Seto[4], Yukio Yoshida[5], Yoichi Hiasa[3], Kazuhiko Koike[2], Ken-ichi Yamamura[9], Ken-ichiro Inoue[4], Toru Miyazaki[1,10,11]*

1 Laboratory of Molecular Biomedicine for Pathogenesis, Center for Disease Biology and Integrative Medicine, Faculty of Medicine, The University of Tokyo, Tokyo, Japan, **2** Department of Gastroenterology, Graduate School of Medicine, The University of Tokyo, Tokyo, Japan, **3** Department of Gastroenterology and Metabology, Ehime University Graduate School of Medicine, Ehime, Japan, **4** Shunkaikai, Inoue Hospital, Nagasaki, Japan, **5** Department of Gastroenterology, Jichi Medical University, Saitama Medical Center, Omiya, Japan, **6** Department of Preventive Medicine and Public Health, School of Medicine, Keio University, Tokyo, Japan, **7** Center for Preventive Medicine, NTT Medical Center Tokyo, Tokyo, Japan, **8** National Center for Global Health and Medicine, Tokyo, Japan, **9** Center for Animal Resources and Development, Kumamoto University, Kumamoto, Japan, **10** Max Planck-The University of Tokyo Center for Integrative Inflammology, Tokyo, Japan, **11** CREST, Japan Science and Technology Agency, Tokyo, Japan

Abstract

Background: Hepatocellular carcinoma (HCC), the fifth most common cancer type and the third highest cause of cancer death worldwide, develops in different types of liver injuries, and is mostly associated with cirrhosis. However, non-alcoholic fatty liver disease often causes HCC with less fibrosis, and the number of patients with this disease is rapidly increasing. The high mortality rate and the pathological complexity of liver diseases and HCC require blood biomarkers that accurately reflect the state of liver damage and presence of HCC.

Methods and Findings: Here we demonstrate that a circulating protein, apoptosis inhibitor of macrophage (AIM) may meet this requirement. A large-scale analysis of healthy individuals across a wide age range revealed a mean blood AIM of 4.99 ± 1.8 μg/ml in men and 6.06 ± 2.1 μg/ml in women. AIM levels were significantly augmented in the younger generation (20s–40s), particularly in women. Interestingly, AIM levels were markedly higher in patients with advanced liver damage, regardless of disease type, and correlated significantly with multiple parameters representing liver function. In mice, AIM levels increased in response to carbon tetrachloride, confirming that the high AIM observed in humans is the result of liver damage. In addition, carbon tetrachloride caused comparable states of liver damage in AIM-deficient and wild-type mice, indicating no influence of AIM levels on liver injury progression. Intriguingly, certain combinations of AIM indexes normalized to liver marker score significantly distinguished HCC patients from non-HCC patients and thus could be applicable for HCC diagnosis.

Conclusion: AIM potently reveals both liver damage and HCC. Thus, our results may provide the basis for novel diagnostic strategies for this widespread and fatal disease.

Editor: Kalpana Ghoshal, The Ohio State University, United States of America

Funding: This work was supported by Grants-in-Aid for Scientific Research (A) (Japan Society for the Promotion of Science), CREST (JST), research grants by ONSENDO Co., Ltd. (to TM), Grants-in-Aid for Scientific Research (B) (Japan Society for the Promotion of Science) (to SA), research grants by The Tokyo Biochemical Research Foundation, Takeda Science Foundation and Ono Medical Research Foundation (to MM). The funders had no role in study design, data collection and analysis, decision to publish, or preparation of the manuscript.

Competing Interests: Although the authors received funding from a commercial source (ONSENDO Co., Ltd), this funding was solely for research activity, and was not used for employment, consultancy, patents, products in development, or marketed products related to either commercial source.

* Email: tm@m.u-tokyo.ac.jp

¤ Current address: Omics Group, Genomic Science Laboratories, Dainippon Sumitomo Pharma Co., Ltd., Osaka, Japan

Introduction

Chronic liver injury is one of the most common and fatal diseases in modern society. It has multiple causes including hepatitis virus infection mostly due to hepatitis C virus (HCV) and to a lesser extent hepatitis B virus (HBV), alcohol injury, autoimmunity, and genetic disorders such as hemochromatosis [1–3]. In addition, the non-alcoholic fatty liver disease (NAFLD), which is associated with obesity, has been observed in a rapidly growing number of patients due to recent and drastic changes in lifestyle. NAFLD comprises a wide variety of disease criteria ranging from benign simple steatosis to progressive inflammation and fibrosis, called non-alcoholic steatohepatitis (NASH) [4,5]. Such chronic liver diseases exhibit continuous inflammation and fibrosis and are a prominent risk for the development of hepatocellular carcinoma (HCC) [6–8]. In contrast to patients with HCV infection, who display a high susceptibility to HCC, only a limited proportion of NAFLD patients progress to carcinoma [9–11]. Intriguingly, recent evidence has revealed that although HCC develops largely on the basis of severe liver fibrosis/cirrhosis, it often occurs without cirrhosis in NAFLD/NASH patients exhibiting mild inflammation and fibrosis [12–18]. However, the mechanism of how each pathological background induces HCC remains to be elucidated. With such increasing risks and complicated pathogenesis, biomarkers that reflect the state of liver damage and the presence of HCC are important, particularly for the early diagnosis of HCC development. Ideally, markers that indicate an individual's susceptibility to HCC may be desirable from the prognostic and preventive views of HCC.

The circulating protein, apoptosis inhibitor of macrophage (AIM), also called CD5L, was initially identified as an apoptosis inhibitor that supports macrophage survival [19]. AIM is produced solely by tissue macrophages under transcriptional regulation by nuclear receptor liver X receptor alpha (LXRα) [20–22], and as a secreted molecule, AIM is detected in both human and mouse blood [19,23]. Interestingly, AIM associates with the immunoglobulin (Ig)M pentamer in the blood, and this association protects AIM from renal excretion, thereby maintaining circulating AIM at a relatively high concentration (approximately 2–5 μg/ml) in mice [23,24]. However, AIM's precise levels in healthy individuals and patients with various diseases remain controversial [25–28].

We recently identified that AIM is incorporated into adipocytes via CD36-mediated endocytosis where it inactivates cytoplasmic fatty acid synthase (FASN) through direct binding. This response reduces the production of lipid droplet-coating proteins such as fat-specific protein 27 (FSP27) and perilipin, thereby decreasing triacylglycerol deposition within adipocytes [29,30]. Consistent with this effect, adipocyte hypertrophy was found to be more advanced with a greater mass of visceral adipose tissue in AIM-deficient ($AIM^{-/-}$) mice than in wild-type ($AIM^{+/+}$) mice fed a high-fat diet (HFD) [29]. We also found that AIM prevents lipid storage in the liver, as in adipocytes [31]. Because a consensus has rapidly emerged that hepatocytic lipid metabolism impacts the pathogenesis of not only NAFLD but also other liver injuries, as well as HCC development, we decided to address the possible relationship in circulating AIM levels, the state of liver damage, and the presence of HCC in humans.

In this study, we first analyzed a large number of healthy individuals to determine the "normal level" of circulating AIM. We then assessed the correlation between circulating AIM levels and the state of liver damage using sera from patients with liver diseases. We also tested whether the difference in AIM levels correlated with the progression of liver damage using a mouse model. Furthermore, we investigated whether the AIM level can be applied for the diagnosis of HCC in humans.

Methods

Human subjects

Serum samples of healthy individuals were collected from volunteers who had annual medical examinations at Inoue Hospitals (Nagasaki, Japan). Serum samples of patients with liver diseases were obtained from Tokyo University Hospital, Ehime University Hospital and Jichi Medical University Hospital.

Ethic

For analysis of human subjects, informed consent in writing was obtained from each healthy volunteer and patient, and the study protocol conformed to the ethical guidelines of the 1975 Declaration of Helsinki as reflected in a priori approval by the Ethics Committee of the University of Tokyo for Medical Experiments (Permission Numbers: #3358 & #2817). In addition, all animal experiments were carried out in strict accordance with the recommendations in the Guide for the Care and Use of Laboratory Animals of the National Institutes of Health. The protocol was approved by the Committee on the Ethics of Animal Experiments of the University of Tokyo (Permit Number: P10-143). All surgery was performed under sodium pentobarbital anesthesia, and all efforts were made to minimize suffering.

Carbon tetrachloride (CCl4) administration

$AIM^{-/-}$ mice [19] had been backcrossed to C57BL/6 (B6) for 15 generations before used for experiments. Mice were intraperitoneally injected with CCl4 (Wako, Osaka, Japan) (1.6 g/kg body weight; dissolved in corn oil) twice a week for 3 or 12 wk. Mice were sacrificed 3 days after the last injection of CCl_4. All mice were maintained under a specific pathogen-free (SPF) condition.

Statistical analysis

Student's *t*-test was performed to compare values from two groups. Correlation coefficients and *p* values were calculated by Excel. Multiple linear regression analysis was performed by backward stepwise approach, with $t>1.5$ for entry and $t<1.5$ or inter-variables correlation coefficient>0.5 or probability $F>0.1$ for removal from the model. Multiple pairwise comparison among groups were performed by ANCOVA using JMP software (version 11).

ELISA assay

Human AIM was measured by an ELISA system using mouse anti-human AIM monoclonal antibodies (clones #6 and #7; established in our laboratory), which is now available from the Trans Genic Inc., Kumamoto, Japan. For ELISA of mouse AIM, we used two different rat anti-mouse AIM monoclonal antibodies (clones #36 and #35; established in our laboratory). Human IgM was measured by Human IgM ELISA Quantification Set (Bethyl Laboratories, Inc. Montgomery, USA).

Histology

Liver specimens were fixed overnight in 4% paraformaldehyde in phosphate buffered saline (PBS) and replaced into 30% sucrose/PBS liquid. Samples were embedded in Tissue-Tek O.C.T. compound (Sakura Finetek Co.,Ltd., Tokyo), cut by 10 μm. For Sirius red staining, sections were washed in PBS for 5 min, counter stained with Mayer's Hematoxylin for 10 min, washed with running water for 2 min and subsequently soaked in hydrochloric acid alcohol (0.5% HCl in 70% EtOH) for 1 min. Sections were then stained with 0.03% Sirius red (Direct red 80, SIGMA-ALDRICH) in saturated picric acid solution for 15 min. HE staining was performed using Mayer's Hematoxylin (MUTO PURE CHEMICALS CO.,LTD., Tokyo) and Eosin (SIGMA-ALDRICH, St. Louis, USA).

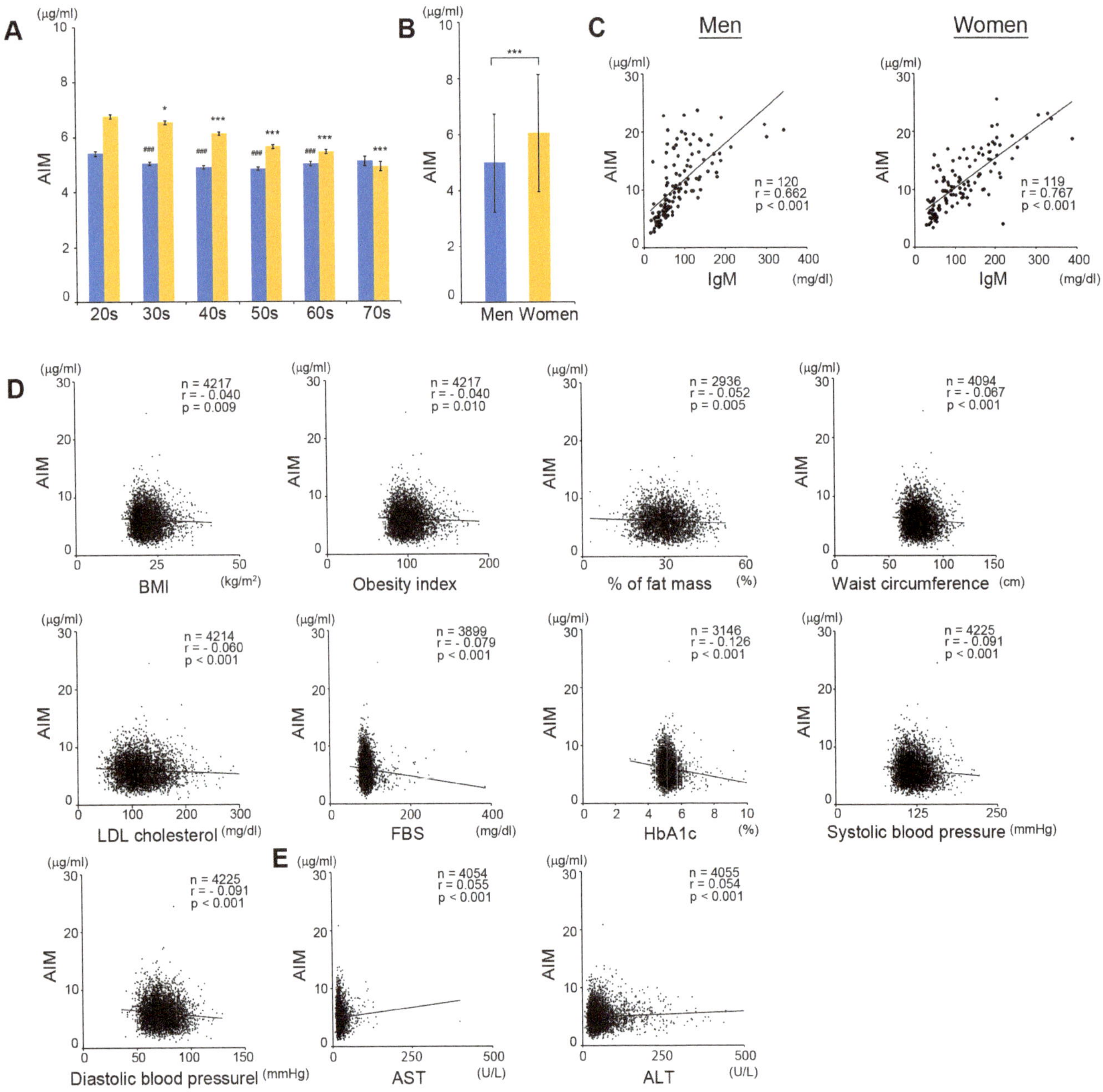

Figure 1. Circulating AIM levels in healthy indivisuals. (A) AIM levels in different generations. Error bar: SEM. ***: $p<0.001$ vs. the value of women in 20s. ###: $p<0.001$ vs. the value of men in 20s. (B) Means ± SD (μg/ml) of AIM levels in whole men and women. AIM levels were significantly higher in women than in men. (C) Correlation of AIM and IgM levels in men and women. IgM levels were analyzed by ELISA in 20 individuals exhibiting a variety of AIM levels in each generation in men and women. (D) Correlation in AIM levels and BMI, obesity index, % of fat mass or waist circumference, LDL cholesterol levels, HbA1C, FBS, systolic or diastolic blood pressure in women. (E) Correlation in AIM and AST or ALT levels in males and females. In C-E, r: correlation coefficients in single linear regression analysis, p: p value, n: number of samples. Blue dots: men, yellow dots: women.

Fibrosis analysis

Fibrosis area determined by Sirius red staining was quantified using NIH Image J software. Five areas for each sample were assessed under a microscope (FSX 100, OLYMPUS, Tokyo).

Quantitative PCR assay

The quantitative evaluation of mRNA was performed by the $\Delta\Delta C_T$ method using a 7500Fast Real-Time PCR system (Life Technologies Japan, Tokyo) and Power SYBR Green PCR Master Mix (Life Technologies). Sequences of the oligonucleotides used are below:

f-GAPDH	5′-AACTTTGGCATTGTGGAAGG-3′
r-GAPDH	5′-GGATGCAGGGATGATGTTCT-3′
f-TNFα	5′-ACGGCATGGATCTCAAAGAC-3′
r-TNFα	5′-AGATAGCAAATCGGCTGACG-3′
f-IL1β	5′-CTGGTGTGTGACGTTCCCATTA-3′
r-IL1β	5′-CCGACAGCACGAGGCTTT-3′
f-IL 6	5′-CCAGTTGCCTTCTTGGGACT-3′

Table 1. The composition of examinees and the AIM level.

	Male		Female	
age	AIM (μg/ml)	n	AIM (μg/ml)	n
10s	5.62±1.66	28	6.39±1.65	15
20s	5.41±1.67	368	6.75±2.05	592
30s	5.04±1.69	806	6.53±2.03	791
40s	4.90±1.76	1153	6.14±2.09	1163
50s	4.84±1.78	988	5.64±1.95	977
60s	5.02±1.80	580	5.45±2.1	579
70s	5.11±1.79	120	4.91±1.57	87
80s	4.69±1.57	9	5.57±2.84	16
90s	7.55±3.60	3	4.22±2.03	5
whole	4.99±1.76	4055	6.06±2.09	4225

The AIM level is presented as mean±SD (μg/ml). n: sample number.

r-IL 6	5′-GGTCTGTTGGGAGTGGTATCC-3′
f-MCP1	5′-ACTGAAGCCAGCTCTCTCTTCCTC-3′
r-MCP1	5′-TTCCTTCTTGGGGTCAGCACAGAC-3′
f-CD11c	5′-GAGCCAGAACTTCCCAACTG-3′
r-CD11c	5′-TCAGGAACACGATGTCTTGG-3′
f-CD163	5′-CCTGGATCATCTGTGACAACA-3′
r-CD163	5′-TCCACACGTCCAGAACAGTC-3′
f-Arg-1	5′-CTCCAAGCCAAAGTCCTTAGAG-3′
r-Arg-1	5′-AGGAGCTGTCATTAGGGACATC-3′
f-MR	5′-CCACAGCATTGAGGAGTTTG-3′
r-MR	5′-ACAGCTCATCATTTGGCTCA-3′
f-TGF β	5′-TGGAGCAACATGTGGAACTC-3′
r-TGF β	5′-CAGCAGCCGGTTACCAAG-3′
f-α SMA	5′-ACTCTCTTCCAGCCATCTTCA-3′
r-α SMA	5′-ATAGGTGGTTTCGTGGATGC-3′
f-Col4a1	5′-TTAAAGGACTCCAGGGACCAC-3′
r-Col4a1	5′-CCCACTGAGCCTGTCACAC-3′
f-CTGF	5′-TGACCTGGAGGAAAACATTAAGA-3′
r-CTGF	5′-AGCCCTGTATGTCTTCACACTG-3′
f-TIMP1	5′-GCAAAGAGCTTTCTCAAAGACC-3′
r-TIMP1	5′-AGGGATAGATAAACAGGGAAACACT-3′
f-mAIM	5′-GAGGACACATGGATGGAATGT-3′
r-mAIM	5′-ACCCTTGTGTAGCACCTCCA-3′

Results

Circulating AIM levels in healthy individuals

To investigate circulating AIM levels in healthy individuals, we performed a large-scale analysis of AIM using more than 8,000 blood samples of volunteers attending annual medical examinations in 2012 and 2013. For this study, we established an ELISA system by generating monoclonal antibodies that accurately estimated human AIM levels in blood. The composition of volunteers and the mean±SD AIM level (μg/ml) are shown in Table 1. AIM levels were highest in both men and women in their 20s and decreased with age (Fig. 1A). In individuals <50 years old, AIM levels were significantly higher in women (Fig. 1A), resulting in an overall higher mean AIM level in women (Fig. 1B). Consistent with our previous report [23], a strong correlation was observed between IgM and AIM levels (Fig. 1C).

The significance of the relationships between AIM levels and various clinical parameters is presented in Table S1. In particular, we focused on obesity-related parameters because AIM has lipolytic function and thus acts as an anti-obese factor in mice [29,30]. The relationship between AIM and various parameters was more significant in women, and AIM levels correlated negatively with body mass index, obesity index, % fat mass, and

Table 2. Number of patients in each type of liver injury.

	HCC		Non HCC	
	Men	Women	Men	Women
Whole	189 (100%)	86 (100%)	90 (100%)	56 (100%)
HBV	36 (19%)	6 (7%)	28 (31%)	14 (25%)
HCV	116 (61%)	61 (71%)	30 (33%)	26 (47%)
HBV and HCV	1 (1%)	1 (1%)	0 (0%)	0 (0%)
Alcoholic hepatitis	21 (11%)	2 (2%)	4 (5%)	3 (5%)
NAFLD	0 (0%)	0 (0%)	21 (23%)	8 (14%)
NASH	3 (2%)	5 (6%)	6 (7%)	4 (7%)
Cryptogenic or other	12 (6%)	11 (13%)	1 (1%)	1 (2%)

The percentage shows the proportion in total number of each gender with or without HCC.

Table 3. Clinical features of patients analyzed for AIM.

	HCC		Non HCC	
	Men	**Women**	**Men**	**Women**
Age (year)	66±10 [32–87]	70±9 [33–87]	55±15 [23–84]	62±13 [31–80]
AIM (μg/ml)	5.7±2.8 [1.7–18.6]	5.8±2.6 [0.8–14.7]	5.1±2.7 [1.5–17.5]	5.8±2.9 [1.8–16.9]
IgM (mg/dl)	144.8±101 [24.2–708.0]	143.4±98.0 [1.6–769.2]	103.3±49.4 [18.7–216.4]	129.4±64.1 [42.8–346.0]
AST (U/L)	56.3±30.7 [14–170]	59.6±42.9 [17–312]	51.8±43.3 [13–287]	44.7±24.5 [14–139]
ALT (U/L)	53.6±37.6 [8–233]	48.0±39.5 [9–315]	60.3±66.8 [6–498]	40.4±26.6 [11–121]
TB (mg/dl)	0.98±0.54 [0.3–3.9]	1.02±0.61 [0.4–3.8]	1.13±0.85 [0.3–5.1]	1.07±1.17 [0.4–9.2]
DB (mg/dl)	0.35±0.32 [0.1–0.7]	0.38±0.32 [0.1–1.6]	0.29±0.28 [0.1–1.6]	0.25±0.13 [0.1–0.5]
ALB (g/dl)	3.69±0.46 [2.3–4.7]	3.64±0.49 [2.2–4.6]	4.06±0.49 [2.5–5.2]	3.89±0.58 [2.2–4.5]
PLT ($x10^4/mm^3$)	12.3±5.29 [3.0–28.3]	11.1±5.43 [4.2–31.9]	16.6±7.32 [2.1–35.6]	13.9±6.57 [2.3–26]
PT (%)	85.4±14.3 [53–100]	84.3±14.7 [42–100]	87.1±17.2 [28–100]	84.0±19.7 [32–100]
Cre (mg/dl)	0.81±0.19 [0.40–1.56]	0.61±0.14 [0.4–1.04]	0.83±0.20 [0.54–1.95]	0.66±0.26 [0.49–2.21]
ICG (%)	23.8±14.4 [2.7–72.4]	24.7±15.6 [0.9–71.2]	-	-

The mean ± SD as well as the range of diversity are presented for each parametric variable. The ICG score was only available in HCC patients.

waist circumference (Fig. 1D). In line with these results, AIM levels also correlated negatively with low-density lipoprotein (LDL) cholesterol levels (Fig. 1D) and several diabetic markers including fasting blood sugar (FBS) and glycated hemoglobin (HbA1C) (Fig. 1D), as well as with blood pressure, in women (Fig. 1D). Thus, consistent with the findings of our previous study in mice [29,30], AIM levels correlated negatively with multiple parameters related to obesity, and these correlations were more prominent in women. Intriguingly however, a weak but significant positive correlation was found between AIM levels and biomarkers of hepatocyte injury, including aspartate aminotransferase (AST) and alanine aminotransferase (ALT), particularly in men (Fig. 1E). Taken together, it is likely that AIM levels increase along with the progression of liver injury. In both men and women, a significant negative correlation was unexpectedly found between AIM levels and red blood cell numbers, but the reason underlying this correlation is unclear (Table S1).

AIM levels correlated strongly with liver function in liver injury

We next analyzed blood samples from patients with chronic hepatitis and liver cirrhosis. As depicted in Table 2, the cause of liver injury in the majority of the patients was hepatitis virus infection, whereas non-infected cases constituted a lower proportion of the patients with alcoholic liver failure and NAFLD/NASH. Patients with or without HCC were investigated. The clinical features of the patients tested are presented in Table 3 focusing on the liver function.

The positive correlation between AIM levels and AST/ALT for liver injury, which was already seen in individuals without severe liver damage (Fig. 1E) was notably more obvious in men and women with advanced liver damage. Highly significant correlations were observed between AIM and multiple biomarkers, thereby reflecting liver function, including total or direct bilirubin (TB or DB), albumin (ALB), platelet count (PLT), % prothrombin time (%PT), and the indocyanine green (ICG) test (Fig. 2). These correlations were obvious in individuals with or without hepatitis virus infection (Table S2) and in the presence or absence of HCC (Fig. 2). In HCC patients, there was no significant correlation in levels of AIM and several HCC markers including alpha fetoprotein (AFP), des-gamma-carboxyprothrombin (DCP, also called prothrombin induced by vitamin K-absence II; PIVKA-II), and AFP fraction L3 (L3) (Fig. S1). As in healthy individuals, a significant correlation was also found between AIM and IgM levels in patients with liver injury (Fig. 3A); namely, IgM levels increased with the progression of liver damage (Fig. S2).

We then addressed which parameters correlated independently with AIM levels. To this end, we performed multiple regression analysis by the backward stepwise method including AIM. Table S3 shows the correlation coefficients between all parameters that reflect liver function and thus were candidates for determinant of AIM level. When confounding factors were eliminated, IgM, TB, ALB, and %PT in men ($R^2 = 54.0\%$) and IgM, TB, and ALB in women ($R^2 = 57.0\%$) were independent determinants of AIM in HCC patients (Table 4). In non-HCC patients, IgM, ALB, and PLT in men ($R^2 = 63.4\%$) and IgM and PLT in women ($R^2 = 53.6\%$) were the independent determinants of AIM (Table 4). In particular, in men, the t-value of TB in HCC patients was 5.39, but was not significant in non-HCC patients. In women, the t-value of ALB was −4.80 in HCC patients, but again was not significant in non-HCC patients (Table 4).

Similar results were obtained for the relationship between AIM and the grade of liver inflammation or fibrosis. Levels in inflammation (0–3) and fibrosis (F0-F4) were evaluated according to the Inuyama classification [32]. The number of patients in each category is presented in Table 5. Clinical information about inflammation and fibrosis were not available in a part of HCC patients and all of non-HCC patients. AIM levels were higher in those with liver inflammation (Fig. 3B). AIM also increased in line with the progression of liver fibrosis (Fig. 3C). Similarly, AIM levels were higher in patients with cirrhosis or ascites (Fig. 3D). Note that all cirrhotic patients tested in this study were under a compensated stage. Since some patients exhibited prominently high or low levels of AIM (>10 μg/ml or <3.0 μg/ml), we assessed relationship in levels of AIM and various parameters in these populations. However, there was no remarkable correlation in AIM and any parameter (Table S4). No significant correlation was observed between AIM levels and alcohol intake (data not shown).

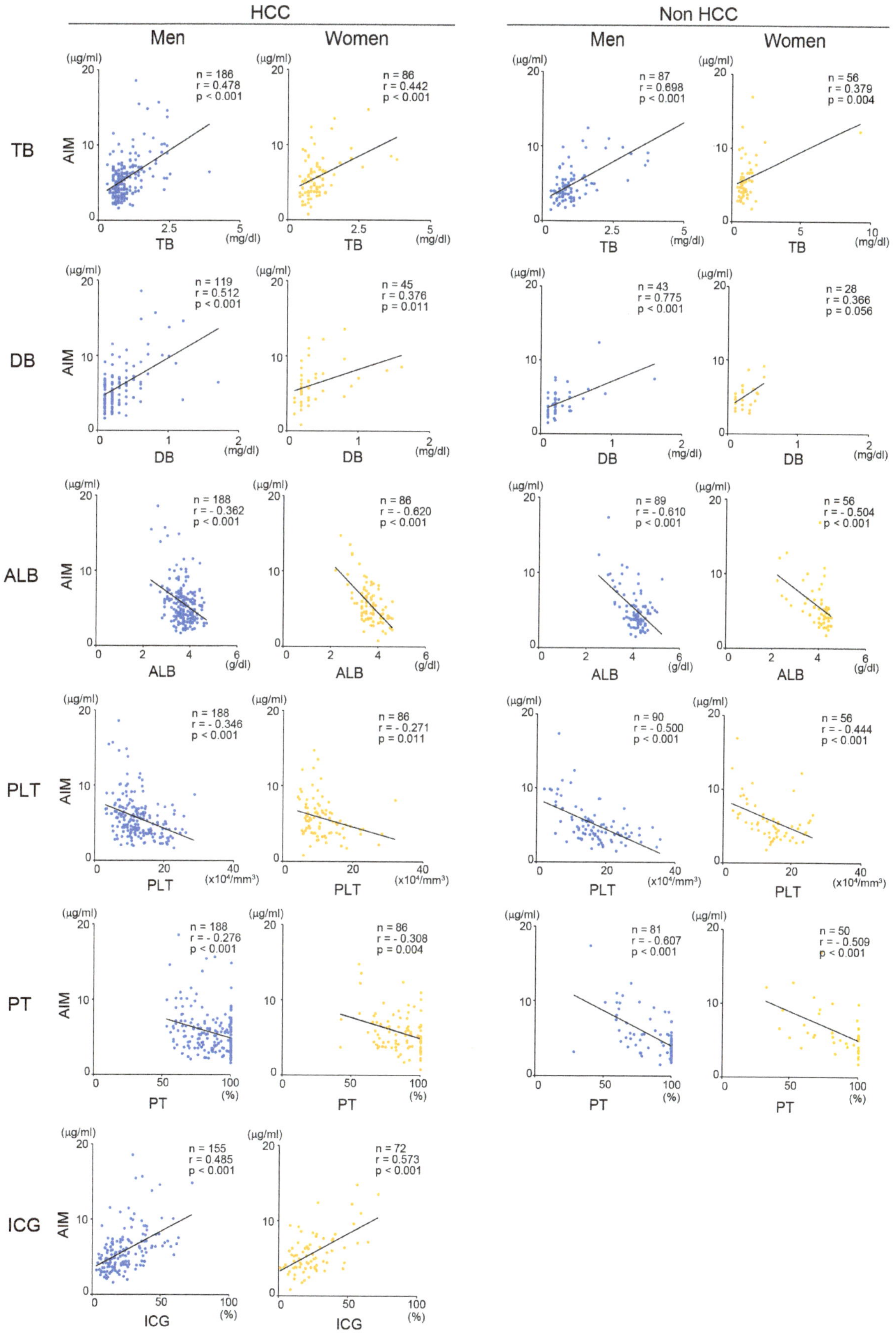
HCC
Non HCC
Men
Women
Men
Women
TB
DB
ALB
PLT
PT
ICG
AIM
(μg/ml)
n = 186
r = 0.478
p < 0.001
n = 86
r = 0.442
p < 0.001
n = 87
r = 0.698
p < 0.001
n = 56
r = 0.379
p = 0.004
(mg/dl)
n = 119
r = 0.512
p < 0.001
n = 45
r = 0.376
p = 0.011
n = 43
r = 0.775
p < 0.001
n = 28
r = 0.366
p = 0.056
n = 188
r = - 0.362
p < 0.001
n = 86
r = - 0.620
p < 0.001
n = 89
r = - 0.610
p < 0.001
n = 56
r = - 0.504
p < 0.001
(g/dl)
n = 188
r = - 0.346
p < 0.001
n = 86
r = - 0.271
p = 0.011
n = 90
r = - 0.500
p < 0.001
n = 56
r = - 0.444
p < 0.001
(x10⁴/mm³)
n = 188
r = - 0.276
p < 0.001
n = 86
r = - 0.308
p = 0.004
n = 81
r = - 0.607
p < 0.001
n = 50
r = - 0.509
p < 0.001
(%)
n = 155
r = 0.485
p < 0.001
n = 72
r = 0.573
p < 0.001

Figure 2. Correlation in the AIM level and the liver function under liver injury. Correlation in AIM levels and various biomarkers representing liver function in men (blue) and women (yellow), with or without HCC. ICG score was only available in HCC patients.

AIM$^{-/-}$ mice had comparable liver damage to wild-type mice in response to CCl4

Next, we assessed whether high AIM levels directly promote liver injury or whether AIM levels increase as a result of liver damage progression. To this end, we employed animal models of progressive liver injury induced by carbon tetrachloride. *AIM*$^{-/-}$ and *AIM*$^{+/+}$ mice were challenged with CCl4 (1.6 g/kg body weight) injected twice a week for 12 weeks, and the state of liver injury was assessed. As demonstrated in Fig. 4A, AST and ALT levels were similar at multiple time points in *AIM*$^{+/+}$ and *AIM*$^{-/-}$ mice, indicating that the liver was comparably damaged in the presence or absence of AIM. Note that the average of circulating AIM levels without CCl4 administration was 3.3 μg/ml in both males and females. Inflammatory states were investigated during the early phase (after 3 weeks of CCl4 challenge) by measuring mRNA levels for various pro-inflammatory cytokines using quantitative RT-PCR (QPCR). No significant differences were observed in the increased expression levels of *TNFα*, *IL-1β*, *IL-6*, and *MCP-1* in both types of mice (Fig. 4B). In line with this result, similar expression profiles of the M1 and M2 macrophage marker genes (*CD11c* for M1; *CD163*, *Arg-1*, and *mannose receptor* (*MR*) for M2) were observed in *AIM*$^{+/+}$ and *AIM*$^{-/-}$ mice (Fig. 4C), suggesting that the absence of AIM did not influence the activation state or the M1/M2 polarity of liver macrophages in response to carbon tetrachloride, resulting in comparable liver inflammation progression in both types of mice. Consistent with this finding, liver fibrosis progressed comparably in *AIM*$^{-/-}$ and *AIM*$^{+/+}$ mice, and Sirius-red staining of liver specimens showed a similar increase in fibrotic areas in both types of mice (Fig. 4D). Accordingly, mRNA levels of various markers of fibrosis progression such as *TGFβ*, *αSMA*, *Col4a1*, and *connective tissue growth factor* (*CTGF*) were also comparable in *AIM*$^{-/-}$ and *AIM*$^{+/+}$ mice (Fig. 4E). Taken together, these results clearly indicate that the presence or absence of AIM did not influence the state of liver injury in response to carbon tetrachloride. Thus, it is likely that the augmented AIM levels observed in humans (Fig. 2) were the result of liver damage. Further supporting this notion is the finding that AIM levels increased markedly with progression of liver damage in *AIM*$^{+/+}$ mice (Fig. 4F, left). However, AIM mRNA levels in the *AIM*$^{+/+}$ liver did not increase in response to CCl4 (Fig. S3), suggesting that the increase in blood AIM was not brought about by enhancement of AIM production in liver Kupffer macrophages, one of the highest AIM-producing cell types [19].

Interestingly, no significant difference in increase in IgM levels was observed in both *AIM*$^{-/-}$ and *AIM*$^{+/+}$ mice, suggesting that the increase in IgM was independent of AIM (Fig. 4F, right). This result is reminiscent of our previous finding of a similar increase in IgM levels in *AIM*$^{-/-}$ and *AIM*$^{+/+}$ mice in response to a HFD [23].

Diagnostic application of AIM for HCC

As demonstrated in Fig. 2, AIM levels increased in line with the progression of liver injury in patients with or without HCC. We then wondered whether HCC and non-HCC patients who show an equivalent score of certain liver biomarkers exhibited different AIM levels. Therefore, we normalized the level of AIM (AIM index) to that of each biomarker. The AIM level was divided by a biomarker score when both correlated positively (*e.g.* AST, ALT, TB, and DB), whereas the scores were multiplied when AIM and

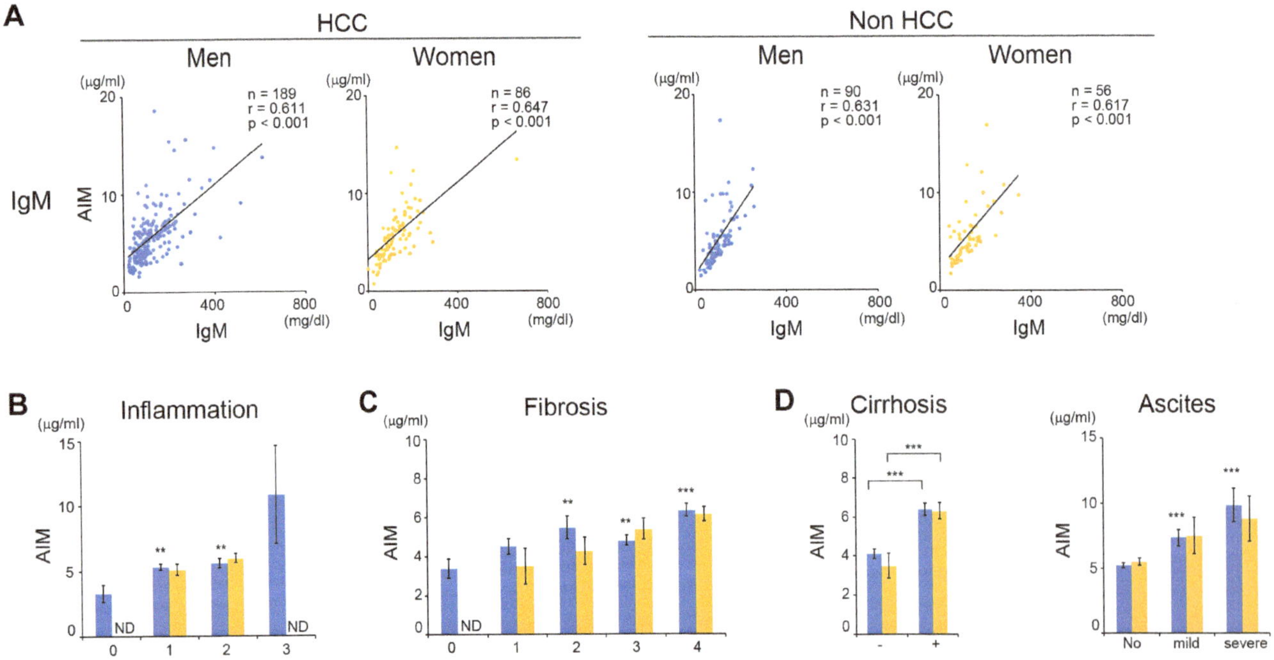

Figure 3. The AIM level increases with progression of liver inflammation and fibrosis. (A) Correlation in AIM and IgM levels in men (blue) and women (yellow), with or without HCC. (B) AIM levels in HCC patients with different inflammatory levels according to the Inuyama classification. (C) AIM levels in HCC patients with different fibrotic scores according to the Inuyama classification. (D) AIM levels in HCC patients with different grades of cirrhosis or ascites. In C-E, AIM levels are presented as means±SEM (μg/ml).

Table 4. Multiple linear regression analysis.

	HCC Men (n = 173)			Non-HCC Men (n = 89)		
	C	*t*	*p*	C	*t*	*p*
R^2	53.98%			63.44%		
Intercept	5.30	2.927	0.004	10.2	6.29	<0.001
IgM	0.0137	9.37	<0.001	0.0266	7.33	<0.001
TB	1.60	5.39	<0.001	_	_	_
ALB	−0.886	−2.53	0.012	−1.41	−3.59	<0.001
PLT	_	_	_	−0.127	−4.88	<0.001
PT	−0.0191	−1.77	0.079	_	_	_
	HCC Women (n = 86)			**Non-HCC Women (n = 56)**		
	C	*t*	*p*	C	*t*	*p*
R^2	57.02%			53.62%		
Intercept	9.58	4.82	<0.001	4.88	5.90	<0.001
IgM	0.0104	4.66	<0.001	0.0265	6.48	<0.001
TB	0.862	2.48	0.016	_	_	_
ALB	−2.17	−4.80	<0.001	_	_	_
PLT	_	_	_	−0.181	−4.53	<0.001

Independent determinants for AIM in men or women with or without HCC. R^2: determination coefficient, C: regression coefficient, *t*: t-value, *p*: p-value, in multiple linear regression models. _: not independent.

the biomarker correlated negatively (*e.g.* ALB, platelets, and %PT). As depicted in Fig. 5A, the ratio of the AIM-TB index to the AIM-ALB index in men was significantly higher in HCC patients than in non-HCC patients by analysis of covariance (ANCOVA), but no significant differences were observed for the ratio of the TB score to the ALB score between HCC and non-HCC patients. Similar results were obtained for the ratio of the AIM-TB index to the AIM-PLT or AIM-AST index, although TB

Table 5. Number of patients showing different levels of inflammation, fibrosis, cirrhosis, or ascites.

		Men	Women
Whole		189	86
Inflammation (in %)	0	6 (3%)	0 (0%)
	1	88 (47%)	36 (42%)
	2	50 (26%)	28 (32%)
	3	2 (1%)	0 (0%)
	unknown	43 (23%)	22 (26%)
Fibrosis (in %)	0	7 (4%)	0 (0%)
	1	14 (7%)	3 (3%)
	2	19 (10%)	13 (15%)
	3	42 (22%)	11(13%)
	4	81 (43%)	42 (49%)
	unknown	26 (14%)	17 (20%)
Cirrhosis (in %)	-	36 (19%)	6 (7%)
	+	82 (43%)	45 (52%)
	unknown	71 (38%)	35 (41%)
Ascites (in %)	No	159 (84%)	77 (90%)
	Mild (1~2L)	18 (10%)	5 (6%)
	Severe (3~5L)	10 (5%)	4 (4%)
	unknown	2 (1%)	0 (0%)

All patients here possessed HCC. The percentage shows the proportion in each level of identical phenotype. Unknown: Information was not available.

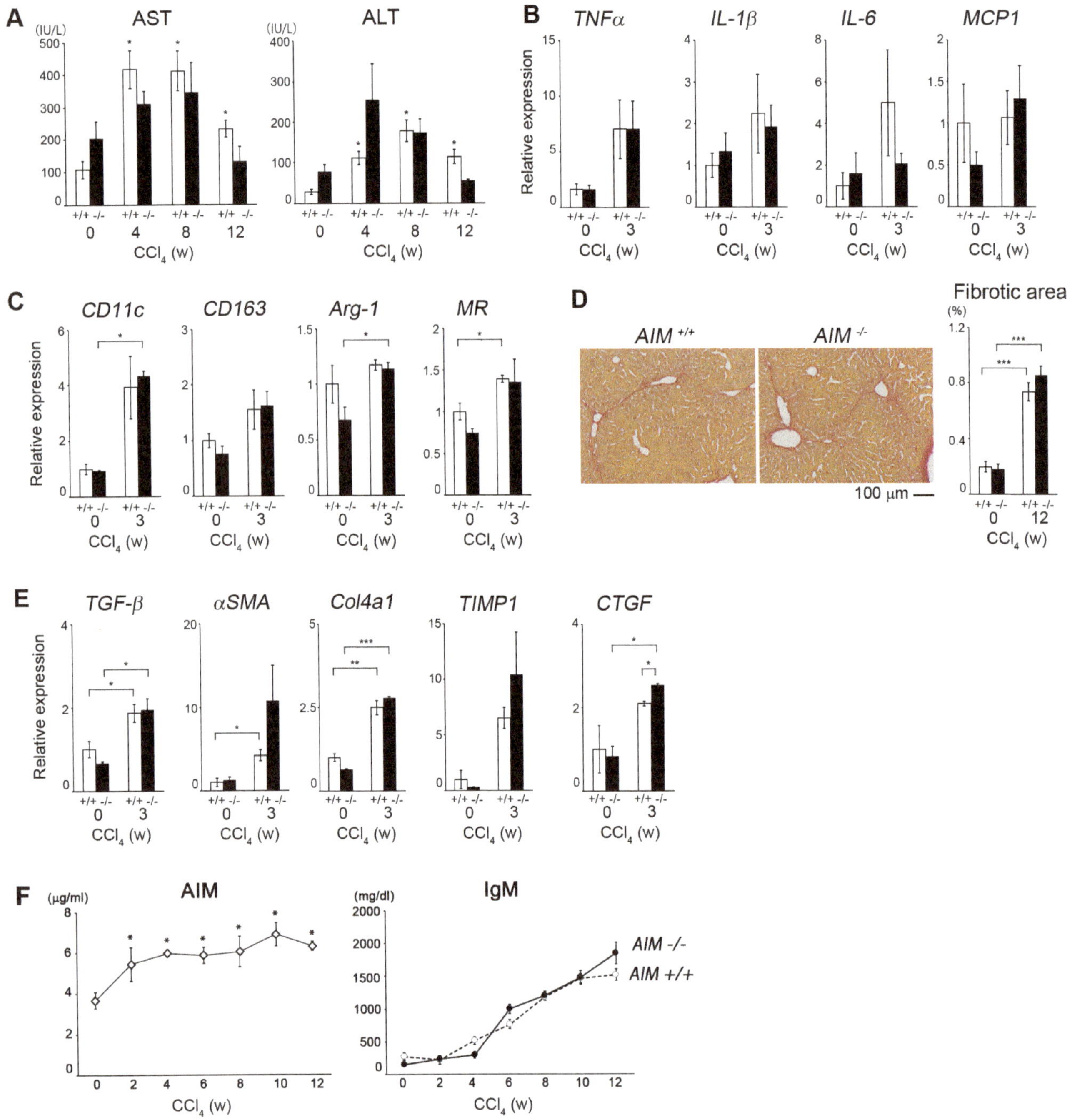

Figure 4. ***AIM***$^{+/+}$ **and** ***AIM***$^{-/-}$ **mice exhibit comparable liver damage in response to** $\mathbf{CCl_4}$**.** (A) AST and ALT at 0, 4, 8, 12 wk after administration of CCl_4 (1.6 g/kg body weight, twice injection per week for 12 weeks) in *AIM*$^{+/+}$ mice (+/+) and *AIM*$^{-/-}$ mice (−/−). n = 3 for each. Error bar: SEM, *: $p<$ 0.05 vs. before CCl4 administration (0 w). (B, C) mRNA levels of *TNFα*, *IL-1β*, *IL-6* and *MCP-1* (B); or *CD11c*, *CD163*, *Arg-1* and *MR* (C) were assessed by QPCR using RNA isolated from liver after administration of CCl_4 for 3 weeks. n = 3 for each. Error bar: SEM, *: $p<0.05$. (D) Sirius-red staining of the liver specimens after administration of CCl_4 for 12 weeks to *AIM*$^{+/+}$ mice (+/+) and *AIM*$^{-/-}$ mice (−/−). Bar: 100 μm. Right graph shows the quantification of fibrotic area. (E) mRNA levels of *TGFβ*, *αSMA*, *Col4a1* and *CTGF* were assessed by QPCR using RNA isolated from liver from mice after administration of CCl_4 for 3 weeks. n = 3 for each. Error bar: SEM; *: $p<0.05$, ***: $p<0.001$. (F) *Left*: Serum AIM levels were measured by ELISA from wild-type mice after administration of CCl_4. n = 6 for each. Error bar: SEM, *: $p<0.05$ vs. before CCl_4 administration (0 w). *Right*: Serum IgM levels were measured by semi-quantitative immunoblotting using sera from *AIM*$^{+/+}$ (+/+) mice and *AIM*$^{-/-}$ (−/−) after administration of CCl_4. Purified mouse IgM clone (3F3) was used as standard. Quantification of signals from immunoblotting was performed by using ImageQuant TL software (GE Healthcare, Little Chalfont, UK). n = 6 for each. Error bar: SEM; *: $p<0.05$, ***: $p<0.01$, vs. before CCl_4 administration (0 w) in *AIM*$^{+/+}$ (+/+) mice; ###: $p<0.001$ vs. before CCl_4 administration in *AIM*$^{-/-}$ mice.

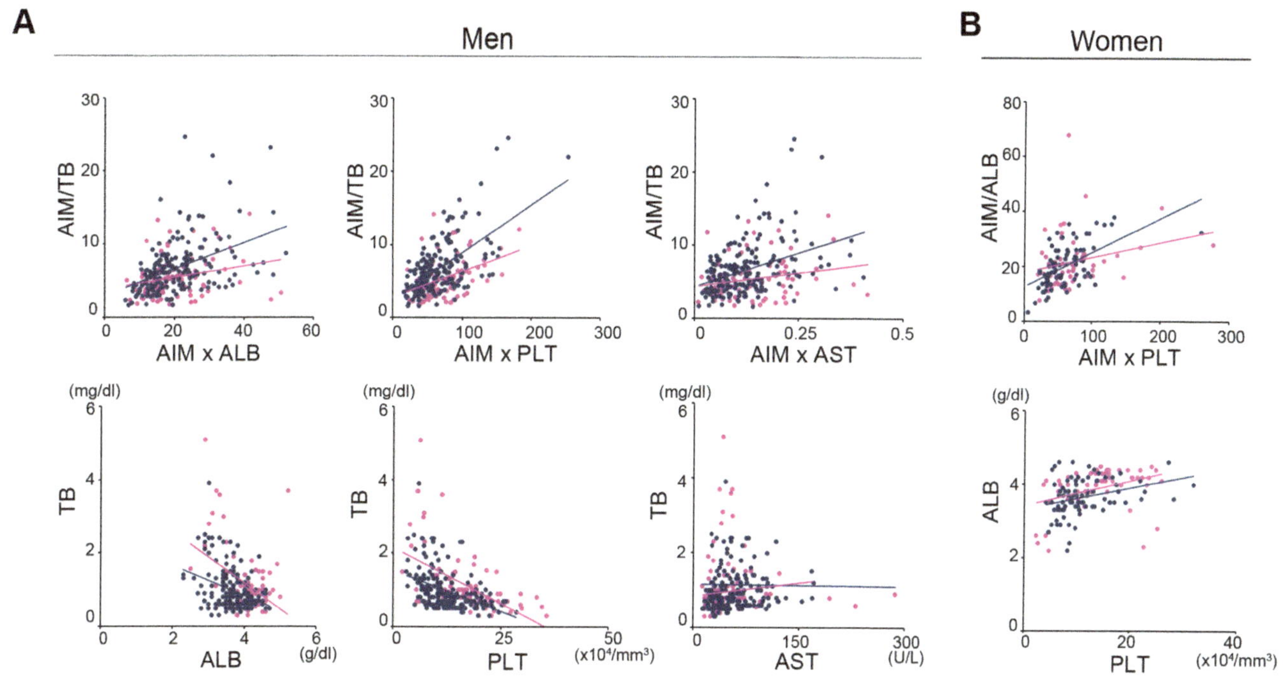

Figure 5. AIM-index distinguishes HCC and non-HCC patients. (A) AIM-TB index vs. AIM-ALB index, AIM-PLT index or AIM-AST index in men with or without HCC. TB vs. ALB, PLT or AST are also presented. (B) AIM-ALB index vs. AIM-%PT index in women with or without HCC. ALB vs. %PT is also presented. r: correlation coefficients; p: p value determined by ANCOVA. Blue dots and bars: HCC patients, red dots and bars: non-HCC patients.

correlated with neither PLT nor AST (Fig. 5A). In women, a comparison of the AIM-ALB and AIM-%PT indexes revealed similar differences between the HCC and non-HCC patients (Fig. 5B). Note that TB in male HCC patients and ALB in female HCC patients produced high t-values in multiple regression analysis when assessing the determinants of AIM (Table 3).

Discussion

This study provides the first large-scale description of the circulating AIM levels in the general population and in the context of liver function parameters in humans. A variety of new findings were obtained as follows. Firstly, relatively higher AIM levels were observed in the younger generation, especially in women, suggesting potential involvement of estrogen in the increase in circulating AIM levels. Accumulating evidence of estrogen-associated physiology including suppression of triacylglycerol (TG) storage in fat and liver tissues [33–36], reduction of expression and enzymatic activity of FASN [37], and preventive effect for foam cell formation and the development of atherosclerosis [38–41], which are all reminiscent of AIM function [20,29,30,42,43]. Although *AIM* mRNA is expressed under transcriptional regulation by LXR [20–22], the impact of estrogen on LXR activation is controversial. For instance, Wang et al. recently reported that E2 activates LXRα [41], whereas suppression of LXRα by E2 was also reported in hepatocytes [34], adipocyte [36], and pancreatic β cells [37]. Alternatively, evidence has shown that estrogen stimulates natural IgM production through B lymphocyte activation [44,45]. This effect certainly increases AIM levels based on the strong correlation between AIM and IgM. However, further studies are required to clarify the precise involvement of estrogen in the regulation of age-dependent AIM levels in humans. It is noteworthy that in individuals without advanced liver damage, AST and ALT showed a weak positive correlation with AIM levels only in men (Fig. 1E and Table S1). It might be possible that the sex-dependent difference of AIM levels obscured the correlation in women.

Secondly, patients with advanced liver damage exhibited high AIM levels. We postulate that the mean±SD AIM level (μg/ml) in each generation in men and women presented in Table 1 can be defined as the "normal range" of AIM levels. Certainly, however, whether AIM levels that are higher or lower than this range mean pathological may depend on the type of disease. At least, patients with progressive liver damage exhibited significantly higher levels than the normal range. Based on the results of mouse experiments demonstrating that the presence or absence of AIM does not influence the state of liver injury in response to CCl4, and that AIM levels increase in response to CCl4 in wild-type mice, it is likely that AIM levels increase as a result of liver damage. Thus, AIM can be used as a novel biomarker for liver injury. The mRNA level of liver *AIM* did not increase in response to CCl4, indicating no enhanced AIM production by liver Kupffer macrophages. It remains possible, however, that inflammatory stimuli caused by carbon tetrachloride will increase *AIM* expression in macrophages in other tissues such as in the peritoneal cavity and splenic marginal zone, but additional experiments are required to assess this possibility. Alternatively, liver damage might increase AIM stability in the blood. Natural IgM is catabolized mainly in the liver [46–48]. Therefore, it is possible that the progression of liver damage prolongs the half-life of IgM, resulting in advanced accumulation of circulating AIM. This scenario can also be applied in humans, and may explain the more profound increase in AIM levels in cirrhotic patients compared with non-cirrhotic patients. A precise assessment of the half-life of IgM and AIM in the presence or absence of liver injury can evaluate this possibility.

More notably, we found that use of the AIM index, which is the blood AIM level normalized to the liver biomarker score, appeared to be useful for distinguishing HCC and non-HCC patients. The AIM-TB index of men with an equivalent AIM-ALB or AIM-PLT index was significantly higher in HCC patients than in non-HCC patients. This is not secondary effect of the correlation in TB and ALB or PLT, as there was no significance in the difference in these correlations in HCC and non-HCC groups. The same conclusion was obtained for the AIM-ALB and AIM-platelets indexes in women. Thus, the presence of HCC may increase the AIM-TB index in men and the AIM-ALB index in women. If this is the case, the AIM index can serve as a novel tumor marker and will be useful for the diagnosis of HCC. Further analysis using HCC-bearing mouse models in the presence or absence of AIM may be appropriate for evaluating this possibility. Alternatively, one could also speculate that individuals who show an enhanced increase in certain AIM indexes (*i.e.* AIM-TB index in men and AIM-ALB index in women) in response to liver injury might be more susceptible to HCC. However, further study such as prospective cohort study of HCC development in patients with similar levels of liver damage and different levels of circulating AIM is certainly needed to assess this possibility. In either case, further investigation will corroborate the applicability of the AIM index for the early detection of HCC.

Since HCC is one of the most common malignant tumors with an increasing incidence, identifying serological biomarkers are extremely needed, especially because most of HCC cases are diagnosed at a late stage. Thus, our study could be the bases of application of circulating AIM level as a diagnostic and/or prognostic marker of HCC, either solo or in combination with other biomarkers.

Supporting Information

Figure S1 Correlation between AIM levels and various HCC markers. Men: blue dots, women: yellow dots. In HCC patients, no significant correlation was observed in levels of AIM and either HCC marker.

Figure S2 Correlation between IgM levels and various biomarkers representing liver function. Men: blue dots, women: yellow dots. ICG score was only available in HCC patients.

Figure S3 *AIM* expression did not increase in the liver in response to CCl_4. mRNA levels of *AIM* in the liver from wild-type mice after administration of CCl_4 for 3 wk. n = 3 for each. Error bar: SEM.

Table S1 Correlation in AIM level and different clinical parameters. Number of samples, and the correlation coefficients and p values in the correlation with AIM levels in separate tested item. n: sample numbers.

Table S2 Correlation between AIM and liver function in patients with or without hepatitis viral infection. Number of samples, and the correlation coefficients and p values in the correlation with AIM levels in the indicated tested item, in patients with or without hepatitis viral infection. n: sample number.

Table S3 Correlation coefficients between all variables that are candidates for determinant of AIM. C: single regression coefficient, *p*: p-value. Cre: creatinine.

Table S4 AIM and various clinical markers in populations who exhibit very high or very low AIM levels. Number of samples (n), and the correlation coefficients and p values in the correlation with AIM levels in identical parameter. Low: patients who exhibited less than 3.0 μg/ml of AIM, High: patients who exhibited more than 10.0 μg/ml of AIM.

Acknowledgments

We particularly thank the staffs in the Center of Health Evaluation and Promotion, Inoue Hospital (Nagasaki) for preparation of a large number of blood samples. We also appreciate S. Jibiki, W. Murasawa and M. Shinohara for technical assistance.

Author Contributions

Conceived and designed the experiments: SA TM. Performed the experiments: TY M. Mori SA AN KA. Analyzed the data: TY TK M. Mori. Contributed reagents/materials/analysis tools: RT MA MB M. Maeda TA K. Izumino JT SH TT TG SO SS YY YH KK KIY K. Inoue. Wrote the paper: TM.

References

1. Jemal A, Bray F, Center MM, Ferlay J, Ward E, et al. (2011) Global cancer statistics. CA Cancer J Clin 61: 69–90.
2. Bosch FX, Ribes J, Cleries R, Diaz M (2005) Epidemiology of hepatocellular carcinoma. Clin Liver Dis 9: 191–211.
3. El-Serag HB, Rudolph KL (2007) Hepatocellular carcinoma: epidemiology and molecular carcinogenesis. Gastroenterology 132: 2557–2576.
4. Baffy G, Brunt EM, Caldwell SH (2012) Hepatocellular carcinoma in non-alcoholic fatty liver disease: an emerging menace. J Hepatol 56: 1384–91.
5. Angulo P (2002) Nonalcoholic fatty liver disease. N Engl J Med 346: 1221–1231.
6. Hytiroglou P, Park YN, Krinsky G, Theise ND (2007) Hepatic precancerous lesions and small hepatocellular carcinoma. Gastroenterol Clin North Am 36: 867–887, vii.
7. He G, Karin M (2011) NF-κB and STAT3 - key players in liver inflammation and cancer. Cell Res 21: 159–168.
8. Park EJ, Lee JH, Yu GY, He G, Ali SR, et al. (2010) Dietary and genetic obesity promote liver inflammation and tumorigenesis by enhancing IL-6 and TNF expression. Cell 140: 197–208.
9. Powell EE, Cooksley WG, Hanson R, Searle J, Halliday JW, et al. (1990) The natural history of nonalcoholic steatohepatitis: a follow-up study of forty-two patients for up to 21 years. Hepatology 11: 74–80.
10. Day CP, Saksena S (2002) Non-alcoholic steatohepatitis: definitions and pathogenesis. J Gastroenterol Hepatol 17: S377–S384.
11. Harrison SA, Torgerson S, Hayashi PH (2003) The natural history of nonalcoholic fatty liver disease: a clinical histopathological study. Am J Gastroenterol 98: 2042–2047.
12. Torres DM, Harrison SA (2012) Nonalcoholic steatohepatitis and noncirrhotic hepatocellular carcinoma: fertile soil. Semin Liver Dis 32: 30–38.
13. Starley BQ, Calcagno CJ, Harrison SA (2010) Nonalcoholic fatty liver disease and hepatocellular carcinoma: a weighty connection. Hepatology 51: 1820–1832.
14. Kawada N, Imanaka K, Kawaguchi T, Tamai C, Ishihara R, et al. (2009) Hepatocellular carcinoma arising from non-cirrhotic nonalcoholic steatohepatitis. J Gastroenterol 44: 1190–1194.
15. Chagas AL, Kikuchi LO, Oliveira CP, Vezozzo DC, Mello ES, et al. (2009) Does hepatocellular carcinoma in non-alcoholic steatohepatitis exist in cirrhotic and non-cirrhotic patients? Braz J Med Biol Res 42: 958–962.
16. Ertle J, Dechêne A, Sowa JP, Penndorf V, Herzer K, et al. (2011) Non-alcoholic fatty liver disease progresses to hepatocellular carcinoma in the absence of apparent cirrhosis. Int J Cancer 128: 2436–2443.
17. Paradis V, Zalinski S, Chelbi E, Guedj N, Degos F, et al. (2009) Hepatocellular carcinomas in patients with metabolic syndrome often develop without significant liver fibrosis: a pathological analysis. Hepatology 49: 851–859.
18. Takuma Y, Nouso K (2010) Nonalcoholic steatohepatitis-associated hepatocellular carcinoma: our case series and literature review. World J Gastroenterol 16: 1436–1441.
19. Miyazaki T, Hirokami Y, Matsuhashi N, Takatsuka H, Naito M (1999) Increased susceptibility of thymocytes to apoptosis in mice lacking AIM, a novel

murine macrophage-derived soluble factor belonging to the scavenger receptor cysteine-rich domain superfamily. J Exp Med 189: 413–422.
20. Arai S, Shelton JM, Chen M, Bradley MN, Castrillo A, et al. (2005) A role of the apoptosis inhibitory factor AIM/Spα/Api6 in atherosclerosis development. Cell Metab 1: 201–213.
21. Joseph SB, Bradley MN, Castrillo A, Bruhn KW, Mak PA, et al. (2004) LXR-dependent gene expression is important for macrophage survival and the innate immune response. Cell 119: 299–309.
22. Valledor AF, Hsu LC, Ogawa S, Sawka-Verhelle D, Karin M, et al. (2004) Activation of liver X receptors and retinoid X receptors prevents bacterial-induced macrophage apoptosis. Proc Natl Acad Sci USA 101: 17813–17818.
23. Arai S, Maehara N, Iwamura Y, Honda S, Nakashima K, et al. (2013) Obesity-associated autoantibody production requires AIM to retain IgM immune complex on follicular dendritic cells. Cell Rep 3: 1187–1198.
24. Tissot JD, Sanchez JC, Vuadens F, Scherl A, Schifferli JA, et al. (2002) IgM are associated to Sp alpha (CD5 antigen-like). Electrophoresis 23: 1203–1206.
25. Gangadharan B, Antrobus R, Dwek RA, Zitzmann N (2007) Novel serum biomarker candidates for liver fibrosis in hepatitis C patients. Clin Chem 53: 1792–1799.
26. Gray J, Chattopadhyay D, Beale GS, Patman GL, Miele L, et al. (2009) A proteomic strategy to identify novel serum biomarkers for liver cirrhosis and hepatocellular cancer in individuals with fatty liver disease. BMC Cancer 9: 271.
27. Kim WK, Hwang HR, Kim do H, Lee PY, In YJ, et al. (2008) Glycoproteomic analysis of plasma from patients with atopic dermatitis: CD5L and ApoE as potential biomarkers. Exp Mol Med 40: 677–685.
28. Mera K, Uto H, Mawatari S, Ido A, Yoshimine Y, et al. (2014) Serum levels of apoptosis inhibitor of macrophage are associated with hepatic fibrosis in patients with chronic hepatitis C. BMC Gastroenterol 13: 14–27.
29. Kurokawa J, Arai S, Nakashima K, Nishijima A, Miyake K, et al. (2010) AIM is endocytosed into adipocytes and decreases lipid droplets via inhibition of fatty acid synthase activity. Cell Metab 11: 479–492.
30. Iwamura Y, Mori M, Nakashima K, Mikami T, Murayama K, et al. (2012) Apoptosis inhibitor of macrophage (AIM) diminishes lipid droplet-coating proteins leading to lipolysis in adipocytes. Biochem Biophys Res Commun 422: 476–481.
31. Arai S, Miyazaki T (2014) Impacts of the apoptosis inhibitor of macrophage (AIM) on obesity-associated inflammatory diseases. Semin Immunopathol 36: 3–12.
32. Ichida F, Tsuji T, Omata M, Ichida T, Inoue K, et al. (1996) New Inuyama classification; new criteria for histological assessment of chronic hepatitis. Int hepatol commun 6: 112–119.
33. Bryzgalova G, Lundholm L, Portwood N, Gustafsson J-Å, Khan A, et al. (2008) Mechanisms of antidiabetogenic and body weight-lowering effects of estrogen in high-fat diet-fed mice. Am J Physiol Endocrinol Metab 295: E904–E912.
34. Gao H, Bryzgalova G, Hedman E, Khan A, Efendic S, et al. (2006) Long-term administration of estradiol decreases expression of hepatic lipogenic genes and improves insulin sensitivity in ob/ob mice: a possible mechanism is through direct regulation of signal transducer and activator of transcription 3. Mol Endocrinol 20: 1287–1299.
35. Han SI, Komatsu Y, Murayama A, Steffensen KR, Nakagawa Y, et al. (2014) Estrogen receptor ligands ameliorate fatty liver through a nonclassical estrogen receptor/Liver X receptor pathway in mice. Hepatology 59: 1791–1802.
36. Lundholm L, Movérare S, Steffensen KR, Nilsson M, Otsuki M, et al. (2004) Gene expression profiling identifies liver X receptor alpha as an estrogen-regulated gene in mouse adipose tissue. J Mol Endocrinol 32: 879–892.
37. Tiano JP, Mauvais-Jarvis F (2012) Molecular mechanisms of estrogen receptors' suppression of lipogenesis in pancreatic β-cells. Endocrinology 153: 2997–3005.
38. Hage FG, Oparil S (2013) Ovarian hormones and vascular disease. Curr Opin Cardiol 28: 411–416.
39. Grodstein F, Manson JE, Colditz GA, Willett WC, Speizer FE, et al. (2000) A prospective, observational study of postmenopausal hormone therapy and primary prevention of cardiovascular disease. Ann Intern Med 133: 933–941.
40. Grady D, Herrington D, Bittner V, Blumenthal R, Davidson M, et al. (2002) Cardiovascular disease outcomes during 6.8 years of hormone therapy: Heart and Estrogen/progestin Replacement Study follow-up (HERS II). JAMA 288: 49–57.
41. Wang H, Liu Y, Zhu L, Wang W, Wan Z, et al. (2014) 17β-estradiol promotes cholesterol efflux from vascular smooth muscle cells through a liver X receptor α-dependent pathway. Int J Mol Med 33: 550–558.
42. Hamada M, Nakamura M, Tran MT, Moriguchi T, Hong C, et al. (2014) MafB promotes atherosclerosis by inhibiting foam-cell apoptosis. Nat Commun 5: 3147.
43. Miyazaki T, Kurokawa J, Arai S (2011) AIMing at Metabolic Syndrome: Towards the development of novel therapies for metabolic diseases via apoptosis inhibitor of macrophage (AIM). Cir J 75: 2522–2531.
44. Xu Y, Fan H, Li X, Sun L, Hou Y (2012) 17β-Estradiol enhances response of mice spleen B cells elicited by TLR9 agonist. Cell Immunol 278: 125–135.
45. Li X, Xu Y, Ma L, Sun L, Fu G, et al. (2009) 17beta-estradiol enhances the response of plasmacytoid dendritic cell to CpG. PLoS One 4: e8412.
46. Bazin H, Malet F (1969) The metabolism of different immunoglobulin classes in irradiated mice. Immunology 17: 345–365.
47. Vieira P, Rajewsky K (1988) The half-lives of serum immunoglobulins in adult mice. Eur J Immunol 18: 313–316.
48. Kai T, Yamazaki T, Arai S, Miyazaki T (2014) Stabilization and augmentation of circulating AIM in mice by synthesized IgM-Fc. PLoS One 9: e97037.

7

FABP7 and HMGCS2 Are Novel Protein Markers for Apocrine Differentiation Categorizing Apocrine Carcinoma of the Breast

Pavel Gromov[1*¶], Jaime A. Espinoza[2¶], Maj-Lis Talman[3], Naoko Honma[4], Niels Kroman[5], Vera Timmermans Wielenga[3], José M. A. Moreira[6], Irina Gromova[1]

1 Danish Cancer Society Research Center, Genome Integrity Unit, Copenhagen, Denmark, **2** Department of Pathology, Center for Investigation in Translational Oncology (CITO), School of Medicine, Pontificia Universidad Católica de Chile, Santiago, Chile, **3** Department of Pathology, the Centre of Diagnostic Investigations, Copenhagen University Hospital, Copenhagen, Denmark, **4** Research Team for Geriatric Pathology, Tokyo Metropolitan Institute of Gerontology, Tokyo, Japan, **5** Department of Breast Surgery, Copenhagen University Hospital, Copenhagen, Denmark, **6** Section of Molecular Disease Biology and Sino-Danish Breast Cancer Research Centre, Department of Veterinary Disease Biology, Faculty of Health and Medical Sciences, University of Copenhagen, Copenhagen, Denmark

Abstract

Apocrine carcinoma of the breast is a distinctive malignancy with unique morphological and molecular features, generally characterized by being negative for estrogen and progesterone receptors, and thus not electable for endocrine therapy. Despite the fact that they are morphologically distinct from other breast lesions, no standard molecular criteria are currently available for their diagnosis. Using gel-based proteomics in combination with mass spectrometry and immunohistochemistry we have identified two novel markers, HMGCS2 and FABP7 that categorize the entire breast apocrine differentiation spectrum from benign metaplasia and cysts to invasive stages. Expression of HMGCS2 and FABP7 is strongly associated with apocrine differentiation; their expression is retained by most invasive apocrine carcinomas (IAC) showing positive immunoreactivity in 100% and 78% of apocrine carcinomas, respectively, as compared to non-apocrine tumors (16.7% and 6.8%). The nuclear localization of FABP7 in tumor cells was shown to be associated with more aggressive stages of apocrine carcinomas. In addition, when added to the panel of apocrine biomarkers previously reported by our group: 15-PGDH, HMGCR and ACSM1, together they provide a signature that may represent a golden molecular standard for defining the apocrine phenotype in the breast. Moreover, we show that combining HMGCS2 to the steroidal profile (HMGCS2+/Androgen Receptor (AR)+/Estrogen Receptor(ER)-/Progesteron Receptor (PR)- identifies IACs with a greater sensitivity (79%) as compared with the steroidal profile (AR+/ER-/PR-) alone (54%). We have also presented a detailed immunohistochemical analysis of breast apocrine lesions with a panel of antibodies against proteins which correspond to 10 genes selected from published transcriptomic signatures that currently characterize molecular apocrine subtype and shown that except for melanophilin that is overexpressed in benign apocrine lesions, these proteins were not specific for morphological apocrine differentiation in breast.

Editor: Masaharu Seno, Okayama University, Japan

Funding: This work was supported by grants from the Danish Cancer Society, the John and Birthe Meyer Foundation, the Kai Lange and Gundhild Kai Lange Fond, and the Lisa and Gudmund JÅrgensens Fond. The ear-marked support of the Marketing Department at the Danish Cancer Society through their fundraising activities on behalf of DCTB is greatly appreciated. The funders had no role in study design, data collection and analysis, decision to publish, or preparation of the manuscript.

Competing Interests: The authors have declared that no competing interests exist.

* Email: psg@cancer.dk

¶ These authors contributed equally to this work.

Introduction

Apocrine carcinoma of the breast exhibits the same histological growth pattern as invasive ductal carcinoma of no special type, and is currently diagnosed on basis of the presence of characteristic apocrine-type epithelial cell morphology observed in more than 90% of tumor cell mass. These tumors represent a relatively rare subtype, constituting less than 5% of all breast cancers [1,2]. Recently, Dellapasqua and coauthors reported a frequency of apocrine carcinoma of 0.8% after analyzing a cohort of 6971 breast cancer patients [3]. This high discrepancy is most likely because there is no consensus on standardized reproducible diagnostic criteria as the current WHO classification of breast malignancies provides an imprecise definition of apocrine carcinoma of the breast [4], a fact that has produced controversial and heterogeneous conclusions in the scientific literature in terms of a precise immunohistochemical profile and molecular classification of invasive apocrine carcinomas (IACs) [1,5,6,7,8,9]. Moreover, apocrine differentiation is detected in several other breast tumor subtypes including papillary, micropapillary, tubular, and lobular carcinoma [9]. In addition to characteristic morphological features IACs are generally accepted to have a distinct hormonal profile, being estrogen receptor (ER) and progesterone receptor (PR) negative, but androgen receptor (AR) positive [10]. Again, it should be noted that throughout the years IACs have been reported as ER positive in 3.8–60% of cases, PR positive in 4.8%–40% and AR positive in 56%–100% [1], underscoring the variability in observation reported for these tumors. There are not much data regarding the clinical outcome of those tumors and the results are not compelling enough partly because of limited numbers of samples selected for the analysis [9]. A comprehensive study published recently has revealed a significantly worse disease free survival for pure IACs as compared with invasive ductal carcinoma (IDC) [3].

A few years ago several transcriptomic studies were performed with the aim to classify these types of breast malignancy at the molecular level. In the gene profiling study carried out by Perou and coauthors, IACs clustered within the basal-like subtype of breast carcinomas [11]. Thereafter, Farmer and colleagues [12] identified a subset of breast tumors characterized by increased androgen signaling and a distinctive expression profile, which they called "molecular apocrine" as these lesions did not exhibit all the histopathological traits that are characteristic of classical apocrine carcinomas. Molecularly defined apocrine carcinomas include tumors that share some common expression characteristics with the HER2+ group (ER-/PR-/HER2+) in the Stanford classification as well as with some lesions that exhibit features of the basal-like/triple negative group (high grade lesions; ER-/PR-/HER2-). It was also shown that it is possible with microarray data to divide mammary tumors into 3 major groups based on steroid hormone status: luminal (ER+/AR+), basal (ER−/AR−), and molecular apocrine (ER−/AR+) with a certain association between apocrine histology and molecular apocrine type [13]. Finally, a meta-analysis study performed by Sanga and colleagues [14] showed that the subgroups described by Farmer and Doane are highly similar and both predict the molecular apocrine subset in other cohorts. To date, however, the relationship between molecular apocrine breast carcinoma and histopathologically defined apocrine tumors remains questionable [15].

With the aim to develop molecular criteria to reproducibly categorize IACs at the protein level we have undertaken a systematic proteomic analysis of well-defined set of apocrine carcinomas aimed at identifying biomarkers that may characterize and subtype these lesions to a greater detail, and to search for targets that may lead to the development of novel targeted therapies and chemoprevention strategies [2,16,17,18,19]. Accordingly, we have identified a number of apocrine protein markers that include 15-prostaglandin dehydrogenase (15-PGDH) and acyl-CoA synthetase medium-chain family member 1 (ACSM1) which together with a set of categorizing markers that are predominantly expressed (AR, CD24) or not expressed (bcl-2, GATA-3) by apocrine metaplastic lesions in benign breast lesions, were proven to be specific for both apocrine ductal carcinoma *in situ* (ADCIS) and IAC [2,16,17,19,20]. This apocrine signature has been shown to identify unambiguously 13 out of 14 ADCIS (92.9%) and 20 out of 33 (60.6%) IACs in a well characterized set of apocrine carcinomas [2] in which more than 90% of the tumor cells exhibited cytological features typical of apocrine cells [21]. Here we describe two additional markers, brain fatty acid binding protein (FABP7) and hydroxymethylglutaryl (HMG)-CoA synthase 2 (HMGCS2), which in combination with markers in the protein signature described previously [19] allowed to identify ADCISs and IACs that failed to be detected in previous studies. Moreover, our results demonstrate that HMGCS2 added to the steroid hormone receptor signature (ER-/PR-/AR+) identifies apocrine tumors from other breast cancer subtypes with greater sensitivity as compared to steroid receptor profile alone. We have also presented a detailed immunohistochemistry (IHC) analysis of a set of proteins corresponding to 10 genes selected from transcriptomic signatures that currently characterize molecular apocrine subtype [12,13,14,22] to evaluate the complementarity of these two approaches.

Results

Determination of the specificity of FABP7 and HMGCS2 antibodies

The sensitivity and specificity of antibodies are critical parameters in the design and development of reliable IHC-based assays for analysis and validation of potential biomarkers. To determine if FABP7 and HMGCS2 antibodies are specific enough in terms of IHC staining to identify benign and malignant apocrine lesions [2,16] we used a three-pronged strategy developed in our laboratory and described in detail elsewhere [23]: (i) analysis of potential cross-reactivity by 2D Western blotting (2D-WB), (ii) mass spectrometry validation of corresponding silver-stained protein spots superimposed with 2D-WB and (iii) IHC experiments with blocking of antibodies with a corresponding protein/epitope. This approach combines the intrinsic sensitivity and cellular resolution of IHC, with the specificity of 2D-WB and MS-based identification, and the overall protein analysis capability of gel-based proteomics [24].

In previous studies we demonstrated overexpression of FABP7 and HMGCS2 by apocrine cells as compared to their normal breast epithelial cell counterparts [2]. 2D-PAGE/MS/2D-WB analyses were performed on tissue lysates obtained from six patients and the results for one matched apocrine cyst/normal epithelia pair are illustrated in Figure 1. As shown, the anti-HMGCS2 antibody detected several train-line protein spots of similar Mw (about 57 kDa) (Figure 1A and C) compatible with multiple post-translational modifications of the protein [25,26]. The identity of these spots as HMGCS2 was confirmed by MS analysis (data not shown). The antibody recognizing FABP7 detected a single spot with Mw ≅15 kDa (Figure 1A and D). No protein spots matched to the positions of FABP7 and HMGCS2 were detected on the 2D gel of normal breast tissue (Figure 1B). The results show that HMGCS2 and FABP7 are recognized by their corresponding antibodies, and, most importantly, cross-reactivity was detected for neither HMGCS2 nor FABP7 with any of the thousands of proteins resolved by 2D PAGE, demonstrating a high specificity for these antibodies. In addition, to exclude the possibility that anti-FABP7 may react with some close homologues from the FABP protein family [27], we performed 2D–WB with protein extracts from several triple-negative breast cancer samples in which we had previously observed aberrant expression of three other FABP protein family members, namely, FABP3, FABP4 and FABP5 [23]. As seen in Figure S1, anti-FABP7 specifically recognized only a single spot corresponding to FABP7 and no cross reactivity was detected with FABP3, FABP4 or FABP5. The identities of all protein spots were determined by mass spectrometry analysis (data not shown). The high specificity of both antibodies was further confirmed by IHC experiments with blocking of antibodies with a corresponding full length recombinant protein (data not shown). Based on these results it can be concluded that the antibodies against FABP7 and HMGCS2 recognize their cognate antigens with high specificity and, thus, can be incorporated into the panel of antibodies used in IHC experiments to distinguish the cell type that express proteins of interest within heterogeneous clinical samples.

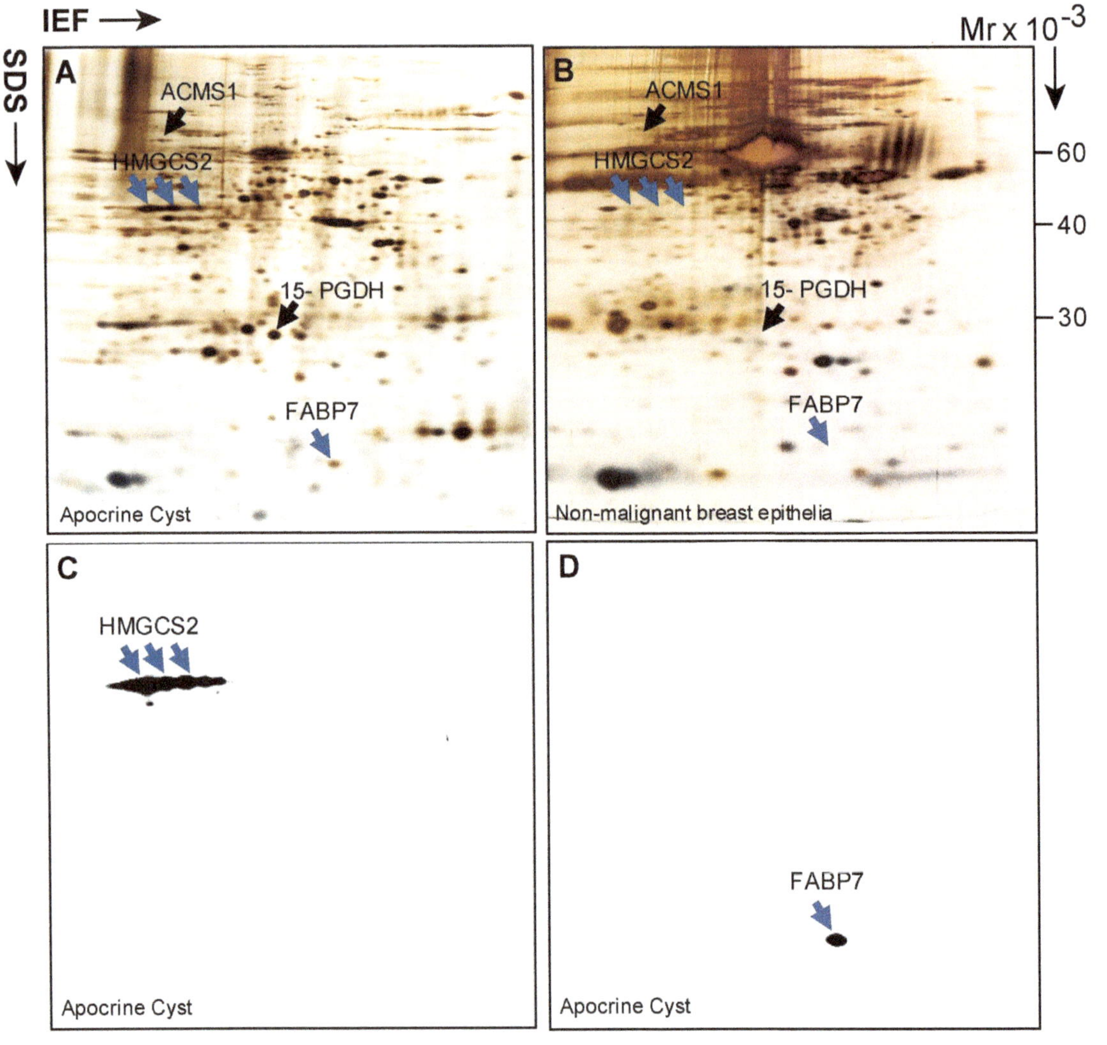

Figure 1. 2D PAGE and 2D Western blot analysis of normal breast lesions and apocrine cyst. (A) 2D silver stained gel of protein lysate from apocrine microcyst excised from tumor biopsy of patient 95 (GrI; $ER^+/PR^+/AR^+/HER2^{1+}$). Positions of FABP7 and HMGCS2 identified by mass spectrometry (MS) are indicated by blue arrows. Positions of apocrine differentiation, markers, 15-PGDH and ACSM1, described in our previous studies are indicated by black arrows for reference. (B) 2D silver stained gel of protein lysate from distant normal (app. 3–4 cm from tumor mass) breast lesion resected from mastectomy of patient 121 (GrII; $ER^+/PR^+/AR^+/HER2^{2+}$). HMGCS2 and FABP7 have been identified by MS and are indicated by blue arrows. Positions of HMGCS2, FABP7 (blue arrow) and 15-PGDH, and ACSM1 (black arrows) are indicated. The positions of HMGCS2 and FABP7 on the 2D gel image (B) are located by matching of corresponding gel images by PDQUEST software. (C and D) 2D Western blot of protein lysate from the same apocrine microcyst as in (A) developed either with anti HMGCS2 or anti FABP7 antibodies.

FABP7 and HMGCS2 are highly expressed in benign breast lesions with apocrine differentiation

Having ascertained the strict specificity of the antibodies recognizing FABP7 and HMGCS2, we investigated their expression profiles by IHC on serial sections of lesions with various forms of benign apocrine metaplasia. Thus, we evaluated the percentage of positivity/negativity for HMGCS2 and FABP7 in 2 sets of breast tissue samples, namely, non-malignant breast tissue dissected from the areas adjacent to tumors (28 patients with various types of breast tumors, Table S1) and 13 benign apocrine microcysts obtained after surgery (Table S2). Expression of cytoplasmic FABP7 and HMGCS2 as well as nuclear FABP7 was considered positive whenever we observed more than 60% of cytoplasmic and above 1% of nuclear staining, respectively. Representative IHC patterns are shown in Figure 2. FABP7 nuclear and cytoplasmic staining was not evaluated independently because of limited number of samples presented in each group. As seen, normal terminal ductal lobular units and normal ducts in breast areas adjacent to tumor showed positivity for both proteins neither in luminal cell nor in basal/myoepithelial cells (Figure 2A and B and Figure 2E and F). However, areas with morphological signs of apocrine differentiation exhibited sporadically positive mosaic staining (Figure 2C and G, respectively). Most notably, apocrine cysts exhibited a high immunoreactivity for both HMGCS2 and FABP7 (Figure 2D and H, respectively). To confirm these observations and to justify intracellular localization of both proteins, we examined the expression pattern of HMGCS2 and FABP7 in apocrine cysts by double immunofluorescence (Figure 3). As expected, normal mammary epithelial cells showed little or no evidence of staining with either antibody (Figure 3, left panel). On the contrary, lesions with apocrine metaplasia (Figure 3, left panel) and apocrine cysts (right panel) were highly positive for both proteins. Taken together these experiments showed a preferential expression of HMGCS2 and FABP7 in benign breast lesions undergoing apocrine differentiation. Additionally, non-apocrine flat cysts (type II) that were detected within analyzed lesions were completely negative for both HMGCS2 and FABP7 in all cases (data not shown).

Based on the IHC scoring we have evaluated the percentage of positivity/negativity of both proteins in apocrine cysts as compared to non-apocrine lesions and shown that FABP7 was positive in 12 out of the 13 apocrine cyst samples and negative in 22 out of the 28 non-apocrine samples (92,3% and 78,6%, respectively; $p<0.0001$). Accordingly 10 out of the 13 apocrine cyst samples (76,9%) and 26 out of 28 non-apocrine ones (92,8%), were classified for HMGCS2 as positive and negative, respectively ($p<0.001$). These results imply that FABP7 and HMGCS2 can be considered as novel biomarkers for breast apocrine differentiation that together with the apocrine biomarker panel reported by us in previous studies, 15-PGDH+ HMG-CoA reductase+ and ACSM1+ [2,16,19,28] may represent the golden standard for defining the breast apocrine phenotype.

Expression of FABP7 and HMGCS2 by apocrine carcinoma

The baseline of expression for HMGCS2 and FABP7 in apocrine carcinomas at the protein level was first evaluated in a selected number of well differentiated IACs (6 samples) using 2D PAGE and PDQUEST-based image analysis as compared to TNBC (6 samples), Luminal B (7 samples) and HER2 (7 samples) subtypes of which there was fresh frozen tissue. The representative 2D images of these breast cancer subtypes are shown in Figure 4. All six of the analyzed IACs expressed both proteins (Figure 4A) as it was determined by MS analysis and confirmed by 2D WB (data not shown). No traces of these proteins were found in any of the 3 other breast cancer subtypes analyzed by 2D PAGE (Figure 4B, C and D). Notably, the acidic isoform of HMGCS2 detected in IACs is co-migrated with the basic variants of alpha-enolase (Figure 4A), a protein that is highly expressed in all tumor subtypes analyzed and, as a result, may mask the identification of HMGCS2 by 2D PAGE in these samples. Hence, we performed IHC analysis of these non-apocrine samples together with ADCIS and IAC and confirmed that both proteins are expressed only by apocrine carcinomas as exemplified in Figure 5. As seen, no positive staining for HMGCS2 and FABP7 was observed in TNBC, Luminal B and HER2 samples (Figure 5E–J). It is noteworthy, that in both apocrine carcinoma types, ADCIS and IAC, HMGCS2 displayed only cytoplasmic staining pattern (Figure 5B and D). FABP7 also exhibited cytoplasmic intracellular localization in both apocrine carcinomas, however, in invasive stages, while retaining in cytoplasm, it was also detected in the nuclei with positivity thresholds more than 1% (Figure 5C).

Based on these results we proceeded to test the putative two-protein signature within the same unique Japanese collection of apocrine carcinomas [21,29,30] that was used to validate the previous protein signature [19]. In this large, well characterized cohort, which is composed of 14 apocrine ductal carcinoma *in situ* (ADCIS) and 33 IACs, more than 90% of the tumor cells exhibited morphological features typical for apocrine cells [19,29]. All 14 ADCIS (100%) stained positively for HMGCS2 and 13 out of 14 (92%) were immunoreactive for FABP7 (Figure 6, Table S3) with weak intensity of cytoplasmic staining (Table S3). As it was shown previously, all samples did not express ER, PR, Bcl2 and GATA3, but were positive for CD24 and AR (with one exception – ADCIS 12) [19]. The frequencies of HMGCS2 and FABP7 in 33 IACs as evaluated by IHC are shown in Figure 6 and Table S4. HMGCS2 and FABP7 were positive in 100% (33/33) and 78% (25/32) of IACs, respectively. Nuclear localization of FABP7 was associated with invasive stage of apocrine carcinomas as it was detected in all 33 IAC samples but was not observed in any of the 14 ADCISs (Table S3 and S4).

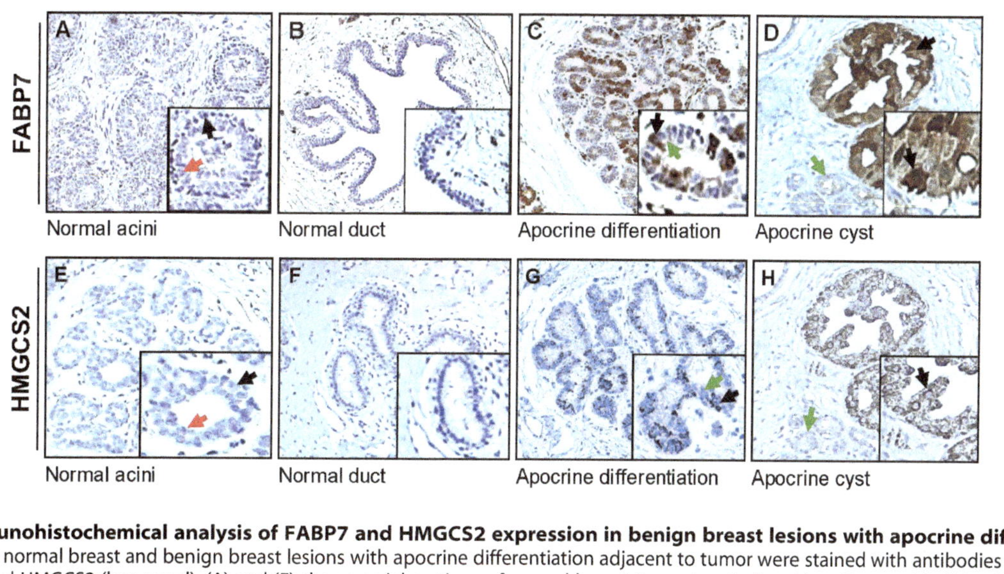

Figure 2. Immunohistochemical analysis of FABP7 and HMGCS2 expression in benign breast lesions with apocrine differentiation. FFPE sections of normal breast and benign breast lesions with apocrine differentiation adjacent to tumor were stained with antibodies against FABP7 (upper panel) and HMGCS2 (low panel). (A) and (E) shows serial sections of normal breast tissue. Luminal and basal/myoepithelial cells are indicated by red and black arrows, respectively. (B) and (F) show sections of large normal ducts. (C) and (G) show serial sections of breast lesions with benign apocrine differentiation (apocrine adenosis). Positive and negative luminal cells are indicated by black and green arrows, respectively. (D) and (H) show serial sections of lesions with apocrine cysts. Apocrine cysts with apical snouts and normal small ducts are indicated with black and green arrows, respectively. Magnification: x10. Representative areas for each staining are shown in higher magnification (x20). The cut-off values for FABP7 and HMGCS2 are specified in Materials and Methods.

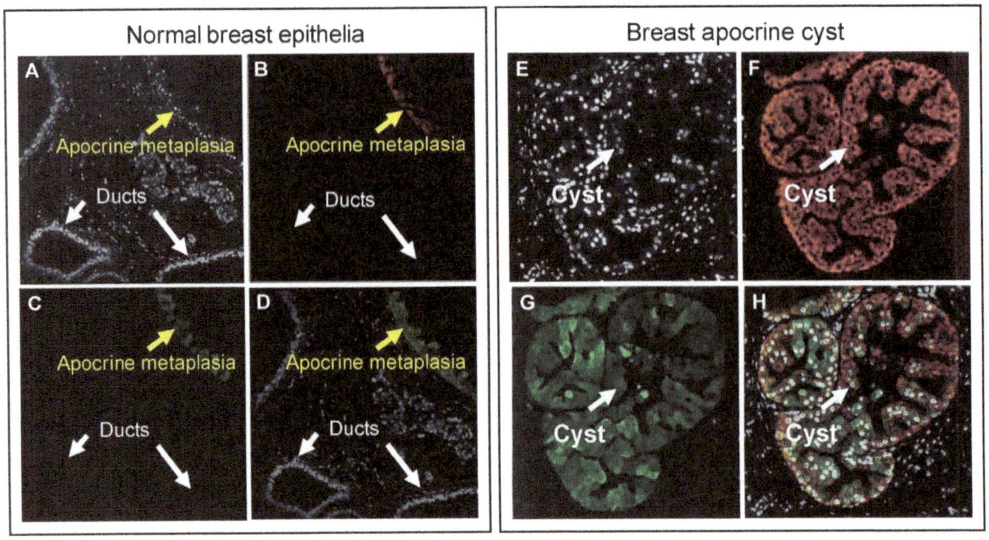

Figure 3. FABP7 and HMGCS2 are colocalized in lesions with apocrine differentiation. Indirect double-label immunofluorescence analysis of normal breast lesion with apocrine metaplasia (left panel) and apocrine cyst sections (right panel) reacted with FABP7 (subpanels B and F) and HMGCS2 (subpanels C and G). Sections were counterstained with the nuclear stain DAPI (blue channel). Merge images are shown on subpanels (D) and (H), respectively.

Expression of FABP7 and HMGCS2 by other breast carcinoma subtypes

To determine whether FABP7 and HMGCS2 are exclusively expressed by apocrine carcinoma we analyzed expression patterns of these putative biomarkers in a set of 205 non-apocrine breast tumors: 42 TNBC (21%), 103 Luminal A (50,2%), 17 Luminal B (8,3%) and 43 HER2+ (20,5%) contained in three commercially available tissue microarrays (BRC1501, 1502, and 1503; Pantomics Inc.) (Figure 6, Table S5). The frequencies of positivity for HMGCS2 and FABP7 as compared to IACs are summarized in Figure 6B. In total, FABP7 positives were detected in 14 out of the 205 breast non-apocrine carcinomas (6,79%): 8 out of the 42 TNBCs (19,04%); 1 out of the 103 Luminal A subtypes (0,97%); in none out of the 17 Luminal B (0%) and in 5 out of the 43 HER2+ (11,62%). HMGCS2 was expressed in 1 out of 42 TNBCs (2,38%); 18 out of 101 Luminal A (17,8%); 4 out of 17 Luminal B (23,5%) and 11 out of 43 HER2+ (25,5%), in total: 34 out of the 203 non-apocrine breast carcinomas (16,7%) (Figure 6B). The Fisher exact test confirmed a statistical significant difference in frequencies of HMGCS2 and FABP7 positives between IACs and Luminal A, Luminal B, HER2+ and TNBC groups ($p<0.0001$ for both proteins). No association was found between HMGCS2 expression and ER or PR status, however, FABP7 is significantly more positive among ER- and PR- breast cancers ($p<0.0001$).

Given that androgen receptor (AR) is widely expressed in various breast cancer types [31] and leaning on our findings that HMGCS2+/AR+/ER-/PR- phenotype is highly frequent in both ADCIS and IAC subgroups (Figure 6A, Tables S3 and S4), we calculated the frequency of this four-protein signature in non-apocrine Pantomics dataset and revealed only 7 samples (3,5%) with a combination of HMGCS2+/AR+/ER-/PR- (Table S5, corresponding rows are highlighted by Thick Box Border). This finding implies the contention that the HMGCS2+/AR+/ER-/PR- profile is associated with breast apocrine malignancy diagnosed by morphological criteria ($p<0.0001$) with a sensitivity of 78,8% and a specificity of 96,6% (using a defined threshold). Thus, HMGCS2+/AR+/ER-/PR- profile exhibited a significantly higher sensitivity as compared with the AR+/ER-/PR- phenotype, which only provides a sensitivity of 54,17% for apocrine tumors. Similar statistical evaluation performed for FABP7 demonstrated that FABP7+/AR+/ER-/PR- phenotype exhibited 75% of sensitivity and 94,7% of specificity, outperforming also the steroidal profile alone.

Interestingly, among 7 non-apocrine samples showing HMGCS2+/AR+/ER-/PR- profile 6 were HER2+ (86%; remaining sample was classified as a borderline) (Table S5), whereas in the entire cohort of 203 samples, HER2 positives were observed in 58 samples (28,6%), indicating that among tumors outside apocrine carcinoma the phenotype HMGCS2+/AR+/ER-/PR- is correlated with HER2 amplification ($p<0.003$). The high percentage of expression of HMGCS2 by HER2+ tumors was further confirmed by IHC using an additional set of 16 samples of HER2+ lesions collected from the department of pathology, Rigshospitalet, Copenhagen University Hospital (data not shown).

Expression of apocrine differentiation markers in the MDA-MB-453 cell line model for apocrine breast carcinoma

The MDA-MB-453 breast cancer cell line obtained from a malignant pleural effusion of a 48-year-old female is characterized by AR+/ER-/PR-/HER2- profile is often used as a model to study the molecular processes underlying apocrine breast malignancy [32,33,34]. In view of this fact, we examined the expression of FABP7 and HMGCS2 together with several other apocrine protein markers in the MDA-MB-453 breast cancer cell line. IHC analysis of MDA-MB-453 cells has been performed using a battery of antibodies against FABP7, HMGCS2, 15-PHGDH, ACSM1 and GCDFP-15. Our data have shown that, in contrast to ADCIS and IACs, MDA-MB-453 cells do not express either the FABP7 or HMGCS2 (Figure S2). This cell line was also negative for 15-PGDH and ACSM1 as well as for GCDFP-15 (Figure S2), which is often considered as an apocrine marker protein in the breast. The latter result is in agreement with the study by Vranic and co-authors [35], who recently updated the molecular profile of the

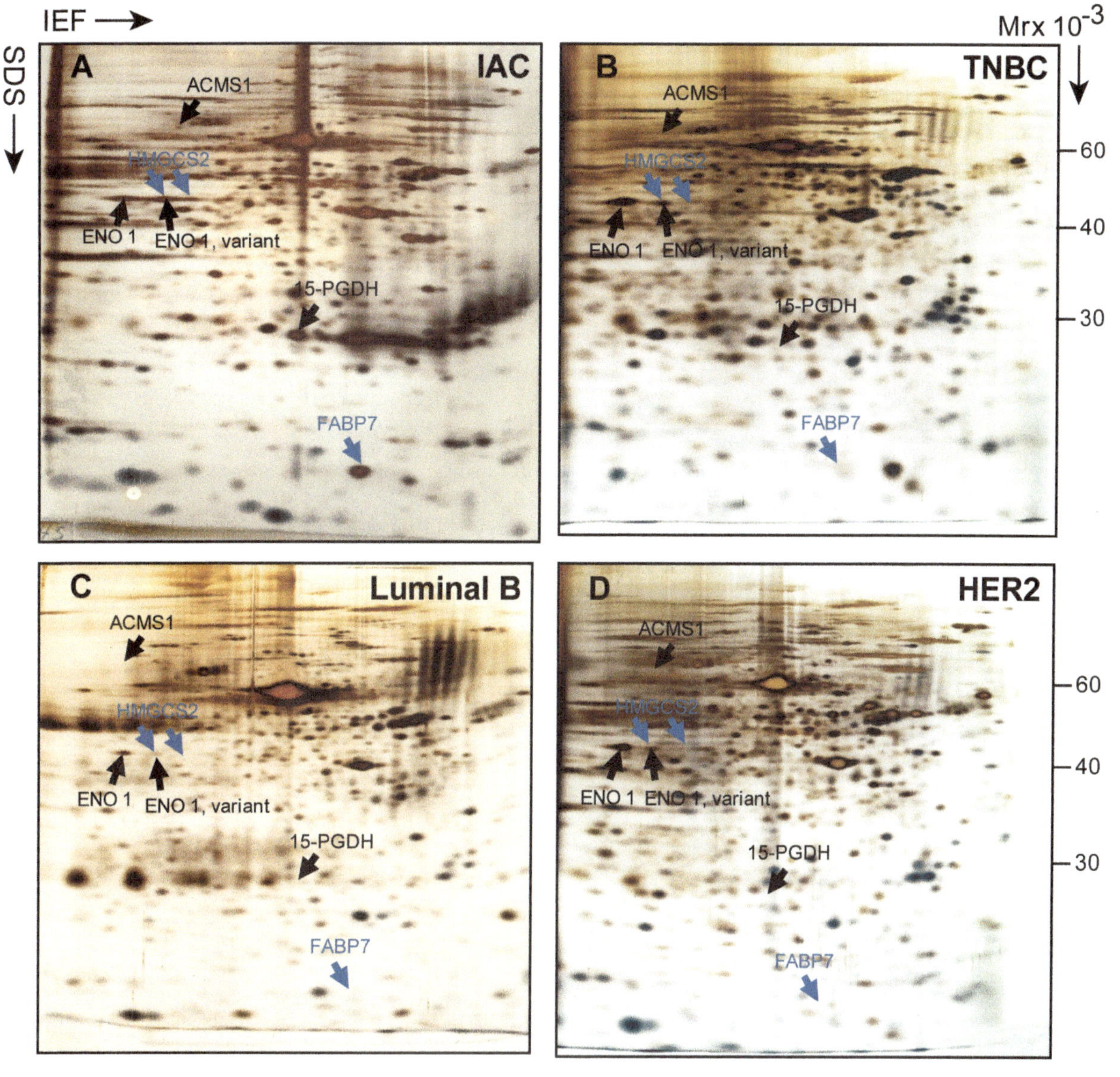

Figure 4. 2D PAGE analysis of FABP7 and HMGCS2 expression among breast cancer subtypes. The representative images of IEF 2D PAGE of protein lysates prepared from frozen sections of 4 breast tumor subtypes: IAC (A), TNBC (B), Luminal B (C) and Her2+(D). HMGCS2 and FABP7 have been identified by MS and indicated by blue arrows. The positions of HMGCS2 and FABP7 on the 2D gels of TNBC, Luminal B and HER2 were determined by matching of corresponding images by PDQUEST software. Alpha-enolase variants, identified by MS, are co-migrated with HMGCS2 and indicated by black arrows. Two other IAC markers, 15-PGDH and ACSMS1 described in our previous studies are shown for reference. IAC = invasive apocrine carcinoma; TNBC = triple negative breast cancer. Tumors have been stratified as specified in Materials and Methods.

MDA-MB-453 cell line and concluded that these cells may not be an ideal model of breast apocrine carcinomas. Consequently, our data also support this output suggesting that, although the MDA-MB-453 cells share certain features with apocrine breast carcinoma their metabolic phenotype remains plastic and may not reproduce certain expression patterns and pathways which are characteristic for apocrine differentiation in breast.

Evaluation of the transcriptomic molecular apocrine signature at the protein level

Recently, a gene expression signature called "molecular apocrine" has been proposed based on transcriptomic studies of breast cancer tumors [12,14]. The molecular apocrine group is AR positive but ER negative, with an increased androgen signaling and some morphological features of apocrine tumors, lacking, however, the strict criteria for diagnosis of classical apocrine carcinomas. To our knowledge, the reliability and significance of the apocrine breast carcinoma molecular signature has not yet been systematically investigated at the protein level. In order to find out to what extend the "molecular apocrine" signature correlates to the expression pattern of corresponding proteins in various breast tumor subtypes we performed a detailed IHC analysis of a 10-protein set selectively chosen from transcriptomic apocrine signature. The selection of the candidate genes was made on the following criteria: (i) their presence in the signatures described by the molecular apocrine meta-analysis as major top candidates [14] and (ii) the availability of specific antibodies to the corresponding proteins suitable for immunohis-

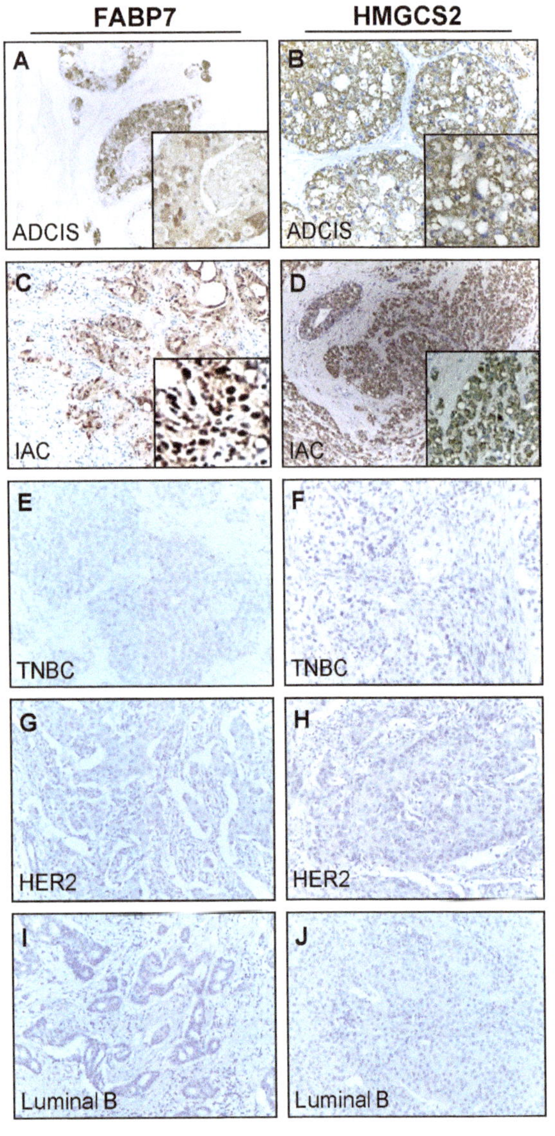

Figure 5 Immunohistochemical expression analysis of FABP7 and HMGCS2 among breast cancer subtypes. The representative IHC images of FFPE sections from 5 breast tumor subtypes immunostained with antibodies against FABP7 (A,C,E,G and I) and HMGCS2 (B,D,F,H and J). ADCIS = apocrine ductal carcinoma *in situ*; IAC= invasive apocrine carcinoma; TNBC= triple negative breast cancer. Magnification: x10. Representative areas are shown in higher magnification (x20) The cut-off values for FABP7 and HMGCS2 are specified in Material and methods. Tumors have been stratified as specified in Materials and Methods.

tochemical detection. Following these landmarks, we have chosen 10 genes consistently associated to the "molecular apocrine" signature: ABCA12 (ATP-binding cassette sub-family A member 12), BLVRA (Biliverdin reductase A), FOXA1 (Hepatocyte nuclear factor 3-alpha), MLPH (Melanophilin), RHOB (Rho-related GTP-binding protein RhoB), SIDT1 (SID1 transmembrane family member 1), SLC2A10 (Glucose transporter type 10), SLC7A8 (L-type amino acid transporter 2), TSC22D3 (TSC22 domain family protein 3) and XBP1 (X-box-binding protein 1). The expression pattern of selected candidates was tested by IHC staining on paraffin sections prepared from selected pairs of benign apocrine cyst and IAC, and representative IHC images are shown in Figure 7. Very low immunoreactivity/negativity was observed in both benign and malignant lesions for SCL2A10, SLC7A8 and MPLH (Figure 7A and B; C and D, E and F, respectively), the latter has a distinct apical expression pattern in apocrine cysts. The other seven proteins displayed positive staining of various intensities and localizations in both types of analyzed apocrine lesions: FOXA1, XBP1, BVLRA and RHOB showed positive cytoplasmic and nuclear staining in both cysts and IAC cells (Figure 7G and H, I and J, K and L, M and N, respectively); TSC22D3 was immunoreactive in nuclei of cysts and in nuclei/cytoplasm of IAC cells (Figure 7O and P), whereas ABCA12 and SIDT1 showed only cytoplasmic localization in both types of lesions (Figure 7Q and R, S and T, respectively).

In order to identify whether or not these proteins are exclusively expressed in breast lesions with apocrine differentiation including IACs, we performed IHC analysis using tissue microarrays (Pantomics Inc.) of non-IAC breast tumor subtypes which we used in our previous experiments (see above). The results are summarized in Figure 8 and demonstrate that the protein expression of 8 genes from the transcriptomic signature, namely, FOXA1, XBP1, BLVRA, ABCA12, SIDT1, RHOB, SLC2A10, TSC22D3 is not apocrine-specific, because those proteins are frequently expressed in other types of breast cancer (Figure 8). Only 2 proteins, MLPH and SLC7A8, displayed low frequencies of positivity in non-apocrine breast tumor subtypes (2,9% and 9,7% respectively; Figure 8). To estimate the value of MLPH and SLC7A8 as putative markers for apocrine differentiation in breast, we screened their expression in the sets of breast normal tissue (the set is presented in Table S1), apocrine cysts (the set is presented in Table S2) and independent set IACs (17 samples) collected from the Department of Pathology, Rigshospitalet Copenhagen University Hospital. The representative IHC sections are shown in Figure 9. All normal ducts and IACs were negative for MLPH. However, 8 out of the 14 apocrine cysts (57%) showed positive immunoreactivity for MLPH with a pattern restricted to the membrane/cytoplasm of luminal cells in apical snouts (Figure 9B). This pattern was also observed in sclerosing adenosis with apocrine differentiation (Figure 9C). Interestingly, MLPH positive expression was still retained by pseudo-glandular structures present in one IAC sample (Figure 9D), suggesting that loss of expression of MLPH protein in IACs may be due to a process of dedifferentiation or loss of the glandular structure. As well, 87% of non-malignant samples and 63% apocrine cysts displayed negative staining with the antibody against SLC7A8. A very weak cytoplasmic staining was observed in 30% of cysts. Notably, all 17 IAC samples were negative for SCL7A8. It is not inconceivable that MLPH and SLC7A8 proteins are expressed and function in apocrine carcinoma at a very low level but, consequently, all oscillations in their expression are below the resolving power of the IHC.

Discussion

The accurate diagnosis of breast apocrine carcinoma remains controversial, mainly due to the rather subjective histopathological criteria and the lack of sensitive and specific biomarkers, which can reliably categorize this subtype of breast carcinoma. The strategy we have employed to generate protein markers to specifically categorize IAC and potentially be used as targets for therapy, is based on the assumption that these lesions arise from apocrine cells, which in turn are derived from normal breast epithelial luminal cells that have undergone apocrine metaplasia [1], i.e. transition from breast epithelial cells into an apocrine sweat-gland type of cells [2,19,28]. Here we report an analysis of

A. IHC profile of HMGCS2, FABP7, steroidal profile and HER2 in breast carcinoma subtypes

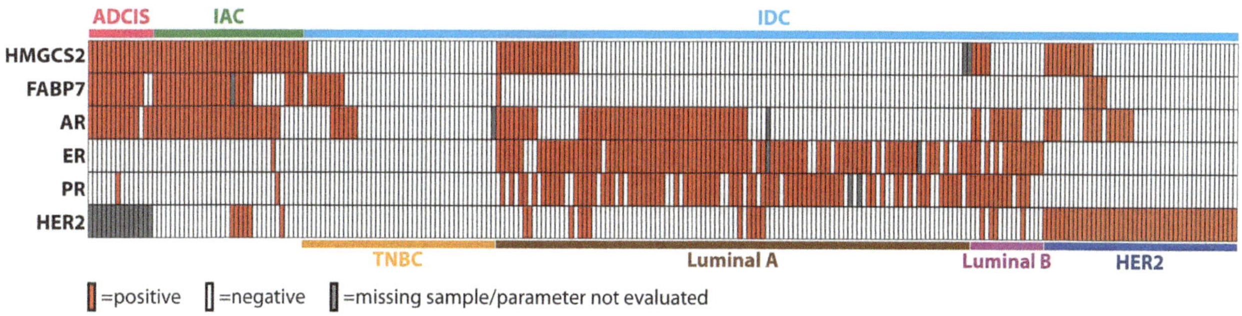

B. Frequencies of HMGCS2 and FABP7 immunoreactivity in breast tumor subtypes presented in (A)

	Tumor subtype					
	ADCIS [a]	IAC [a]	TNBC [b]	Luminal A [b]	Luminal B [b]	HER2 [b]
HMGCS2 positives/total (%)	14/14 (100%)	33/33 (100%)	1/42 (2.3%)	18/101 [c] (17.8%)	4/17 (23.5%)	11/43 (25.5%)
			In total: 34 positives out of 203 non-IACs (16.7%)			
FABP7 positives/total (%)	13/14 (92%)	25/32 [d] (78%)	8/42 (19%)	1/103 (0.97%)	0/17 (0%)	5/43 (11.6%)
			In total: 14 positives out of 205 non-IACs (6.8%)			

[a] FFPE sections of apocrine carcinomas from Cancer Institute Hospital, Tokyo (Honma et al., 2005; 2006; 2007)
[b] Three breast cancer tissue microarrays (BRC1501, 1502, and 1503; Pantomics Inc., USA)
[c] 2 cores from 103 were missed
[d] 1 section from 33 was missed

Figure 6. Expression profile of FABP7, HMGCS2 and other markers among breast cancer subtypes. (A) The diagram presents immunohistochemical profiles of ADCIS, IACs and invasive ductal carcinomas (TNBC, Luminal A Luminal B and HER2) reacted with antibodies against HMGCS2, FABP7, AR, ER, PR and HER2. The rows indicate the expression of particular protein in every core in breast cancer TMA (BRC1501, 1502 and 1503; Pantomics INC, USA): red box – positive staining, white box – negative staining, grey box – parameter was not determined. (B) Frequencies of positives for HMGCS2 and FABP7 among breast cancer subtypes. ADCIS = apocrine ductal carcinoma *in situ*; IAC = apocrine carcinoma; IDC = invasive ductal carcinoma; TNBC = triple negative breast cancer. The cut-off values for HMGCS2 and FABP7 are specified in Materials and Methods. The cut-off values for ER, PR, AR and HER2 are specified in the Table S3 and S4.

the expression of two novel putative protein biomarkers, FABP7 and HMGCS2, in breast lesions undergoing apocrine differentiation: from benign apocrine metaplasia to invasive apocrine carcinoma.

We have found that the lesions with apocrine metaplasia as well as apocrine cysts in breast were highly positive for both HMGCS2 and FABP7 as compared to normal non-apocrine mammary epithelial cells ($p<0.001$ and $p<0.0001$, respectively), implying their value as novel biomarkers for breast apocrine differentiation. HMGCS2 and FABP7 in combination with the panel published in our previous studies, 15-PGDH+, HMGCR+ and ACSM1+ [2,16,19,28] may represent the golden standard for defining the breast apocrine phenotype. Expression of FABP7 and HMGCS2 by invasive apocrine cancer was further demonstrated by IHC using a well characterized set of apocrine carcinomas [2] in which more than 90% of the tumor cells exhibited cytological features typical of apocrine cells [21]. FABP7 positives were found in 78% of all IAC cases and in 96% of ADCIS and only in 14 out of the 210 non-IAC breast tumor subtypes (6,6%). Tang and coauthors [36] reported that FABP7 overexpression exhibited a strong relationship with triple-negative cases (45,8%, $p=0.001$) and the basal-like subtype (37,5%, $p=0.001$). Our results confirmed partially a higher frequency of FABP7 positives in TNBC group (~19%) as compared to the other subtypes of breast tumors (Figure 6B). These findings are also in the line with the studies showing that FABP7 is associated with the basal phenotype and patient outcome in human breast cancer [37,38]. Importantly, our data have demonstrated various sub-cellular localization of FABP7 in apocrine carcinomas and have shown that, unlike ADCIS, in which FABP7 was detected mainly in the cytoplasm, in IACs FABP7 was also observed in nuclei, which is in the line with recent data demonstrating that nuclear location is associated with a more aggressive phenotype of breast cancer [37,38]. It was also shown, that FABP7 overexpression is correlated with pure glioblastoma histology and that nuclear expression of FABP7 is more specifically associated with more invasive tumors [39,40]. Taken together these data support the contention that translocation of FABP7 between nuclei and cytoplasm may play a role in tumor progression and further investigation should be undertaken to understand roles of FABP7 signaling and intracellular traffic in tumor biology.

To our knowledge, there are no data available on the expression and activity on the protein level of HMGCS2, the gene that controls the anabolic ketogenic pathway in breast cancer. Here we have shown for the first time that HMGCS2 was up-regulated in ADCIS and IAC and only rarely found in non-apocrine breast carcinoma (Figure 6). Notably, HMGCS2 expression is retained by all the IACs from our morphologically-defined cohort. This stresses the potential value of HMGCS2 as a breast apocrine cancer biomarker, since other apocrine differentiation markers such as 15-PGDH, ACSM1 and HMGCR reported by us previously, are expressed consistently in benign apocrine lesions

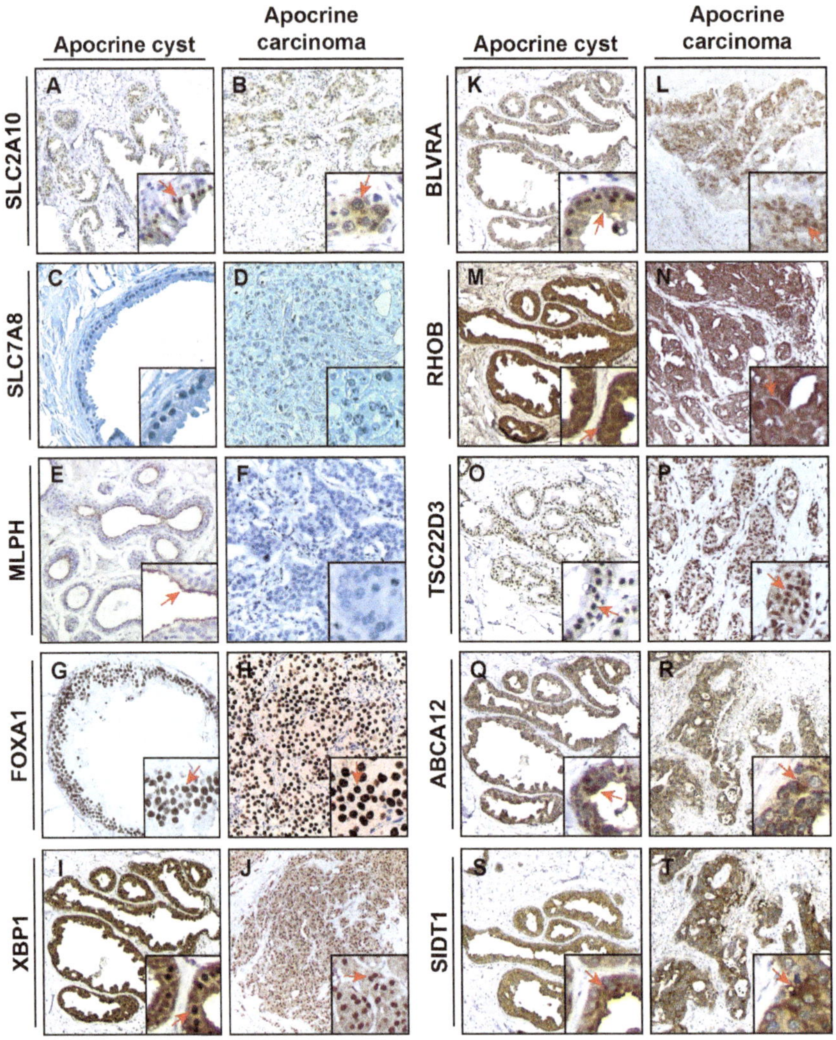

Figure 7. Immunohistochemical analysis of molecular apocrine markers derived from trancriptomics data within the apocrine cyst and carcinoma dataset. Representative staining of FFPE of apocrine cysts and IACs with antibodies against SLC2A10 (Glucose transporter type 10, sections A and B) - cytoplasmic immunoreactivity; SLC7A8 (L-type amino acid transporter 2, sections C and D) - mainly cytoplasmic and membranous immunereactivity; MLPH (Melanophilin, sections E and F) - cytoplasmic and luminal membranous immunoreactivity; FOXA1 (Hepatocyte nuclear factor 3-alpha, sections G and H) – nuclear staining; XBP1 (X-box-binding protein 1, sections I and J) – mainly nuclear and cytoplasmic immunereactivity; BLVRA (Biliverdin reductase A, sections K and L) - cytoplasmic immunoreactivity which combined with rare nuclear positivity; RHOB (Rho-related GTP-binding protein RhoB, sections M and N) - cytoplasmic immunoreactivity; TSC22D3 (TSC22 domain family protein 3, sections O and P) - mainly nuclear and cytoplasmic immunereactivity; ABCA12 (ATP-binding cassette sub-family A member 12, sections Q and R) - cytoplasmic immunoreactivity and SIDT1 (SID1 transmembrane family member 1, sections I and G) - cytoplasmic immunoreactivity. Magnification: x10. Representative areas are shown in higher magnification (x20) and examples of positive staining are indicated by red arrows.

but are conserved at lower frequencies or even negative in the invasive stages [19]. Recently, Wang and co-authors using Illumina expression array/RT PCR analysis sought to identify risk biomarkers that are specific to ER status of breast cancer and among several others revealed a significant overexpression of HMGCS2 in ER- cases [41]. However, our data did not confirm overexpression of HMGCS2 in ER negative tumors at the protein level: the group of TNBCs displayed only ~2% positives for HMGCS2 (Table S4).

IAC as defined by morphological criteria is often characterized by a specific hormone receptor signature: AR+/ER-/PR- [9,42,43,44,45] that has been proposed as a marker for apocrine–type tumors by Tsutsumi and coauthors, who suggested to include androgen receptor to immunohistochemical criteria [46]. However, several studies reported a significant proportion of AR+/ER-/PR- phenotypes outside breast apocrine malignancy: 59% in HER2+ type and 32% in basal-like tumors [31]; 39% in ER- [47]; 10% in TNBC [10]. Our IHC data revealed only 22 AR+ER-PR- phenotypes out of the 205 non-apocrine samples (10.7%) present almost exclusively in TNBC patients (6) and HER2+ (14) samples. These discrepancies could be in part due to the lack of consistent application of the morphological criteria and the use of different methods and cut-offs values for positivity [9] suggesting that hormonal status AR+/ER-/PR- may not be sufficient to discriminate IAC from other breast cancer subtypes. The results presented here demonstrate for the first time a very high frequency of HMGCS2+/AR+/ER-/PR- phenotype (78,8%) in IAC diagnosed by classical morphological criteria as compared with the non-IAC control set (3%). We suggest that this four-protein signature can categorize breast apocrine carcinoma more

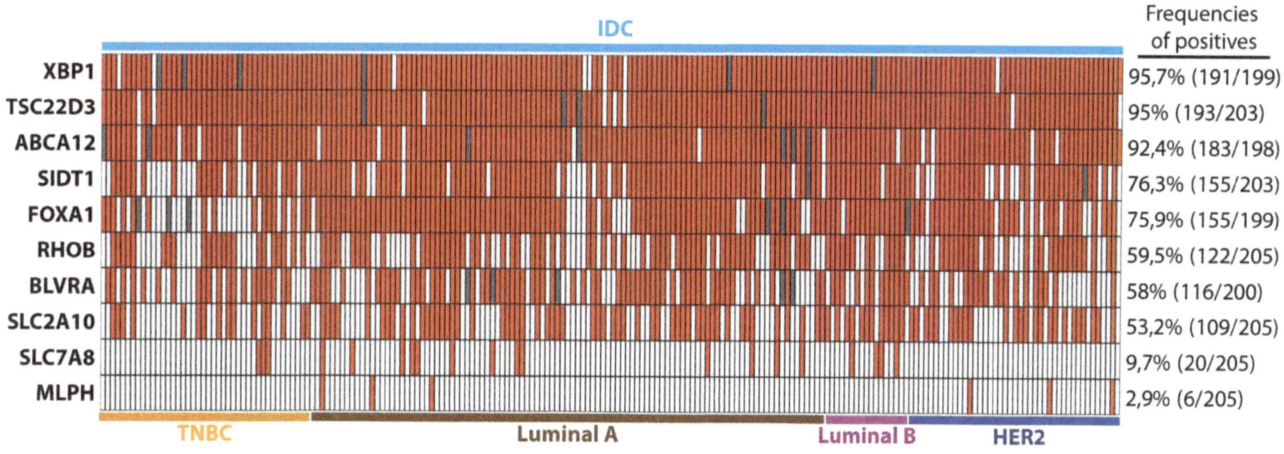

Figure 8. Protein expression profile of transcriptome-derived apocrine markers among breast cancer subtypes. The diagram presents immunohistochemical profiles of four breast tumor subtypes, TNBC, Luminal A Luminal B and HER2, reacted with antibodies against ten transcriptome-derived apocrine markers: XBP1, TSC22D3, ABCA12, SIDT1, FOXA1, RHOB, BLVRA, SLC2A10, SLC7A8 and MLPH. The rows indicate the expression of particular protein in every core in breast cancer TMA (BRC1501, 1502 and 1503; Pantomics INC, USA): red box – positive staining, white box – negative staining grey box – parameter was not determined. Corresponding frequencies of positives are shown on the right side of the diagram. Samples were considered as positive if 10% or more of the cells showed a clear positive staining with the antibodies. IDC = invasive ductal carcinoma; TNBC = triple negative breast cancer. Tumors have been stratified as specified in Materials and Methods.

confidently and supports the contention of a strict definition of pure apocrine carcinomas as it was suggested previously [48].

The identification of differentially expressed proteins that characterize the progression from early benign apocrine lesions to invasive stages opens a window of opportunity for designing and testing new approaches for pharmacological intervention as, for example, 15-hydroxyprostaglandin dehydrogenase (15-PGDH) and 3-hydroxymethylglutaryl-CoA reductase (HMGCR) are currently being targeted for chemoprevention strategies in various malignancies [49,50,51]. HMGCS2 is one of the rate-limiting enzymes controlling generation and re-utilization of ketone bodies [52]. Recently it was shown that ketone bodies support the driving of neoplastic growth which is often accompanied by starvation of all components of tumor environment and it has been speculated that ketone inhibitors can be designed as novel therapeutics to effectively treat advanced cancer patients [53,54]. Consequently, HMGCS2, the enzymes associated with ketone body production and re-utilization, might be considered as new "druggable" targets

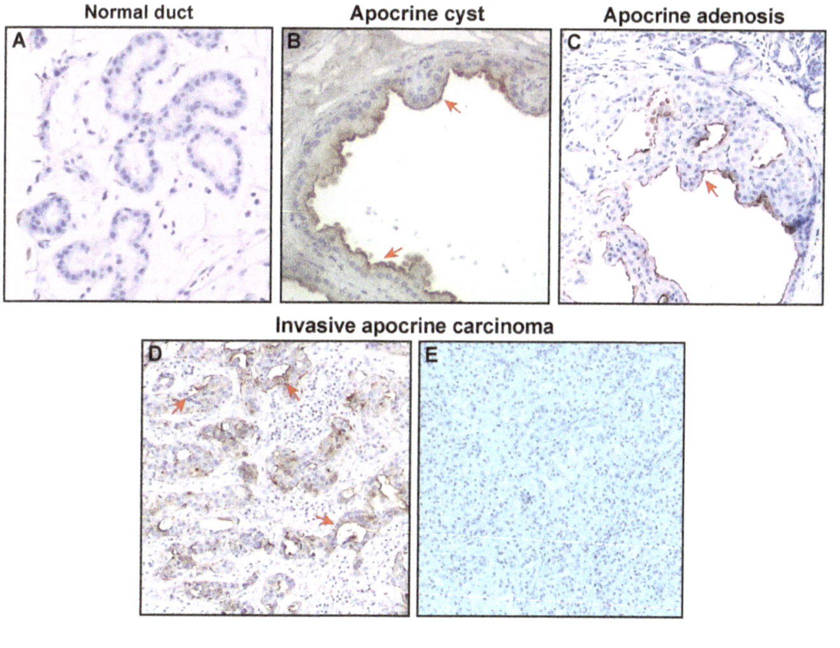

Figure 9. MLPH is expressed by non-malignant apocrine cells but is lost in IACs. Representative images of FFPE sections immunostained with antibody against MLPH. (A) normal ducts, (B) benign apocrine cysts (mainly luminal membranous immunoreactivity), (C) sclerosing adenosis with apocrine differentiation, (D) IAC showing positive immunostaining in pseudo-glands structures (cytoplasmic and luminal membranous immunoreactivity) and (E) IAC with negative immunostaining. Magnification: x20.

for anticancer therapy. Our finding that IACs are characterized by an overexpression of HMGCS2, suggests that the patients diagnosed with apocrine carcinoma might benefit from therapy with HMGCS2 inhibitors. In addition, the high levels of AR expression in the IACs makes this receptor a promising anticancer therapeutic target for this type of breast cancer, but the ability to exploit AR for therapy remains to be challenging [55,56,57,58]. Given that AR and HMGCS2 are both overexpressed in IAC, the use of the dual therapy targeting two parallel AR and HMGCS2 pathways may provide an additional benefit for therapeutic attack of breast apocrine carcinoma. HMGCS2 is the only gene from the breast apocrine protein marker panel identified in our studies that has been included in the molecular apocrine transcriptomic signature [14], and was also found among the genes which transcription was affected by modulation of AR/FOXA1 axis in apocrine cells [59]. It is plausible, based on these findings, to consider this enzyme as a "marker" to indicate an active AR, which can be used to predict which tumors are driven by this receptor and, therefore, capable of being treated with anti-androgen therapy.

To date, there is uncertainty regarding the relationship between molecular apocrine tumors identified by mRNA-array studies [12,13,14] and histopatologically-diagnosed apocrine malignancies. Thus, Lehman-Che and co-authors found only 4 tumors that meet morphological criteria for apocrine tumors among 58 patients diagnosed as "molecular apocrine" [15], suggesting that molecular apocrine subtype is much broader than initially reported by Farmer and co-authors [12]. Apocrine transcriptomic signatures contain several genes related to signaling pathways (RHOB and SIDT1), transcription factors (FOXA1, XBP1, TSC22D3) and transporters (ABCA12, SLC2A10 and SCL7A8) that are not observed in our proteomic signature and therefore were of interest to study. Our reciprocal IHC analysis of a set of 10 proteins selected from the major top candidates of molecular apocrine signature: FOXA1, XBP1, BLVRA, ABCA12, SIDT1, MLPH, RHOB, TSC22D3, SLC2A10 and SLC7A8 has revealed only one protein, melanopholin (MLPH), an adapter protein involved in melanosome transport to cell periphery [60], which expression was specific for benign apocrine lesions, but was lost in invasive stages. Most of other selected candidates were expressed on protein level at different frequencies among non-IAC samples, presumably because their function is related to housekeeping tasks. The differences in concentration of mRNAs and proteins within a cell is on average from 17 to over 50,000 copies, respectively [61], and most studies agree that mRNA levels can explain only about 30–60% of protein abundance, so regulation of post-transcription, translation and protein processing contribute as much to variation in protein concentrations as transcription and transcript degradation do [62]. On the contrary, as we have seen for HMGCS2 and FABP7, and previously for 15-PGDH, HMGCR, ACSM1 and other proteins [2,16], the secondary metabolism of lipids, amino acids and carbohydrates is strongly represented in apocrine cells, providing a clear cut differentiation from other cell types of the breast. Therefore, the unique metabolic identity of the apocrine cells has offered so far the best candidates to identify IAC biomarkers.

In conclusion, HMGCS2 and FABP7 are novel protein markers for apocrine differentiation that are highly conserved among apocrine breast tumors retaining their expression during tumor progression. Inclusion of these markers into the protein signature described previously: 15-PGDH, ACSM1 as well as markers that are consistently expressed (AR, CD24) or not present (ER alpha, PR, Bcl-2, and GATA-3) in benign apocrine lesions [19,28] may categorize ADCISs and IACs with far more accuracy. Combination of HMGCS2 with steroidal profile (AR+/ER-/PR-) offers greater sensitivity to detect breast apocrine tumors compared to steroidal profile alone. Moreover, HMGCS2 widespread expression among IACs makes it a candidate to be studied as potential therapeutic target for this malignancy. Integration of proteomic and transcriptomic technologies applied to apocrine breast cancers may offer complementary information about the particular biology of this tumor subtype and the identification of biomarkers and therapeutic targets of clinical importance.

Materials and Methods

Sample collection and handling

Tissue samples from 412 high risk breast cancer patients that underwent breast surgery were obtained from the Department of Pathology, Rigshospitalet, Copenhagen University Hospital between 2003 and 2014. The criteria for high risk cancer applied by the Danish Cooperative Breast Cancer Group (www.dbcg.dk) are age below 35 years old, and/or tumor diameter of more than 20 mm, and/or histological malignancy grade 2 or 3, and/or negative estrogen and progesterone receptor status, and/or positive axillary status. All patients did not receive preoperative treatment. The samples were routinely collected within about 30–45 min from the time of surgical excision. To evaluate the content of tumor cells and the ration of tumor/stroma the hematoxylin/eosin stained slides were prepared and reviewed by two researches (IIG and M-L T). The age range was 32–84 with a mean average of 59 years. All 412 samples collected during the above period were subjected to 2D PAGE analysis. The samples were placed in dry ice and were rapidly transported to the Danish Cancer Society Research Center where they were stored at −80°C. Apocrine carcinoma was morphologically defined as a carcinoma in which more than 90% of the tumor cells showed typical apocrine features. TNBC, Luminal B and HER2+ tumor subtypes were defined in accordance with St. Galen classification [63]. The project was approved (KF 01-069/03) by the Copenhagen and Frederiksberg regional division of the Danish National Committee on Biomedical Research Ethics. The written informed consent from the donor was obtained for the use of the samples in research. In addition, one set of specific samples comprising 14 ADCISs and 33 IACs diagnosed between 1997 and 2001 used in this study have been described in previous publications [21,29]. Breast cancer tissue microarray slides were obtained from Pantomics (BRC1501, BRC1502 and BRC1503 Pantomics Inc., CA, USA). The TMAs contain of 210 non overlapping breast tumors in total.

Antibodies

The polyclonal antibody raised against synthetic peptides of human FABP7 (HPA028825), BLVRA (HPA042865), ABCA12 (HPA043194), SIDT1 (HPA035862), MLPH (HPA014685) were purchased from Atlas Antibodies and were used in IHC at a dilution of 1:200, 1:100, 1:500, 1:50 and 1:100 respectively in accordance to the manufacturer instructions. The polyclonal antibody against HMGCS2 (XW-7255) was obtained from BioSite (Sweden) and was used in IHC at a dilution of 1:500. The polyclonal antibody raised against synthetic peptides of human FOXA1 (ab23738), XBP1 (ab37152) and RHOB (ab75064) were purchased from Abcam and were used in IHC at a dilution of 1:400, 1:300 and 1:2000 respectively. The polyclonal antibody against SLC2A10 (LS-B1622) and monoclonal antibodies against TSC22D3 (LS-B4313) were purchased from LSBio and were used in IHC at a dilution 1:2000 and 1:2000 respectively. The polyclonal antibody raised against synthetic peptide of human SLC7A8 (BMP041) was obtained from MBL and was used in IHC at a dilution 1:500. All dilutions were used according to the manufacturer's instruction. The antibodies against 15-PGDH, ACSM1, GCDRP15, ER, PR, AR, HER2, 15-PGDH, ASCM1, CD24, Bcl2 and GATA3 are described in our previous studies [19,28].

2D PAGE and 2D Western immunoblotting

Twenty to thirty, 6 µm cryostat sections of frozen tissues were resuspended in 0.1 ml lysis solution [64] or CLB1 buffer [65]. The resulting lysates were frozen and kept at −20°C until used [66]. Twenty to forty µl were applied to the gels and each sample was run at least in duplicate. The first and last sections of each sample were used for IHC analysis using cytokeratin 19 (CK19) antibodies to trace possible changes in epithelial cell pattern during tissue sectioning. (CK19 is ubiquitously expressed by mammary epithelial cells [67,68] and can serve as an additional control for the sample quality. 2D PAGE (isoelectric focusing, IEF), silver staining and 2D gel Western blotting were performed as previously described [69].

Image analysis

For comparative proteomic analysis 2D gels were scanned and analyzed using the PDQUEST software package from BioRad (version 8.0.1). All detected proteins were identified by mass spectrometry (see below), selected for the comparative analysis and added to the master image.

Mass spectrometry analysis

Protein spots were excised from silver stained dry gels and the gel pieces were re-hydrated in water. Gel pieces were detached from the cellophane film and cut into 1 mm^2 pieces followed by "in-gel" digestion as previously described [70] followed by a procedure that has been reported previously [71]. Briefly, MALDI-TOF-TOF data were acquired using an Ultraflex III 200 time-of-flight mass spectrometer (Bruker Daltonik, Germany) equipped with a Smart beam laser and a LIFT-TOF/TOF unit. Data acquisition and data processing were performed by the Flex Control 3.0 and Flex Analysis 3.0 software (Bruker Daltonik, Germany). All of the spectra were obtained using reflector positive mode with an acceleration voltage of 25 kV, reflector voltage of 26.38 kV and detection suppressed up to 450 Da. A total of 2000 shots in steps of 200 shots were added to one spectrum in the mass range of *m/z* 600–4000. Spectral analysis and protein identification were performed as described previously. Protein identifications were considered to be confident when the protein score of the hit exceeded the threshold significance score of 65 ($p<0.05$) and no less than 6 peptides were recognized.

Immunohistochemistry

The procedures for IHC have been described in detail in previous publications [2,21,29]. For FABP7 and HMGCS2 we used the following cut-off values: ADCIS: positive if 60% or more of the CIS contained at least 30% of the cells reacting with the antibodies. IACs: positive if 30% or more of the invasive cells reacted with the antibodies. The cut-off values for ER, PR, AR, HER2, 15-PGDH, ASCM1, CD24, Bcl2 and GATA3 are used as described previously [19]. For XBP1, TSC22D3, ABCA12, SIDT1, FOXA1, RHOB, BLVRA, SLC2A10, SLC7A8 and MLPH we used the following cut-off values: positive if 10% or more of the cells showed a clear positive staining with the antibodies. TMAs were analysed by scoring of up to 5 separate areas per single core and the intensities were averaged to generate a summary score (percentage of cells stained, intensity). Frequency distribution analyses were performed on GraphPad Prism 5 software (GraphPad Software, Inc, San Diego, CA, USA) using Fisher's exact test, considering a P value <0.05 as statistically significant. Immunohistochemical profiles were constructed using Multiexperiment Viewer MeV [72].

Immunofluorescence on paraffin sections

Five-µm sections cut from paraffin blocks of breast tissue samples were mounted on Super Frost Plus slides (Menzel-Gläser, Braunschweig, Germany), baked at 60°C for 60 min, deparaffinized, and rehydrated through graded alcohol rinses. Heat induced antigen retrieval was performed by immersing the slides in Tris/EDTA pH 9.0 buffer (10 mM Tris, 1 mM EDTA) and microwaving in a 750 W microwave oven for 8 min. Following antigen retrieval sections were treated with Image-iT FX signal enhancer (Molecular Probes, USA) to block non-specific staining and subsequently incubated with the relevant primary antibodies at appropriate dilutions. Detection of immune complexes was done with species specific secondary antibodies conjugated to Alexa Fluor 488 and Alexa Fluor 594 (Molecular Probes, OR, USA). Nuclear material was counterstained with TO-PRO-3. The sections were washed three times with cold phosphate-buffered saline (PBS) between incubations. Normal rabbit or mouse serum instead of primary antibody was used as a negative control. Sections were imaged using a laser scanning microscope (Zeiss LSM510Meta) as previously described [73].

IHC blocking with recombinant FABP7 and HMGCS2

The human recombinant FABP7 (H00002173) and HMGCS2 (H00003158) proteins were purchased from Abnova (USA). The appropriate amount of corresponding antibodies (see above) were diluted in TBS buffer to the final volume needed for staining of two section slides and divided equally. The blocking recombinant proteins FABP7 and HMGCS2 were added to a final concentration 5 µg/ml providing approximately 5-fold molar excess of blocking peptide. Tubes containing either pure antibody or the antibody mixed with corresponding recombinant protein were incubated at room temperature for 1 hr with agitation. Two identical tissue sections were probed with the blocked antibody and antibody alone as described in the Immunohistochemistry section.

Breast cancer cell lines

Human breast cancer cell line MDA-MB-453 was obtained from the American Type Culture Collection (ATCC, Manassas, VA, USA). Cells were cultured in Dulbecco's modified Eagle's medium (DMEM, Gibco-BRL, Invitrogen, Carlsbad, CA, USA) supplemented with 10% fetal bovine serum (FBS) at 37°C in a humidifed CO_2 incubator. The cell pellet from exponentially growing breast cancer cells was collected by centrifugation at 1000 g to prepare the FFPE block. IHC staining was performed as described above.

Supporting Information

Figure S1 Validation of anti-FABP7 antibodies specificity towards highly homologous members of human fatty acid-binding protein family. (A) 2D silver stained gel of proteins extracted from tumor tissue obtained from TNBC patient

22. (B) Zoomed fraction of area shown in (A) by dash rectangle. Four members of FABP family, namely, FABP3, FABP4, FABP5 and FABP7 are indicated by red. Several other neighboring proteins are indicated as references. The identity of all proteins was determined by mass spectrometry analysis. (C) 2D Western blot of 2D gel shown in (A). Only the fraction of blot image corresponding to the area shown in (B) is presented. The antibodies recognize only FABP7 but do not cross react with FABP3, FABP4 and FABP5.

Figure S2 Immunohistochemical expression analysis of FABP7 and HMGCS2 in MDA-MB-453 cell line. The FFPE sections from breast cancer cell line MDA-MB-453 were immunostained with antibodies against FABP7, HMGCS2, 15-PGDH, ACSM1 and GCDFP-15. Magnification: x20.

Table S1 Expression of FABP7 and HMGCS2 in 28 normal breast lesions adjacient to tumor.

Table S2 Expression of FABP7 and HMGCS2 in 13 breast apocrine cysts.

Table S3 Expression of FABP7, HMGCS2 and several other markers by 14 ADCISs.

Table S4 Expression of FABP7, HMGCS2 and several other markers by 33 IACs.

Table S5 Expression of FABP7, HMGCS 2 and several other markers in various nonapocrine breast tumors as determined by IHC of TMA array (Pantomics 1501, 1502 and 1503).

Acknowledgments

We would like to thank Anni Handesten and Maria Grønvig Nielsen for expert technical assistance.

Author Contributions

Conceived and designed the experiments: PG JAE JMAM IG. Performed the experiments: PG JAE JMAM MLT IG. Analyzed the data: PG JAE MLT NH NK IG. Contributed reagents/materials/analysis tools: MLT NH NK VTW. Wrote the paper: PG JAE NK VTW MLT JMAM IG.

References

1. O'Malley FP, Bane A (2008) An update on apocrine lesions of the breast. Histopathology 52: 3–10.
2. Celis JE, Gromov P, Cabezon T, Moreira JM, Friis E, et al. (2008) 15-prostaglandin dehydrogenase expression alone or in combination with ACSM1 defines a subgroup of the apocrine molecular subtype of breast carcinoma. Mol Cell Proteomics 7: 1795–1809.
3. Dellapasqua S, Maisonneuve P, Viale G, Pruneri G, Mazzarol G, et al. (2013) Immunohistochemically defined subtypes and outcome of apocrine breast cancer. Clin Breast Cancer 13: 95–102.
4. Lakhani SR, Ellis IO, Schnitt SJ, Tan PH, van de Vijver MJ (2012) World Helath Organisation Classification of Tumours of the Breast. 4th edn, Lyon, France: IARC Press.
5. Japaze H, Emina J, Diaz C, Schwam RJ, Gercovich N, et al. (2005) 'Pure' invasive apocrine carcinoma of the breast: a new clinicopathological entity? Breast 14: 3–10.
6. Page DL (2005) Apocrine carcinomas of the breast. Breast 14: 1–2.
7. Wells CA, El-Ayat GA (2007) Non-operative breast pathology: apocrine lesions. J Clin Pathol 60: 1313–1320.
8. Tanaka K, Imoto S, Wada N, Sakemura N, Hasebe K (2008) Invasive apocrine carcinoma of the breast: clinicopathologic features of 57 patients. Breast J 14: 164–168.
9. Vranic S, Schmitt F, Sapino A, Costa JL, Reddy S, et al. (2013) Apocrine carcinoma of the breast: A comprehensive review. Histol Histopathol 28: 1393–1409.
10. Niemeier LA, Dabbs DJ, Beriwal S, Striebel JM, Bhargava R (2010) Androgen receptor in breast cancer: expression in estrogen receptor-positive tumors and in estrogen receptor-negative tumors with apocrine differentiation. Mod Pathol 23: 205–212.
11. Perou CM, Sorlie T, Eisen MB, van de Rijn M, Jeffrey SS, et al. (2000) Molecular portraits of human breast tumours. Nature 406: 747–752.
12. Farmer P, Bonnefoi H, Becette V, Tubiana-Hulin M, Fumoleau P, et al. (2005) Identification of molecular apocrine breast tumours by microarray analysis. Oncogene 24: 4660–4671.
13. Doane AS, Danso M, Lal P, Donaton M, Zhang L, et al. (2006) An estrogen receptor-negative breast cancer subset characterized by a hormonally regulated transcriptional program and response to androgen. Oncogene 25: 3994–4008.
14. Sanga S, Broom BM, Cristini V, Edgerton ME (2009) Gene expression meta-analysis supports existence of molecular apocrine breast cancer with a role for androgen receptor and implies interactions with ErbB family. BMC Med Genomics 2: 59.
15. Lehmann-Che J, Hamy AS, Porcher R, Barritault M, Bouhidel F, et al. (2013) Molecular apocrine breast cancers are aggressive estrogen receptor negative tumors overexpressing either HER2 or GCDFP15. Breast Cancer Res 15: R37.
16. Celis JE, Gromov P, Moreira JM, Cabezon T, Friis E, et al. (2006) Apocrine cysts of the breast: biomarkers, origin, enlargement, and relation with cancer phenotype. Mol Cell Proteomics 5: 462–483.
17. Celis JE, Gromova I, Cabezon T, Gromov P, Shen T, et al. (2007) Identification of a subset of breast carcinomas characterized by expression of cytokeratin 15: relationship between CK15+ progenitor/amplified cells and pre-malignant lesions and invasive disease. Mol Oncol 1: 321–349.
18. Celis JE, Moreira JM, Gromova I, Cabezon T, Gromov P, et al. (2007) Characterization of breast precancerous lesions and myoepithelial hyperplasia in sclerosing adenosis with apocrine metaplasia. Mol Oncol 1: 97–119.
19. Celis JE, Cabezon T, Moreira JM, Gromov P, Gromova I, et al. (2009) Molecular characterization of apocrine carcinoma of the breast: validation of an apocrine protein signature in a well-defined cohort. Mol Oncol 3: 220–237.
20. Elayat G, Selim AG, Wells CA (2009) Alterations of the cell cycle regulators cyclin D1, cyclin A, p27, p21, p16, and pRb in apocrine metaplasia of the breast. Breast J 15: 475–482.
21. Honma N, Takubo K, Akiyama F, Sawabe M, Arai T, et al. (2005) Expression of GCDFP-15 and AR decreases in larger or node-positive apocrine carcinomas of the breast. Histopathology 47: 195–201.
22. Guedj M, Marisa L, de Reynies A, Orsetti B, Schiappa R, et al. (2011) A refined molecular taxonomy of breast cancer. Oncogene 31: 1196–1206.
23. Cabezon T, Gromova I, Gromov P, Serizawa R, Timmermans Wielenga V, et al. (2013) Proteomic profiling of triple-negative breast carcinomas in combination with a three-tier orthogonal technology approach identifies Mage-A4 as potential therapeutic target in estrogen receptor negative breast cancer. Mol Cell Proteomics 12: 381–394.
24. Rogowska-Wrzesinska A, Le Bihan MC, Thaysen-Andersen M, Roepstorff P (2013) 2D gels still have a niche in proteomics. J Proteomics 88: 4–13.
25. Kostiuk MA, Keller BO, Berthiaume LG (2010) Palmitoylation of ketogenic enzyme HMGCS2 enhances its interaction with PPARalpha and transcription at the Hmgcs2 PPRE. FASEB Journal 24: 1914–1924.
26. Grimsrud PA, Carson JJ, Hebert AS, Hubler SL, Niemi NM, et al. (2012) A quantitative map of the liver mitochondrial phosphoproteome reveals post-translational control of ketogenesis. Cell Metabolism 16: 672–683.
27. Smathers RL, Petersen DR (2011) The human fatty acid-binding protein family: evolutionary divergences and functions. Human genomics 5: 170–191.
28. Celis JE, Gromova I, Gromov P, Moreira JM, Cabezon T, et al. (2006) Molecular pathology of breast apocrine carcinomas: a protein expression signature specific for benign apocrine metaplasia. FEBS Letters 580: 2935–2944.
29. Honma N, Takubo K, Akiyama F, Kasumi F, Sawabe M, et al. (2007) Expression of oestrogen receptor-beta in apocrine carcinomas of the breast. Histopathology 50: 425–433.
30. Honma N, Takubo K, Arai T, Younes M, Kasumi F, et al. (2006) Comparative study of monoclonal antibody B72.3 and gross cystic disease fluid protein-15 as markers of apocrine carcinoma of the breast. APMIS 114: 712–719.
31. Collins LC, Cole KS, Marotti JD, Hu R, Schnitt SJ, et al. (2011) Androgen receptor expression in breast cancer in relation to molecular phenotype: results from the Nurses' Health Study. Mod Pathol 24: 924–931.
32. Naderi A, Hughes-Davies L (2008) A functionally significant cross-talk between androgen receptor and ErbB2 pathways in estrogen receptor negative breast cancer. Neoplasia 10: 542–548.
33. Chia KM, Liu J, Francis GD, Naderi A (2011) A feedback loop between androgen receptor and ERK signaling in estrogen receptor-negative breast cancer. Neoplasia 13: 154–166.
34. de Longueville F, Lacroix M, Barbuto AM, Bertholet V, Gallo D, et al. (2005) Molecular characterization of breast cancer cell lines by a low-density microarray. International journal of oncology 27: 881–892.

35. Vranic S, Gatalica Z, Wang ZY (2011) Update on the molecular profile of the MDA-MB-453 cell line as a model for apocrine breast carcinoma studies. Oncology letters 2: 1131–1137.
36. Tang XY, Umemura S, Tsukamoto H, Kumaki N, Tokuda Y, et al. (2010) Overexpression of fatty acid binding protein-7 correlates with basal-like subtype of breast cancer. Pathol Res Pract 206: 98–101.
37. Zhang H, Rakha EA, Ball GR, Spiteri I, Aleskandarany M, et al. (2010) The proteins FABP7 and OATP2 are associated with the basal phenotype and patient outcome in human breast cancer. Breast Cancer Res Treat 121: 41–51.
38. Alshareeda AT, Rakha EA, Nolan CC, Ellis IO, Green AR (2012) Fatty acid binding protein 7 expression and its sub-cellular localization in breast cancer. Breast Cancer Res Treat 134: 519–529.
39. Liang Y, Bollen AW, Aldape KD, Gupta N (2006) Nuclear FABP7 immunoreactivity is preferentially expressed in infiltrative glioma and is associated with poor prognosis in EGFR-overexpressing glioblastoma. BMC Cancer 6: 97.
40. Kaloshi G, Mokhtari K, Carpentier C, Taillibert S, Lejeune J, et al. (2007) FABP7 expression in glioblastomas: relation to prognosis, invasion and EGFR status. Journal of neuro-oncology 84: 245–248.
41. Wang J, Scholtens D, Holko M, Ivancic D, Lee O, et al. (2013) Lipid metabolism genes in contralateral unaffected breast and estrogen receptor status of breast cancer. Cancer Prev Res (Phila) 6: 321–330.
42. Gatalica Z (1997) Immunohistochemical analysis of apocrine breast lesions. Consistent over-expression of androgen receptor accompanied by the loss of estrogen and progesterone receptors in apocrine metaplasia and apocrine carcinoma in situ. Pathol Res Pract 193: 753–758.
43. Sapp M, Malik A, Hanna W (2003) Hormone receptor profile of apocrine lesions of the breast. Breast J 9: 335–336.
44. Iggo RD (2011) New insights into the role of androgen and oestrogen receptors in molecular apocrine breast tumours. Breast Cancer Res 13: 318.
45. Sasahara M, Matsui A, Ichimura Y, Hirakata Y, Murata Y, et al. (2014) Overexpression of Androgen Receptor and Forkhead-box A1 Protein in Apocrine Breast Carcinoma. Anticancer Res 34: 1261–1267.
46. Tsutsumi Y (2012) Apocrine carcinoma as triple-negative breast cancer: novel definition of apocrine-type carcinoma as estrogen/progesterone receptor-negative and androgen receptor-positive invasive ductal carcinoma. Jpn J Clin Oncol 42: 375–386.
47. Moinfar F, Okcu M, Tsybrovskyy O, Regitnig P, Lax SF, et al. (2003) Androgen receptors frequently are expressed in breast carcinomas: potential relevance to new therapeutic strategies. Cancer 98: 703–711.
48. Vranic S, Tawfik O, Palazzo J, Bilalovic N, Eyzaguirre E, et al. (2010) EGFR and HER-2/neu expression in invasive apocrine carcinoma of the breast. Mod Pathol 23: 644–653.
49. Edwards TL, Shrubsole MJ, Cai Q, Li G, Dai Q, et al. (2012) A study of prostaglandin pathway genes and interactions with current nonsteroidal anti-inflammatory drug use in colorectal adenoma. Cancer Prev Res (Phila) 5: 855–863.
50. Vainio P, Gupta S, Ketola K, Mirtti T, Mpindi JP, et al. (2011) Arachidonic acid pathway members PLA2G7, HPGD, EPHX2, and CYP4F8 identified as putative novel therapeutic targets in prostate cancer. Am J Pathol 178: 525–536.
51. Yeganeh B, Wiechec E, Ande SR, Sharma P, Moghadam AR, et al. (2014) Targeting the mevalonate cascade as a new therapeutic approach in heart disease, cancer and pulmonary disease. Pharmacol Ther.
52. Girard J, Ferre P, Pegorier JP, Duee PH (1992) Adaptations of glucose and fatty acid metabolism during perinatal period and suckling-weaning transition. Physiol Rev 72: 507–562.
53. Martinez-Outschoorn UE, Lin Z, Whitaker-Menezes D, Howell A, Lisanti MP, et al. (2012) Ketone bodies and two-compartment tumor metabolism: stromal ketone production fuels mitochondrial biogenesis in epithelial cancer cells. Cell Cycle 11: 3956–3963.
54. Martinez-Outschoorn UE, Lin Z, Whitaker-Menezes D, Howell A, Sotgia F, et al. (2012) Ketone body utilization drives tumor growth and metastasis. Cell Cycle 11: 3964–3971.
55. Garay JP, Park BH (2012) Androgen receptor as a targeted therapy for breast cancer. Am J Cancer Res 2: 434–445.
56. Gasparini P, Fassan M, Cascione L, Guler G, Balci S, et al. (2014) Androgen receptor status is a prognostic marker in non-basal triple negative breast cancers and determines novel therapeutic options. PLoS ONE 9: e88525.
57. Lakis S, Kotoula V, Eleftheraki AG, Batistatou A, Bobos M, et al. (2014) The androgen receptor as a surrogate marker for molecular apocrine breast cancer subtyping. Breast 23: 234–243.
58. Safarpour D, Pakneshan S, Tavassoli FA (2014) Androgen receptor (AR) expression in 400 breast carcinomas: is routine AR assessment justified? Am J Cancer Res 4: 353–368.
59. Robinson JL, Macarthur S, Ross-Innes CS, Tilley WD, Neal DE, et al. (2011) Androgen receptor driven transcription in molecular apocrine breast cancer is mediated by FoxA1. The EMBO journal 30: 3019–3027.
60. Sckolnick M, Krementsova EB, Warshaw DM, Trybus KM (2013) More than just a cargo adapter, melanophilin prolongs and slows processive runs of myosin Va. J Biol Chem 288: 29313–29322.
61. Schwanhausser B, Busse D, Li N, Dittmar G, Schuchhardt J, et al. (2011) Global quantification of mammalian gene expression control. Nature 473: 337–342.
62. Vogel C, Marcotte EM (2012) Insights into the regulation of protein abundance from proteomic and transcriptomic analyses. Nature reviews Genetics: 227–232.
63. Goldhirsch A, Wood WC, Coates AS, Gelber RD, Thurlimann B, et al. (2011) Strategies for subtypes—dealing with the diversity of breast cancer: highlights of the St. Gallen International Expert Consensus on the Primary Therapy of Early Breast Cancer 2011. Annals of oncology: official journal of the European Society for Medical Oncology/ESMO 22: 1736–1747.
64. O'Farrell PH (1975) High resolution two-dimensional electrophoresis of proteins. J Biol Chem 250: 4007–4021.
65. Gromov P, Celis JE, Gromova I, Rank F, Timmermans-Wielenga V, et al. (2008) A single lysis solution for the analysis of tissue samples by different proteomic technologies. Mol Oncol 2: 368–379.
66. Celis JE, Trentemølle S, Gromov P (2006) Gel-Based Proteomics: High-Resolution Two-Dimensional Gel Electrophoresis of Proteins. Isoelectric Focusing (IEF) and Nonequilibrium pH Gradient Electrophoresis (NEPHGE). In: Celis JE, Carter N, Hunter T, Simons K, Small JV, et al., editors. A Cell Biology Laboratory Handbook. 3rd Edition ed: Elsevier. pp. 165–174.
67. Moll R (1998) Cytokeratins as markers of differentiation in the diagnosis of epithelial tumors. Subcell Biochem 31: 205–262.
68. Bartek J, Bartkova J, Taylor-Papadimitriou J (1990) Keratin 19 expression in the adult and developing human mammary gland. Histochem J 22: 537–544.
69. Gromova I, Celis JE (2006) Protein Detection in Gels by Silver Staining: A procedure Compatible with Mass Spectrometry. In: Celis JE, Carter N, Hunter T, Simons K, Small JV, et al., editors. A Cell Biology Laboratory Handbook. 3rd Edition ed: Elsevier. pp. 219–223.
70. Shevchenko A, Wilm M, Vorm O, Mann M (1996) Mass spectrometric sequencing of proteins silver-stained polyacrylamide gels. Anal Chem 68: 850–858.
71. Gromov P, Gromova I, Bunkenborg J, Cabezon T, Moreira JM, et al. (2010) Up-regulated proteins in the fluid bathing the tumour cell microenvironment as potential serological markers for early detection of cancer of the breast. Mol Oncol 4: 65–89.
72. Saeed AI, Bhagabati NK, Braisted JC, Liang W, Sharov V, et al. (2006) TM4 microarray software suite. Methods in enzymology 411: 134–193.
73. Moreira JM, Ohlsson G, Rank FE, Celis JE (2005) Down-regulation of the tumor suppressor protein 14-3-3sigma is a sporadic event in cancer of the breast. Mol Cell Proteomics 4: 555–569.

8

Blood Levels of S-100 Calcium-Binding Protein B, High-Sensitivity C-Reactive Protein, and Interleukin-6 for Changes in Depressive Symptom Severity after Coronary Artery Bypass Grafting: Prospective Cohort Nested within a Randomized, Controlled Trial

Daniel M. Pearlman[1,2], Jeremiah R. Brown[2,3,4], Todd A. MacKenzie[2,3,4], Felix Hernandez Jr.[5], Souhel Najjar[1]*

1 Neuroinflammation Research Group, Epilepsy Center Division, Department of Neurology, NYU School of Medicine, New York, New York, United States of America, **2** The Dartmouth Institute for Health Policy and Clinical Practice, Audrey and Theodor Geisel School of Medicine at Dartmouth, Hanover, New Hampshire, United States of America, **3** Section of Epidemiology and Biostatistics, Department of Community and Family Medicine, Audrey and Theodor Geisel School of Medicine at Dartmouth, Hanover, New Hampshire, United States of America, **4** Section of Cardiology, Department of Medicine, Audrey and Theodor Geisel School of Medicine at Dartmouth, Hanover, New Hampshire, United States of America, **5** Cardiothoracic Surgery, Eastern Maine Medical Center, Bangor, Maine, United States of America

Abstract

Background: Cross-sectional and retrospective studies have associated major depressive disorder with glial activation and injury as well as blood–brain barrier disruption, but these associations have not been assessed prospectively. Here, we aimed to determine the relationship between changes in depressive symptom severity and in blood levels of S-100 calcium-binding protein B (S-100B), high-sensitivity C-reactive protein, and interleukin-6 following an inflammatory challenge.

Methods: Fifty unselected participants were recruited from a randomized, controlled trial comparing coronary artery bypass grafting procedures performed with versus without cardiopulmonary bypass for the risk of neurocognitive decline. Depressive symptom severity was measured at baseline, discharge, and six-month follow-up using the Beck Depression Inventory II (BDI-II). The primary outcome of the present biomarker study was acute change in depressive symptom severity, defined as the intra-subject difference between baseline and discharge BDI-II scores. Blood biomarker levels were determined at baseline and 2 days postoperative.

Results: Changes in S-100B levels correlated positively with acute changes in depressive symptom severity (Spearman ρ, 0.62; $P = 0.0004$) and accounted for about one-fourth of their observed variance (R^2, 0.23; $P = 0.0105$). This association remained statistically significant after adjusting for baseline S-100B levels, age, weight, body-mass index, or β-blocker use, but not baseline BDI-II scores ($P = 0.064$). There was no statistically significant association between the primary outcome and baseline S-100B levels, baseline high-sensitivity C-reactive protein or interleukin-6 levels, or changes in high-sensitivity C-reactive protein or interleukin-6 levels. Among most participants, levels of all three biomarkers were normal at baseline and markedly elevated at 2 days postoperative.

Conclusions: Acute changes in depressive symptom severity were specifically associated with incremental changes in S-100B blood levels, largely independent of covariates associated with either. These findings support the hypothesis that glial activation and injury and blood–brain barrier disruption can be mechanistically linked to acute exacerbation of depressive symptoms in some individuals.

Editor: Malú G. Tansey, Emory University, United States of America

Funding: DMP received funding from the Audrey and Theodor Geisel School of Medicine (Hanover, New Hampshire, United States). JRB was supported in part by a grant from the Agency for Healthcare Research and Quality (K01HS018443). For the original randomized, controlled trial (Scarecrow trial, 2001–2004), FH received donated funds, donated supplies, biomarker assays, and loaned equipment from Medtronic Inc. (Minneapolis, Minnesota, United States), Genzyme Surgical (Fall River, Massachusetts, United States), and Somanetics Corporation (Troy, Michigan, United States). FH also received biomarker assays from the Northern New England Cardiovascular Disease Study Group (Hanover, New Hampshire, United States). Loaned equipment included the Genzyme Off-Pump Coronary Artery Bypass (OPCAB) Elite apparatus and the Medtronic Octopus system, both of which used to stabilize target vessels during off-pump coronary artery bypass grafting procedures performed in the trial. The funders had no role in study design, data collection and analysis, decision to publish, or preparation of the manuscript.

Competing Interests: FH discloses that he has a financial relationship with Genzyme Surgical (Fall River, Massachusetts, United States).

* Email: mna1024231@aol.com

Introduction

A large body of evidence substantiates the association between inflammation and major depressive disorder [1–13]. Cross-sectional and retrospective studies of depression have documented microglial activation and proliferation [3,4,14] as well as astroglial loss in biopsied and post-mortem brain tissue [15–18], and increased Th1 proinflammatory cytokines in cerebrospinal fluid (CSF) and blood samples [6–12] (recently reviewed in [1]). In addition, population-level studies identify autoimmune diseases and severe infections as risk factors for depression [19,20]. Prospective etiologic [5,21–31] and treatment studies [3,32–35] have provided some of the most direct evidence supporting the hypothesis that inflammation can be causally related to depressive symptoms. The prototypical etiologic studies in this regard are the so-called inflammation-challenge paradigms, such as interferon-α administration [36]. Among those treated with interferon-α, typically for hepatitis C or cancer, about half experience acute-onset depression in association with systemic inflammatory and neuroimaging abnormalities [5,21–31]. These inflammation-challenge paradigms have also been extended to include orthopedic surgery [37], and more recently–cardiac surgery [38,39], in which the occurrence of a robust systemic inflammatory response is well-established [40].

A related and emerging area of research in psychoimmunology has focused on elucidating the connections among inflammatory abnormalities as well as glial activation and injury and blood–brain barrier disruption in depression [2,3]. Like inflammation, evidence of glial activation and injury in depression has been extensively documented [1]. Despite this, however, and notwithstanding the necessary functions of astroglial–endothelial interactions in maintaining blood–brain barrier integrity [35], only recently has evidence linking blood–brain barrier disruption to depression begun to accumulate [2,3]. Evidence to this effect includes histological and ultrastructural findings in biopsied and post-mortem brain tissue [3,41]; elevated CSF-to-serum albumin ratios [42–44]; reduced flow-mediated dilation (a surrogate of endothelial dysfunction) [45]; increased vascular disease comorbidity [46,47]; and elevated blood levels of endothelial dysfunction biomarkers (e.g., intercellular adhesion molecule 1, vascular adhesion molecule 1, E-selectin, and P-selectin) [48–61].

S-100 calcium-binding protein B (S-100B) is a 10 kDa protein, consisting of 92 amino acids and two EF-hand domains, that is implicated in the pathophysiology of major depressive disorder [55,59,62–71] and various neurological disorders [72–74]. S-100B is produced and secreted by both intracerebral (i.e., mainly astrocytes, and to a lesser degree, oligodendrocytes) and extracerebral sources (e.g., adipocytes and myocytes) [72], and is involved in numerous regulatory and immune pathways [75,76]. Elevated blood S-100B levels are considered a marker of glial activation and injury [72,74,77–87] as well as blood–brain barrier disruption [72,81,88–93], and have been associated with suicidality [56], lower Glasgow Coma Scale scores [73], greater post-concussive symptom severity [74], ictal events [72], and greater risk of postoperative cognitive decline [94–97] (in addition to numerous other clinically significant outcomes). To date, however, no studies have simultaneously assessed the relationships between depression and glial activation and injury, blood–brain barrier disruption, and inflammation using a prospective design. Here, we aimed to address this gap in the literature by evaluating perioperative changes in blood levels of S-100B, high-sensitivity C-reactive protein (hs-CRP), and interleukin-6 for changes in depressive symptom severity in the inflammation-challenge paradigm of cardiac surgery.

Materials and Methods

Design, setting, and participants

This is a prospective cohort study nested within a randomized, controlled trial. An unselected group of 50 participants was recruited from among 201 patients undergoing coronary artery bypass grafting in the context of a randomized, controlled trial comparing conventional vs off-pump procedures for the risk of neurocognitive decline (Scarecrow trial, 2001–2004) [98]. Inclusion criteria were ages 40 to 80 years, clinical indication for urgent or elective coronary artery bypass grafting, referral to the Cardiothoracic Surgery service at Eastern Maine Medical Center (Bangor, Maine, United States), and capacity to provide written informed consent. Exclusion criteria were concomitant surgical procedures, severe calcification of the ascending aorta or deep intra-myocardial left anterior descending coronary artery, recent administration of an inotropic agent in excess of 3 μg/kg/min, requiring a cardiac-assist device for hemodynamic instability, and not providing written informed consent. Details of the surgical and anesthesia protocols used in the trial have been described previously [98]. All participants provided written informed consent. The Institutional Review Board of Eastern Maine Medical Center approved this study.

Biochemical measurements

Blood samples were collected by standard venipuncture at baseline and approximately 2 days postoperative. Upon collection, samples were stored at −80°C and then transferred on dry ice to the Laboratory for Clinical and Biochemical Research (Colchester, Vermont, United States) where S-100B, hs-CRP, and interleukin-6 blood levels were determined in either plasma or serum. Enzyme-linked immunosorbent assays were used to determine S-100B (#364701D, DiaSorin, Bromma, Sweden) and interleukin-6 blood levels (#HS600B, R&D Systems, Minnesota, United States). An automated BNII nephelometer was used to perform an

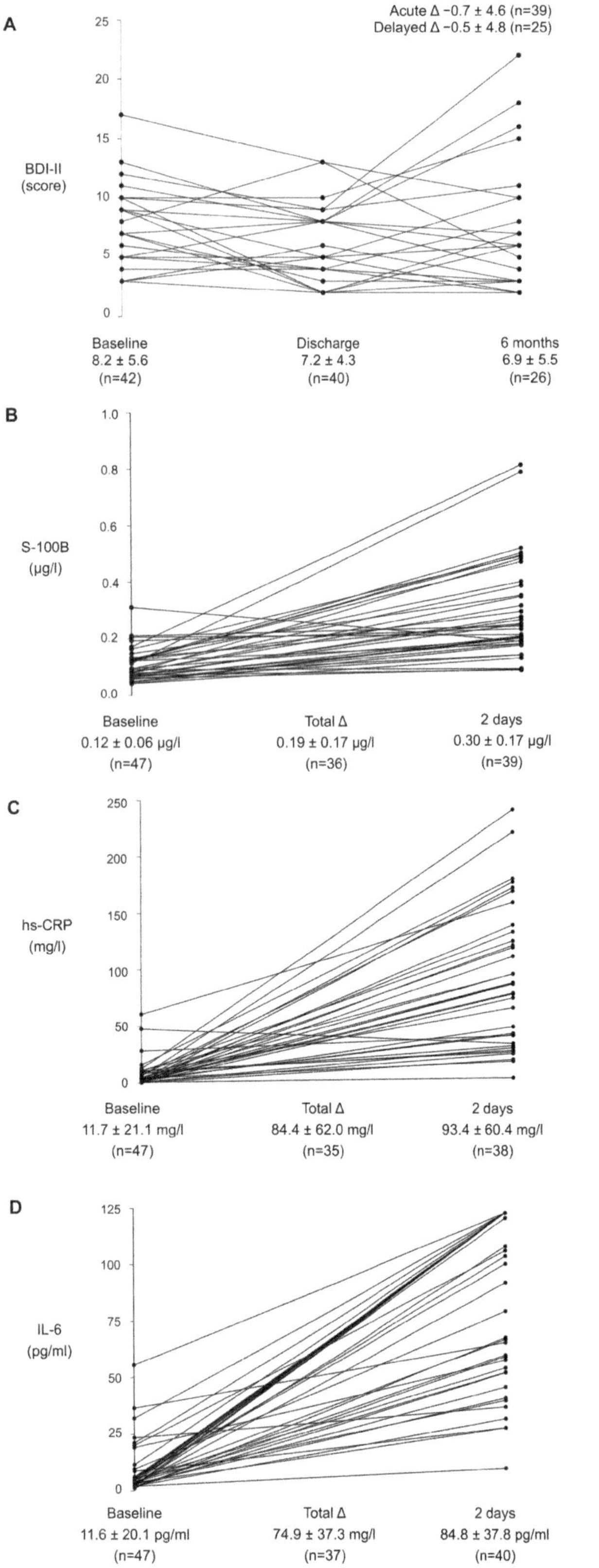

Figure 1. Paired distributions of Beck Depression Inventory II scores and blood biomarker measures. (A) Beck Depression Inventory II scores at baseline, discharge, six-month follow-up; (B) S-100 calcium-binding protein B levels at baseline, 2 days postoperative, and the total change between them; (C) high-sensitivity C-reactive protein levels at baseline 2 days postoperative, and the total change between them; (D) inteleukin-6 levels at baseline 2 days postoperative, and the total change between them. Values given below the x-axis are arithmetic mean ± standard deviation. BDI-II = Beck Depression Inventory II. hs-CRP = high-sensitivity C-reactive protein. IL-6 = interleukin-6. S-100B = S-100 calcium-binding protein B.

immunonephelometric assay to determine hs-CRP blood levels (Siemens Healthcare Diagnostics, Illinois, United States). All laboratory personnel were blinded to participant characteristics and clinical information.

Lower limits of detection were 0.02 µg/l for S-100B, 0.16 mg/l for hs-CRP, and 0.16 pg/ml for interleukin-6. Inter-assay coefficients of variance at baseline and 2 days postoperative were 6.01% and 3.31% for S-100B, 2.93% and 1.82% for hs-CRP, and 7.95% and 8.71% for interleukin-6. In determining S-100B and interleukin-6 blood levels, each sample was run twice, the arithmetic mean of which was taken as the final value. In determining hs-CRP blood levels, each sample was run once, as the assays were automated. The approximate upper limits of normal blood levels for each biomarker are 0.15 µg/l for S-100B, 10.0 mg/l for hs-CRP, and 5.0 pg/ml for interleukin-6. hs-CRP levels less than or equal to 1.0 mg/l are indicative of low risk for ischemic heart disease, 1.0 to 3.0 mg/l moderate risk, and 3.0 to 10.0 mg/l high risk. hs-CRP levels greater than or equal to 10.0 mg/l are indicative of acute systemic inflammation of a non-cardiac origin (e.g., as occurs with infection or cardiac surgery). The change (i.e., intra-subject difference) between blood levels of each biomarker at baseline and 2 days postoperative was computed for each participant. Instances where 2-day postoperative blood levels were greater than baseline levels (for a given biomarker and participant), were considered a positive change (i.e., perioperative increases). Likewise, when 2-day postoperative blood levels were less than baseline levels, this was considered a negative change (i.e., perioperative decreases).

Main outcomes

Depressive symptom severity was assessed at baseline, discharge, and six-month month follow-up using the Beck Depression Inventory II (BDI-II). Scores ranging from 0 to 13 indicate subclinical or minimal depressive symptom severity, 14 to 19 mild, 20 to 28 moderate, and 29 to 63 severe [99]. Participants, family members, treating clinicians, BDI-II test examiners, and all other trial staff in contact with participants were blinded to the results of blood biomarker levels. The primary outcome of the present biomarker study, acute change in depressive symptom severity, was defined as the intra-subject difference between baseline and discharge BDI-II scores. The secondary outcome, delayed change in depressive symptom severity, was defined as the intra-subject difference between baseline and six-month follow-up BDI-II scores.

Statistical analysis

Analyses were done using Stata version 12.1 for Mac (StataCorp, LP. College Station, Texas, United States). Participant characteristics were summarized as the arithmetic mean ± standard deviation for continuous data and frequency and percentage for categorical data. These descriptive statistics were then compared between the biomarker and non-biomarker cohorts that comprised the Scarecrow trial with the use of two-

Table 1. Prospective biomarker cohort, nested within the Scarecrow trial (2001–2004).

	Biomarker cohort (n = 50)	Non-biomarker cohort (n = 151)	P Value*
Age (years)	63.0±8.3	64.2±9.5	0.43
Female	6 (12.0)	34 (22.5)	0.11
Weight (kg)	87.7±12.9	88.3±14.9	0.83
Height (cm)	172.5±9.3	172.8±8.8	0.87
Body-mass index (kg/m^2)	29.5±3.8	29.5±4.2	0.95
History of vascular disease	8 (16.0)	34 (22.5)	0.33
History of diabetes mellitus	17 (34.0)	49 (32.5)	0.84
History of COPD	3 (6.0)	13 (8.6)	0.56
History of smoking	10 (20.0)	28 (18.5)	0.82
Charlson comorbidity index	0.62±0.70	0.77±0.92	0.28
Myocardial infarction†	8 (16.0)	17 (11.3)	0.38
Unstable angina at admission	35 (70.0)	88 (58.3)	0.14
Two-vessel disease	18 (36.0)	43 (28.5)	0.32
Three-vessel disease	27 (54.0)	85 (56.3)	0.78
Left-ventricular ejection fraction (%)‡	61.4±10.8	58.9±13.3	0.25
Troponin T at 24 hours (ng/dl)	0.62±0.61	0.58±1.01	0.77
NYHA class (I-IV)§	1.70±0.83	1.75±0.85	0.75
Serum creatinine (mg/dl)	1.05±0.24	1.15±0.73	0.33
β-blocker	39 (78.0)	112 (74.2)	0.59
ACE-inhibitor	11 (22.0)	49 (32.5)	0.16
Ca^{2+} channel blocker	11 (22.0)	24 (15.9)	0.32
Acetylsalicylic acid†	39 (78.0)	106 (70.2)	0.29
Randomized to off-pump procedure	23 (46.0)	76 (50.3)	0.60
Underwent off-pump procedure	21 (42.0)	70 (46.4)	0.59
Urgent priority procedure	30 (60.0)	95 (62.9)	0.71
Time from baseline to procedure (days)	3.1±3.6	2.6±3.3	0.34
Time from procedure to discharge (days)	6.0±2.6	7.3±4.9	0.08
BDI-II (score), baseline (n = 42; n = 145)	8.2±5.6	9.6±6.9	0.23
BDI-II (score), discharge (n = 40; n = 121)	7.2±4.3	9.8±6.7	0.026
BDI-II (score), 6 months (n = 26; n = 105)	6.9±5.5	7.8±7.4	0.59
BDI-II (score), acute Δ (n = 39; n = 120)‖	−0.7±4.6	0.0±5.4	0.43
BDI-II (score), delayed Δ (n = 25; n = 104)¶	−0.5±4.8	−1.8±5.7	0.29

Values are arithmetic mean ± standard deviation for continuous data, and frequency (percentage) for categorical data. The Scarecrow trial compared CABG performed with vs. without cardiopulmonary bypass for the risk of postoperative neurocognitive decline (defined as a ≥20% reduction on ≥20% of 19 psychometrics) among 201 patients at Eastern Maine Medical Center. Abbreviations: ACE = angiotensin-converting enzyme. CABG = coronary artery bypass grafting. COPD = chronic obstructive pulmonary disease. hs-CRP = high-sensitivity C-reactive protein. NYHA = New York Heart Association. S-100B = S-100 calcium-binding protein B.

*Two-tailed Student t test for continuous data; χ^2 test for categorical data.

†Within 7 days before the index procedure.

‡Missing data for: n = 3; n = 19.

§Missing data for: n = 3; n = 3.

‖Acute Δ refers to the primary outcome, acute change in depressive symptom severity, defined as the intra-subject difference between BDI-II scores at baseline and discharge.

¶Delayed Δ refers to the secondary outcome, delayed change in depressive symptom severity, defined as the intra-subject difference between BDI-II scores at baseline and six-month follow-up.

tailed Student t tests for continuous data and Cochran–Mantel–Haenszel χ^2 tests for categorical data. To identify covariates of blood biomarker measures at baseline and their differences between baseline and postoperative assessments and/or the main outcomes, Spearman rank correlation coefficients (Spearman ρ) were calculated for all possible two-term combinations, applying the pairwise deletion method for comparisons involving missing data. Participant characteristics that yielded statistically significant

Table 2. Spearman rank correlation coefficients for comparisons between participant characteristics and main outcomes as well as blood biomarker levels.

	BDI-II (score)		S-100B (μg/l)		hs-CRP (mg/l)		IL-6 (pg/ml)	
	Acute Δ	Delayed Δ	Baseline	Total Δ	Baseline	Total Δ	Baseline	Total Δ
	(n = 39)†	(n = 25)‡	(n = 47)	(n = 36)§	(n = 47)	(n = 35)§	(n = 47)	(n = 37)§
Age (years)	0.30	0.04	0.23	0.39*	0.15	–0.35*	0.23	–0.22
Female	0.07	0.05	0.14	0.16	0.08	0.13	0.08	0.12
Weight (kg)	–0.14	–0.05	–0.21	–0.38*	–0.04	0.07	0.00	0.16
Height (cm)	–0.01	0.15	–0.12	–0.06	–0.07	0.10	–0.01	0.10
Body-mass index (kg/m^2)	–0.22	–0.21	–0.15	–0.34*	0.05	–0.01	0.06	0.06
History of vascular disease	–0.04	–0.11	0.07	0.10	–0.08	0.12	0.00	0.08
History of diabetes mellitus	0.03	–0.19	–0.16	–0.07	–0.33*	–0.05	–0.05	–0.10
History of COPD	0.04	0.16	0.11	0.20	–0.21	0.04	–0.08	–0.12
History of smoking	–0.06	0.00	–0.11	0.03	0.08	–0.09	0.10	0.12
Charlson comorbidity index	–0.03	–0.14	–0.06	0.16	–0.37*	0.05	–0.05	0.01
Myocardial infarction‖	–0.15	0.39	–0.04	–0.10	0.34*	0.14	0.42**	0.24
Unstable angina at admission	0.11	–0.09	–0.08	0.15	0.36*	0.14	0.40**	0.23
Two-vessel disease	0.07	–0.20	–0.01	–0.26	0.07	0.02	0.15	0.13
Three-vessel disease	–0.18	0.22	–0.10	0.26	0.02	0.06	–0.14	0.03
Left-ventricular ejection fraction (%)††	–0.08	–0.06	0.17	–0.23	–0.09	–0.19	–0.24	–0.28
Troponin T at 24 hours (ng/dl)	–0.10	0.02	0.30*	0.21	0.30*	–0.21	0.16	–0.14
NYHA class (I-IV)‡‡	0.04	–0.19	0.21	0.29	–0.14	–0.25	0.04	–0.24
Serum creatinine (mg/dl)§§	0.05	–0.05	0.09	–0.02	0.06	–0.08	0.15	–0.09
β-blocker	–0.05	–0.13	0.07	–0.39*	–0.30*	–0.17	–0.20	–0.15
ACE-inhibitor	–0.21	0.04	–0.21	–0.01	–0.22	0.19	–0.06	0.19
Ca^{2+} channel blocker	0.10	0.23	–0.13	0.15	0.20	0.24	–0.21	0.45**
Acetylsalicylic acid†	0.29	0.01	0.12	0.12	–0.05	–0.30	–0.26	–0.21
Randomized to off-pump procedure	0.21	–0.16	–0.39**	–0.01	–0.01	0.50**	–0.05	0.54***
Underwent off-pump procedure	0.26	–0.06	–0.41**	0.02	–0.07	0.50**	–0.09	0.53***
Urgent priority procedure	0.01	0.24	0.19	0.29	0.23	0.00	0.59***	0.10
Time from baseline to procedure (days)	0.02	0.24	0.18	0.34*	0.19	0.00	0.41**	0.16
Time from procedure to discharge (days)	0.20	–0.15	–0.06	0.09	–0.02	0.14	0.31*	0.05

Pairwise case deletion was used for missing observations. Abbreviations: ACE = angiotensin-converting enzyme. BDI-II = Beck Depression Inventory II. CABG = coronary artery bypass grafting. COPD = chronic obstructive pulmonary disease. hs-CRP = high-sensitivity C-reactive protein. IL-6 = interleukin-6. NYHA = New York Heart Association. S-100B = S-100 calcium-binding protein B.

*$P<0.05$; **$P<0.01$; ***$P<0.001$.

†Acute Δ refers to the primary outcome, acute change in depressive symptom severity, defined as the intra-subject difference between BDI-II scores at baseline and discharge.

‡Delayed Δ refers to the secondary outcome, delayed change in depressive symptom severity, defined as the intra-subject difference between BDI-II scores at baseline and six-month follow-up.

§Total Δ refers to the intra-subject difference in blood biomarker levels between baseline and 2 days postoperative.

‖Within 7 days before the index procedure.

††Missing data (from left to right): n = 3; n = 1; n = 3; n = 2; n = 2; n = 3; n = 2; n = 3; n = 2.

‡‡Missing data (from left to right): n = 0; n = 1; n = 3; n = 2; n = 2; n = 3; n = 2; n = 3; n = 3.

§§Missing data (from left to right): n = 0; n = 1; n = 0; n = 0; n = 0; n = 0; n = 0; n = 0; n = 0.

Table 3. Spearman rank correlation coefficients for comparisons between and among Beck Depression Inventory II scores and blood biomarker measures.

		BDI-II (score)					S-100B (μg/l)			hs-CRP (mg/l)			IL-6 (pg/ml)		
		Baseline	Discharge	6 months	Acute Δ	Delayed Δ	Baseline	2 days	Total Δ	Baseline	2 days	Total Δ	Baseline	2 days	Total Δ
BDI-II (score)	Baseline	.	0.46**	0.66***	−0.52***	−0.03	0.02	−0.31	−0.43*	−0.01	−0.01	−0.21	0.24	−0.26	−0.22
		.	39	25	39	25	39	33	30	39	39	29	39	34	31
	Discharge	0.46**	.	0.48*	0.46**	0.34	−0.01	0.11	0.18	0.10	0.04	−0.10	0.13	0.06	0.07
		39	.	26	39	25	37	31	28	37	30	27	37	32	29
	6 months	0.66***	0.48*	.	−0.14	0.67***	−0.13	−0.06	0.03	0.28	−0.01	−0.12	0.26	0.14	0.13
		25	26	.	25	25	25	22	21	25	21	20	25	23	22
	Acute Δ	−0.52***	0.46**	−0.14	.	0.40*	0.02	0.55**	0.62***	0.21	0.05	−0.00	0.06	0.34	0.29
		39	39	25	.	25	36	31	28	36	30	27	36	32	29
	Delayed Δ	−0.03	0.34	0.67***	0.40*	.	0.10	0.47*	0.42	0.32	−0.03	−0.07	0.10	0.29	0.26
		25	25	25	25	.	24	22	21	24	21	20	24	23	22
S-100B (μg/l)	Baseline	0.02	−0.01	−0.13	0.02	0.10	.	0.51**	0.10	−0.09	−0.56***	−0.53**	0.02	0.39*	−0.42**
		39	37	25	36	24	.	36	36	47	35	35	47	37	37
	2 days	−0.31	0.11	−0.06	0.55**	0.47*	0.51**	.	0.89***	0.41*	−0.22	−0.25	0.25	0.21	0.07
		33	31	22	31	22	36	.	36	36	38	35	36	39	36
	Total Δ	−0.43*	0.18	0.03	0.62***	0.42	0.10	0.89***	.	0.54***	0.02	−0.05	0.28	0.37*	0.24
		30	28	21	28	21	36	36	.	36	35	35	36	36	36
hs-CRP (mg/l)	Baseline	−0.01	0.10	0.28	0.21	0.32	−0.09	0.41*	0.54***	.	0.23	0.05	0.59***	0.29	0.10
		39	37	25	36	24	47	36	36	.	35	35	47	37	37
	2 days	−0.11	0.04	−0.01	0.05	−0.03	−0.56***	−0.22	0.02	0.23	.	0.97***	−0.02	0.52***	0.63***
		32	30	21	30	21	35	38	35	35	.	35	35	38	35
	Total Δ	−0.21	−0.10	−0.12	−0.00	−0.07	−0.53**	−0.25	−0.05	0.05	0.97***	.	−0.15	0.54***	0.62***
		29	27	20	27	20	35	35	35	35	35	.	35	35	35
IL-6 (pg/ml)	Baseline	0.24	0.13	0.26	0.06	0.10	0.02	0.25	0.28	0.59***	−0.02	−0.15	.	0.21	−0.08
		39	37	25	36	24	47	36	36	47	35	35	.	37	37
	2 days	−0.26	0.06	0.14	0.34	0.29	0.39*	0.21	0.37*	0.29	0.52***	0.54***	0.21	.	0.93***
		34	32	23	32	23	37	39	36	37	38	35	37	.	37
	Total Δ	−0.22	0.07	0.13	0.29	0.26	−0.42**	0.07	0.24	0.10	0.63***	0.62***	−0.08	0.93***	.
		31	29	22	29	22	37	36	36	37	35	35	37	37	.

Values in the cells for each comparison are (from top to bottom): the Spearman rank correlation coefficient (Spearman ρ) and number of observations. Pairwise case deletion was used for missing observations. Abbreviations: ACE = angiotensin-converting enzyme. BDI-II = Beck Depression Inventory II. CABG = coronary artery bypass grafting. COPD = chronic obstructive pulmonary disease. hs-CRP = high-sensitivity C-reactive protein. NYHA = New York Heart Association. S-100B = S-100 calcium-binding protein B.

*$P<0.05$; **$P<0.01$; ***$P<0.001$.

[†]Acute Δ refers to the primary outcome, acute change in depressive symptom severity, defined as the intra-subject difference between BDI-II scores at baseline and discharge.

[‡]Delayed Δ refers to the secondary outcome, delayed change in depressive symptom severity, defined as the intra-subject difference between BDI-II scores at baseline and six-month follow-up.

[§]Total Δ refers to the intra-subject difference in blood biomarker levels between baseline and 2 days postoperative.

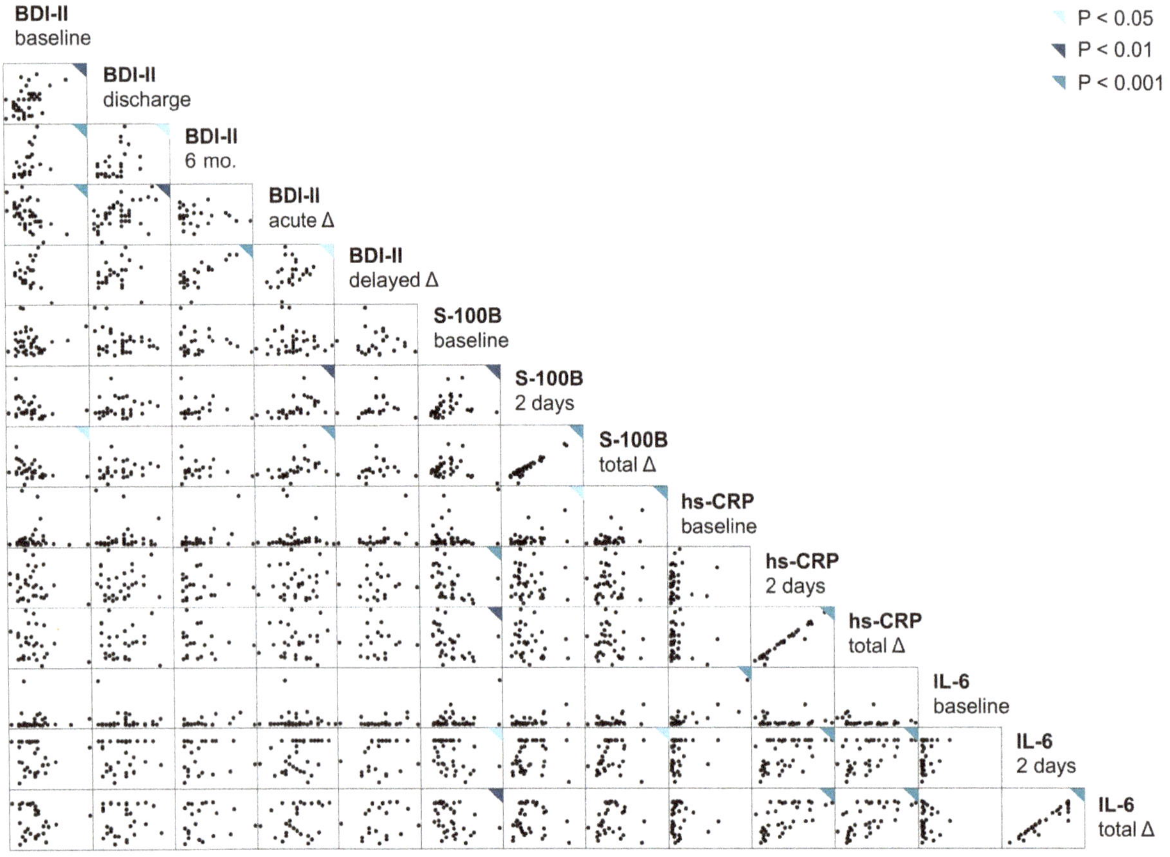

Figure 2. Scatterplot matrix of all possible combinations between and among Beck Depression Inventory II scores and blood biomarker measures. BDI-II scores were assessed at baseline, discharge, and 6 months. Differences between baseline and discharge BDI-II scores (primary outcome) and baseline and 6-month BDI-II scores (secondary outcome) were computed for each participant. Biomarker levels were determined at baseline and 2 days postoperatively, and change scores computed. BDI-II = Beck Depression Inventory II. hs-CRP = high-sensitivity C-reactive protein. IL-6 = interleukin-6. S-100B = S-100 calcium-binding protein B.

correlations were entered into the relevant multiple linear regression models (see below).

Spearman ρ values were calculated and scatterplots generated for all possible two-term combinations between and among blood biomarker measures at baseline and postoperative assessments, and the difference between them and BDI-II scores at baseline, discharge, six-month follow-up, the difference between baseline and discharge BDI-II scores (primary outcome), and the difference between baseline and six-month follow-up BDI-II scores (secondary outcome). For statistically significant correlations between blood biomarker measures and the main outcomes, we did sensitivity analysis by recalculating Spearman ρ values using Bonferroni-adjusted significance levels and again using Sidak-adjusted significance levels. Last, the main outcomes were regressed on blood biomarker measures at baseline and the difference between blood biomarker levels at baseline and postoperative assessments using ordinary-least squares simple and multiple linear regressions. Before entering terms into the models, variable transformations were first applied to all variables that did not have a normal distribution. The transformation used for a given variable was based on the lowest χ^2 value yielded by a ladder of powers analysis [100].

Results

Biomarker cohort

The pairwise distributions of BDI-II scores and blood biomarker levels are displayed in Figure 1. Participant characteristics and BDI-II scores were generally similar among those comprising the biomarker cohort relative to the remaining participants in the Scarecrow trial (Table 1). One exception was discharge BDI-II scores, which were lower on average among those in the biomarker cohort (Table 1).

Covariate assessment

Spearman ρ values for comparisons between participant characteristics and the main outcomes and blood biomarker measures are displayed in Table 2. None of the participant characteristics showed a statistically significant correlation with either outcome (Table 2). Intra-subject differences between baseline and postoperative S-100B levels correlated positively with age and negatively with weight and body-mass index, and were significantly lower on average among those taking β-blockers (Table 2). Perioperative increases in hs-CRP levels correlated negatively with age. Perioperative increases in hs-CRP and

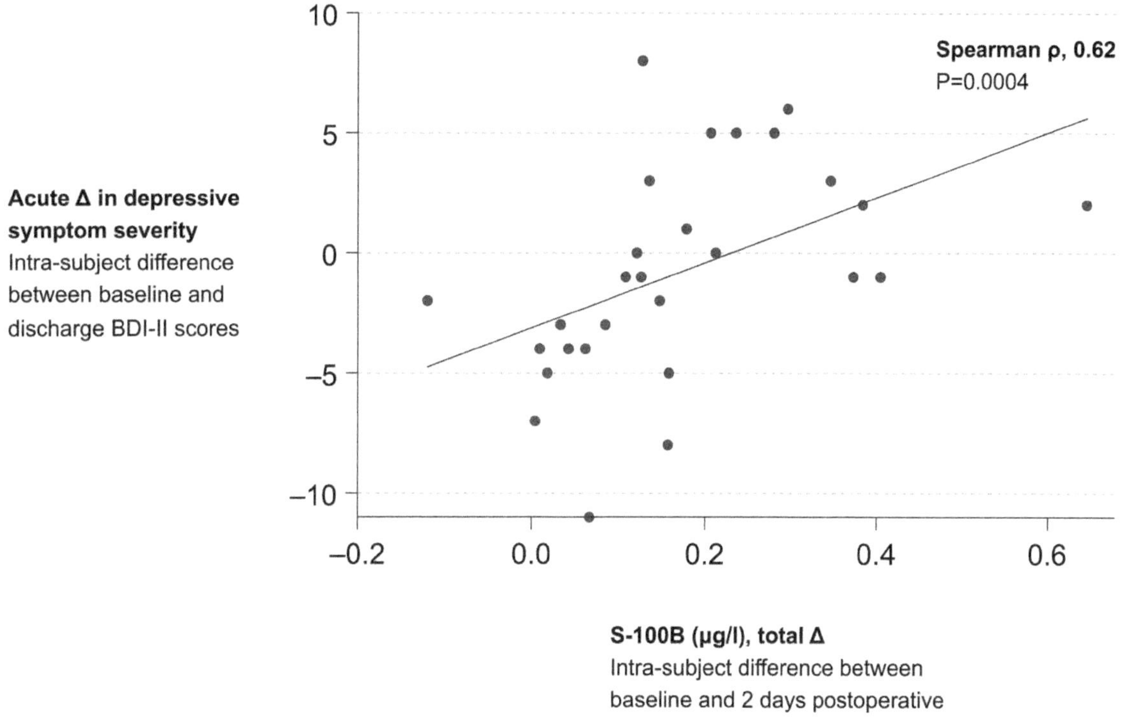

Figure 3. Association between perioperative increases in blood levels of S-100 calcium-binding protein B and acute changes in depressive symptom severity. The x-axis refers to the intra-subject difference between S-100 calcium binding protein B (S-100B) levels measured at baseline and 2 days postoperative. The y-axis refers to the primary outcome, acute change in depressive symptom severity, defined as the intra-subject difference between baseline and discharge Beck Depression inventory II (BDI-II) scores. BDI-II = Beck Depression Inventory II. S-100B = S-100 calcium-binding protein B. Spearman rho = Spearman rank correlation coefficient.

interleukin-6 levels were significantly greater on average among participants randomized to (intention-to-treat) and having undergone (as-treated) off-pump procedures, as compared with those randomized to and having undergone conventional procedures (Table 2). Spearman ρ values and scatterplots for all possible two-term combinations between and among BDI-II scores and blood biomarker measures are displayed in Table 3 and Figure 2.

Acute change in depressive symptom severity

Intra-subject differences between baseline and postoperative S-100B levels exhibited a strong positive correlation with intra-subject differences between baseline and discharge BDI-II scores (Spearman ρ, 0.62; P = 0.0004; Table 3; Figure 3). Neither the strength nor the statistical significance of this correlation was affected by Bonferroni- or Sidak-adjusted significance levels (for both adjustments: Spearman ρ, 0.62; P = 0.0004). There were no other statistically significant correlations between blood biomarker measures and the primary outcome (Table 3). Significant negative correlations were observed between baseline BDI-II scores and changes in S-100B levels and between baseline BDI-II scores and acute changes in depressive symptom severity (Table 3).

The results of simple and multiple linear regressions of the primary outcome on blood biomarker measures are displayed in Table 4. A simple linear regression model showed that each 0.10-µg/l increase in intra-subject differences between baseline and postoperative S-100B levels was associated with a 1.36-point increase in intra-subject differences between baseline and discharge BDI-II scores (regression coefficient $[R] = 13.60$, coefficient of determination $[R^2] = 0.23$, $t = 2.76$, $P = 0.010$, standardized regression coefficient $[\beta] = 0.48$, $F_{(1,26)} = 7.61$, $P = 0.0105$; Table 4; Figure 3). This association remained statistically significant after individual adjustments for baseline S-100B levels, age, weight, body-mass index, and β-blocker use, but not baseline BDI-II scores ($R = 9.18$, $R^2 = 0.40$, $t = 1.94$, $P = 0.064$) adjusting for which improved the explanatory power of the model overall ($\beta = 0.32$, $R^2_{\text{adjusted}} = 0.35$, $F_{(2,25)} = 8.29$, P model = 0.0017; Table 4). There were no statistically significant associations between the primary outcome and the remaining blood biomarker measures (Table 3; Table 4).

Delayed change in depressive symptom severity

Spearman ρ values and scatterplots for all possible two-term combinations between the secondary outcome and blood biomarker measures are displayed in Table 3 and Figure 2. There were no statistically significant correlations between blood biomarker levels and the secondary outcome (Table 3). The results of simple and multiple linear regressions of the secondary outcome on blood biomarker levels are displayed in Table 5. None of these models, unadjusted or adjusted, yielded a statistically significant relationship between blood biomarker levels and delayed change in depressive symptom severity (Table 5).

Discussion

This is the first study, to our knowledge, to have prospectively assessed the relationships between blood biomarkers of glial

Table 4. Linear regression of the primary outcome on blood biomarker measures and covariates.

Independent variables		Acute Δ in depressive symptom severity*					
Biomarker measures	**Covariates**	**β**	***n***	**R^2**	**$R^2_{adjusted}$**	**RMSE**	**P Value**†
S-100B (μg/l), baseline	Unadjusted	−0.02	36	0.00	−0.03	4.72	0.92
	BDI-II (scores), baseline	−0.16	36	0.30	0.25	4.02	0.91
	Underwent off-pump procedure	0.22	36	0.15	0.09	4.43	0.07
	Urgent priority procedure	−0.03	36	0.01	−0.05	4.76	0.82
	Troponin T at 24 hours (ng/dl)	0.07	36	0.05	−0.01	4.68	0.47
S-100B (μg/l), total Δ	Unadjusted	0.48	28	0.23	0.20	4.03	0.010
	S-100B (μg/l), baseline	0.47	28	0.24	0.18	4.09	0.012
	BDI-II (scores), baseline	0.32	28	0.40	0.35	3.63	0.06
	Age (years)	0.42	28	0.26	0.20	4.02	0.030
	Weight (kg)	0.40	28	0.25	0.20	4.04	0.046
	Body-mass index (kg/m^2)	0.44	28	0.23	0.17	4.09	0.025
	β-blocker	0.53	28	0.24	0.18	4.08	0.011
hs-CRP (mg/l), baseline	Unadjusted	0.07	36	0.01	−0.02	4.71	0.67
	BDI-II (scores), baseline	0.08	36	0.30	0.26	4.00	0.58
	Charlson comorbidity index	0.13	36	0.02	−0.04	4.73	0.48
	Myocardial infarction†	0.07	36	0.01	−0.05	4.77	0.69
	Troponin T at 24 hours (ng/dl)	0.12	36	0.05	−0.00	4.66	0.50
hs-CRP (mg/l), total Δ	Unadjusted	0.03	27	0.00	−0.04	4.67	0.87
	hs-CRP (mg/l), baseline	0.05	27	0.09	0.02	4.55	0.79
	BDI-II (scores), baseline	−0.03	27	0.31	0.25	3.96	0.86
	Age (years)	0.15	27	0.13	0.05	4.46	0.47
	Underwent off-pump procedure	−0.17	27	0.06	−0.02	4.63	0.52
	Urgent priority procedure	−0.02	27	0.13	0.06	4.45	0.92
IL-6 (pg/ml), baseline	Unadjusted	−0.05	36	0.00	−0.03	4.71	0.76
	BDI-II (scores), baseline	−0.10	36	0.31	0.26	3.99	0.50
	Myocardial infarction‡	−0.05	36	0.01	−0.05	4.77	0.77
	Unstable angina at admission	0.04	36	0.03	−0.02	4.71	0.82
IL-6 (pg/ml), total Δ	Unadjusted	0.23	29	0.06	0.02	4.37	0.22
	IL-6 (pg/ml), baseline	0.23	29	0.08	0.01	4.41	0.23
	BDI-II (scores), baseline	0.13	29	0.32	0.27	3.77	0.44
	Acetylsalicylic acid‡	0.27	29	0.08	0.01	4.39	0.18

Table 4. Cont.

Independent variables		Acute Δ in depressive symptom severity*					
Biomarker measures	**Covariates**	β	n	R^2	$R^2_{adjusted}$	**RMSE**	**P Value**†
	Underwent off-pump procedure	0.18	29	0.06	−0.01	4.44	0.47
	Urgent priority procedure	0.19	29	0.16	0.09	4.21	0.31

BDI-II = Beck Depression Inventory II. β = standardized regression coefficient. hs-CRP = high-sensitivity C-reactive protein. IL-6 = interleukin-6. R^2 = coefficient of determination. $R^2_{adjusted}$ = adjusted coefficient of determination. RMSE = root-mean-square error. S-100B = S-100 calcium-binding protein B.
*Acute Δ refers to the primary outcome, acute change in depressive symptom severity, defined as the intra-subject difference between BDI-II scores at baseline and discharge
†Corresponds to the blood biomarker term in the model.
‡Within 7 days before the index procedure.

activation and injury, blood–brain barrier disruption, and depressive symptom severity in the context of the systemic inflammatory challenge paradigm of coronary artery bypass grafting. We found that perioperative increases in the glial activation and injury and blood–brain barrier-disruption biomarker, S-100B, exhibited a strong positive correlation with acute changes in depressive symptom severity, largely independent of covariates associated with either. Given the magnitude of the test statistic for this correlation (P = 0.0004), the statistical significance of this finding cannot readily be attributed to the fact that we did multiple pre-specified comparisons that included assessing the relationship between depressive symptoms and two other biomarkers besides S-100B (α/comparisons = [0.05]/[3] = 0.001 > 0.0004). We also found that baseline BDI-II scores correlated negatively with both perioperative increases in S-100B levels as well as acute changes in depressive symptom severity, and that adjusting for baseline BDI-II scores diminished the strength and statistical significance of their association (the term for perioperative increases in S-100B levels still approached statistical significance at P = 0.064). Adjusting for baseline BDI-II scores also increased the proportion of variance in the primary outcome explained by the model (from 23% to 35%). Exploratory analyses indicated that the association between perioperative increases in S-100B levels and acute changes in depressive severity remained statistically significant after adjusting for baseline BDI-II scores among participants with BDI-II scores greater than or equal to 5 at baseline (Spearman ρ, 0.66; P = 0.0007). This was not the case, however, among those with BDI-II scores less than 5 at baseline (Spearman ρ, 0.15; P = 0.15).

Two earlier studies assessed relationships between depression and inflammation in the context of coronary artery bypass grafting [38,39]. In the first of these, Yang and colleagues found that mean levels of hs-CRP at baseline were significantly higher among those with clinical depression at six-month follow-up (defined as a Patient Health Questionnaire (PHQ-9) score ≥9) compared with those who were not [38]. By comparison, the correlation between baseline blood levels of hs-CRP blood levels and six-month BDI-II scores in the present study was not statistically significant. A possible explanation for this apparent discrepancy is that six-month follow-up depressive symptom severity was defined as a dichotomous outcome in Yang and colleagues' study, whereas it was defined as a continuous outcome in the present study. Supporting this interpretation, results of an exploratory analysis we performed showed that baseline hs-CRP blood levels were significantly higher among participants who were clinically depressed at six-month follow-up (defined as a BDI-II score ≥ 14), as compared with participants who were not (26.9±41.1 mg/l (n = 4) vs 5.6±6.3 mg/l (n = 21); mean difference, 21.3 mg/l; 95% confidence interval, 3.3 to 39.3 mg/l; P = 0.022). The same between-group comparison for interleukin-6 blood levels at baseline approached statistical significance (16.0±15.4 pg/ml (n = 4) vs 7.0±7.9 pg/ml (n = 21); mean difference, 8.5 pg/ml; 95% confidence interval, 1.4 to 19.4 pg/ml; P = 0.09). In the second study, Poole and colleagues found that elevated hs-CRP levels at postoperative day four mediated the association between depression and an increased length of stay [39]. Differences in the aims and designs of this study compared with the present one limit the ability to directly compare and contrast their findings.

The present study has limitations. First, some studies have shown that cardiopulmonary bypass can produce a transient elevation in blood S-100B levels, potentially confounding the

Table 5. Linear regression of the secondary outcome on blood biomarker measures and covariates.

Independent variables		Delayed Δ in depressive symptom severity*					
Biomarker measures	**Covariates**	**β**	**n**	**R^2**	**$R^2_{adjusted}$**	**RMSE**	**P Value†**
S-100B (μg/l), baseline	Unadjusted	−0.04	24	0.00	−0.04	5.01	0.86
	BDI-II (scores), baseline	−0.39	24	0.02	−0.08	5.09	0.85
	BDI-II (scores), acute Δ	−0.10	24	0.12	0.03	4.83	0.63
	Underwent off-pump procedure	−0.12	24	0.02	−0.07	5.08	0.64
	Urgent priority procedure	−0.07	24	0.05	−0.04	5.01	0.74
	Troponin T at 24 hours (ng/dl)	−0.04	24	0.00	−0.09	5.13	0.88
S-100B (μg/l), total Δ	Unadjusted	0.22	21	0.05	−0.00	4.63	0.35
	S-100B (μg/l), baseline	0.21	21	0.05	−0.05	4.74	0.37
	BDI-II (scores), baseline	0.12	21	0.07	−0.03	4.69	0.64
	BDI-II (scores), acute Δ	0.03	21	0.15	−0.05	4.49	0.90
	Age (years)	0.21	21	0.05	−0.06	4.75	0.38
	Weight (kg)	0.16	21	0.08	−0.02	4.66	0.50
	Body-mass index (kg/m^2)	0.18	21	0.06	−0.04	4.71	0.46
	β-blocker	0.25	21	0.05	−0.06	4.74	0.25
hs-CRP (mg/l), baseline	Unadjusted	0.28	24	0.08	0.04	4.81	0.18
	BDI-II (scores), baseline	0.29	24	0.10	0.01	4.88	0.18
	BDI-II (scores), acute Δ	0.21	24	0.15	0.07	4.74	0.31
	Charlson comorbidity index	0.29	24	0.08	−0.01	4.93	0.20
	Myocardial infarction†	0.31	24	0.15	0.07	4.74	0.14
	Troponin T at 24 hours (ng/dl)	0.30	24	0.09	−0.00	4.91	0.18
hs-CRP (mg/l), total Δ	Unadjusted	−0.07	20	0.00	−0.05	4.77	0.78
	hs-CRP (mg/l), baseline	−0.07	20	0.00	−0.11	4.91	0.79
	BDI-II (scores), baseline	−0.08	20	0.06	−0.05	4.77	0.73
	BDI-II (scores), acute Δ	0.00	20	0.16	0.06	4.51	0.99
	Age (years)	−0.05	20	0.01	−0.11	4.90	0.85
	Underwent off-pump procedure	−0.10	20	0.01	−0.11	4.91	0.77
	Urgent priority procedure	−0.07	20	0.01	−0.11	4.90	0.78
IL-6 (pg/ml), baseline	Unadjusted	−0.10	24	0.01	−0.04	4.99	0.64
	BDI-II (scores), baseline	−0.15	24	0.04	−0.06	5.04	0.50
	BDI-II (scores), acute Δ	−0.13	24	0.12	0.04	4.81	0.54
	Myocardial infarction‡	−0.13	24	0.07	−0.02	4.96	0.54
	Unstable angina at admission	−0.25	24	0.08	−0.01	4.94	0.32
IL-6 (pg/ml), total Δ	Unadjusted	0.16	22	0.03	−0.02	4.89	0.47
	IL-6 (pg/ml), baseline	0.17	22	0.03	−0.07	5.01	0.47

Table 5. Cont.

Independent variables		Delayed Δ in depressive symptom severity*					
Biomarker measures	**Covariates**	β	n	R^2	$R^2_{adjusted}$	**RMSE**	**P Value**†
	BDI-II (scores), baseline	0.14	22	0.06	−0.04	4.94	0.54
	BDI-II (scores), acute Δ	0.11	22	0.15	0.06	4.69	0.63
	Acetylsalicylic acid‡	0.17	22	0.03	−0.07	5.01	0.46
	Underwent off-pump procedure	0.31	22	0.06	−0.04	4.92	0.28
	Urgent priority procedure	0.15	22	0.04	−0.06	4.97	0.52

BDI-II = Beck Depression Inventory II. β = standardized regression coefficient. hs-CRP = high-sensitivity C-reactive protein. IL-6 = interleukin-6. R^2 = coefficient of determination. $R^2_{adjusted}$ = adjusted coefficient of determination. RMSE = root-mean-square error. S-100B = S-100 calcium-binding protein B.

*Delayed Δ refers to the secondary outcome, delayed change in depressive symptom severity, defined as the intra-subject difference between BDI-II scores at baseline and six-month follow-up

†Corresponds to the blood biomarker term in the model.

‡Within 7 days before the index procedure.

observed correlation between perioperative increases in S-100B levels and acute changes in depressive symptom severity [101]. However, subsequent studies, which performed serial assays of blood S-100B levels among patients undergoing coronary artery bypass grafting found that increases in blood S-100B levels due to cardiopulmonary bypass are no longer apparent after 24 hours [102,103]. Accordingly, because we collected postoperative blood samples at about 48 hours, it is unlikely that perioperative increases in S-100B levels in our study were related to cardiopulmonary bypass. Supporting this interpretation, perioperative increases in S-100B levels among participants in our study did not differ significantly between patients who had cardiopulmonary bypass and those who did not. Second, whether the observed perioperative increases in blood S-100B levels are reliably attributable to glial activation and injury and blood-brain barrier disruption rather than non-cardiac extracerebral sources remains subject to interpretation. This concern arises primarily in the context of two animal model studies having shown a disconnect between S-100B levels in blood and those in CSF or brain parenchyma [68], and one recent cross-sectional study that found a negative correlation between CSF levels of S-100B and depressive symptom severity among patients with non-inflammatory neurological disorders [62]. Arguing in the opposite direction, however, other studies have shown that extracerebral sources do not influence blood S-100B levels [104]. In addition, a recent study of patients undergoing coronary artery bypass grafting found that S-100B levels in both blood and CSF increased together with those of the quintessential astroglial marker glial fibrillary acidic protein as well as CSF-to-serum albumin ratios [81]. Last, since data on antidepressant and statin use were not collected for the original Scarecrow trial, the effect of these drugs on the observed correlation between changes in S-100B levels and acute changes in depressive symptom severity cannot be excluded.

In conclusion, perioperative increases in S-100B levels exhibited a strongly positive correlation with acute changes in depressive symptom severity in the systemic inflammatory challenge paradigm of cardiac surgery. There were no significant associations between either acute or delayed changes in depressive symptom severity and baseline S-100B levels, baseline hs-CRP or interleukin-6 levels, or perioperative changes in hs-CRP or interleukin-6 levels. Among most participants, levels of all three biomarkers were normal at baseline and markedly elevated at 2 days postoperative. Taken together, these findings are consistent with the hypothesis that depression can be mechanistically linked to glial activation and injury as well as blood-brain barrier disruption in the context of systemic inflammation challenge paradigms, to include cardiac surgery. Large prospective cohort studies that can inform the reproducibility of these findings are warranted.

Acknowledgments

We thank all participants and staff involved in the Scarecrow trial.

Author Contributions

Conceived and designed the experiments: DMP SN JRB. Performed the experiments: DMP SN JRB. Analyzed the data: DMP SN TAM JRB. Contributed reagents/materials/analysis tools: JRB FH. Contributed to the writing of the manuscript: DMP SN. Contributed the Scarecrow trial dataset, including Beck Depression Inventory II scores and biomarker blood levels: JRB FH. Revised the paper for important intellectual content: DMP JRB TAM SN FH.

References

1. Najjar S, Pearlman DM, Alper K, Najjar A, Devinsky O (2013) Neuroinflammation and psychiatric illness. J Neuroinflammation 10: 43.
2. Najjar S, Pearlman DM, Devinsky O, Najjar A, Zagzag D (2013) Neurovascular unit dysfunction with blood-brain barrier hyperpermeability contributes to major depressive disorder: a review of clinical and experimental evidence. J Neuroinflammation 10: 142.
3. Najjar S, Pearlman DM, Hirsch S, Friedman K, Strange J, et al. (2014) Brain biopsy findings link major depressive disorder to neuroinflammation, oxidative stress, and neurovascular dysfunction: a case report. Biol Psychiatry 75: e23–26.
4. Steiner J, Walter M, Gos T, Guillemin GJ, Bernstein HG, et al. (2011) Severe depression is associated with increased microglial quinolinic acid in subregions of the anterior cingulate gyrus: evidence for an immune-modulated glutamatergic neurotransmission? J Neuroinflammation 8: 94.
5. Dantzer R, O'Connor JC, Freund GG, Johnson RW, Kelley KW (2008) From inflammation to sickness and depression: when the immune system subjugates the brain. Nat Rev Neurosci 9: 46–56.
6. Howren MB, Lamkin DM, Suls J (2009) Associations of depression with C-reactive protein, IL-1, and IL-6: a meta-analysis. Psychosom Med 71: 171–186.
7. Kuo HK, Yen CJ, Chang CH, Kuo CK, Chen JH, et al. (2005) Relation of C-reactive protein to stroke, cognitive disorders, and depression in the general population: systematic review and meta-analysis. Lancet Neurol 4: 371–380.
8. Dowlati Y, Herrmann N, Swardfager W, Liu H, Sham L, et al. (2010) A meta-analysis of cytokines in major depression. Biol Psychiatry 67: 446–457.
9. Hiles SA, Baker AL, de Malmanche T, Attia J (2012) Interleukin-6, C-reactive protein and interleukin-10 after antidepressant treatment in people with depression: a meta-analysis. Psychol Med 42: 2015–2026.
10. Liu Y, Ho RC, Mak A (2012) Interleukin (IL)-6, tumour necrosis factor alpha (TNF-alpha) and soluble interleukin-2 receptors (sIL-2R) are elevated in patients with major depressive disorder: a meta-analysis and meta-regression. J Affect Disord 139: 230–239.
11. Ford DE, Erlinger TP (2004) Depression and C-reactive protein in US adults: data from the Third National Health and Nutrition Examination Survey. Arch Intern Med 164: 1010–1014.
12. Hickman RJ, Khambaty T, Stewart JC (2014) C-reactive protein is elevated in atypical but not nonatypical depression: data from the National Health and Nutrition Examination Survey (NHANES) 1999–2004. J Behav Med 37: 621–629.
13. Raison CL, Capuron L, Miller AH (2006) Cytokines sing the blues: inflammation and the pathogenesis of depression. Trends Immunol 27: 24–31.
14. Steiner J, Bielau H, Brisch R, Danos P, Ullrich O, et al. (2008) Immunological aspects in the neurobiology of suicide: elevated microglial density in schizophrenia and depression is associated with suicide. J Psychiatr Res 42: 151–157.
15. Miguel-Hidalgo JJ, Baucom C, Dilley G, Overholser JC, Meltzer HY, et al. (2000) Glial fibrillary acidic protein immunoreactivity in the prefrontal cortex distinguishes younger from older adults in major depressive disorder. Biol Psychiatry 48: 861–873.
16. Altshuler LL, Abulseoud OA, Foland-Ross L, Bartzokis G, Chang S, et al. (2010) Amygdala astrocyte reduction in subjects with major depressive disorder but not bipolar disorder. Bipolar Disord 12: 541–549.
17. Webster MJ, O'Grady J, Kleinman JE, Weickert CS (2005) Glial fibrillary acidic protein mRNA levels in the cingulate cortex of individuals with depression, bipolar disorder and schizophrenia. Neurosci 133: 453–461.
18. Johnston-Wilson NL, Sims CD, Hofmann JP, Anderson L, Shore AD, et al. (2000) Disease-specific alterations in frontal cortex brain proteins in schizophrenia, bipolar disorder, and major depressive disorder. The Stanley Neuropathology Consortium. Mol Psychiatry 5: 142–149.
19. Benros ME, Waltoft BL, Nordentoft M, Ostergaard SD, Eaton WW, et al. (2013) Autoimmune diseases and severe infections as risk factors for mood disorders: a nationwide study. JAMA Psychiatry 70: 812–820.
20. Kayser M (2014) Severe infection and autoimmune disease are associated with increased risk of mood disorders. Evid Based Ment Health 17: 20.
21. Capuron L, Raison CL, Musselman DL, Lawson DH, Nemeroff CB, et al. (2003) Association of exaggerated HPA axis response to the initial injection of interferon-alpha with development of depression during interferon-alpha therapy. Am J Psychiatry 160: 1342–1345.
22. Raison CL, Borisov AS, Woolwine BJ, Massung B, Vogt G, et al. (2010) Interferon-alpha effects on diurnal hypothalamic-pituitary-adrenal axis activity: relationship with proinflammatory cytokines and behavior. Mol Psychiatry 15: 535–547.
23. Raison CL, Borisov AS, Broadwell SD, Capuron L, Woolwine BJ, et al. (2005) Depression during pegylated interferon-alpha plus ribavirin therapy: prevalence and prediction. J Clin Psychiatry 66: 41–48.
24. Raison CL, Broadwell SD, Borisov AS, Manatunga AK, Capuron L, et al. (2005) Depressive symptoms and viral clearance in patients receiving interferon-alpha and ribavirin for hepatitis C. Brain Behav Immun 19: 23–27.
25. Raison CL, Borisov AS, Majer M, Drake DF, Pagnoni G, et al. (2009) Activation of central nervous system inflammatory pathways by interferon-alpha: relationship to monoamines and depression. Biol Psychiatry 65: 296–303.
26. Dereure O, Raison-Peyron N, Larrey D, Blanc F, Guilhou JJ (2002) Diffuse inflammatory lesions in patients treated with interferon alfa and ribavirin for hepatitis C: a series of 20 patients. Br J Dermatol 147: 1142–1146.
27. Udina M, Castellvi P, Moreno-Espana J, Navines R, Valdes M, et al. (2012) Interferon-induced depression in chronic hepatitis C: a systematic review and meta-analysis. J Clin Psychiatry 73: 1128–1138.
28. Musselman DL, Lawson DH, Gumnick JF, Manatunga AK, Penna S, et al. (2001) Paroxetine for the prevention of depression induced by high-dose interferon alfa. N Engl J Med 344: 961–966.
29. Musselman DL, Miller AH, Porter MR, Manatunga A, Gao F, et al. (2001) Higher than normal plasma interleukin-6 concentrations in cancer patients with depression: preliminary findings. Am J Psychiatry 158: 1252–1257.
30. Raison CL, Woolwine BJ, Demetrashvili MF, Borisov AS, Weinreib R, et al. (2007) Paroxetine for prevention of depressive symptoms induced by interferon-alpha and ribavirin for hepatitis C. Aliment Pharmacol Ther 25: 1163–1174.
31. Raison CL, Rye DB, Woolwine BJ, Vogt GJ, Bautista BM, et al. (2010) Chronic interferon-alpha administration disrupts sleep continuity and depth in patients with hepatitis C: association with fatigue, motor slowing, and increased evening cortisol. Biol Psychiatry 68: 942–949.
32. Martins JG (2009) EPA but not DHA appears to be responsible for the efficacy of omega-3 long chain polyunsaturated fatty acid supplementation in depression: evidence from a meta-analysis of randomized controlled trials. J Am Coll Nutr 28: 525–542.
33. Bloch MH, Hannestad J (2012) Omega-3 fatty acids for the treatment of depression: systematic review and meta-analysis. Mol Psychiatry 17: 1272–1282.
34. Na KS, Lee KJ, Lee JS, Cho YS, Jung HY (2014) Efficacy of adjunctive celecoxib treatment for patients with major depressive disorder: a meta-analysis. Prog Neuropsychopharmacol Biol Psychiatry 48: 79–85.
35. Müller N, Schwarz MJ, Dehning S, Douhe A, Cerovecki A, et al. (2006) The cyclooxygenase-2 inhibitor celecoxib has therapeutic effects in major depression: results of a double-blind, randomized, placebo controlled, add-on pilot study to reboxetine. Mol Psychiatry 11: 680–684.
36. Eisenberger NI, Berkman ET, Inagaki TK, Rameson LT, Mashal NM, et al. (2010) Inflammation-induced anhedonia: endotoxin reduces ventral striatum responses to reward. Biol Psychiatry 68: 748–754.
37. Cremeans-Smith JK, Soehlen S, Greene K, Alexander T, Delahanty DL (2009) In-hospital levels of C-reactive protein and IL-6 predict post-operative depressive symptoms among patients undergoing total knee replacement surgery. Brain Behav Immun 23: 1096–1103.
38. Yang L, Wang J, Zhang L, Hou J, Yuan X, et al. (2012) Preoperative high-sensitivity C-reactive protein predicts depression in patients undergoing coronary artery bypass surgery: a single-center prospective observational study. J Thorac Cardiovasc Surg 144: 500–505.
39. Poole L, Kidd T, Leigh E, Ronaldson A, Jahangiri M, et al. (2014) Depression, C-reactive protein and length of post-operative hospital stay in coronary artery bypass graft surgery patients. Brain Behav Immun 37: 115–121.
40. Newman MF, Mathew JP, Grocott HP, Mackensen GB, Monk T, et al. (2006) Central nervous system injury associated with cardiac surgery. Lancet 368: 694–703.
41. Miguel-Hidalgo JJ, Overholser JC, Jurjus GJ, Meltzer HY, Dieter L, et al. (2011) Vascular and extravascular immunoreactivity for intercellular adhesion molecule 1 in the orbitofrontal cortex of subjects with major depression: age-dependent changes. J Affect Disord 132: 422–431.
42. Gudmundsson P, Skoog I, Waern M, Blennow K, Palsson S, et al. (2007) The relationship between cerebrospinal fluid biomarkers and depression in elderly women. Am J Geriatr Psychiatry 15: 832–838.
43. Bechter K, Reiber H, Herzog S, Fuchs D, Tumani H, et al. (2010) Cerebrospinal fluid analysis in affective and schizophrenic spectrum disorders: identification of subgroups with immune responses and blood-CSF barrier dysfunction. J Psychiatr Res 44: 321–330.
44. Niklasson F, Agren H (1984) Brain energy metabolism and blood-brain barrier permeability in depressive patients: analyses of creatine, creatinine, urate, and albumin in CSF and blood. Biol Psychiatry 19: 1183–1206.
45. Lavoie KL, Pelletier R, Arsenault A, Dupuis J, Bacon SL (2010) Association between clinical depression and endothelial function measured by forearm hyperemic reactivity. Psychosom Med 72: 20–26.
46. Valkanova V, Ebmeier KP (2013) Vascular risk factors and depression in later life: a systematic review and meta-analysis. Biol Psychiatry 73: 406–413.
47. Serlin Y, Levy J, Shalev H (2011) Vascular pathology and blood-brain barrier disruption in cognitive and psychiatric complications of type 2 diabetes mellitus. Cardiovasc Psychiatry Neurol 2011: 609202.
48. Permoda-Osip A, Dorszewska J, Skibinska M, Chlopocka-Wozniak M, Rybakowski JK (2013) Hyperhomocysteinemia in bipolar depression: clinical and biochemical correlates. Neuropsychobiology 68: 193–196.
49. Zill P, Baghai TC, Schule C, Born C, Frustuck C, et al. (2012) DNA methylation analysis of the angiotensin converting enzyme (ACE) gene in major depression. PLoS ONE 7: e40479.
50. Do DP, Dowd JB, Ranjit N, House JS, Kaplan GA (2010) Hopelessness, depression, and early markers of endothelial dysfunction in U.S. adults. Psychosom Med 72: 613–619.

51. Dimopoulos N, Piperi C, Salonicioti A, Mitsonis C, Liappas I, et al. (2006) Elevation of plasma concentration of adhesion molecules in late-life depression. Int J Geriatr Psychiatry 21: 965–971.
52. Schaefer M, Horn M, Schmidt F, Schmid-Wendtner MH, Volkenandt M, et al. (2004) Correlation between sICAM-1 and depressive symptoms during adjuvant treatment of melanoma with interferon-alpha. Brain Behav Immun 18: 555–562.
53. Thomas AJ, Perry R, Kalaria RN, Oakley A, McMeekin W, et al. (2003) Neuropathological evidence for ischemia in the white matter of the dorsolateral prefrontal cortex in late-life depression. Int J Geriatr Psychiatry 18: 7–13.
54. Thomas AJ, Ferrier IN, Kalaria RN, Woodward SA, Ballard C, et al. (2000) Elevation in late-life depression of intercellular adhesion molecule-1 expression in the dorsolateral prefrontal cortex. Am J Psychiatry 157: 1682–1684.
55. Gos T, Schroeter ML, Lessel W, Bernstein HG, Dobrowolny H, et al. (2013) S100B-immunopositive astrocytes and oligodendrocytes in the hippocampus are differentially afflicted in unipolar and bipolar depression: a postmortem study. J Psychiatr Res 47: 1694–1699.
56. Falcone T, Fazio V, Lee C, Simon B, Franco K, et al. (2010) Serum S100B: a potential biomarker for suicidality in adolescents? PLoS ONE 5: e11089.
57. Schroeter ML, Abdul-Khaliq H, Sacher J, Steiner J, Blasig IE, et al. (2010) Mood disorders are glial disorders: evidence from in vivo studies. Cardiovasc Psychiatry Neurol 2010: 780645.
58. Schroeter ML, Abdul-Khaliq H, Krebs M, Diefenbacher A, Blasig IE (2008) Serum markers support disease-specific glial pathology in major depression. J Affect Disord 111: 271–280.
59. Arolt V, Peters M, Erfurth A, Wiesmann M, Missler U, et al. (2003) S100B and response to treatment in major depression: a pilot study. Eur Neuropsychopharmacol 13: 235–239.
60. Rajkowska G, Stockmeier CA (2013) Astrocyte pathology in major depressive disorder: insights from human postmortem brain tissue. Curr Drug Targets 14: 1225–1236.
61. Rajkowska G, Hughes J, Stockmeier CA, Javier Miguel-Hidalgo J, Maciag D (2013) Coverage of blood vessels by astrocytic endfeet is reduced in major depressive disorder. Biol Psychiatry 73: 613–621.
62. Uher T, Bob P (2012) Cerebrospinal fluid S100B levels reflect symptoms of depression in patients with non-inflammatory neurological disorders. Neurosci Lett 529: 139–143.
63. Zhang Y, Rothermundt M, Peters M, Wiesmann M, Hoy L, et al. (2009) S100B serum levels and word memory processing in remitted major depression as reflected by brain potentials. Neuropsychobiology 59: 172–177.
64. Yang K, Xie GR, Hu YQ, Mao FQ, Su LY (2008) The effects of gender and numbers of depressive episodes on serum S100B levels in patients with major depression. J Neural Transm 115: 1687–1694.
65. Jang BS, Kim H, Lim SW, Jang KW, Kim DK (2008) Serum S100B Levels and Major Depressive Disorder: Its Characteristics and Role in Antidepressant Response. Psychiatry Investig 5: 193–198.
66. Dietrich DE, Hauser U, Peters M, Zhang Y, Wiesmann M, et al. (2004) Target evaluation processing and serum levels of nerve tissue protein S100B in patients with remitted major depression. Neurosci Lett 354: 69–73.
67. Goncalves FM, Freitas AE, Peres TV, Rieger DK, Ben J, et al. (2013) Vatairea macrocarpa lectin (VML) induces depressive-like behavior and expression of neuroinflammatory markers in mice. Neurochem Res 38: 2375–2384.
68. Luo KR, Hong CJ, Liou YJ, Hou SJ, Huang YH, et al. (2010) Differential regulation of neurotrophin S100B and BDNF in two rat models of depression. Prog Neuropsychopharmacol Biol Psychiatry 34: 1433–1439.
69. Ye Y, Wang G, Wang H, Wang X (2011) Brain-derived neurotrophic factor (BDNF) infusion restored astrocytic plasticity in the hippocampus of a rat model of depression. Neurosci Lett 503: 15–19.
70. Veena J, Srikumar BN, Raju TR, Shankaranarayana Rao BS (2009) Exposure to enriched environment restores the survival and differentiation of new born cells in the hippocampus and ameliorates depressive symptoms in chronically stressed rats. Neurosci Lett 455: 178–182.
71. Rothermundt M, Arolt V, Wiesmann M, Missler U, Peters M, et al. (2001) S-100B is increased in melancholic but not in non-melancholic major depression. J Affect Disord 66: 89–93.
72. Bargerstock E, Puvenna V, Iffland P, Falcone T, Hossain M, et al. (2014) Is peripheral immunity regulated by blood-brain barrier permeability changes? PLoS ONE 9: e101477.
73. Mondello S, Müller U, Jeromin A, Streeter J, Hayes RL, et al. (2011) Blood-based diagnostics of traumatic brain injuries. Expert Rev Mol Diagn 11: 65–78.
74. Shahim P, Tegner Y, Wilson DH, Randall J, Skillback T, et al. (2014) Blood biomarkers for brain injury in concussed professional ice hockey players. JAMA Neurol 71: 684–692.
75. Ponath G, Schettler C, Kaestner F, Voigt B, Wentker D, et al. (2007) Autocrine S100B effects on astrocytes are mediated via RAGE. J Neuroimmunol 184: 214–222.
76. Beer C, Blacker D, Bynevelt M, Hankey GJ, Puddey IB (2010) Systemic markers of inflammation are independently associated with S100B concentration: results of an observational study in subjects with acute ischaemic stroke. J Neuroinflammation 7: 71.
77. Szelenyi A, Heukamp C, Seifert V, Marquardt G (2014) S100B, intraoperative neuromonitoring findings and their relation to clinical outcome in surgically treated intradural spinal lesions. Acta Neurochir (Wien) 156: 733–739.
78. Blennow K, Jonsson M, Andreasen N, Rosengren L, Wallin A, et al. (2011) No neurochemical evidence of brain injury after blast overpressure by repeated explosions or firing heavy weapons. Acta Neurol Scand 123: 245–251.
79. Derkach DN, Okamoto H, Takahashi S (2000) Neuronal and astroglial injuries in patients undergoing coronary artery bypass grafting and aortic arch replacement during hypothermic cardiopulmonary bypass. Anesth Analg 91: 1066–1072.
80. Kinoshita H, Iranami H, Fujii K, Yamazaki A, Shimogai M, et al. (2003) The use of bone cement induces an increase in serum astroglial S-100B protein in patients undergoing total knee arthroplasty. Anesth Analg 97: 1657–1660.
81. Reinsfelt B, Ricksten SE, Zetterberg H, Blennow K, Freden-Lindqvist J, et al. (2012) Cerebrospinal fluid markers of brain injury, inflammation, and blood-brain barrier dysfunction in cardiac surgery. Ann Thorac Surg 94: 549–555.
82. Ashraf S, Bhattacharya K, Tian Y, Watterson K (1999) Cytokine and S100B levels in paediatric patients undergoing corrective cardiac surgery with or without total circulatory arrest. Eur J Cardiothorac Surg 16: 32–37.
83. Sellner J, Davies NW, Howard RS, Petzold A (2014) Neurofilament heavy chain as a marker of neuroaxonal pathology and prognosis in acute encephalitis. European Journal of Neurology 21: 845–850.
84. Skold MK, Risling M, Holmin S (2006) Inhibition of vascular endothelial growth factor receptor 2 activity in experimental brain contusions aggravates injury outcome and leads to early increased neuronal and glial degeneration. Eur J Neurosci 23: 21–34.
85. Shore PM, Thomas NJ, Clark RS, Adelson PD, Wisniewski SR, et al. (2004) Continuous versus intermittent cerebrospinal fluid drainage after severe traumatic brain injury in children: effect on biochemical markers. J Neurotrauma 21: 1113–1122.
86. Laskowitz DT, Grocott H, Hsia A, Copeland KR (1998) Serum markers of cerebral ischemia. J Stroke Cerebrovasc Dis 7: 234–241.
87. Kessler FH, Woody G, Portela LV, Tort AB, De Boni R, et al. (2007) Brain injury markers (S100B and NSE) in chronic cocaine dependents. Revista Brasileira de Psiquiatria 29: 134–139.
88. Marchi N, Angelov L, Masaryk T, Fazio V, Granata T, et al. (2007) Seizure-promoting effect of blood-brain barrier disruption. Epilepsia 48: 732–742.
89. Reiber H (1998) Cerebrospinal fluid–physiology, analysis and interpretation of protein patterns for diagnosis of neurological diseases. Mult Scler 4: 99–107.
90. Reiber H (2001) Dynamics of brain-derived proteins in cerebrospinal fluid. Clin Chim Acta 310: 173–186.
91. Marchi N, Fazio V, Cucullo L, Kight K, Masaryk T, et al. (2003) Serum transthyretin monomer as a possible marker of blood-to-CSF barrier disruption. J Neurosci 23: 1949–1955.
92. Marchi N, Rasmussen P, Kapural M, Fazio V, Kight K, et al. (2003) Peripheral markers of brain damage and blood-brain barrier dysfunction. Restor Neurol Neurosci 21: 109–121.
93. Zongo D, Ribereau-Gayon R, Masson F, Laborey M, Contrand B, et al. (2012) S100-B protein as a screening tool for the early assessment of minor head injury. Ann Emerg Med 59: 209–218.
94. Johnsson P, Lundqvist C, Lindgren A, Ferencz I, Alling C, et al. (1995) Cerebral complications after cardiac surgery assessed by S-100 and NSE levels in blood. J Cardiothorac Vasc Anesth 9: 694–699.
95. Grocott HP, Arrowsmith JE (2001) Serum S100 protein as a marker of cerebral damage during cardiac surgery. Br J Anaesth 86: 289–290.
96. Bayram H, Hidiroglu M, Cetin L, Kucuker A, Iriz E, et al. (2013) Comparing S-100 beta protein levels and neurocognitive functions between patients undergoing on-pump and off-pump coronary artery bypass grafting. J Surg Res 182: 198–202.
97. Whitaker DC, Green AJ, Stygall J, Harrison MJ, Newman SP (2007) Evaluation of an alternative S100b assay for use in cardiac surgery: relationship with microemboli and neuropsychological outcome. Perfusion 22: 267–272.
98. Hernandez F, Jr., Brown JR, Likosky DS, Clough RA, Hess AL, et al. (2007) Neurocognitive outcomes of off-pump versus on-pump coronary artery bypass: a prospective randomized controlled trial. Ann Thorac Surg 84: 1897–1903.
99. Beck AT, Steer RA, Garbin MG (1988) Psychometric properties of the Beck Depression Inventory: Twenty-five years of evaluation. Clin Psychol Rev 8: 77–100.
100. Tukey JW (1977) Exploratory data analysis. Reading, MA: Addison-Wesley.
101. Fazio V, Bhudia SK, Marchi N, Aumayr B, Janigro D (2004) Peripheral detection of S100beta during cardiothoracic surgery: what are we really measuring? Ann Thorac Surg 78: 46–52; discussion 52–43.
102. Jonsson H, Johnsson P, Alling C, Westaby S, Blomquist S (1998) Significance of serum S100 release after coronary artery bypass grafting. Ann Thorac Surg 65: 1639–1644.
103. Baufreton C, Allain P, Chevailler A, Etcharry-Bouyx F, Corbeau JJ, et al. (2005) Brain injury and neuropsychological outcome after coronary artery surgery are affected by complement activation. Ann Thorac Surg 79: 1597–1605.
104. Pham N, Fazio V, Cucullo L, Teng Q, Biberthaler P, et al. (2010) Extracranial sources of S100B do not affect serum levels. PLoS ONE 5: e12691.

9

Systems Level Analysis and Identification of Pathways and Networks Associated with Liver Fibrosis

Mohamed Diwan M. AbdulHameed[1], Gregory J. Tawa[1], Kamal Kumar[1], Danielle L. Ippolito[2], John A. Lewis[2], Jonathan D. Stallings[2], Anders Wallqvist[1]*

1 Department of Defense Biotechnology High Performance Computing Software Applications Institute, Telemedicine and Advanced Technology Research Center, U.S. Army Medical Research and Materiel Command, Fort Detrick, Maryland, United States of America, **2** U.S. Army Center for Environmental Health Research, Fort Detrick, MD, United States of America

Abstract

Toxic liver injury causes necrosis and fibrosis, which may lead to cirrhosis and liver failure. Despite recent progress in understanding the mechanism of liver fibrosis, our knowledge of the molecular-level details of this disease is still incomplete. The elucidation of networks and pathways associated with liver fibrosis can provide insight into the underlying molecular mechanisms of the disease, as well as identify potential diagnostic or prognostic biomarkers. Towards this end, we analyzed rat gene expression data from a range of chemical exposures that produced observable periportal liver fibrosis as documented in DrugMatrix, a publicly available toxicogenomics database. We identified genes relevant to liver fibrosis using standard differential expression and co-expression analyses, and then used these genes in pathway enrichment and protein-protein interaction (PPI) network analyses. We identified a PPI network module associated with liver fibrosis that includes known liver fibrosis-relevant genes, such as tissue inhibitor of metalloproteinase-1, galectin-3, connective tissue growth factor, and lipocalin-2. We also identified several new genes, such as perilipin-3, legumain, and myocilin, which were associated with liver fibrosis. We further analyzed the expression pattern of the genes in the PPI network module across a wide range of 640 chemical exposure conditions in DrugMatrix and identified early indications of liver fibrosis for carbon tetrachloride and lipopolysaccharide exposures. Although it is well known that carbon tetrachloride and lipopolysaccharide can cause liver fibrosis, our network analysis was able to link these compounds to potential fibrotic damage before histopathological changes associated with liver fibrosis appeared. These results demonstrated that our approach is capable of identifying early-stage indicators of liver fibrosis and underscore its potential to aid in predictive toxicity, biomarker identification, and to generally identify disease-relevant pathways.

Editor: Christina Chan, Michigan State University, United States of America

Funding: The authors were supported by the Military Operational Medicine Research Program and the U.S. Army's Network Science Initiative, U.S. Army Medical Research and Materiel Command (USAMRMC, http://mrmc.amedd.army.mil), Ft. Detrick, MD. This research was supported in part by an appointment to the Postgraduate Research Participation Program at the U.S. Army Center for Environmental Health Research (USACEHR, http://usacehr.amedd.army.mil) administered by the Oak Ridge Institute for Science and Education through an interagency agreement between the U.S. Department of Energy and USAMRMC. The funders had no role in study design, data collection and analysis, decision to publish, or preparation of the manuscript.

Competing Interests: The authors have declared that no competing interests exist.

* Email: awallqvist@bhsai.org

Introduction

Exposure to toxic chemicals can lead to liver injury through a variety of mechanisms, such as oxidative stress, the immune response, activation of apoptotic pathways, and necrosis [1]. Liver fibrosis is a common pathologic feature observed in a wide spectrum of liver injuries [2,3] and is marked by inflammation and excessive accumulation of extracellular matrix (ECM) components [4]. Liver fibrosis results in scar formation and, if unresolved, leads to cirrhosis, portal hypertension, and liver failure [4]. Liver fibrosis typically starts with apoptosis or necrosis of hepatocytes, which causes reactive oxygen species generation. This process leads to the release of inflammatory mediators and ultimately results in activation of hepatic stellate cells [3], the main ECM-producing cells in the liver. This activation of hepatic stellate cells is the key pathogenic mechanism of liver fibrosis [3–6]. Activated hepatic stellate cells lead to further inflammation and ECM generation, which results in the replacement of liver parenchymal cells with ECM [5]. Despite recent progress, our understanding of the molecular mediators of liver fibrosis remains incomplete, and we are still in the process of identifying such mediators [7,8].

Although fibrotic damage is reversible, there are no approved drugs or treatments for liver fibrosis. Key in understanding damage and control of fibrosis is accurate diagnosis or early indicators of damage. The gold standard for diagnosing fibrosis is currently via liver biopsy. This invasive method has many limitations, such as inter- and intra-observer variations and sampling variability [9]. Thus, there is a need to identify sensitive, specific, and non-invasive biomarkers of liver fibrosis. Identification of such biomarkers will improve diagnosis and allow better clinical management of the disease. In the military, this capability would aid in field assessment and potentially enable timely evacuation or guide return-to-duty

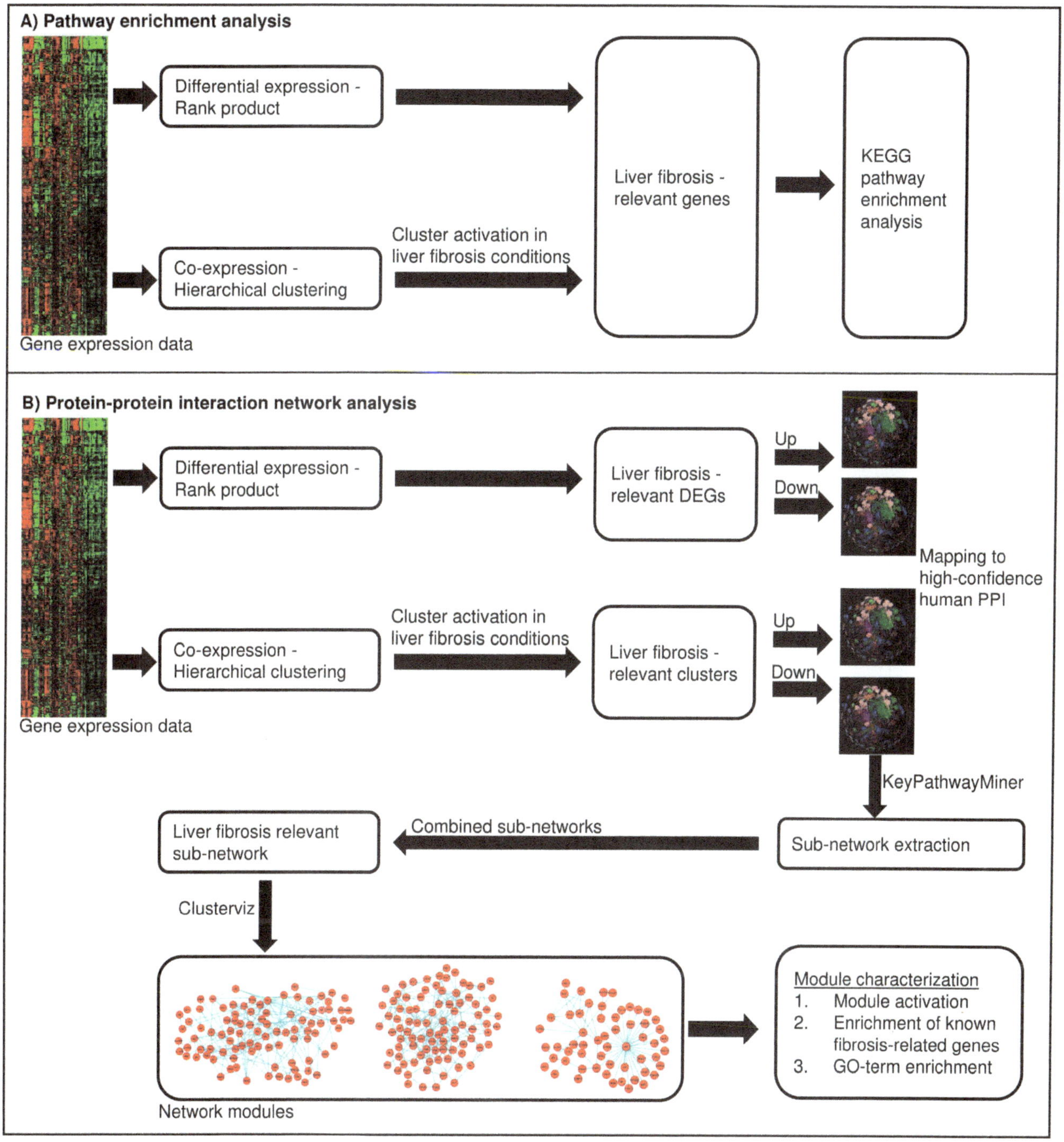

Figure 1. Workflow used in this study to identify pathways and networks associated with liver fibrosis.

decisions. Elucidation of the pathways and networks associated with liver fibrosis will provide insight into the molecular mechanisms of this disease and, importantly, help us to identify mechanism-based biomarkers of liver damage.

Computational systems biology approaches are now routinely used to analyze gene expression data and to gain insight into the molecular mechanisms of many diseases [10–15]. Pathway enrichment analysis provides a biological interpretation of gene lists obtained from microarray data using manually curated pathway databases, such as the Kyoto Encyclopedia of Genes and Genomes (KEGG) and Reactome [16,17]. The BioSystems database [18,19] provides an integrated resource of pathways from several major pathway databases, including KEGG and Reactome. Huang et al. [20] have summarized the various tools and statistical methods available for pathway enrichment analysis and their utility in elucidating the mechanisms of diseases [21–23]. In literature related to liver fibrosis, the work of Affo et al. [24] utilizes KEGG pathway analysis in identifying the role of focal adhesion and cytokine-cytokine receptor interaction pathways in alcoholic hepatitis. Although widely used, pathway analysis has

Table 1. Chemical exposure conditions that produced periportal liver fibrosis.

Chemical	Dose (mg/kg)	Duration (days)	Histopathology (severity score)
1-Naphthylisothiocyanate	30	7	2
1-Naphthylisothiocyanate	60	7	2
4,4′-Methylenedianiline	81	5	2
N-Nitrosodimethylamine	10	5	2

some limitations [25]. Foremost, pathway analysis relies exclusively on experimentally confirmed, curated data. Only a small fraction of human genes map to curated pathway collections (e.g., KEGG [14]); thus, pathway analysis is inherently biased against the discovery of new molecular mediators. For example, we found that only 5,870 of the ~21,000 human genes mapped to the 229 KEGG pathways [26]. Moreover, the gene networks comprising the pathway maps are not mutually exclusive, and the same gene can occur in many pathways [25]. Integrated analyses of gene expression data with protein-protein interaction (PPI) networks enable us to partly overcome the limitations associated with pathway analysis. The potential of this integrated approach has been shown in identifying biomarkers for breast cancer [27] and in understanding the molecular mechanisms of dilated cardiomyopathy [28], hepatitis C virus infection [29], and cancer and heart disease [30–34]. However, to the best of our knowledge, no such integrated analysis has been reported for liver fibrosis.

Thus, our goal in this study was to identify liver fibrosis-relevant pathways and networks based on an integrated gene expression and PPI network analysis. We analyzed the gene expression data from a range of chemical exposure conditions that produced periportal liver fibrosis in DrugMatrix, a publicly available toxicogenomics database [35]. We carried out differential expression and co-expression analysis using rank product and hierarchical clustering, respectively, to identify genes associated with liver fibrosis [36]. We then examined these genes in two separate analyses. In the first analysis, we identified the KEGG pathways associated with liver fibrosis. In the second analysis, we integrated the gene expression data with the high-confidence human PPI network to obtain liver fibrosis-relevant sub-networks [37]. We identified a PPI network module associated with liver fibrosis that includes known liver fibrosis-relevant genes like *Timp1*, *Lgals3*, *Ctgf*, and *Lcn2*, along with several new genes. We further analyzed the expression pattern of the genes in the PPI network across a wide range of 640 chemical exposure conditions in DrugMatrix and linked compounds such as carbon tetrachloride to potential fibrotic damage before histopathological evidence of liver fibrosis appeared. These results illustrate the potential of our approach to aid in toxicity prediction and biomarker discovery.

Materials and Methods

Figure 1 shows the overall workflows used in this study to identify liver fibrosis-relevant pathways and interaction networks. We used two separate but complementary approaches to map the overall gene transcriptional response to liver fibrosis via *1*) enrichment analysis of knowledge-based pathways association, and *2*) integration of gene expression data with PPI networks to identify interaction networks. These fibrosis-relevant interaction networks can be considered as *de novo* pathways.

Data collection and processing

We used DrugMatrix, a publicly available toxicogenomics database [35,38], for our analyses. DrugMatrix is a large collection of gene expression, hematology, histopathology, and clinical chemistry data obtained from Sprague-Dawley rats after exposure to a range of chemicals, including industrial chemicals, toxicants, and drugs with multiple time intervals, dose ranges, and tissues for each chemical [35]. A chemical exposure condition in DrugMatrix data refers to exposure to a particular chemical at a particular dose and time. We downloaded the DrugMatrix liver gene expression data generated using Affymetrix GeneChip Rat Genome 230 2.0 Arrays from the National Institute of Environmental Health Sciences (NIEHS) server (https://ntp.niehs.nih.gov/drugmatrix/index.html). Of the 2,218 microarray CEL files in this database, 1,941 were chemical exposures and 277 were controls. We performed background correction, quantile normalization, and summarization using the robust multi-array average method in R/BioConductor package *affy* [26,39–41]. We then used the BioConductor package *ArrayQualityMetrics* to assess the quality of the microarray data and removed 155 outlier arrays [42]. We reprocessed the remaining arrays using the robust multi-array average method and used this final normalized data for all our analyses. With the BioConductor package *genefilter*, we carried out non-specific filtering of the genes [43]. We removed probe sets without Entrez ID or with low variance across chemical exposures based on inter-quartile range. We additionally filtered probe sets based on "Present" calls using the BioConductor package *affy*, retaining only the probe sets for which at least 25% of the chemical exposures had "Present" calls for all replicates within the chemical exposure condition. After calculating the average intensity between the replicates of a chemical exposure condition, we computed log-ratios for each gene between treatments and their corresponding controls. Our final log-ratio matrix contained 7,826 genes and 640 chemical exposure conditions.

Identifying genes relevant to liver fibrosis

The DrugMatrix database provides histopathology data associated with each chemical exposure condition. There were five chemical exposure conditions that produced liver periportal fibrosis with a histopathology score >1 (**Figure S1**). We carried out a quality check by clustering the replicates of these five chemical exposures, along with their respective controls. Ideally, the chemical exposures and controls would have clustered separately. But all replicates of 5-day exposures to Crotamiton-750 mg/kg clustered with controls rather than with other treatments (**Figure S1**). Hence, we excluded this condition from the liver fibrosis-producing condition set. **Table 1** lists the four chemical exposure conditions that were used in this study as the liver fibrosis-producing condition set. All replicates of the four chemical exposure conditions had a histopathology score of 2. We used the rank product method to identify differentially expressed genes (DEG) [36]. Rank product is a non-parametric, permutation-based method that has been widely used in many studies [36,44,45]. With this method, the fold-change values were converted into rank, and then the significance of the obtained rank, including the false discovery rate (FDR) p-value, was calculated. We used the BioConductor package *RankProd* for this analysis [44]. This method produces separate lists of up-regulated and down-regulated genes. We considered all genes with an FDR <0.05 to be significantly differentially expressed. We carried out the rank product analysis separately for each of the four chemical exposure conditions; the genes that were significantly differentially expressed in at least two of the four chemical exposure conditions that produced periportal liver fibrosis were considered as fibrosis-relevant DEGs.

We carried out hierarchical clustering using the R package *hclust* to identify co-expressed genes [21]. We clustered the genes in the log-ratio matrix using their $\log_2$ ratio values across 640 chemical exposure conditions. We used the Pearson correlation and the average linkage method to perform the clustering, and the R package *dynamicTreeCut* for automated extraction of clusters [46]. The dynamic tree cut algorithm implements an automated iterative process to identify and split sub-clusters from a dendrogram until the minimum cluster size threshold is reached [46]. We used the *cutreeDynamic* function in this package with *minimum cluster size* set to *16, method* set to *hybrid*, and *deepsplit* set to *True*.

We calculated cluster activation scores to identify liver fibrosis-relevant clusters in order to identify clusters whose constituent genes show altered gene expression (either up- or down-regulation) in chemical exposure conditions that produce periportal liver fibrosis. To calculate a cluster activation score, we first normalized the log-ratio values of each gene across 640 chemical exposure conditions by converting them into Z-scores. The Z-score of gene i under chemical exposure condition j is given by

$$Z_{i,j} = \frac{X_{i,j} - \mu_i}{\sigma_i}, \tag{1}$$

where $X_{i,j}$ is the log-ratio value for gene i under chemical exposure condition j, μ_i is the average log ratio for gene i across all 640 chemical exposure conditions, and σ_i is the standard deviation of the log ratio for gene i across all 640 chemical exposure conditions. Next, we obtained the cluster activation scores for liver fibrosis by averaging the Z-scores of all genes within a cluster and across all chemical exposure conditions that produced periportal liver fibrosis. The activation score A_c of cluster c in liver fibrosis is given by

$$A_c = \frac{1}{N_c N_f} \sum_{i \in c}^{N_c} \sum_{j}^{N_f} Z_{i,j}, \tag{2}$$

where N_c is the number of genes associated with cluster c, N_f is the number of chemical exposure conditions that produce periportal liver fibrosis, and $Z_{i,j}$ is the Z-score of gene i under chemical exposure conditions that produce periportal liver fibrosis j. We used an absolute cluster activation score cutoff of 2, corresponding to the 95th percentile of the probability density distribution, and selected genes in clusters above this threshold as liver fibrosis-relevant co-expressed genes.

In general, to find disease-relevant genes, either differential expression or co-expression analysis is commonly used. Utilization of both approaches together will allow us to overcome the limitation associated with each approach. Hence, we combined the gene list from both approaches, i.e., differential expression and co-expression, to form the liver fibrosis-relevant gene set.

Pathway enrichment analysis

We used the Database for Annotation, Visualization, and Integrated Discovery (DAVID) tool to perform KEGG pathway enrichment analysis [47]. The pathways below a Benjamini-Hochberg FDR <0.05 were considered to be significantly enriched. We used the liver fibrosis-relevant gene set, i.e., the combined list of genes determined by differential expression and co-expression analysis to be relevant to liver fibrosis, for the pathway enrichment analysis. Then we separately used the up-regulated genes and down-regulated genes in this set and carried out pathway enrichment analysis.

PPI network analysis

Yu et al. [37] used the interaction detection based on shuffling (IDBOS) approach to generate a high-confidence PPI network and showed that the resulting high-confidence PPIs reduce the noise inherent in aggregated PPIs. In their work, they created experimentally derived high-confidence PPI networks for both rats and humans [37]. The rat high-confidence PPI network contained 1,001 nodes, whereas the human high-confidence PPI network consisted of 14,230 nodes. We chose to use the human high-confidence PPI network due to its much larger coverage. The rat probe-set identifiers were mapped to their corresponding human gene identifiers using orthology mapping tools [26,48,49]. This approach followed the work by Zhang et al. [50] for mapping other species' gene expression data to a human PPI network. We utilized the KeyPathwayMiner program in Cytoscape 2.8 to obtain the liver fibrosis-relevant sub-network [51–53]. KeyPathwayMiner attempts to find maximally connected sub-networks for the input query genes with gene expression data using the ant-colony optimization algorithm [51]. We used KeyPathwayMiner with *ant-colony optimization algorithm*, *node exceptions (K)* set to *100*, and *case exceptions (L)* set to *0*. The *node exception (K)* value provided the allowance for genes that were not present in the input gene set and the *case exception (L)* defined the number of conditions in which the input gene may not be active. We separately ran KeyPathwayMiner using the up-regulated and down-regulated genes in liver fibrosis-relevant DEGs and co-expressed genes and extracted the sub-networks. We then combined the four sub-networks into one final liver fibrosis-relevant sub-network. This sub-network was created by the union of the four sub-networks. We did not use the intersection of the four sub-networks, as it contained only two nodes. Finally, we clustered this liver fibrosis-relevant sub-network using the topology-based network clustering program in Cytoscape, Clusterviz. We used the *EAGLE algorithm* in Clusterviz with default parameters [54]. As implemented, Clusterviz generated 11 network modules.

Module characterization

We mapped the proteins in the PPI network modules to the rat gene expression Z-score matrix. We calculated the activation scores (**Equation 2**) for the 11 network modules under conditions that caused periportal liver fibrosis. The method is the same as described above, except that here we used the genes in the module instead of cluster. We collected 28 known liver fibrosis-relevant genes from literature (*Set 1*) [3,5,55,56]. Of these 28 genes, 26 mapped to the high-confidence human PPI network. We also collected genes that are known to be associated with liver cirrhosis from the Comparative Toxicogenomics Database (CTD) (*Set 2*) [57]. Of the 126 genes with direct evidence of an association with

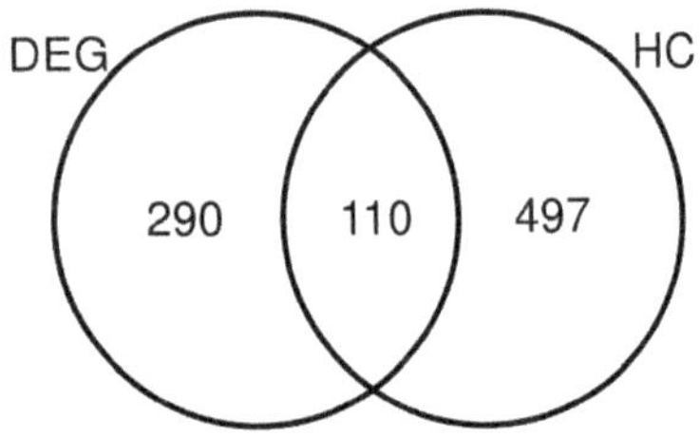

Figure 2. Number of fibrosis-relevant genes from differential and co-expression analysis. Number of genes in the liver fibrosis-relevant differentially expressed gene list and liver fibrosis-relevant co-expressed gene list and the overlap between them.

liver cirrhosis, 95 mapped to the high-confidence human PPI network. We used the Fisher exact test to calculate the enrichment of these genes (*Set 1* and *Set 2*) in each PPI network module. The module genes were also characterized by gene ontology (GO) biological process-term enrichment using the DAVID tool. We used the Revigo tool to visualize the GO enrichment results [58] and analyzed the network modules in terms of activation in liver fibrosis, enrichment with known liver fibrosis-relevant genes, and enrichment of liver fibrosis-relevant GO terms. Based on this analysis, we prioritized one PPI network module (M5) as a liver fibrosis-relevant network module.

We used two statistical significance tests to analyze whether the network module M5 was obtained by random chance. Our null hypothesis was that the observed number of nodes ($M5_{nodes}$) and edges ($M5_{edges}$) in module M5 were obtained by random chance. In the first analysis, we randomly selected 92 proteins from the human PPI network and counted the number of nodes (R_{nodes}) and edges (R_{edges}) of the largest connected component. This process was repeated 1,000 times. We computed the number of times $R_{nodes} \geq M5_{nodes}$, denoted as $N_{randnode}$. Similarly, we computed the number of times $R_{edges} \geq M5_{edges}$, denoted as $N_{randedge}$. Then we computed the probability of obtaining a similar number of nodes by random chance using $P = N_{randnode}/1{,}000$, and the probability of obtaining a similar number of edges by random chance using $P = N_{randedge}/1{,}000$. In the second analysis, we shuffled the human PPI network and then mapped the proteins in the M5 network to this randomized network. We preserved the average node degree during network shuffling. Similar to the first analysis, we extracted the largest connected component, counted the number of nodes and edges, and calculated the probability of obtaining M5 parameters by random chance. We analyzed the overall robustness of the M5 module by comparing the modules generated from a reduced number of samples to those generated from the full dataset. We left out one quarter of the samples from the differential gene expression dataset and analyzed the remaining samples, repeating this procedure four times and leaving out each quarter of the data once. We then compared the overlap of the final module proteins from these four analyses with the module M5 proteins and found an average overlap of 72%. This showed that our method identified roughly the same genes even when samples were missing. We analyzed the expression of genes in module M5 in chemical exposures that produced periportal liver fibrosis across different time periods of exposures. Among the four chemical exposure conditions that produced periportal liver fibrosis, earlier time points were not available for exposure with N-nitroso dimethylamine at 10 mg/kg. Data were available for exposures to 1-naphthyl isothiocyanate at 30 mg/kg and 60 mg/kg at all time points, i.e., 0.25 day, 1 day, and 3 days, and for exposures to 4,4'-methylene dianiline at 1 day and 3 days. We mapped the expression profile of genes in module M5 across different time periods using the average $\log_2$ ratio of the available chemical exposure data at that time point. Finally, the genes in the prioritized network module M5 were used to cluster the 640 chemical exposure conditions in the DrugMatrix database. We used the clustering software *cluster3* for this purpose [59]. We

Table 2. KEGG[a] pathway enrichment for all genes relevant to liver fibrosis.

Pathway	Count	BH[b]
Prion diseases	11	0.003
Leukocyte transendothelial migration	19	0.008
Focal adhesion	26	0.007
Fc gamma R-mediated phagocytosis	16	0.006
Pyruvate metabolism	10	0.010
Viral myocarditis	15	0.011
Antigen processing and presentation	14	0.035
Systemic lupus erythematosus	14	0.037
Chemokine signaling pathway	21	0.035
Complement and coagulation cascades	12	0.033
Regulation of actin cytoskeleton	24	0.031
ECM[c]-receptor interaction	13	0.030
PPAR[d] signaling pathway	12	0.029
Arginine and proline metabolism	10	0.035
Glycerolipid metabolism	9	0.035

[a]Kyoto Encyclopedia of Genes and Genomes
[b]Benjamini-Hochberg false discovery rate
[c]Extracellular matrix
[d]Peroxisome proliferator-activated receptor

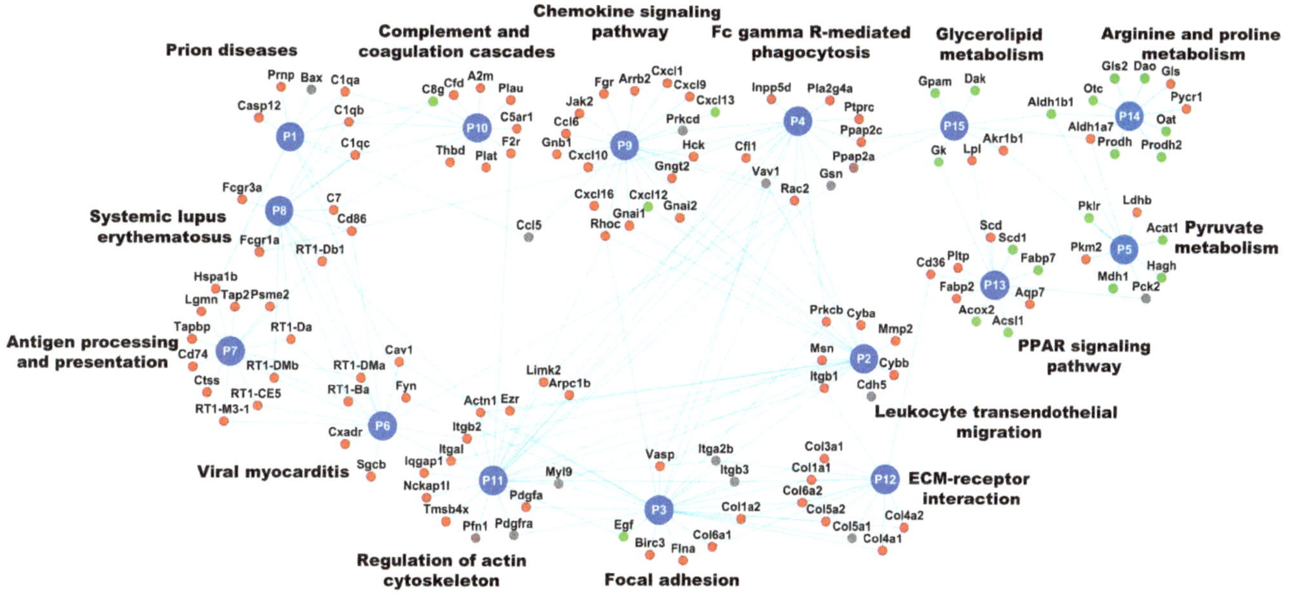

Figure 3. Genes that mapped to the enriched Kyoto Encyclopedia of Genes and Genomes (KEGG) pathways. The average $\log_2$ fold-change ratio across chemical exposures that produced periportal liver fibrosis was used as the gene expression value. Genes with average $\log_2$ fold-change ratios >0.6 are colored in red. Genes with average $\log_2$ fold-change ratios <−0.6 are colored in green. Genes whose average $\log_2$ fold-change ratios are between 0.6 and −0.6 are colored in grey.

evaluated the specificity of network module M5 using the average Z-score across the genes in M5 for each of the 640 chemical exposure conditions.

External validation

In order to further demonstrate the relevance of network module M5 in liver fibrosis, we evaluated the M5 genes in two external datasets (GSE13747 and GSE6929) from the Gene Expression Omnibus (GEO). Both datasets used Affymetrix GeneChip Rat Genome 230 2.0 Arrays. In GSE13747, liver fibrosis was produced by bile duct ligation [60]. Six replicates of liver fibrosis samples and six controls were available. In GSE6929, liver cirrhosis was induced by inhalation of carbon tetrachloride [13]. Four replicates of liver cirrhosis controls and four replicates of sunitinib (SU11248)-treated samples were available. We used the same steps described above for the DrugMatrix database to preprocess these two external datasets and calculated the $\log_2$ ratio between the treatment and controls. Finally, we matched the genes in module M5 and calculated the correlation between the average $\log_2$ ratios in the four chemical exposure conditions that produced periportal liver fibrosis from the DrugMatrix database with the $\log_2$ ratio from external datasets.

Results and Discussion

Identification of liver fibrosis-relevant genes

We used differential gene expression and co-expression analysis to identify liver fibrosis-relevant genes. As outlined in the Materials and Methods section, we analyzed the chemical exposures in the DrugMatrix data that produced periportal liver fibrosis with a histopathological score >1. We used the rank product approach and identified 400 liver fibrosis-relevant DEGs, of which 192 genes were significantly up-regulated, and 208 genes were significantly down-regulated. Here, we used an FDR <0.05 as the cutoff value to select DEGs. This cutoff-based approach knowingly excludes DEGs to minimize false positives and may not capture the complete picture of the disease or processes being studied [61–63]. For example, many genes that do not meet the cutoff criteria can be involved in the same pathway as the DEGs and provide insights into the altered disease process [63]. Identifying co-expressed genes by means of gene clustering is an alternative approach that does not use cutoffs or thresholds at the individual gene level. Instead, genes are clustered based on their expression profiles across a wide range of exposures in order to identify gene sets that are expected to have similar functions, i.e., participate in related pathways [64]. We used hierarchical clustering to cluster 7,826 genes based on their log-ratio values across 640 chemical exposure conditions, which yielded 210 gene clusters containing an average of 37 genes each. Unlike differential expression analysis, these co-expressed genes were not linked or associated with liver fibrosis or any other particular disease. We used the cluster activation scores defined in **Equation 2** to establish the connection between the gene clusters and liver fibrosis. We found 565 genes in the nine clusters with activation scores >2 and 42 genes in the two clusters with activation scores <−2. The genes in these clusters were used as liver fibrosis-relevant co-expressed genes. Finally, we combined the differentially expressed and co-expressed gene lists to create a liver fibrosis-relevant gene set with 897 genes. There were 110 genes in common between the differentially expressed and co-expressed genes, and we show the overlap between these two sets as a Venn diagram (**Figure 2**). **Table S1** provides the list of 897 genes, along with log-ratio values, in the four chemical exposure conditions that produced periportal liver fibrosis.

Pathway enrichment analysis

Table 2 lists the significantly enriched KEGG pathways derived from the liver fibrosis-relevant gene set. These pathways include leukocyte transendothelial migration, focal adhesion, chemokine signaling, regulation of the actin cytoskeleton pathway, and ECM-receptor interaction, and they mainly represent liver fibrosis-related processes. These processes are consistent with previous reports for liver fibrosis. Injured liver cells and activated

Table 3. Activation of network modules and enrichment of known genes relevant to liver fibrosis.

Module	Activation score in Liver fibrosis	No. of genes in module	No. of fibrosis genes (*set 1*)[a]	*p*-value (*set 1*)[a]	No. of cirrhosis genes (*set 2*)[b]	*p*-value (*set 2*)[b]
M1	1.47	150	1	0.24	1	1
M2	0.95	144	3	0.002	5	0.003
M3	1.67	127	2	0.02	0	1
M4	1.92	110	1	0.18	1	0.52
M5	2.12	92	6	1.28E-08	13	3.25E-14
M6	0.77	81	1	0.14	2	0.10
M7	1.09	58	-	1	1	0.32
M8	1.38	49	-	1	2	0.04
M9	0.36	46	-	1	1	0.27
M10	0.87	40	-	1	1	0.24
M11	1.38	34	-	1	1	0.20

[a]Liver fibrosis-relevant genes collected from literature [3,5,55,56]
[b]Liver cirrhosis-relevant genes collected from the Comparative Toxicogenomics Database (CTD)

hepatic stellate cells release chemokines that recruit leukocytes to the site of injury [65]. An elevated expression of chemokines and chemokine receptors has been reported in both animal models and clinical cases of liver fibrosis [66]. Hepatic stellate cell migration is an essential process in fibrosis [67]. Hepatic stellate cells are also known to express adhesion molecules and α-smooth muscle actin

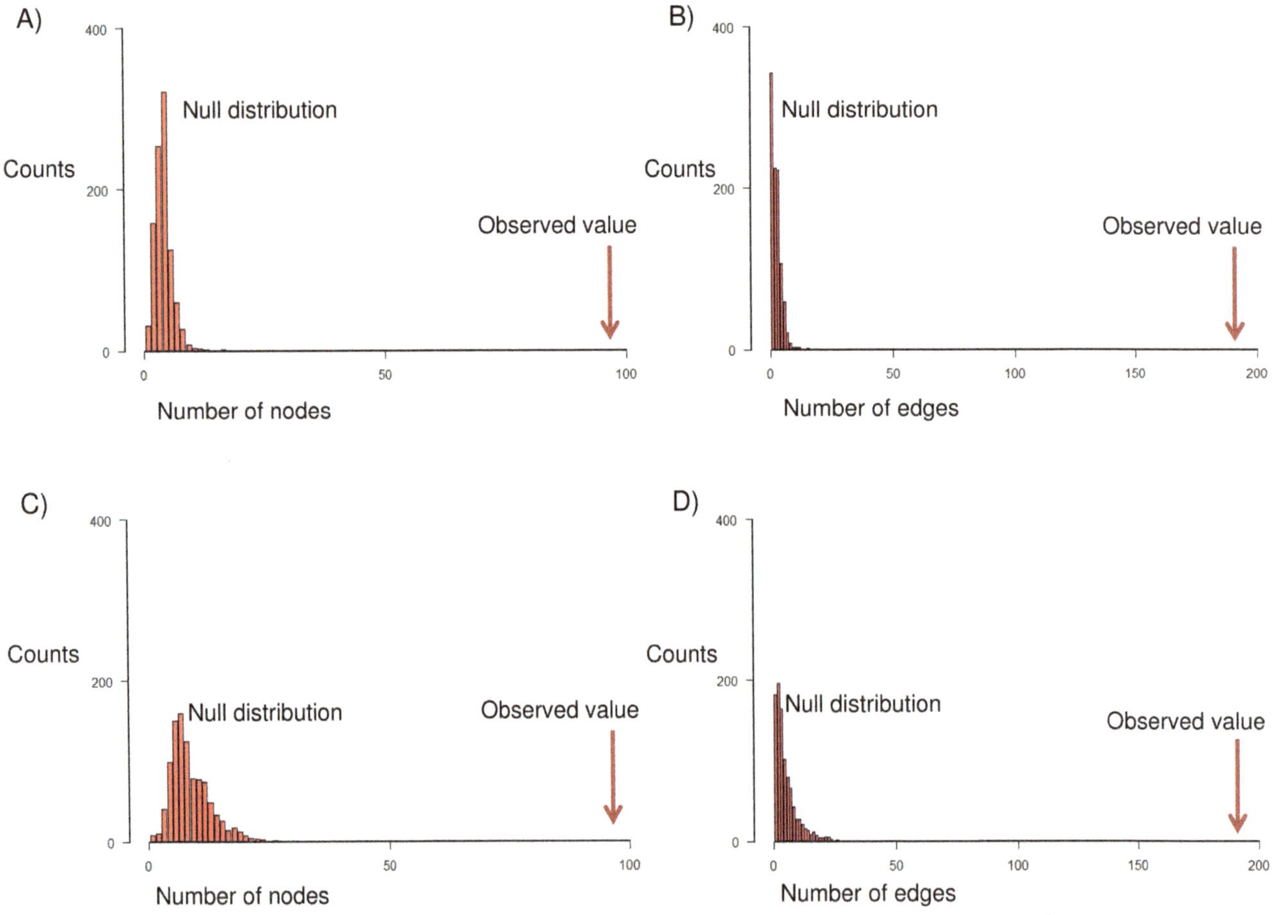

Figure 4. Statistical significance analysis of network module M5. A) The comparison of number of nodes in M5 to that from random sampling analysis. B) The comparison of number of edges in M5 to that from random sampling analysis. C) The comparison of number of nodes in M5 to the number present in shuffled protein-protein interaction (PPI) networks. D) The comparison of number of edges in M5 to the number present in shuffled PPI networks.

(SMA) [4]. Activated hepatic stellate cells are known to secrete prion protein [68,69]. Innate immunity and adaptive immunity play a major role in hepatic stellate cell activation and propagation of liver fibrosis [70]. Anticoagulant drugs and peroxisome proliferator-activated receptor (PPAR)-γ agonists were reported to have an anti-fibrotic effect in experimental liver fibrosis, which is consistent with the enriched pathways, such as complement and coagulation cascades, and the PPAR signaling pathway [70].

We analyzed genes involved in the enriched pathways to ascertain whether we could provide new, testable hypotheses. Genes were mapped to the enriched KEGG pathways (**Figure 3**) and **Table S2** provides the complete list of these genes with pathway information, and their average $\log_2$ ratio in chemical exposures that produced periportal liver fibrosis. The $\log_2$ ratio is commonly used in microarray data analysis, and a value of 0.6 corresponds to a ~1.5 fold-change (up-regulation) in gene expression. *Col1a1*, *Col1a2*, *Col4a1*, *Col4a2*, *Col5a2*, *Itgb1*, *Plat*, *Plau*, *Pdgfa*, *Ezr*, and *Msn* were up-regulated and have an average $\log_2$ ratio >0.6. These genes are known to be altered in liver fibrosis [4,67,71]. We also analyzed the gene list (**Table S2**) for potential new candidates and found genes such as *Lgmn* and *Limk2*, which were up-regulated in all four chemical exposure conditions that produced periportal liver fibrosis. These genes are potential candidates for further exploration. Next, we carried out pathway enrichment analyses using the up- and down-regulated genes separately (**Tables S3** and **S4**). The significantly up-regulated pathways were related to liver fibrosis-relevant processes, whereas the significantly down-regulated pathways were related to metabolism. The down-regulation of metabolism-related pathways could either be related to external factors, such as altered food intake, or could also be an indication of reduced liver function.

Although pathway enrichment analyses are useful and provide an overview of biological processes associated with our gene list, the method has some well-known limitations. Pathway analysis is based on curated data and is limited to the information present in the underlying knowledge database. Moreover, the pathway enrichment based on an over-representation analysis approach treats pathways as simple gene lists without accounting for network connectivity [72]. As such, pathway analysis has limited utility in identifying new molecular mediators or new pathways. Using the connectivity information or pathway topology may provide us with alternative approaches to capture the most relevant pathways associated with a disease.

PPI network analysis

Based on the premise that proteins that are closely connected to each other in a network are more likely to be involved in similar processes, an integration of gene expression with PPI networks has been used to identify disease-specific networks [73]. Such networks have been proposed as *de novo* pathways and partly remedy the limitations of KEGG pathway analysis [25]. Consequently, we mapped the liver fibrosis-relevant genes to a high-confidence human PPI network. Out of 897 fibrosis-relevant genes, 606 mapped to the human PPI network. We extracted a liver fibrosis-relevant sub-network with 902 nodes (proteins) and 2,527 edges using KeyPathwayMiner. Out of the 606 fibrosis-relevant genes,

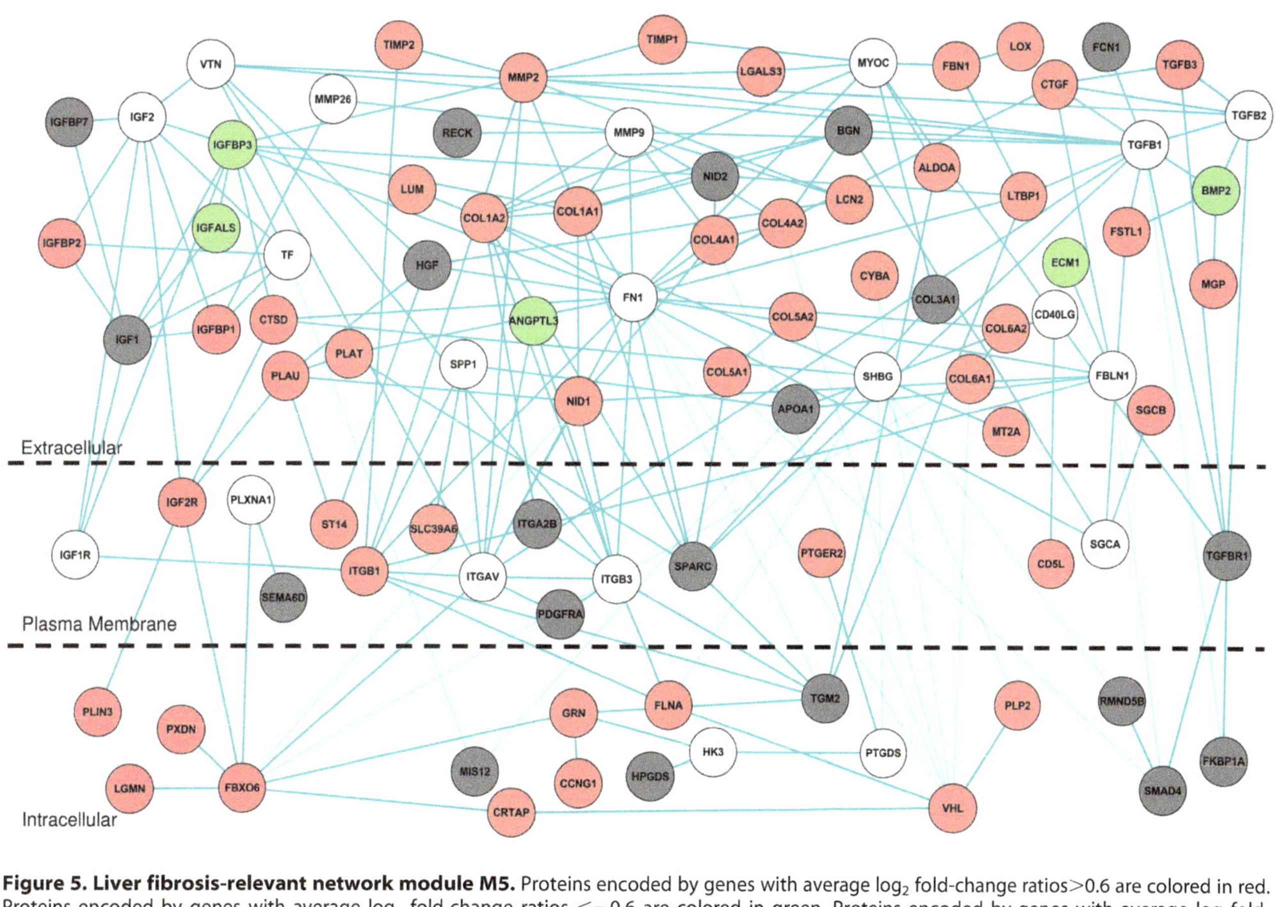

Figure 5. Liver fibrosis-relevant network module M5. Proteins encoded by genes with average $\log_2$ fold-change ratios>0.6 are colored in red. Proteins encoded by genes with average $\log_2$ fold-change ratios <−0.6 are colored in green. Proteins encoded by genes with average $\log_2$fold-change ratios between 0.6 and −0.6<−0.6 are colored in grey. Proteins without corresponding gene expression data are shown as white circles.

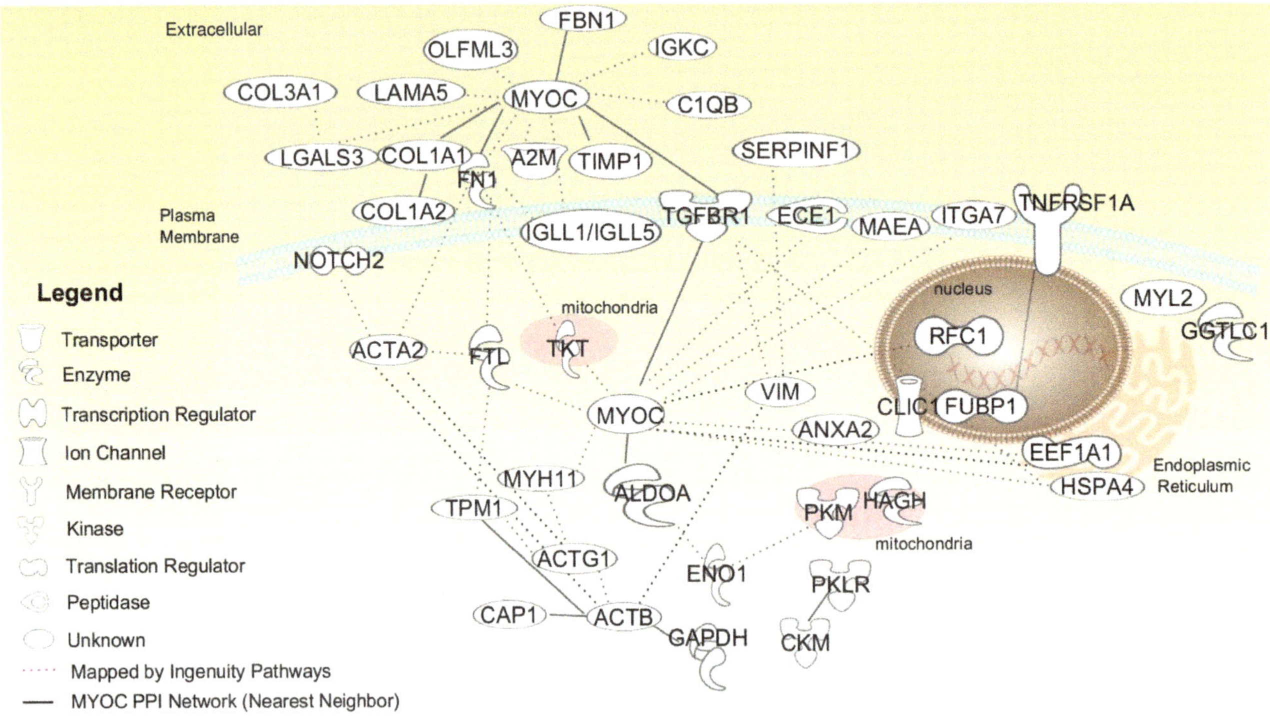

Figure 6. Myocilin interaction network. First neighbors of myocilin (MYOC) in the entire high-confidence human protein-protein interaction (PPI) network.

573 were present in this sub-network. Finally, we clustered the 902 proteins in the liver fibrosis-relevant sub-network into 11 PPI network modules. **Data S1 – S3** provides all the input and Cytoscape session files associated with PPI network analysis. **Table S5** provides the mapping of rat probe IDs to human gene IDs, and **Table S6** provides the protein membership in the PPI network modules, along with their gene expression data.

Module characterization and potential application

We further analyzed the 11 network modules in terms of activation in chemical exposure conditions that produced periportal liver fibrosis, enrichment with known liver fibrosis-relevant genes, and enrichment of GO terms. **Table 3** shows the module activation scores $|A|_c$ calculated using **Equation 2** for chemical exposure conditions that produced periportal liver fibrosis. Module M5 with 92 genes coding for proteins was the highest activated module with an activation score of 2.12. Next, we analyzed the enrichment of known fibrosis-relevant genes collected from the literature (**Table S7**) [3,5,55,56]. **Table 3** shows the p-values for enrichment of known fibrosis-relevant genes in the network modules. Modules M2, M3, and M5 were enriched with liver fibrosis-relevant genes with p-values <0.05. Module M5 had the lowest enrichment p-value with six known fibrosis-associated genes coding for proteins mapped to this module: TIMP1, APOA1, CTGF, LGALS3, TGFB1, and MMP-2. CTD provides curated information on genes associated with a disease [57]. Liver fibrosis was not curated in CTD, but genes associated with liver cirrhosis, the final stage of liver fibrosis, were available. We further analyzed the enrichment of genes associated with liver cirrhosis collected from CTD (**Table S8**) and found module M5 to be the module most enriched with liver cirrhosis-related genes (**Table 3**). We also characterized the 11 modules using the GO biological process-term enrichment analysis. We found that module M5 was enriched with liver fibrosis-relevant GO terms such as *ECM organization* and *Wound healing*. **Figure S2** shows the enriched GO biological process-terms for module M5, and **Table S9** provides the entire list of enriched GO terms for all modules. Based on activation in liver fibrosis-producing conditions, enrichment of known liver fibrosis-relevant genes, and liver fibrosis-relevant GO terms, we selected module M5 as the top liver fibrosis-relevant network module identified from this analysis.

First, we ascertained whether the network module M5 could be observed by random chance. As outlined in the Materials and Methods section, we carried out two statistical significance tests based on random sampling and permutation of the network. The average node degree of the network was 12.76 and it was preserved during network shuffling. Our null hypothesis was that the number of nodes and edges in M5 could be obtained by random chance. In both tests, M5 was significantly different from random occurrence, and the probability of finding this module by random chance was essentially zero (**Figure 4**).

Second, we plotted the PPI network for the protein products encoded by the genes in module M5 (**Figure 5**). Many of the molecular interactions captured were already reported to be associated with liver fibrosis, validating the computational approach. For example, the network map shows connectivity between the genes coding for matrix metalloproteinases and the up-regulated genes encoding TIMP1, COLs and FBN1 (**Figure 5**) [4]. This network map supports a published disease mechanism where increased expression of the gene coding for TIMP1, the negative regulator of matrix metalloproteinases, leads to an increased accumulation of ECM proteins, e.g., collagens (COLs). The network module M5 included other genes encoding the proteins implicated in the pathogenesis of fibrosis (e.g., LUM, CTGF, LGALS3, LCN2, PDGFR, PLAT, and LOX) [4,74–76]. Genes coding for the integrin receptors (ITG) in this network

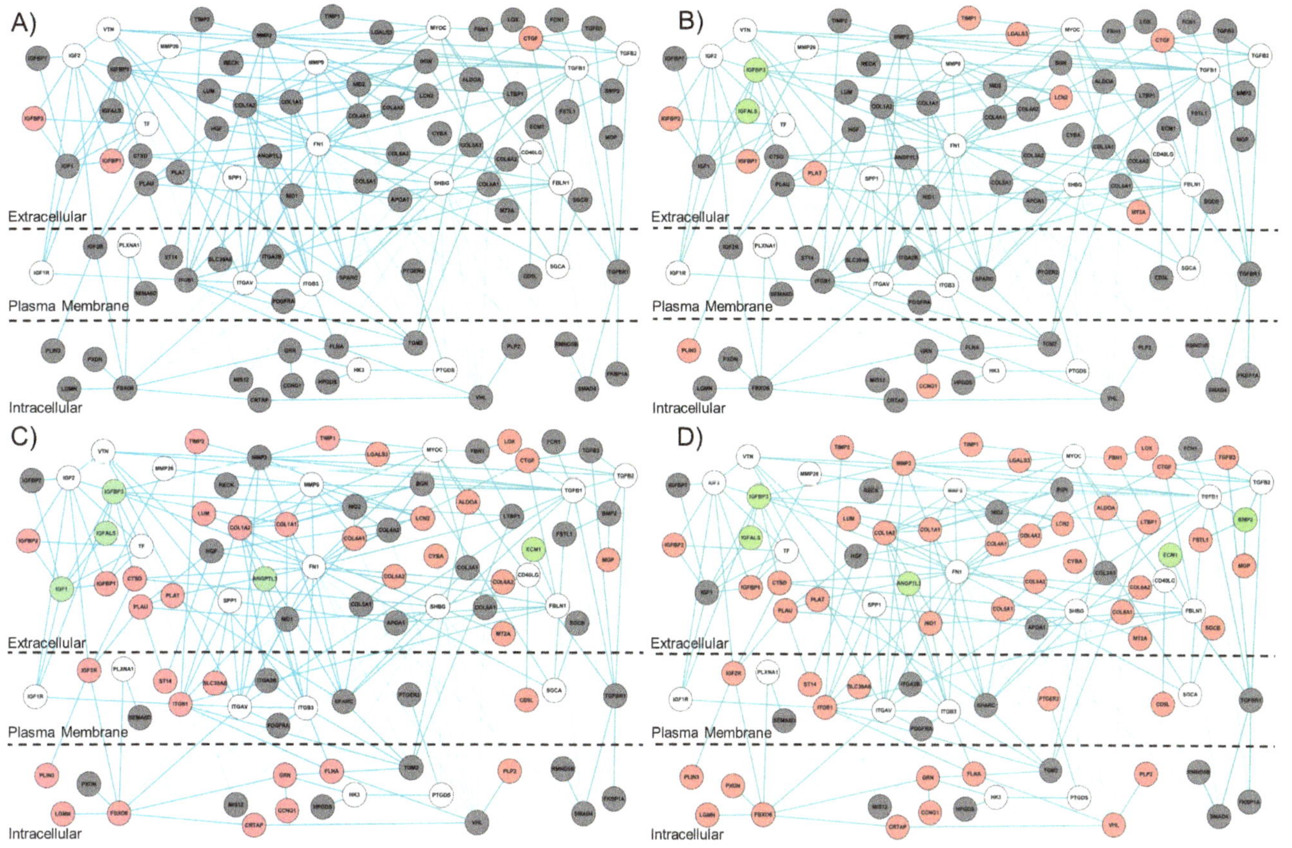

Figure 7. Activation of genes encoding proteins in liver fibrosis-relevant network module M5 at different time points. Genes encoding proteins with average $\log_2$ fold-change ratios$>$0.6 are colored in red. Genes encoding proteins with average $\log_2$ fold-change ratios <-0.6 are colored in green. Genes encoding proteins with average $\log_2$fold-change ratios between 0.6 and $-0.6<-0.6$ are colored in grey. A) Activation at 0.25-day exposure. The mapped expression profile is the average $\log_2$ ratio in 1-naphthyl isothiocyanate 30 mg/kg and 60 mg/kg, at 0.25-day exposure. B) Activation at 1 day of exposure. The mapped expression profile is the average $\log_2$ ratio in 1-naphthyl isothiocyanate 30 mg/kg and 60 mg/kg, and 4,4′-Methylenedianiline 81 mg/kg, at 1 day of exposure. C) Activation at 3 days of exposure. The mapped expression profile is the average $\log_2$ ratio in 1-naphthyl isothiocyanate 30 mg/kg and 60 mg/kg, and 4,4′-Methylenedianiline 81 mg/kg, at 3 days of exposure. D) Activation at $>$3 days of exposure. The mapped expression profile is the average $\log_2$ ratio across chemical exposures that produced liver fibrosis.

interact with ECM proteins that support their known role as mediators of pro-fibrogenic signaling of ECM proteins [77]. In addition to retrieving genes coding for proteins that are already known to be associated with liver fibrosis, this network module also retrieved some potential new candidate protein products. One such candidate is LGMN (average $\log_2$ ratio of 1.24), a cysteine protease that functions in ECM remodeling, but has no known associations with liver fibrosis [78]. Another candidate is the gene encoding PLIN3 (mannose-6-phosphate receptor binding protein), with an average $\log_2$ ratio of 1.29; it interacts with IGF2R in the M5 network. PLIN3 is known to play a role in the pathogenesis of steatosis, and is also reported to play a role in PGE2 production [79,80].

Third, we used the network analysis to identify proteins encoded by genes that do not change in expression, but may form PPI networks. Among the 92 proteins in M5, 30 are K-node exceptions obtained using KeyPathwayMiner, based on their connection to fibrosis-relevant proteins. In protein network analysis, the concept of guilt by association is well known [14]. If a protein is known to be associated with many proteins involved in a biological process, it can be hypothesized to play a role or to be related to the biological process associated with these proteins. For example, the genes encoding osteopontin (SPP1) and vitronectin (VTN) are known to be associated with liver fibrosis [4,81]. These genes did not reach the fold-change threshold in our preprocessed expression dataset, but the network interactions with other fibrosis-relevant protein products that did change in expression predicted them to be fibrosis-relevant (**Figure 5**). In addition to retrieving known proteins, the network analysis also identified MYOC, a protein with no reported association with liver fibrosis. MYOC is a secreted glycoprotein involved in the pathogenesis of glaucoma [82]. MYOC interacts with many up-regulated genes in the high-confidence human PPI network, including genes that encode TIMP1, LGALS3, FBN1, COL1A2, and COL3A1 (**Figure 6**). Based on its connection with many liver fibrosis-relevant proteins, MYOC is a new testable candidate in fibrosis diagnosis and/or pathogenesis. We also analyzed the expression profile of genes in module M5 in chemical exposures that produced periportal liver fibrosis across different time periods of exposures (**Figure 7**). Only a few genes were activated (i.e., $\log_2$ ratio $>$0.6) after 0.25 day and 1 day, but at $\geq$3 days, most of the genes exhibited increased expression (**Figure 7**).

We performed hierarchical clustering of the 640 chemical exposure conditions present in the DrugMatrix database using the expression data for the genes in module M5. We identified a single cluster that included all four chemical exposure conditions that

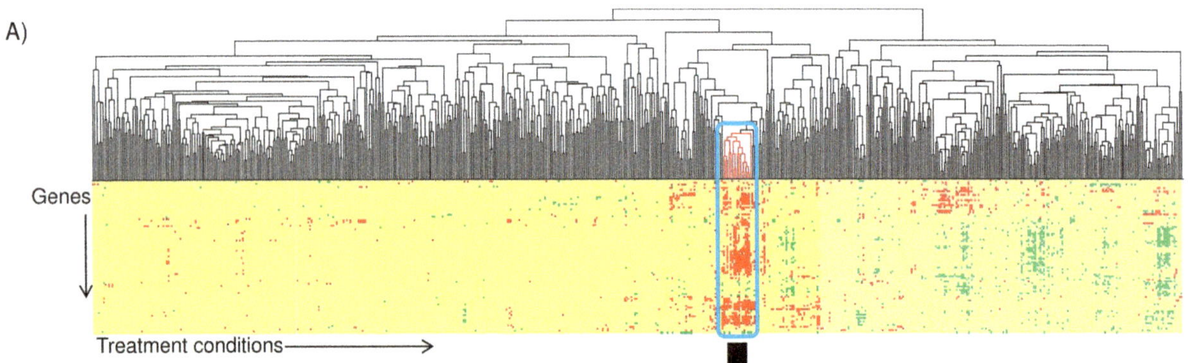

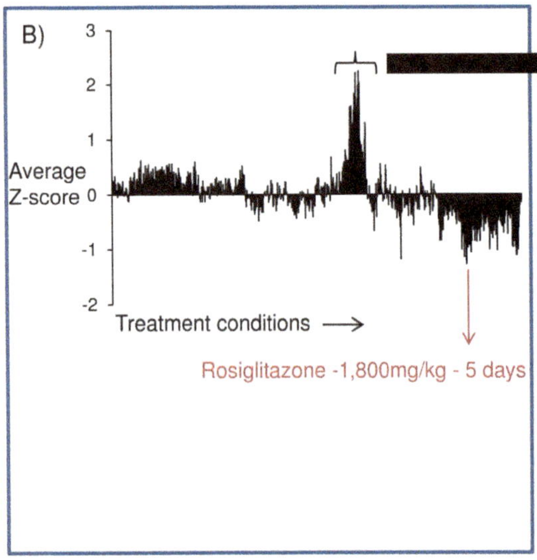

No.	Chemical	Dose (mg/kg)	Duration (days)	Histopathology (severity score)
1	Vinblastine	0.3	5	0
2	Carmustine	16	3	1
3	Carmustine	16	5	1
4	Carbontetrachloride	1175	7	0
5	Carbontetrachloride	400	7	0
6	Carbontetrachloride	400	3	0
7	Lipopolysaccharide ecoli o55B5	1.25	3	0
8	Lipopolysaccharide ecoli o55B5	1.25	5	0
9	N,N-Dimethylformamide	1400	3	NA
10	N-Nitrosodimethylamine	10	5	2
11	Allylalcohol	32	3	NA
12	1-Naphthylisothiocyanate	60	3	1
13	1-Naphthylisothiocyanate	30	3	0
14	4,4-Methylenedianiline	81	5	2
15	1-Naphthylisothiocyanate	30	7	2
16	1-Naphthylisothiocyanate	60	7	2
17	Lipopolysaccharide ecoli o55B5	1.25	1	0

Figure 8. Analysis of genes in liver fibrosis-relevant network module M5. A) Hierarchical clustering of 640 chemical exposures using genes in liver fibrosis-relevant network module M5. The conditions that clustered with four liver fibrosis-producing conditions are highlighted and listed. Genes with Z-scores>2 are colored in red. Genes with Z-scores <−2 are colored in green. Genes with Z-scores between 2 and -2 are colored in yellow. NA in the table represents that histopathological data was not available for that chemical exposure condition. B) Average Z-scores across the genes in module M5 for each of the 640 chemical exposure conditions.

were initially identified with grade 2 periportal liver fibrosis (**Figure 8a**). Most of the 17 conditions in the cluster were associated with compounds that cause fibrosis. Vinblastine, carmustine, and allyl alcohol all had conditions within the drug matrix dataset that caused periportal fibrosis, but they did not meet the histopathology grade 2 threshold used for our initial

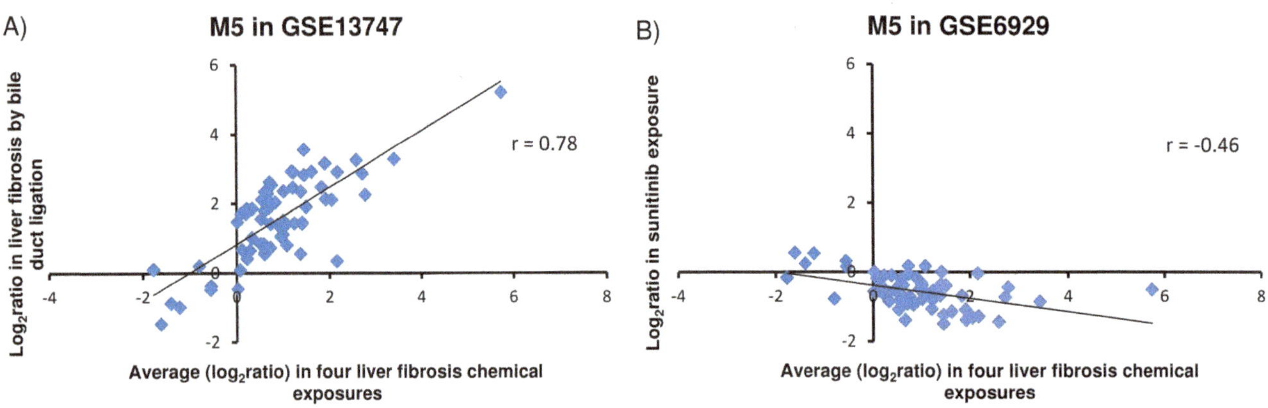

Figure 9. Validation with external datasets. M5 gene expression compared with external datasets. A) GSE13747 represents liver fibrosis produced by bile duct ligation. B) GSE6929 represents sunitinib (SU11248) treatment in liver cirrhosis.

analysis. Carbon tetrachloride and lipopolysaccharide exposures were present in this cluster (**Figure 8a**). Analysis of the literature shows that both carbon tetrachloride and lipopolysaccharide are well known agents that cause liver fibrosis [66]. In the DrugMatrix database, a 28-day exposure study with carbon tetrachloride showed histopathological evidence of liver fibrosis; however, gene expression data were not available for this time point. Furthermore, all but one (crotamiton-750 mg/kg exposure) of the chemicals in the DrugMatrix database that caused periportal fibrosis and had Affymetrix arrays for the liver were identified in this cluster. The data associated with the crotamiton-750 mg/kg exposure most likely represents an outlier in the underlying dataset. Thus, our analysis has the potential to generate gene sets that could predict the early onset of liver fibrosis, consistent with earlier reports that gene expression analysis of liver biopsy samples could complement histopathological data [83].

To evaluate whether network module M5 activation was specific for liver fibrosis, we plotted the average Z-scores of M5 genes in each of the 640 chemical exposure conditions (**Figure 8b**). The M5 genes were mostly activated in liver fibrosis-related chemical exposure conditions and showed very low activation in other chemical exposure conditions (**Figure 8b**). Exposure to rosiglitazone, a PPAR-γ agonist, produced an opposing effect on expression of the genes encoding the protein products in M5 (i.e., down-regulation as measured by $\log_2$ ratio values; **Figure S3**). This result was consistent with the evidence that PPAR-γ agonists prevented liver fibrosis in experimental models [70].

Finally, we used two external gene expression datasets (GEO datasets GSE13747 and GSE6929) to evaluate the relevance of module M5 in liver fibrosis. The overlap of genes between the M5 module and the processed GSE13747 and GSE6929 datasets was 66 and 65, respectively. In the study associated with the GSE13747 dataset, liver fibrosis was induced using bile duct ligation. We observed the predicted positive correlation of gene expression data between the DEGs in this dataset and the genes in module M5 ($r = 0.78$, **Figure 9a**). In the GSE6929 dataset, sunitinib, a multi-kinase inhibitor, was used to treat experimental liver cirrhosis. As expected, we observed a negative correlation ($r = -0.46$) between $\log_2$ ratio gene expression data from GSE6929 and M5 (**Figure 9b**). Thus, the external dataset further supports the validity of M5 genes in liver fibrosis.

In this work, we showed the utility of integrating gene expression and PPI network analyses to understand the molecular-level details of liver fibrosis and to identify biomarker candidates. The presented computational approach has general applicability for characterizing adverse health effects. For example, our approach can be used to computationally predict toxicity pathways associated with specific diseases. Recent work has suggested that the body's response to toxic exposures and the resulting disease progression proceed through a finite set of toxicity pathways [84]. As stated earlier, the available knowledge-based pathway databases are limited in coverage and susceptible to annotation biases towards well-studied diseases. The computational approach presented in this work enabled us to partly overcome these limitations and develop *de novo* pathways linked to a specific disease. In particular, we believe that our approach could be used to further understand the molecular basis of adverse health effects such as acute kidney injury, liver cholestasis, liver steatosis, and myocardial infarction. More recently, the concept of adverse outcome pathways (AOPs) has been proposed as a novel tool in mechanism-based predictive toxicology [85]. The AOPs provide a flow-chart-like mechanistic representation of adverse health effects and consist of a molecular initiating event and a series of intermediate key events that lead to the final adverse outcome [85]. Our computational approach will be applicable to the development of novel AOPs; we believe that network modules, such as the liver fibrosis module (M5) identified in this work, could be used either as a key molecular event or used to quantify the reversibility or point of departure of key events in AOPs.

Conclusion

We have carried out systems-level analyses of gene expression data for periportal liver fibrosis. We found that both pathway and network analyses provided insights into the molecular mechanisms of liver fibrosis. Network analyses allowed us to generate *de novo* pathways and overcome the limitations of analyses based on KEGG pathways. We identified a liver fibrosis-relevant network module that was enriched with known liver fibrosis-relevant genes predictive of liver fibrosis and validated it with external data. The systems approach used in this study allowed us to generate liver fibrosis-relevant pathways and have the potential to predict mechanism-based biomarker candidates.

Supporting Information

Figure S1 Dendrogram from the clustering of chemical exposure conditions that produced periportal liver fibrosis with histopathological scores >1 and their controls.

Figure S2 Treemap view of gene ontology (GO) biological process-term enrichment for genes in the network module M5.

Figure S3 Activation of proteins in liver fibrosis-relevant network module M5 in rosiglitazone-1,800 mg/kg, at 5 days of exposure.

Table S1 The list of fibrosis-relevant genes from differential expression and co-expression analysis.

Table S2 The list of genes that mapped to enriched Kyoto Encyclopedia of Genes and Genomes (KEGG) pathways and their gene expression data in chemical exposures that produced liver fibrosis.

Table S3 The list of enriched up-regulated pathways for the liver fibrosis-relevant gene set.

Table S4 The list of enriched down-regulated pathways for the liver fibrosis-relevant gene set.

Table S5 Mapping of rat probe IDs to human gene IDs.

Table S6 Protein membership in the protein-protein interaction (PPI) network modules and their gene expression data.

Table S7 List of 28 fibrosis-relevant genes collected from literature.

Table S8 List of 126 experimental liver cirrhosis-relevant genes collected from the Comparative Toxicogenomics Database (CTD).

Table S9 List of enriched gene ontology (GO) terms for the protein-protein interaction (PPI) network modules, M1-M11.

Data S1 Cytoscape session file associated with network module generation. The Cytoscape session file includes 1) high-confidence human PPI network data, 2) the liver fibrosis-relevant parent sub-network, and 3) 11 modules obtained by clustering the liver fibrosis-relevant parent sub-network.

Data S2 KeyPathwayMiner input gene list.

Data S3 Cytoscape session file associated with generation of the liver fibrosis-relevant parent sub-network. The Cytoscape session file includes 1) four sub-networks obtained from KeyPathwayMiner, 2) merged nodes of four sub-networks, 3) high-confidence human PPI network data, and 4) the final liver fibrosis-relevant parent sub-network.

Acknowledgments

We thank Drs. Xueping Yu and Nela Zavaljevski for valuable discussions and comments on the manuscript. *Disclaimer*: The opinions and assertions contained herein are the private views of the authors and are not to be construed as official or as reflecting the views of the U.S. Army or of the U.S. Department of Defense. Citations of commercial organizations or trade names in this report do not constitute an official Department of the Army endorsement or approval of the products or services of these organizations. This paper has been approved for public release with unlimited distribution.

Author Contributions

Conceived and designed the experiments: MDMA GJT DLI JAL JDS AW. Performed the experiments: MDMA. Analyzed the data: MDMA GJT DLI AW. Contributed reagents/materials/analysis tools: KK. Wrote the paper: MDMA GJT DLI JAL JDS AW.

References

1. Malhi H, Gores GJ (2008) Cellular and molecular mechanisms of liver injury. Gastroenterology 134: 1641–1654.
2. Sebastiani G (2012) Serum biomarkers for the non-invasive diagnosis of liver fibrosis: the importance of being validated. Clin Chem Lab Med 50: 595–597.
3. Brenner DA (2009) Molecular pathogenesis of liver fibrosis. Trans Am Clin Climatol Assoc 120: 361–368.
4. Bataller R, Brenner DA (2005) Liver fibrosis. J Clin Invest 115: 209–218.
5. Baranova A, Lal P, Birerdinc A, Younossi ZM (2011) Non-invasive markers for hepatic fibrosis. BMC Gastroenterology 11: 91.
6. Kisseleva T, Brenner DA (2008) Mechanisms of fibrogenesis. Exp Biol Med (Maywood) 233: 109–122.
7. Mukhopadhyay P, Rajesh M, Cao Z, Horváth B, Park O, et al. (2014) Poly (ADP-ribose) polymerase-1 is a key mediator of liver inflammation and fibrosis. Hepatology 59: 1998–2009.
8. Qiu L, Lin J, Ying M, Chen W, Yang J, et al. (2013) Aldose reductase is involved in the development of murine diet-induced nonalcoholic steatohepatitis. PLOS ONE 8: e73591.
9. Adams LA (2011) Biomarkers of liver fibrosis. J Gastroenterol Hepatol 26: 802–809.
10. Miller JA, Oldham MC, Geschwind DH (2008) A systems level analysis of transcriptional changes in Alzheimer's disease and normal aging. J Neurosci 28: 1410–1420.
11. Afshari CA, Hamadeh HK, Bushel PR (2011) The evolution of bioinformatics in toxicology: advancing toxicogenomics. Toxicol Sci 120 Suppl 1: S225–S237.
12. Shi Z, Derow CK, Zhang B (2010) Co-expression module analysis reveals biological processes, genomic gain, and regulatory mechanisms associated with breast cancer progression. BMC Syst Biol 4: 74.
13. Tugues S, Fernandez-Varo G, Munoz-Luque J, Ros J, Arroyo V, et al. (2007) Antiangiogenic treatment with sunitinib ameliorates inflammatory infiltrate, fibrosis, and portal pressure in cirrhotic rats. Hepatology 46: 1919–1926.
14. Feala JD, Abdulhameed MD, Yu C, Dutta B, Yu X, et al. (2013) Systems biology approaches for discovering biomarkers for traumatic brain injury. J Neurotrauma 30: 1101–1116.
15. Tawa GJ, AbdulHameed MD, Yu X, Kumar K, Ippolito DL, et al. (2014) Characterization of chemically induced liver injuries using gene co-expression modules. PLOS ONE 9: e107230.
16. Kanehisa M, Goto S, Sato Y, Furumichi M, Tanabe M (2012) KEGG for integration and interpretation of large-scale molecular data sets. Nucleic Acids Res 40: D109–D114.
17. Matthews L, Gopinath G, Gillespie M, Caudy M, Croft D, et al. (2009) Reactome knowledgebase of human biological pathways and processes. Nucleic Acids Res 37: D619–D622.
18. Geer LY, Marchler-Bauer A, Geer RC, Han L, He J, et al. (2010) The NCBI BioSystems database. Nucleic Acids Res 38: D492–D496.
19. Pan Y, Cheng T, Wang Y, Bryant SH (2014) Pathway analysis for drug repositioning based on public database mining. J Chem Inf Model 54: 407–418.
20. Huang da W, Sherman BT, Lempicki RA (2009) Bioinformatics enrichment tools: paths toward the comprehensive functional analysis of large gene lists. Nucleic Acids Res 37: 1–13.
21. Kim MJ, Pelloux V, Guyot E, Tordjman J, Bui LC, et al. (2012) Inflammatory pathway genes belong to major targets of persistent organic pollutants in adipose cells. Environ Health Perspect 120: 508–514.
22. Smid M, Wang Y, Zhang Y, Sieuwerts AM, Yu J, et al. (2008) Subtypes of breast cancer show preferential site of relapse. Cancer Res 68: 3108–3114.
23. Huang L, Heinloth AN, Zeng ZB, Paules RS, Bushel PR (2008) Genes related to apoptosis predict necrosis of the liver as a phenotype observed in rats exposed to a compendium of hepatotoxicants. BMC Genomics 9: 288.
24. Affo S, Dominguez M, Lozano JJ, Sancho-Bru P, Rodrigo-Torres D, et al. (2013) Transcriptome analysis identifies TNF superfamily receptors as potential therapeutic targets in alcoholic hepatitis. Gut 62: 452–460.
25. Lehne B, Schlitt T (2012) Breaking free from the chains of pathway annotation: de novo pathway discovery for the analysis of disease processes. Pharmacogenomics 13: 1967–1978.
26. Gentleman RC, Carey VJ, Bates DM, Bolstad B, Dettling M, et al. (2004) Bioconductor: open software development for computational biology and bioinformatics. Genome Biol 5: R80.
27. Chuang HY, Lee E, Liu YT, Lee D, Ideker T (2007) Network-based classification of breast cancer metastasis. Mol Syst Biol 3: 140.
28. Zhu W, Yang L, Du Z (2009) Layered functional network analysis of gene expression in human heart failure. PLOS ONE 4: e6288.
29. Reiss DJ, Avila-Campillo I, Thorsson V, Schwikowski B, Galitski T (2005) Tools enabling the elucidation of molecular pathways active in human disease: application to hepatitis C virus infection. BMC Bioinformatics 6: 154.
30. Camargo A, Azuaje F (2007) Linking gene expression and functional network data in human heart failure. PLOS ONE 2: e1347.
31. Azuaje F, Devaux Y, Wagner DR (2010) Coordinated modular functionality and prognostic potential of a heart failure biomarker-driven interaction network. BMC Syst Biol 4: 60.
32. Azuaje FJ, Dewey FE, Brutsaert DL, Devaux Y, Ashley EA, et al. (2012) Systems-based approaches to cardiovascular biomarker discovery. Circ Cardiovasc Genet 5: 360–367.
33. Xiao Y, Xu C, Xu L, Guan J, Ping Y, et al. (2012) Systematic identification of common functional modules related to heart failure with different etiologies. Gene 499: 332–338.
34. Huan J, Wang L, Xing L, Qin X, Feng L, et al. (2014) Insights into significant pathways and gene interaction networks underlying breast cancer cell line MCF-7 treated with 17beta-estradiol (E2). Gene 533: 346–355.
35. Ganter B, Snyder RD, Halbert DN, Lee MD (2006) Toxicogenomics in drug discovery and development: mechanistic analysis of compound/class-dependent effects using the DrugMatrix database. Pharmacogenomics 7: 1025–1044.
36. Breitling R, Armengaud P, Amtmann A, Herzyk P (2004) Rank products: a simple, yet powerful, new method to detect differentially regulated genes in replicated microarray experiments. FEBS Lett 573: 83–92.
37. Yu X, Wallqvist A, Reifman J (2012) Inferring high-confidence human protein-protein interactions. BMC Bioinformatics 13: 79.
38. DrugMatrix (nd) National Institute of Environmental Health Sciences. Available: https://ntp.niehs.nih.gov/drugmatrix/index.html.
39. Irizarry RA, Bolstad BM, Collin F, Cope LM, Hobbs B, et al. (2003) Summaries of Affymetrix GeneChip probe level data. Nucleic Acids Res 31: e15.
40. Gautier L, Cope L, Bolstad BM, Irizarry RA (2004) Affy – analysis of Affymetrix GeneChip data at the probe level. Bioinformatics 20: 307–315.
41. R Development Core Team (2011) R: A language and environment for statistical computing. Vienna, Austria: R Foundation for Statistical Computing. Available: http://www.R-project.org/.

42. Kauffmann A, Gentleman R, Huber W (2009) ArrayQualityMetrics – a bioconductor package for quality assessment of microarray data. Bioinformatics 25: 415–416.
43. Gentleman R, Carey V, Huber W, Hahne F (2013) genefilter: methods for filtering genes from microarray experiments, R. package version 1.40.0. Seattle, WA: Bioconductor. Available: http://bioc.ism.ac.jp/2.11/bioc/html/genefilter.html.
44. Hong F, Breitling R, McEntee CW, Wittner BS, Nemhauser JL, et al. (2006) RankProd: a bioconductor package for detecting differentially expressed genes in meta-analysis. Bioinformatics 22: 2825–2827.
45. Vinuela A, Snoek LB, Riksen JA, Kammenga JE (2010) Genome-wide gene expression analysis in response to organophosphorus pesticide chlorpyrifos and diazinon in *C. elegans*. PLOS ONE 5: e12145.
46. Langfelder P, Zhang B, Horvath S (2008) Defining clusters from a hierarchical cluster tree: the Dynamic Tree Cut package for R. Bioinformatics 24: 719–720.
47. Huang DW, Sherman BT, Lempicki RA (2009) Systematic and integrative analysis of large gene lists using DAVID bioinformatics resources. Nat Protoc 4: 44–57.
48. Yu C, Desai V, Cheng L, Reifman J (2012) QuartetS-DB: a large-scale orthology database for prokaryotes and eukaryotes inferred by evolutionary evidence. BMC Bioinformatics 13: 143.
49. Eppig JT, Blake JA, Bult CJ, Kadin JA, Richardson JE, et al. (2012) The Mouse Genome Database (MGD): comprehensive resource for genetics and genomics of the laboratory mouse. Nucleic Acids Res 40: D881–D886.
50. Zhang J, Yang Y, Wang Y, Zhang J, Wang Z, et al. (2011) Identification of hub genes related to the recovery phase of irradiation injury by microarray and integrated gene network analysis. PLOS ONE 6: e24680.
51. Alcaraz N, Friedrich T, Kotzing T, Krohmer A, Muller J, et al. (2012) Efficient key pathway mining: combining networks and OMICS data. Integr Biol (Camb) 4: 756–764.
52. Baumbach J, Friedrich T, Kotzing T, Krohmer A, Muller J, et al. (2012) Efficient algorithms for extracting biological key pathways with global constraints. Proceedings of the 14th Annual Conference on Genetic and Evolutionary Computation. Philadelphia, Pennsylvania, USA: Association for Computing Machinery. pp. 169–176.
53. Saito R, Smoot ME, Ono K, Ruscheinski J, Wang PL, et al. (2012) A travel guide to Cytoscape plugins. Nat Methods 9: 1069–1076.
54. Shen H (2009) Detect overlapping and hierarchical community structure in networks. Physica A 388: 1706–1712.
55. Henderson NC, Mackinnon AC, Farnworth SL, Poirier F, Russo FP, et al. (2006) Galectin-3 regulates myofibroblast activation and hepatic fibrosis. Proc Natl Acad Sci U S A 103: 5060–5065.
56. Page S, Birerdinc A, Estep M, Stepanova M, Afendy A, et al. (2013) Knowledge-based identification of soluble biomarkers: hepatic fibrosis in NAFLD as an example. PLOS ONE 8: e56009.
57. Davis AP, Murphy CG, Johnson R, Lay JM, Lennon-Hopkins K, et al. (2013) The Comparative Toxicogenomics Database: update 2013. Nucleic Acids Res 41: D1104–1114.
58. Supek F, Bosnjak M, Skunca N, Smuc T (2011) REVIGO summarizes and visualizes long lists of gene ontology terms. PLOS ONE 6: e21800.
59. de Hoon MJ, Imoto S, Nolan J, Miyano S (2004) Open source clustering software. Bioinformatics 20: 1453–1454.
60. Moreno M, Chaves JF, Sancho-Bru P, Ramalho F, Ramalho LN, et al. (2010) Ghrelin attenuates hepatocellular injury and liver fibrogenesis in rodents and influences fibrosis progression in humans. Hepatology 51: 974–985.
61. Subramanian A, Tamayo P, Mootha VK, Mukherjee S, Ebert BL, et al. (2005) Gene set enrichment analysis: a knowledge-based approach for interpreting genome-wide expression profiles. Proc Natl Acad Sci U S A 102: 15545–15550.
62. Pan KH, Lih CJ, Cohen SN (2005) Effects of threshold choice on biological conclusions reached during analysis of gene expression by DNA microarrays. Proc Natl Acad Sci U S A 102: 8961–8965.
63. Nam D, Kim SY (2008) Gene-set approach for expression pattern analysis. Brief Bioinform 9: 189–197.
64. Lee HK, Hsu AK, Sajdak J, Qin J, Pavlidis P (2004) Coexpression analysis of human genes across many microarray data sets. Genome Res 14: 1085–1094.
65. Friedman SL (2000) Molecular regulation of hepatic fibrosis, an integrated cellular response to tissue injury. J Biol Chem 275: 2247–2250.
66. Liedtke C, Luedde T, Sauerbruch T, Scholten D, Streetz K, et al. (2013) Experimental liver fibrosis research: update on animal models, legal issues and translational aspects. Fibrogenesis Tissue Repair 6: 19.
67. Li L, Wang JY, Yang CQ, Jiang W (2012) Effect of RhoA on transforming growth factor beta1-induced rat hepatic stellate cell migration. Liver Int 32: 1093–1102.
68. Ikeda K, Kawada N, Wang YQ, Kadoya H, Nakatani K, et al. (1998) Expression of cellular prion protein in activated hepatic stellate cells. Am J Pathol 153: 1695–1700.
69. Kitada T, Seki S, Ikeda K, Nakatani K, Sakaguchi H, et al. (2000) Clinicopathological characterization of prion: a novel marker of activated human hepatic stellate cells. J Hepatol 33: 751–757.
70. Wynn TA, Ramalingam TR (2012) Mechanisms of fibrosis: therapeutic translation for fibrotic disease. Nat Med 18: 1028–1040.
71. Okayama T, Kikuchi S, Ochiai T, Ikoma H, Kubota T, et al. (2008) Attenuated response to liver injury in moesin-deficient mice: impaired stellate cell migration and decreased fibrosis. Biochim Biophys Acta 1782: 542–548.
72. Khatri P, Sirota M, Butte AJ (2012) Ten years of pathway analysis: current approaches and outstanding challenges. PLOS Comput Biol 8: e1002375.
73. Ulitsky I, Krishnamurthy A, Karp RM, Shamir R (2010) DEGAS: de novo discovery of dysregulated pathways in human diseases. PLOS ONE 5: e13367.
74. Krishnan A, Li X, Kao WY, Viker K, Butters K, et al. (2012) Lumican, an extracellular matrix proteoglycan, is a novel requisite for hepatic fibrosis. Lab Invest 92: 1712–1725.
75. Schuppan D, Kim YO (2013) Evolving therapies for liver fibrosis. J Clin Invest 123: 1887–1901.
76. Zhang LP, Takahara T, Yata Y, Furui K, Jin B, et al. (1999) Increased expression of plasminogen activator and plasminogen activator inhibitor during liver fibrogenesis of rats: role of stellate cells. J Hepatol 31: 703–711.
77. Mallat A, Lotersztajn S (2013) Cellular mechanisms of tissue fibrosis. 5. Novel insights into liver fibrosis. Am J Physiol Cell Physiol 305: C789–C799.
78. Morita Y, Araki H, Sugimoto T, Takeuchi K, Yamane T, et al. (2007) Legumain/asparaginyl endopeptidase controls extracellular matrix remodeling through the degradation of fibronectin in mouse renal proximal tubular cells. FEBS Lett 581: 1417–1424.
79. Okumura T (2011) Role of lipid droplet proteins in liver steatosis. J Physiol Biochem 67: 629–636.
80. Nose F, Yamaguchi T, Kato R, Aiuchi T, Obama T, et al. (2013) Crucial role of perilipin-3 (TIP47) in formation of lipid droplets and PGE2 production in HL-60-derived neutrophils. PLOS ONE 8: e71542.
81. Koukoulis GK, Shen J, Virtanen I, Gould VE (2001) Vitronectin in the cirrhotic liver: an immunomarker of mature fibrosis. Hum Pathol 32: 1356–1362.
82. Tamm ER (2002) Myocilin and glaucoma: facts and ideas. Prog Retin Eye Res 21: 395–428.
83. Heinloth AN, Boorman GA, Foley JF, Flagler ND, Paules RS (2007) Gene expression analysis offers unique advantages to histopathology in liver biopsy evaluations. Toxicol Pathol 35: 276–283.
84. Hartung T, McBride M (2011) Food for Thought… on mapping the human toxome. ALTEX 28: 83–93.
85. Vinken M (2013) The adverse outcome pathway concept: a pragmatic tool in toxicology. Toxicology 312: 158–165.

10

Holding Thermal Receipt Paper and Eating Food after Using Hand Sanitizer Results in High Serum Bioactive and Urine Total Levels of Bisphenol A (BPA)

Annette M. Hormann[1], Frederick S. vom Saal[1], Susan C. Nagel[2], Richard W. Stahlhut[1], Carol L. Moyer[1], Mark R. Ellersieck[3], Wade V. Welshons[4], Pierre-Louis Toutain[5,6], Julia A. Taylor[1]*

1 Division of Biological Sciences, University of Missouri, Columbia, Missouri, United States of America, **2** Department of Obstetrics, Gynecology and Women's Health, University of Missouri, Columbia, Missouri, United States of America, **3** Department of Statistics, University of Missouri, Columbia, Missouri, United States of America, **4** Department of Biomedical Sciences, University of Missouri, Columbia, Missouri, United States of America, **5** Université de Toulouse, INPT, ENVT, UPS, UMR1331, F- 31062 Toulouse, France, **6** INRA, UMR1331, Toxalim, Research Centre in Food Toxicology, F-31027 Toulouse, France

Abstract

Bisphenol A (BPA) is an endocrine disrupting environmental contaminant used in a wide variety of products, and BPA metabolites are found in almost everyone's urine, suggesting widespread exposure from multiple sources. Regulatory agencies estimate that virtually all BPA exposure is from food and beverage packaging. However, free BPA is applied to the outer layer of thermal receipt paper present in very high (~20 mg BPA/g paper) quantities as a print developer. Not taken into account when considering thermal paper as a source of BPA exposure is that some commonly used hand sanitizers, as well as other skin care products, contain mixtures of dermal penetration enhancing chemicals that can increase by up to 100 fold the dermal absorption of lipophilic compounds such as BPA. We found that when men and women held thermal receipt paper immediately after using a hand sanitizer with penetration enhancing chemicals, significant free BPA was transferred to their hands and then to French fries that were eaten, and the combination of dermal and oral BPA absorption led to a rapid and dramatic average maximum increase (Cmax) in unconjugated (bioactive) BPA of ~7 ng/mL in serum and ~20 μg total BPA/g creatinine in urine within 90 min. The default method used by regulatory agencies to test for hazards posed by chemicals is intra-gastric gavage. For BPA this approach results in less than 1% of the administered dose being bioavailable in blood. It also ignores dermal absorption as well as sublingual absorption in the mouth that both bypass first-pass liver metabolism. The elevated levels of BPA that we observed due to holding thermal paper after using a product containing dermal penetration enhancing chemicals have been related to an increased risk for a wide range of developmental abnormalities as well as diseases in adults.

Editor: David O. Carpenter, Institute for Health & the Environment, United States of America

Funding: This work was supported by a grant from The Passport Foundation (no URL available) and by NIEHS grant ES018764 to FvS (NIEHS website http://www.niehs.nih.gov). The funders had no role in study design, data collection and analysis, decision to publish, or preparation of the manuscript.

Competing Interests: The authors have declared that no competing interests exist.

* Email: TaylorJA@missouri.edu

Introduction

Bisphenol A [BPA; bis(4-hydroxyphenyl)propane; CAS #80-05-7] is one of the highest volume chemicals in commerce with 15-billion pounds produced per year [1], and based on the presence of BPA metabolites in urine, it can be concluded that virtually everyone is exposed [2,3]. BPA has estrogenic and other endocrine disrupting activities [4,5]. BPA molecules are polymerized to make polycarbonate plastic used for food and beverage containers, epoxy resins used to line cans, and dental composites and sealants, but free (unpolymerized) BPA is also used as an additive (plasticizer), such as in polyvinyl chloride (PVC) products. Our interest is in the use of BPA in thermal paper, which is used for airline ticket, gas, ATM, cash register and other types of receipts (Figure 1). The print surface of thermal paper is coated with milligrams of free BPA per gram paper as a heat-activated print developer [6], and it appears that free BPA is readily transferred to other materials that the thermal paper contacts [7].

While small lipophilic compounds such as BPA (logP = 3.4; molecular weight 228 Da) can pass through skin [8,9], regulatory agencies have assumed that this route of human BPA exposure should not be significant in spite of the lack of data and acknowledged "significant uncertainties" around the issue of human exposure to BPA from thermal paper [10]. However, a factor that has not been considered in estimating transdermal exposure to BPA from thermal paper is that hand sanitizers are now commonly used, particularly in fast-food restaurants where people may handle thermal receipts before eating or ordering food. Hand sanitizer and other skin care products may also be used by cashiers while working. Exposure to BPA from thermal paper goes beyond just transdermal exposure and consumption of food that is picked up and eaten with a BPA-contaminated hand.

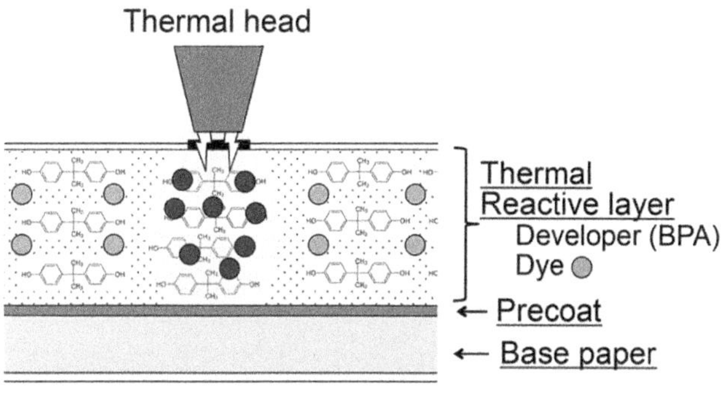

Figure 1. Schematic diagram of thermal receipt paper identifying the thermal reactive layer that contains BPA as a developer and a leuco dye, as well as stabilizers and binders (not shown).

The transfer of a chemical directly from hand-to-mouth (mouthing behavior) has been proposed to be an important variable for estimating total chemical exposure in humans [11], particularly in young children [12].

The use of hand sanitizers and other skin-care products, including soaps, lotions and sunscreens, is significant because some contain mixtures of chemicals that are also used as dermal penetration enhancers to increase the transdermal delivery of drugs. Drugs and chemicals that are suitable for transdermal delivery and are impacted by dermal penetration enhancers have a LogP>1.5 and a molecular weight <500 Da [9]. There are many factors that impact the ability of compounds to pass through skin in addition to molecular weight and lipophilicity, including differences arising from the location of skin on the body, gender and age [13]. Mixtures of dermal penetration enhancing chemicals can act synergistically to increase by up to 100 fold the dermal penetration of small lipophilic molecules such as estradiol [8,9], with which BPA shares physical-chemical and biological properties [4]. For example, Purell hand sanitizer (Gojo Industries), which we used in the current study, contains a number of dermal penetration enhancers, such as isopropyl myristate and propylene glycol, and is (63% w/w) ethanol. The use of hand sanitizers has increased in recent years and is now about a 200 million dollar a year industry just in the USA [14]. The impact of the use of personal care products such as moisturizing lotions that contain dermal penetration enhancing chemicals on exposure to environmental chemicals has been identified as a concern [15].

To assess the relevance of this research to real-world behavior, we conducted a preliminary observational study in fast-food restaurants, food courts and shopping malls in Columbia Missouri. Receipt contact time varied widely, but was sometimes substantial. In one restaurant, we found that receipt contact time ranged up to 65 sec for people purchasing food that was eaten in the restaurant; the 75th percentile for time holding the receipt was >12 sec, and the 90th percentile >32 sec. In a fast-food restaurant that is part of an international chain, take-out food was placed into a bag and the top of the bag was folded, then the thermal receipt was stapled to the top of the bag; the result was that the print surface of the receipt (coated with BPA) was grabbed when the bag was picked up. The contact time between the hand and thermal receipt was thus considerably longer than would be the case for food eaten in the restaurant. In a food court we observed that some fast-food restaurants had hand sanitizer dispensers available for use by customers next to the cash register, and customers were observed using the hand sanitizer before handling the thermal receipt. The estimate is that 50 million people eat in a fast-food establishment every day in the USA [16]. Finally, our experiments here are also relevant to occupational exposures, because we observed in a national chain big-box store that all cash registers had a hand sanitizer dispenser next to them for use by the cashiers.

Our objectives were to examine the impact of having dry hands vs. wet hands due to using a popular hand sanitizer that contains dermal penetration enhancing chemicals on extraction of BPA from the surface of thermal receipt paper coated with BPA. We also measured (using a LC/MSMS assay) unconjugated, bioactive BPA (uBPA) and its conjugated metabolites, BPA-glucuronide (BPA-G) and BPA-monosulfate (BPA-S), in serum and urine in adult male and female subjects after holding a thermal receipt. To determine the proportion of thermal receipts that contained BPA, we examined receipt papers for the presence and amount of BPA. We also examined receipts for the most commonly used BPA replacement chemical, bisphenol S [bis(4-hydroxyphenyl)sulfone; BPS; CAS #80-09-1].

Methods

Ethics statement

The University of Missouri School of Medicine Institutional Review Board approved all procedures involving human subjects, and sample collection was conducted by licensed personnel in the Clinical Research Center (CRC) within the University of Missouri School of Medicine. Subjects were informed of the procedures, and provided written consent. The signed consent forms were retained. The University IRB approved the consent procedure.

Subjects

Participants for the different experiments in this study were recruited through a weekly University of Missouri campus-wide email newsletter. Candidates (men and women) were pre-screened by age, height, weight, and health status. Participants selected were 20–40 years old (average 27.0 yrs), and an attempt was made to select those with average height, weight and normal-range body-mass index. Participants selected were not taking any prescription or non-prescription medication other than oral contraceptives; the type of oral contraceptive used was recorded. To ensure that pregnant women were excluded from the study, all women were administered a pregnancy test when they arrived at the CRC.

For all studies participants were asked to refrain from touching thermal paper receipts, consuming food or beverages stored in polycarbonate or other types of plastic containers as well as canned food and beverages during the 48 hr prior to participating in the study, in order to reduce background BPA levels in body fluids as much as possible. The participants also filled out a questionnaire concerning their activities during the prior 48 hr (see Section S3 in File S1 for questionnaire).

For experiments in which there was hand contact with thermal receipt paper, subjects were required to wash their hands with soap and water, rinse thoroughly, and then dry using Kimwipes (Kimberly-Clark, Irving, TX). A number of soaps were screened for BPA content and/or chromatographic interference prior to the start of the study, and the soap chosen was Softsoap "Aquarium series" (Colgate Palmolive Company, Manhattan, NY), which showed no detectable BPA or chromatographic interference with the assay of BPA. Standard brown laboratory paper towels were tested and found to contain BPA at around 6 μg/towel. Because of this, Kimwipes, which tested negative for BPA, were used throughout for drying hands. Water from faucets used in the CRC was tested and found to be below the limit of detection (LOD) for BPA content (detection limit was 10 pg/mL by HPLC with CoulArray detection based on C-18 extraction of 250 ml of water).

Sample analysis

Analysis of BPA in extracted samples occurred within an accredited facility (Veterinary Medicine Diagnostic Laboratory) within the College of Veterinary Medicine at the University of Missouri.

Reagents. Solvents (methanol, acetonitrile) and water were HPLC grade, and were obtained from Fisher Scientific. BPA, bisphenol S (BPS), and BPA monosulfate (BPA-S) were obtained from Sigma-Aldrich (St. Louis MO; purity >99%, 98% and 95% respectively). C^{13}-BPA was obtained from Cambridge Isotope Laboratories Inc. (Andover, MA; purity 99%), and both BPA-G (purity 98%) and BPA D-glucuronide (BPA-DG; purity >99%) were provided by the National Institute of Environmental Health Sciences (NIEHS), Research Triangle Park, NC. Ethanol (200 proof) used for hand swipes was obtained from Decon Labs, Inc. (King of Prussia, PA).

Total receipt BPA and BPS content. Weighed samples of each receipt (3×3 cm) were incubated overnight in methanol at room temperature. The methanol extracts were diluted in methanol, typically to a final dilution of 1/10,000, and BPA content was analyzed by HPLC with CoulArray detection (see Section S1 in File S1 for details). We also analyzed the same receipt sample extracts for BPS using LC/MSMS (see Section S1 in File S1 for details).

BPA levels in Kimwipe hand swipes. Kimwipe swipes were incubated in methanol at room temperature overnight, and aliquots were taken from the methanol extract for analysis. BPA in the methanol extract was determined by HPLC with CoulArray detection.

BPA levels in French fries. French fries were incubated individually in methanol overnight. The fries were then removed, and the samples centrifuged briefly to separate any solid and/or oily matter, and a sample of the clear methanol extract was assayed. Equal volumes from the 10 extracts from the 10 French fries touched by each participant were pooled, and a single measurement was made for each participant. Quantitation was made by HPLC with CoulArray detection.

Serum sample collection and extraction. Multiple-point blood samples were collected via IV catheter into 10 mL syringes, and the syringes were emptied into the same uncoated vacutainer tubes (for details and catalog numbers of collection materials Section S1 in File S1). Single point blood samples were collected by venipuncture into uncoated glass vacutainer tubes (Becton Dickinson, Franklin Lakes, NJ). All blood samples were allowed to clot at room temperature for 15–30 min and then refrigerated until centrifugation at 4°C for 15 min. The serum was transferred with glass Pasteur pipets into 15 mL centrifuge tubes and then frozen at −20°C. Samples were extracted using C18 SPE as previously described [17]; see Section S1 in File S1. Procedural blanks were also run alongside the samples to monitor for reagent contamination or interference. Serum extracts were analyzed by LC/MSMS.

Urine sample collection and extraction. All urine samples were collected directly into Samco polypropylene specimen cups (Fisher Scientific, Waltham, MA) and were immediately refrigerated (4°C for 2–5 hours) until they could be transferred to the research laboratory, at which point they were frozen at −20°C. The total BPA concentration (representing a combined measure of unconjugated and conjugated BPA) was measured by LC/MSMS (see Section S1 in File S1).

Assay of creatinine in urine. To calculate creatinine-corrected urine BPA concentrations, urine creatinine was measured using an ELISA kit (R&D Systems Inc., Minneapolis, MN), according to manufacturer's instructions. Sensitivity of this assay is 0.02 mg/dL.

Field blanks. The possibility of BPA leaching from each piece of equipment used in the collection or processing of samples identified above was determined by passing BPA-free water through all collection equipment, which was then handled and assayed for BPA as described below for the actual samples. All equipment and sample handling was determined to not leach detectable BPA before any sample collections occurred.

Statistical methods and calculation of pharmacokinetic parameters

For both uBPA and BPA-G, the area under the concentration-time curve (AUC) up to the last measured serum concentration above the LOQ, i.e. AUC (0–90 min), was calculated by using the linear trapezoidal rule. The average AUC (0–90 min) (ng/mL) was calculated by dividing AUC (0–90 min ng/mL)/90 min. Time (Tmax) of maximal plasma BPA concentration (Cmax) was directly obtained from the raw data. Comparisons of men and women were conducted using the Mann-Whitney U test or ANOVA. Statistical significance was set a $P<0.05$, two-tailed test. All data are presented as mean±SEM.

Experiment 1: Measurement of BPA and BPS in 50 used thermal receipt papers

The objective of this experiment was to determine the amount of BPA and BPS in thermal receipt paper and to determine the proportion of receipts that contained BPA or BPS, which is the most commonly used BPA replacement chemical. Thermal paper sales receipts were obtained by purchasing items from 41 different vendors in Columbia, MO and from a further 9 vendors in Southern Missouri (50 receipts total). Weighed portions of each paper were extracted and assayed for BPA by HPLC with CoulArray detection and for BPS by LC/MSMS. After screening, an unused roll was obtained from a vendor from which a BPA-positive receipt had been identified. The BPA content of paper from this roll was confirmed prior to being used for testing with human subjects in Experiments 2, 3 and 4.

Experiment 2: BPA transferred to a hand with and without using hand sanitizer due to holding a thermal receipt for different lengths of time

The objective of this experiment was to determine the amount of BPA extracted by a hand from a standard piece of thermal receipt paper immediately after using Purell hand sanitizer (Experiment 2-A) or with dry hands (Experiment 2-B). Subjects in both experiments cleaned and dried their hands prior to the experiment and between each trial. For Experiment 2-A the subjects (2 men and one woman) each held the thermal paper for different lengths of time: 2, 15, 30, 45, 60 or 240 sec (in 6 separate trials for each subject). Both hands were wetted by applying three "squirts" of Purell to each hand, and the hands were then briefly rubbed together to distribute the hand sanitizer evenly across both palms and fingers, but the sanitizer was not allowed to dry prior to holding the receipt paper. In experiment 2-B the subjects (2 men and 2 women) held the receipt with dry hands for 60 or 240 sec (2 separate trials for each subject). In both experiments an 8×12 cm portion of thermal paper cut from an unused receipt roll that was obtained from a local merchant (previously identified as containing 27.2 mg BPA/g paper) was placed BPA-coated (print surface) side down into the right hand. The hand was swiped 3 times each with 3 ethanol-soaked Kimwipes, and BPA was extracted from the Kimwipes with methanol and measured by HPLC with CoulArray detection.

Experiment 3: Serum and urine BPA in men and women before and after transdermal and oral exposure to BPA from thermal receipt paper after using hand sanitizer

The objective of this experiment was to measure the transfer of BPA from thermal paper receipts to hands, and the amount of BPA remaining on the surface of a hand 90-min later, after using Purell hand sanitizer (as described in the prior experiment) in 5 male and 5 female subjects. In addition, we measured the amount of BPA transferred from a BPA-contaminated hand to 10 French fries, and measured blood and urine concentrations of uBPA, BPA-G and BPA-S before and after ingestion of the French fries and BPA absorption through skin. The design of the study is shown in Figure 2.

The background level of BPA on the dominant hand was determined when the subjects first arrived at the CRC. The dominant hand was swiped 3 times with 3 separate Kimwipes soaked with ethanol, from which we extracted BPA for analysis by HPLC with CoulArray detection, and the hands were then cleaned. The subjects' weight and height were determined, after which they provided a baseline urine specimen, an IV port was inserted into the cubital vein, and a baseline blood sample was collected. Purell hand sanitizer was applied to the hands as described in Experiment 2. An 8×12 cm piece of thermal paper cut from an unused receipt roll (used in Experiment 2) was then placed BPA-coated side down into each hand with the hands still wet. The subjects held the receipt papers for 4 min in each hand. The dominant arm of each subject was determined based on whether the person was right or left handed, and in this experiment the non-dominant hand remained contaminated with BPA for the duration of the experiment. Blood was collected from the cubital vein in the contaminated arm of one set of subjects ($N = 7$) and from the cubital vein in the non-contaminated arm of other subjects ($N = 3$). We note that the phlebotomist did not handle the thermal paper for either Experiment 3 or Experiment 4. The study coordinator who did handle the paper wore gloves to do so and did not touch the blood tubes of other equipment. A separate person swiped the subjects' hands after thermal paper exposure and wore fresh gloves for each swipe session and discarded them immediately afterwards.

French fries that had been purchased from a local fast food restaurant and had been found to not contain detectable BPA were briefly warmed in a toaster oven. Immediately after holding the thermal receipts in each hand, the subjects picked up a French fry in each hand, and held both fries for 10 sec. The fry held in the dominant hand was placed into a labeled glass tube, and the fry that was held in the non-dominant hand was eaten. A total of 10 French fries was handled by each hand and either placed in a test tube or eaten using this same procedure. Approximately 4 min elapsed between removal of the receipt paper from the hand and consumption of the last French fry. Thus, it took about 8 min from the time that the thermal receipt paper was first touched and consumption of the last French fry.

After the last French fry was consumed, the subject's dominant hand was swiped with 3 ethanol-soaked Kimwipes to clean BPA off the hand and for determination (by extracting BPA from the Kimwipes) of the amount of BPA remaining on the hand immediately after holding the 10 French fries that were placed into test tubes. The non-dominant hand was not cleaned after holding the receipt paper and eating French fries, and thus was a continuing source of transdermal BPA exposure over the following 90-min period of blood collection.

Blood samples were collected from the cubital vein from the still contaminated arm of 7 subjects, 4 males and 3 females, and from the uncontaminated arm of 3 subjects, one male and 2 females. The blood collected from the BPA-contaminated arm provided direct information about BPA absorbed from the hand on which BPA remained for 90 min, since the cubital vein is one of the major veins draining the hand; this blood is not subject to first-pass liver metabolism prior to going to the heart and being transported in the arterial circulation to tissues. The blood collected from the uncontaminated arm provided information about BPA in the systemic (mixed) circulation.

Blood was collected from the IV port before holding the thermal paper (baseline) and at 15, 30, 60 and 90 min after consumption of the last French fry. The non-dominant contaminated hand (from which the French fries were eaten) was not allowed to touch anything during the 90-min after holding the receipt paper and then picking up the 10 French fries; this hand was swiped with 3 ethanol-soaked Kimwipes after the final 90-min blood collection at the end of the study. After these swipes were obtained, both hands were thoroughly cleaned and a second urine sample was collected.

Experiment 4: Serum and urine BPA in men and women before and after transdermal exposure to BPA from thermal receipt paper with dry hands

The objective of this study was to examine the amount of BPA transferred to a clean dry hand and then present in serum and urine without using hand sanitizer. In this study we examined 12 adult men and 12 adult women subjects. The subjects washed and dried their hands and provided a baseline blood and urine sample as described in Experiment 3. The non-dominant hand was swiped 3 times each with 3 ethanol-soaked Kimwipes to obtain a baseline measure of BPA on the hand prior to holding a thermal receipt. After the hand was dry, subjects held an 8×12 cm piece of thermal receipt paper (from the roll used in Experiment 1) with the non-dominant dry hand for 4 min. Thirty minutes later a second blood sample was collected from the contaminated arm, after which the BPA was swiped from the contaminated hand with ethanol-soaked Kimwipes as described previously. As above, the contaminated hand was not allowed to touch anything during the 30-min period prior to the second blood collection. The hands were washed, and a second urine sample was collected 60 min after holding the receipt paper.

Results

Experiment 1: Measurement of BPA and BPS in thermal receipt paper

Thermal receipts were collected at stores, bars and restaurants in mid-Missouri. Of the 50 receipts, 22 (44%) contained high levels of BPA (Table 1). High levels of the BPA replacement chemical BPS were found in 26 (52%) of the receipts, and 2 receipts contained an unidentified chemical as the print developer [18]; see Section S2 in File S1 for individual values. These findings suggest that BPS is now as commonly used as BPA as a developer in thermal receipt paper. Note that these receipts had been obtained with purchases, while the receipt paper used in Experiments 2, 3 and 4 came from an unused roll of thermal paper that we determine contained BPA as the developer.

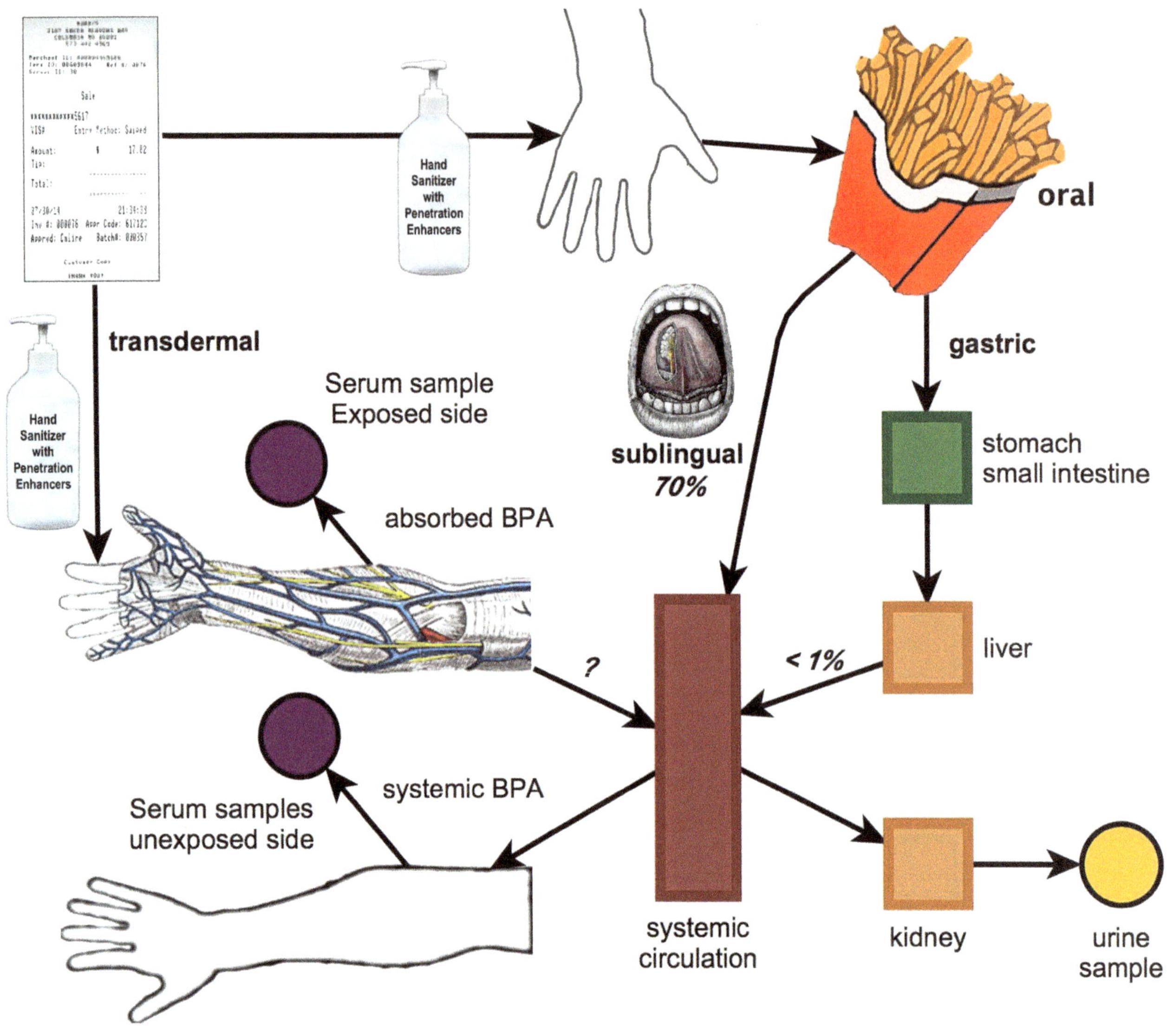

Figure 2. Schematic diagram of the protocol for Experiment 3 in which thermal receipt paper containing BPA was held with a hand wet from using Purell hand sanitizer, after which the subjects picked up 10 French fries and ate them, resulting in both oral and transdermal routes of exposure. Of the 5 male and 5 female subjects, 7 subjects had serum collected from the cubital vein in the arm with a contaminated hand that contained the BPA from holding thermal paper. Three subjects had blood collected from the cubital vein in the unexposed arm that did not have BPA on the hand throughout the 90-min test period during which blood was collected. Urine samples were obtained before and at the end of the test period.

Table 1. BPA and BPS concentrations in 50 thermal paper receipt samples.

Chemical in paper	mg/g receipt	mg/8×12 cm receipt
BPA-positive (44%)	19.6±1.0	9.0±0.4
	(11.5–26.3)	(6.1–11.3)
BPS-positive (52%)	23.5±0.7	10.8±0.3
	(15.2–30.1)	(7.1–13.2)

Two (4%) of 50 papers tested did not contain either BPA or BPS and did not show any estrogenic activity in a MCF-7 breast cancer cell proliferation assay (data not shown). Values are mean±SEM, with the range of measured values given in parentheses. See Section S2 in File S1 for individual receipt data.

Experiment 2: BPA transferred to a hand with and without using hand sanitizer due to holding a thermal receipt for different lengths of time

The data shown in Figure 3-A reveal that after using Purell hand sanitizer with the hand still wet, the maximum amount of BPA swiped from the palm and fingers of the hand (581 µg BPA) occurred after holding a receipt for 45 sec. After holding a receipt for 2 sec, 40% (235 µg BPA) of maximum was recovered from the hand, and within 15 sec 58% (339 µg BPA) of maximum was recovered from the hand. The decrease in BPA swiped from the hand between 45 sec and 4 min to 73% of maximum (425 µg BPA) may have been due to absorption into skin occurring at a greater rate than transfer to the skin from the thermal receipt.

The data in Figure 3-B show that holding a thermal receipt with dry hands resulted in dramatically lower amounts of BPA being extracted from the receipt relative to the amounts extracted immediately after using hand sanitizer. The ratio of the extracted BPA swiped from the wet vs. dry hand was higher at 60 sec (ratio = 185) than at 240 sec (ratio = 51), reflecting the fact that while the amount of BPA swiped from a wet hand decreased between 60 and 240 sec, the levels increased over this time when the hand was dry, likely due to a reduced rate of absorption with dry relative to wet hands.

Experiment 3: Serum and urine BPA before and after transdermal and oral exposure to BPA from thermal receipt paper after using hand sanitizer

We measured the amount of BPA swiped from the dominant hand after using hand sanitizer, holding a receipt and then eating 10 French fries, which took 8 min. BPA levels were not significantly different for the 5 males (mean±SEM: 126±19 µg) and the 5 females (mean±SEM: 128±10 µg). These levels measured at about 8-min after first touching the thermal receipt paper were lower than levels measured at 45 sec and 4 min in Experiment 2 (Figure 3-A), which likely reflects rapid transdermal absorption of BPA due to the use of hand sanitizer as well as some of the BPA having been transferred to the French fries. Importantly, females transferred significantly more (58±19 µg) BPA from their dominant hand to the 10 French fries than males (15±3 µg; Mann-Whitney U; $P<0.05$), resulting in females having a significantly higher oral BPA dose than males between 4–8 min after applying the hand sanitizer.

Since the participants had been instructed to avoid known sources of BPA, such as canned products, and instructed not to touch thermal paper, 9 of the 10 subjects had undetectable BPA on their dominant hand prior to washing their hands when they first arrived at the Clinical Research Center; none of the subjects was a cashier. However, one female had 0.9 µg of BPA extracted from her hand upon arriving at the CRC, and she was also found to have a very high background concentration of serum uBPA (14.3 ng/mL) prior to holding the thermal receipt paper (subject #3; Figure 4-B). This was the only female subject who was menstruating and thus using products to control menstrual flow, and she also indicated use of hand and body lotion 7–9 times in the prior 48 hr, which was more than any other female or male subject (see Section S3 in File S1). However, even though female #3 (Figure 4-B) had very high background serum uBPA, she showed a dramatic 9.5 ng/mL increase relative to baseline in serum uBPA after holding the thermal receipt and eating 10 contaminated fries at the 15 min blood collection time (15 min after consuming the last French fry). The increase relative to baseline in serum uBPA for female #3 was thus virtually identical to the maximum increase (relative to baseline) found for the other 2 females who had low baseline serum uBPA levels and that were tested in the same way (blood was collected from the BPA contaminated arm; Figure 4-A; Table 1).

Experiment 3-A: Collection of blood from the cubital vein in the contaminated arm with BPA remaining on the hand throughout the 90-min test period

The data for female subject #3 are not included in the pharmacokinetic data (Table 2) calculated for the remaining 6 subjects that had blood collected from their contaminated arm but who had undetectable baseline levels of BPA on their hands when they first entered the CRC and also had very low baseline uBPA in serum (0.23±0.15 ng/mL; N = 6]. These 6 subjects showed a dramatic increase in serum uBPA after holding the thermal receipt

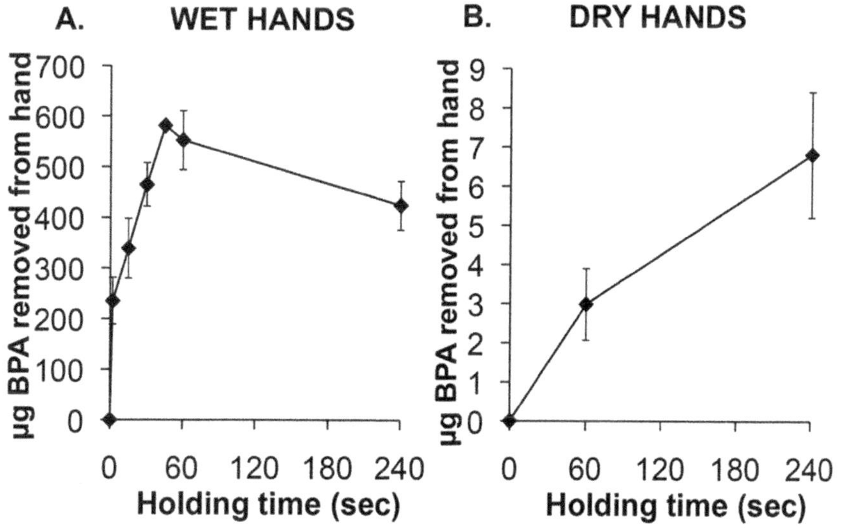

Figure 3. Effect of length of time holding an 8×12 cm thermal receipt on the amount of BPA (µg) swiped from the hand, when hands were pre-wetted with hand sanitizer (Panel A) or left dry (Panel B). The hand was swiped with KimWipes wetted with ethanol to remove the BPA from the surface of the palm and fingers.

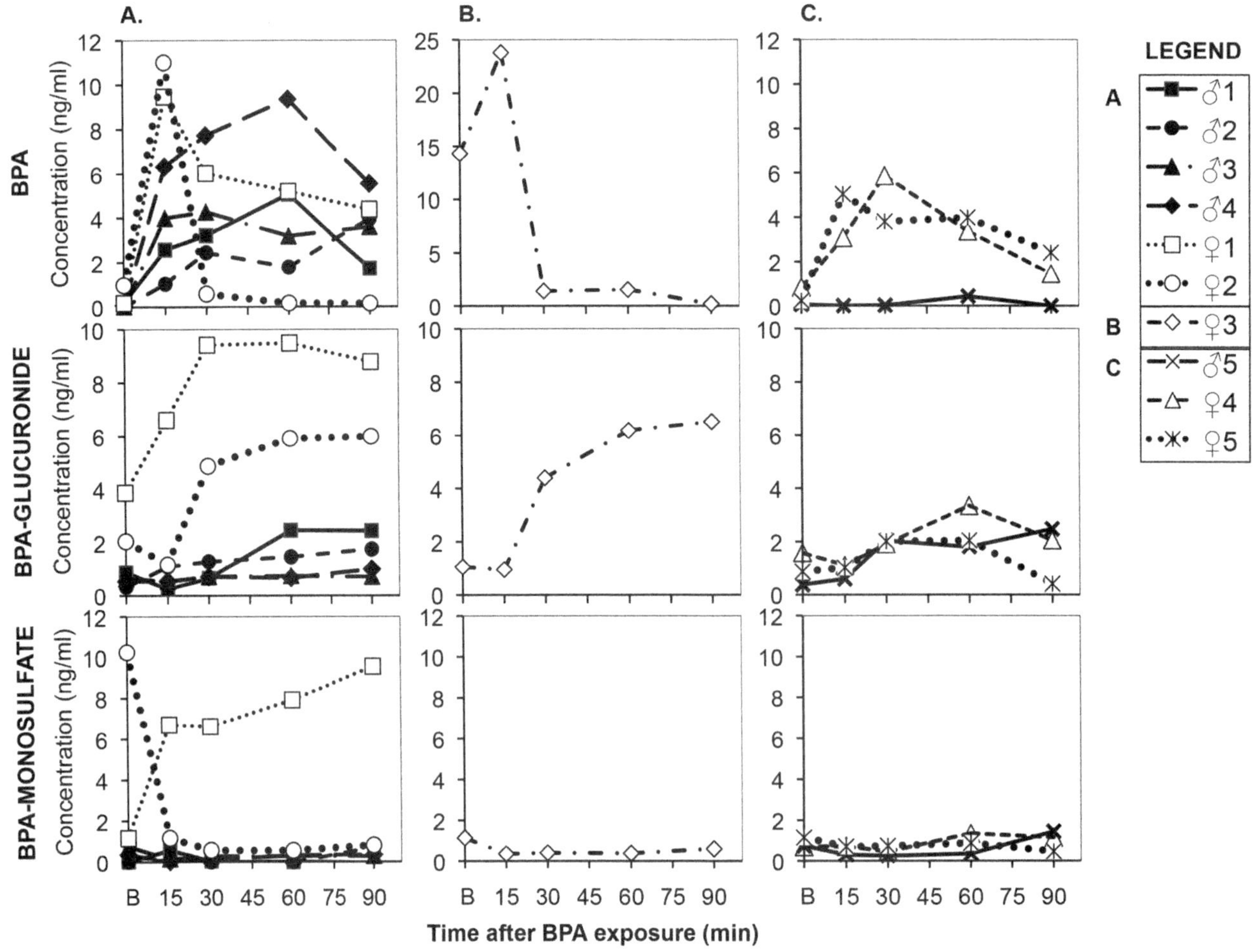

Figure 4. Individual serum profiles of BPA, BPA-G and BPA-MS in men and women prior to (B = baseline levels) and after holding BPA-containing receipt paper for 4 min followed by picking up and eating 10 French fries over about 4 min with a BPA-contaminated hand. The BPA then remained on the contaminated hand throughout the following 90-min period of blood collection (blood was collected between 15–90 min after eating the last French fry). Panel A: data for serum BPA collected from the contaminated arm with BPA remaining on the hand for 4 males and 2 females that had very low baseline serum uBPA. Panel B: serum BPA data collected from the contaminated arm from Female #3 who had a high baseline serum concentration of uBPA. Panel C: serum BPA data for one male and 2 females who had systemic blood collected from the uncontaminated arm.

and eating 10 contaminated fries. Females had a greater Cmax and maximum increase relative to baseline in serum uBPA and BPA-G than males after holding the thermal paper, while males reached peak levels of uBPA (Tmax) later than females. The average uBPA value, based on the area under the concentration-time curve [AUC (0–90 min)] did not differ between males and females, while for BPA-G, the AUC (0–90 min) was greater for females than males. The ratio of BPA-G/uBPA based on the average AUC (0–90 min) was very low (0.35±0.12 for males and 1.82±0.30 for females), consistent with routes of absorption of BPA (dermal and sublingual) that bypass first pass metabolism [19,20].

Only female #1 (Figure 4-A) showed a marked increase in serum BPA-S relative to baseline, revealing that while BPA-G is the major conjugated metabolite of BPA in most men and non-pregnant women, some individuals do form significant amounts of BPA-S. Urine total BPA (unconjugated and conjugated) increased dramatically between baseline and 90 min after handling thermal paper, although unlike the serum data, there was no difference between males and females (Table 2).

Experiment 3-B: Collection of blood from the cubital vein in the uncontaminated arm to measure BPA in mixed systemic blood throughout the 90-min test period

We also obtained data from 3 subjects who had the same procedures described above except that they had blood collected from the cubital vein in the opposite uncontaminated arm that did not have BPA remaining on the hand during the 90-min period of blood collection. The 3 subjects consisted of one male and 2 females (age 22.3±0.9 yrs, BMI 26.0±0.9). While the baseline serum uBPA levels were very low (Figure 4-C; Table 3), the average serum uBPA AUC (0–90 min) for the two female subjects (Table 3) was similar to the data from the other 7 subjects discussed in Experiment 3-A (Table 2). Even for the male subject with low serum uBPA after holding thermal receipt paper, BPA-G in serum increased between baseline and 90 min (Figure 4-C), and urine total BPA increased dramatically over the 90-min test, similar to the increase in total urine BPA in the women (Table 3). These findings show that high levels of uBPA could be detected in the systemic circulation of subjects after holding thermal receipt paper and eating 10 French fries. Levels of total BPA in urine at

Table 2. Unconjugated BPA (uBPA) and glucuronidated BPA (BPA-G) pharmacokinetic parameters for 4 male and 2 female subjects who held thermal receipt paper and ate French fries after using hand sanitizer (shown in Figure 5-A).

Analyte	Parameter	Male	Female	All
Serum uBPA	Baseline (ng/ml)	0.06±0.04	0.57±0.28	0.23±0.15
	Cmax (ng/ml)	5.66±1.25	10.24±0.77	7.19±1.26
	Maximum increase (ng/ml)	5.60±1.24	9.66±0.37	6.95±1.17
	Range of increase (ng/ml)	3.96–9.28	9.29–10.03	3.96–10.03
	Tmax (min)	60.00±12.25	15.00±0.00	45.00±12.25
	Range of Tmax	30.00–90.00	15.00	15.00–90.00
	Average AUC (0–90 min) (ng/ml)	3.92±1.08	3.85±0.04	3.90±0.75
Serum BPA-G	Baseline (ng/ml)	0.60±0.10	2.95±0.91	1.38±0.55
	Cmax (ng/ml)	1.49±0.39	7.74±1.75	3.57±1.42
	Maximum increase (ng/ml)	0.89±0.36	4.79±0.85	2.19±0.88
	Range of increase (ng/ml)	0.09–1.58	3.94–5.63	0.09–5.63
	Tmax (min)	75.00±8.66	75.00±15.00	75.00±6.71
	Range of Tmax	60.00–90.00	60.00–90.00	60.00–90.00
	Average AUC (0–90 min) (ng/ml)	1.05±0.21	6.48±1.93	2.86±1.25
	BPA-G/uBPA AUC (0–90 min) (ng/mL)	0.35±0.12	1.82±0.30	0.84±0.33
Urine Total BPA	Baseline (ng/ml)	0.15±0.04	1.10±0.58	0.46±0.24
	Baseline (µg/g creatinine)	0.20±0.09	1.22±0.24	0.54±0.19
	90 min (ng/ml)	23.36±6.66	10.62±3.16	19.11±4.32
	90 min (µg/g creatinine)	18.20±5.33	40.93±22.56	25.77±8.56

For these subjects blood was collected from the arm draining the hand that remained contaminated with BPA throughout the 90-min period of blood collection. Urine total BPA at baseline and at 90 min are presented as both actual concentration (ng/ml) and creatinine adjusted (µg BPA/g creatinine) values.
For the one female (Female #3; Figure 5-B) who had very high baseline serum uBPA (data not included in this table), the average serum AUC (0–90) values for uBPA and BPA-G were 6.05 and 4.49 ng/ml, respectively, and urine total BPA levels at baseline and at 90 min were 0.41 and 41.41-µg/g creatinine, respectively.

baseline or 90 min in these 3 subjects (Table 3) were similar to levels measured in the other 7 subjects (Table 2).

Experiment 4: Serum and urine BPA in men and women before and after transdermal exposure to BPA from thermal receipt paper with dry hands

We conducted this study with 12 male (age 27.7±1.6 yrs, BMI 26.9±0.9) and 12 female (age 25.8±1.6 yrs, BMI 25.2±1.5) subjects. Male and females subjects held a single 8×12 cm piece of thermal receipt paper in the non-dominant hand for 4 min, but unlike the prior experiment, no hand sanitizer was used prior to holding the thermal paper with a dry hand. No BPA was detected on the hands of any subject after washing and drying the hands prior to holding the thermal receipt paper. We did not determine the amount of BPA transferred to the hand immediately after holding the thermal receipt paper, since we had previously examined this (Figure 3-B). However, 30 min after holding the thermal paper BPA was swiped from the surface of the hand: for men (5.5±1.7 µg; range: 0.8–22.5 µg) and women (6.1±0.8 µg; range: 1.3–10.6 µg). There was no difference between males and females in the urine total BPA concentration at baseline or at 60 min, and there was also no difference between total urine BPA at baseline vs. 60 min for either males or females (Figure 5-A). There was a tendency (based on 2-tailed t-tests) for males to have higher serum uBPA at baseline ($P = 0.08$) and after 30 min ($P = 0.06$) relative to females (Figure 5-B). While there was no sex difference in conjugated BPA (cBPA), consisting of both BPA-G and BPA-S, at the baseline blood collection (Figure 5-C), at 30 min after holding the thermal receipt males had significantly higher serum conjugated BPA than females (ANOVA; $P<0.001$).

Discussion

Our data provide the first evidence that the use of very large amounts of free BPA as a developer on the print surface of thermal paper (~20 mg BPA/g paper) could be an important factor in accounting for the high levels of bioactive serum uBPA and urine total excreted BPA reported previously in various human populations [21]. We conducted this study to mimic aspects of the behavior of people in a fast-food restaurant where we have observed people using hand sanitizer and handling a thermal receipt for variable periods of time prior to picking up and eating food with their hands. In Figure 3 we show that holding a receipt for 45 sec immediately after using hand sanitizer containing dermal penetration enhancing chemicals resulted in the maximum amount of BPA that was swiped from the palm and fingers (581 µg BPA). After holding the receipt for 2 sec 40% of maximum was recovered from the hand, and within 15 sec 58% of maximum was recovered. Between 45 sec and 4 min, the amount of BPA recovered from the surface of the hand decreased, which may have been due to absorption into skin occurring at a greater rate than transfer to the skin from the thermal receipt. These findings show that a very large amount of BPA is transferred from thermal paper to a hand as a result of holding a thermal receipt for only a few seconds immediately after using a product with dermal penetration enhancing chemicals. The data in Figure 3-A also suggest that transdermal BPA absorption is very rapid due to the penetration enhancing chemicals in the hand sanitizer that we used, and thus

Table 3. Unconjugated BPA (uBPA) and glucuronidated BPA (BPA-G) pharmacokinetic parameters for one male and two female subjects who held thermal receipt paper and ate French fries after using hand sanitizer (shown in Figure 5-C).

Analyte	Parameter	Male	Female	All
Serum uBPA	Baseline (ng/ml)	0.06	0.53±0.30	0.37±0.24
	Cmax (ng/ml)	0.42	5.44±0.42	3.77±1.69
	Maximum increase (ng/ml)	0.37	4.91±0.13	3.40±1.53
	Range of increase (ng/ml)	0.37	4.80–5.03	0.37–5.03
	Tmax (min)	60.00	22.50±7.50	35.00±13.23
	Range of Tmax	60.00	15.00–30.00	15.00–60.00
	Average AUC (0–90 min) (ng/ml)	0.15	3.47±0.06	2.36±1.11
Serum BPA-G	Baseline (ng/ml)	0.38	1.22±0.36	0.94±0.35
	Cmax (ng/ml)	2.47	2.69±0.65	2.62±0.39
	Maximum increase (ng/ml)	2.09	1.47±0.30	1.68±0.27
	Range of increase (ng/ml)	2.09	1.18–1.77	1.18–2.09
	Tmax (min)	90.00	60.00	70.00±10.00
	Range of Tmax	90.00	60.00	60.00–90.00
	Average AUC (0–90 min) (ng/ml)	1.65	1.87±0.38	1.80±0.23
	BPA-G/uBPA AUC (0–90 min) (ng/mL)	11.00	0.54±0.12	4.03±3.49
Urine Total BPA	Baseline (ng/ml)	1.92	0.38±0.15	0.89±0.52
	Baseline (μg/g creatinine)	1.17	0.21±0.08	0.53±0.40
	90 min (ng/ml)	27.86	29.34±0.35	28.85±0.54
	90 min (μg/g creatinine)	27.35	14.11±1.16	18.53±4.46

For these subjects mixed systemic blood was collected from the uncontaminated arm over the 90 min after BPA exposure. Urine total BPA at baseline and at 90 min are presented as both actual concentration (ng/ml) and creatinine adjusted (μg/g creatinine) values.

measurement of BPA swiped from the surface of the hand likely underestimates the actual amount of free BPA transferred from the print surface of thermal paper. We note that since the thermal receipt paper is sold in rolls, the non-print surface has BPA transferred to it from the print surface (Figure 1). By swiping the two surfaces with ethanol on Kimwipes, the print surface was found to contain an 8.7-fold greater amount of BPA relative to the non-print surface of the thermal receipt paper roll used in these experiments (data not shown).

In both men and women there was a dramatic increase in serum uBPA after using hand sanitizer with dermal penetration enhancing chemicals and then holding thermal receipt paper and eating French fries with the BPA-contaminated hand (Figure 4-A and 4-B). While the sample size was small, our data suggest higher maximum serum levels (Cmax) for females and a greater maximum increase relative to baseline for both uBPA and BPA-G (the primary conjugated BPA metabolite) for females relative to males (Table 2). This finding was related to a greater transfer of BPA from the hand to the French fries and thus a greater oral dose (by about 4 fold) in females relative to males. However, we cannot rule out that the skin of females also allows greater transdermal transport of BPA relative to males due to sex differences in skin permeability [13]. In fact, our data are consistent with the hypothesis that a combination of both transdermal and buccal/sublingual absorption (Figure 2) resulted in the dramatic increase in both serum uBPA (Figure 4-A and 4-B) and total BPA excreted in urine (Table 2). The profile of serum uBPA suggests that females absorbed BPA more rapidly than

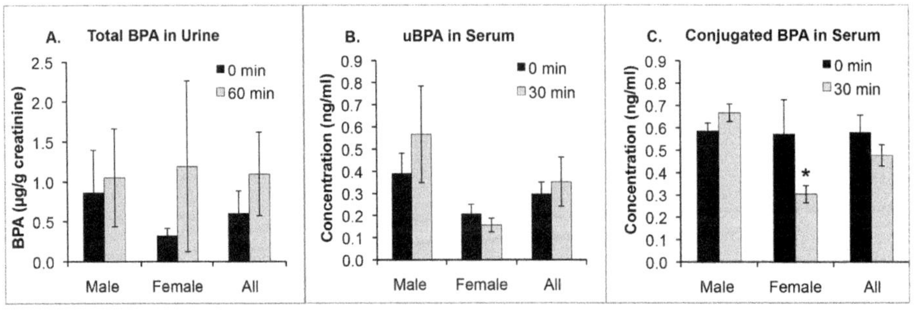

Figure 5. BPA in urine and serum of 12 men and 12 women who held thermal receipt paper with dry hands for 4 min, Panel A: the total concentration of BPA in urine (expressed relative to creatinine) at baseline and 60-min after holding the thermal receipt. Panel B: unconjugated BPA (uBPA) in serum at baseline and 30 min after holding the thermal receipt. Panel C: conjugated BPA (BPA-G and BPA-S) in serum at baseline and 30 min after holding the thermal receipt paper. * = significant difference between males and females (P<0.001).

males (Figure 4-A), consistent with females having a shorter time to reach the maximum serum level (Tmax) of uBPA (Table 2). The later Tmax in men than in women is consistent with men having a thicker stratum corneum (the outermost layer of the epidermis) relative to women [22,23]. In addition to skin thickness, another possible explanation for the sex differences we observed (Table 2) would be a greater use of skin moisturizers in females than in males, which could impact both the transfer of BPA to the hand from the surface of thermal paper as well as transdermal absorption of BPA. Our finding that males tended to have higher serum uBPA and had significantly higher serum conjugated BPA than women at 30 min after holding a receipt with a dry hand (Figure 5-B and 5-C) requires further study, since the more rapid absorption of BPA found for women after using hand sanitizer (Figure 4-A and 4-B) would have been missed at the 30-min blood collection time.

For the 3 females that had blood collected from the cubital vein in the same arm with the BPA contaminated hand (Figure 4-A and 4-B; Table 2), the maximum increase in serum uBPA relative to baseline (~10 ng/mL) was about two-times greater than the maximum increase found in the other two females whose blood was collected from the opposite uncontaminated arm (~5 ng/mL; Table 3; Figure 4-C). This difference between blood collected from a vein draining the contaminated hand vs. blood from the opposite uncontaminated arm (reflecting uBPA in the systemic circulation) suggests that a substantial amount of uBPA in blood from the contaminated arm was due to the BPA that was transdermally absorbed before its mixing in the general circulation. Our data from the cubital vein draining the contaminated hand that had BPA remaining on it for 90 min thus support the hypothesis of a higher arterial than mixed venous blood BPA concentration during the dermal absorption phase in the framework of a physiologically based pharmacokinetic (PBPK) model [24]. The hypothesis that served as the basis for collecting blood from the same arm in which BPA was being absorbed is that a portion of the BPA contaminated blood would be transported from the contaminated hand through the cubital vein and then to the heart. Subsequently, the contaminated blood would enter the arterial circulation and be transported to the tissues in the body, including endocrine target tissues. This leads to the prediction that during the dermal absorption of BPA, the BPA concentration in arterial blood is likely more relevant to consider in terms of exposure than the BPA concentration in the mixed venous blood, because blood in a vein draining the contaminated hand is not subjected to clearance by enzymes in the liver prior to reaching endocrine target tissues in arterial blood.

When examining all of our data for serum unconjugated and conjugated BPA, we show significant inter-subject variability in the absorption and clearance of BPA (Figure 4), which was also previously found for the estrogenic drug used in oral contraceptives, ethinylestradiol [25]. A particular concern is that there are individuals who have limited capacity to excrete BPA or other estrogenic compounds; one population at risk is patients with early-stage or advanced kidney disease [26,27].

The default method of administration of chemicals to animals by regulatory agencies is by intra-gastric gavage, regardless of how the chemical is used or whether there are known non-oral routes of exposure [28]. It is thus not surprising that US and European regulatory agencies [29,30] have modeled human exposure to BPA based on results from intra-gastric gavage administration of BPA to animals, which results in direct transport of BPA to the liver via the mesenteric vessels and extensive first-pass metabolism (detoxification) in the liver (Figure 2); the result is less than 1% of the gavage administered dose being bioavailable in blood [19,31]. However, Gayrard et al. [19] found high absorption and bioavailability (~70%) of BPA following sublingual administration that was dramatically different than the much lower bioavailability (<1%) of BPA following gavage administration in a parallel experiment. These findings directly challenge predictions that it is not possible to find the high blood levels of biologically active uBPA that have actually been measured in numerous human biomonitoring studies [21,32] but are currently being rejected for use in risk assessments by the US-Food and Drug Administration (US-FDA) as not plausible [31].

In contrast to the extremely high ratio of BPA-G to uBPA (> 100:1) predicted by gavage exposure studies due to rapid phase 2 metabolism in the liver, the average ratio of BPA-G to uBPA in our Experiment 3 was 0.84±0.33 based on the average AUC (0–90 min) for the 6 subjects with blood collected from the arm with the contaminated hand (Figure 5-A; Table 2); this ratio was also low for the subjects with systemic blood collected from the uncontaminated arm (Table 3). These findings indicate that the primary route of BPA exposure was not via gastrointestinal absorption after eating the BPA-contaminated French fries, since this ratio would be predicted to exceed 100:1 [31,33]. One reason may have been that, in addition to transdermal absorption, the BPA transferred to the French fries would have been on the surface of the fries and thus easily absorbed by the highly vascularized epithelium in the mouth [19].

In the present study we measured total BPA in urine to be able to relate our findings to a very large epidemiological literature showing BPA in urine to be correlated with abnormal development and diseases in children and adults [5,34]. The geometric mean for adults in the 95th percentile for total BPA in urine reported in NHANES 2003/4 was about 11 μg/g creatinine [2] and the range of values at the 95th percentile include values we measured here. Periodically, BPA levels exceeding those we found are reported in studies that measured BPA in urine [21], and it is possible that those assays are of people who had very recently been exposed to BPA in a manner similar to our experiment.

Our findings thus provide evidence regarding how some people could be found to have very high urine levels of BPA. Importantly, the amount of total BPA in urine was ~20 μg BPA/g creatinine (~20 ng/mL urine uncorrected for creatinine). This high level of urine total BPA collected 90 min after using hand sanitizer and holding a thermal receipt (Table 2 and Table 3) has been associated with a significant increase in the likelihood of developing cardiovascular disease and type 2 diabetes [35,36]. BPA levels in human urine have also been related to a wide range of other diseases in over 60 human epidemiological studies [5,34]. Published findings include: reproductive effects in women (polycystic ovary syndrome, altered ovarian response to hormones, reduced fertilization success, implantation failure, endometrial disorders, reduced embryo quality, miscarriage, premature delivery and breast cancer), reproductive effects in men (reduced libido, sperm quality, altered sex hormone concentrations and embryo quality), altered thyroid hormone concentrations, obesity, impaired liver function, impaired immune and kidney function, inflammation, and neurobehavioral deficits such as aggressiveness, hyperactivity and impaired learning [5,34]. The estimate of the costs per year of additional cases of just cardiovascular disease in the USA attributable to BPA is 1.5 billion dollars [37].

In a study that involved handling thermal receipts (without using hand sanitizer) continuously for 2 hr, which would be relevant for a cashier, there was a significant increase in urine total BPA relative to baseline [38]. This finding is consistent with prior data that cashiers have higher levels of BPA in urine than the general public [39]. Blood concentrations of BPA were not determined in these studies, and they also did not take into account that perhaps 50% of the receipts handled may have contained BPS rather than BPA (Table 1). The results of these studies indicate that with repeated handling of thermal receipts in an occupational setting, even without the use of hand sanitizer, there is a significant increase in BPA exposure. Future studies involving handling of thermal paper need to include analysis of the thermal paper to determine if the developer used is BPA or some other chemical. Related to the issue of occupational exposure to BPA is our observation that at least one big-box store in Columbia, Missouri provides hand sanitizer dispensers for use by all cashiers, and our data suggest this can not only markedly increase transfer of BPA from the thermal paper to hands but also increase transdermal absorption of BPA.

Our findings that thermal receipt paper is a potential source of high exposure to BPA are supported by data showing that BPA readily leaches from thermal receipts and thus likely contaminates anything that a receipt contacts. Thus, environmental contamination caused by the use of unpolymerized (free) BPA in thermal paper is widespread [7]. The dermal penetration enhancing chemicals present in personal care products as well as hand sanitizers cause a breakdown of the dermal barrier leading to an increase in transdermal absorption [8,9]. While BPA was reported to be absorbed through pig and human skin *in vitro* [40], our data show after holding a receipt for 60 sec, there was 185-times more BPA transferred to a wet hand due to holding thermal receipt paper immediately after using hand sanitizer with penetration enhancing chemicals as opposed to when the hands were dry (Figure 3). The specific mixtures of chemicals used in products will impact transdermal exposure to environmental chemicals such as BPA [8,9], and additional research is needed to determine the degree to which alcohols and other chemicals impact exposures. This is important because when soap and water are not available, hand sanitizers are recommended to reduce infectious disease transmission [http://www.cdc.gov/handwashing/when-how-handwashing.html]. It is also important to determine the length of time after using skin-care products with dermal penetration enhancing chemicals that there is an impact on absorption of environmental contaminants.

The issue of assay performance is obviously very important and was examined using a round robin validation process in Europe for a number of chemicals, including BPA, which identified that some laboratories were able to accurately assay uBPA and other chemicals without contamination, while other laboratories were unable to assay uBPA or other chemicals accurately [41]. Importantly, our findings reported here are based on measurement of uBPA with a sensitive, validated, contamination-free LC/MSMS assay. Specifically, our laboratory is one of three in the U.S. that recently successfully completed a NIH-sponsored round-robin measuring uBPA in human serum [17]. In addition, in the present experiment, the time course of blood uBPA concentrations after a controlled BPA exposure in our university Clinical Research Center (Figure 4) is not consistent with any spurious contamination; this conclusion was also supported by the use of field blanks. It is thus clear that the prediction that any finding of uBPA in human serum must be due to sample contamination [31] is not valid, even though a few investigators report being unable to control BPA contamination in their assays [42,43]. Supporting our conclusion is a report from the CDC in which sources of contamination were identified and systematically eliminated during the successful development of assays for BPA and three other chemicals [44]. The issue of the potential for assay contamination is thus not unique to BPA and simply requires the use of standard assay procedures and appropriate controls that should be routinely employed.

Conclusions

Thermal paper requires a chemical in the surface coating as a print developer. The current preferred developers, BPA and BPS, have both been shown to have estrogenic activity [45,46]. This is leading to widespread exposure to both of these endocrine-disrupting chemicals [7,47], and BPS is more persistent in the environment relative to BPA and is thus an unacceptable replacement for BPA [18,48]. A recent EPA report examined 19 alternative chemicals, including BPS, that could potentially replace BPA as a developer in thermal paper and concluded that "No clearly safer alternatives to BPA were identified in this report; most alternatives have Moderate or High hazard designations for human health or aquatic toxicity endpoints" [18]. The report identified that "decision makers may wish to consider alternative printing systems". Two of the papers screened for our current study employed a developer other than BPA or BPS that was not estrogenic in a MCF-7 human breast cancer cell proliferation assay (data not shown), but lack of estrogenic activity does not imply safety, as indicated in the EPA report.

Thermal paper is a major source of BPA contamination in recycled paper, and its use results in the widespread contamination of other products and the environment [49] due to the presence of large amounts of free, unpolymerized BPA in the surface coating of thermal paper (Figure 1). Further, our findings are consistent with other data reporting that BPA can be transferred from the surface of thermal paper to items it contacts. Because no safe alternatives to the use of BPA or its primary replacement chemical BPS in thermal paper have been identified, our findings provide support for the EPA's recommendation that thermal paper should be replaced with other safer technologies [18].

Our study provides the first data that thermal paper may be a significant factor in accounting for high levels of bioactive BPA in human serum and total BPA in urine that have been associated with diseases that are increasing in frequency in human populations [21,34]. Our findings also suggest that the impact of the use of dermal penetration enhancing chemicals in skin care products on transdermal absorption of environmental contaminants should be taken into consideration in risk assessments and should be a priority for future research.

Supporting Information

File S1 Section S1: Sample handling, extraction and assay methods. Section S2: Table of individual BPA and BPS values for 50 thermal receipt papers. Section S3: List of questions asked each subject.

Author Contributions

Conceived and designed the experiments: FVS AMH JAT. Performed the experiments: AMH JAT CLM. Analyzed the data: JAT PLT RWS MRE FVS. Contributed reagents/materials/analysis tools: FVS. Contributed to the writing of the manuscript: FVS AMH CLM JAT SCN WVW PLT RWS.

References

1. GrandViewResearch (2014) Global bisphenol A (BPA) market by appliation (appliances, automotive, consumer, construction, electrical & electronics) expected to reach USD 20.03 billion by 2020. http://www.digitaljournal.com/pr/2009287, Accessed June 24, 2014. http://www.digitaljournal.com/pr/2009287, Accessed June 24, 2014.
2. Calafat AM, Ye X, Wong LY, Reidy JA, Needham LL (2008) Exposure of the U.S. population to bisphenol A and 4-tertiary-octylphenol: 2003–2004. Environ Health Perspect 116: 39–44.
3. Liao C, Kannan K (2012a) Determination of free and conjugated forms of bisphenol a in human urine and serum by liquid chromatography-tandem mass spectrometry. Environ Sci Technol 46: 5003–5009.
4. Welshons WV, Thayer KA, Judy BM, Taylor JA, Curran EM, et al. (2003) Large effects from small exposures. I. Mechanisms for endocrine-disrupting chemicals with estrogenic activity. Environ Health Perspect 111: 994–1006.
5. Vandenberg LN, Ehrlich S, Belcher SM, Ben-Jonathan N, Dolinoy DC, et al. (2013a) Low Dose Effects of Bisphenol A: An Integrated Review of In Vitro, Laboratory Animal and Epidemiology Studies. Endocrine Disruption 1: E1–E20.
6. Mendum T, Stoler E, VanBenschoten H, Warner JC (2011) Concentration of bisphenol A in thermal paper. Green Chemistry Letters and Reviews 4: 81–86.
7. Liao C, Kannan K (2011) Widespread Occurrence of Bisphenol A in Paper and Paper Products: Implications for Human Exposure. Environ Sci Technol 45: 9372–9739.
8. Funke AP, Schiller R, Motzkus HW, Gunther C, Muller RH, et al. (2002) Transdermal delivery of highly lipophilic drugs: in vitro fluxes of antiestrogens, permeation enhancers, and solvents from liquid formulations. Pharm Res 19: 661–668.
9. Karande P, Mitragotri S (2009) Enhancement of transdermal drug delivery via synergistic action of chemicals. Biochim Biophys Acta 1788: 2362–2373.
10. EFSA (2013) Draft scientific opinion on the risks to public health related to the presence of bisphenol A (BPA) in foodstuffs – exposure assessment; EFSA Panel on Food Contact Materials, Enzymes, Flavourings and Processing Aids; European Food Safety Authority (EFSA), Parma, Italy, July 1.
11. Xue J, Zartarian V, Moya J, Freeman N, Beamer P, et al. (2007) A meta-analysis of children's hand-to-mouth frequency data for estimating nondietary ingestion exposure. Risk Anal 27: 411–420.
12. Heffernan AL, Aylward LL, Samidurai AJ, Davies PS, Toms LM, et al. (2014) Short term variability in urinary bisphenol A in Australian children. Environ Int 68C: 139–143.
13. Singh I, Morris AP (2011) Performance of transdermal therapeutic systems: Effects of biological factors. Int J Pharm Investig 1: 4–9.
14. IBISWorld (2012) Hand sanitizer manufacturing in the US: Market research report. Feb 2012. http://www.ibisworld.com/industry/hand-sanitizer-manufacturing.html.
15. Brand RM, Charron AR, Sandler VL, Jendrzejewski JL (2007) Moisturizing lotions can increase transdermal absorption of the herbicide 2,4-dichlorophenoxacetic acid across hairless mouse skin. Cutan Ocul Toxicol 26: 15–23.
16. StatisticsBrain (2014) Fast food statistics, http://www.statisticbrain.com/fast-food-statistics/, Accessed March 26.Statistic Brain.
17. Vandenberg LN, Gerona RR, Kannan K, Taylor JA, van Breemen RB, et al. (2014a) A round robin approach to the analysis of bisphenol a (BPA) in human blood samples. Environ Health 13: 25.
18. EPA (2014) Bisphenol A alternatives in thermal paper. United States Environmental Protection Agency, Final document, January 2014. http://www.epa.gov/dfe/pubs/projects/bpa/bpa-report-complete.pdf. Accessed 9/9/14.
19. Gayrard V, Lacroix MZ, Collet SH, Viguie C, Bousquet-Melou A, et al. (2013) High bioavailability of bisphenol a from sublingual exposure. Environ Health Perspect 121: 951–956.
20. vom Saal FS, Vandevoort CA, Taylor JA, Welshons WV, Toutain PL, et al. (2014) Bisphenol A (BPA) pharmacokinetics with daily oral bolus or continuous exposure via silastic capsules in pregnant rhesus monkeys: Relevance for human exposures. Reprod Toxicol 45: 105–116.
21. Vandenberg LN, Chahoud I, Heindel JJ, Padmanabhan V, Paumgartten FJ, et al. (2010a) Urinary, circulating, and tissue biomonitoring studies indicate widespread exposure to bisphenol A. Environ Health Perspect 118: 1055–1070.
22. Fitzmaurice S, Maibach HI (2010) Gender differences in skin. In: M.A F, Miller KM, Maibach HI, editors. Textbook of Aging Skin. New York: Springer. 999–1017.
23. Polak S, Ghobadi C, Mishra H, Ahamadi M, Patel N, et al. (2012) Prediction of concentration-time profile and its inter-individual variability following the dermal drug absorption. J Pharm Sci 101: 2584–2595.
24. Levitt DG (2004) Physiologically based pharmacokinetic modeling of arterial - antecubital vein concentration difference. BMC Clin Pharmacol 4: 2–7.
25. Goldzieher JW, Stanczyk FZ (2008) Oral contraceptives and individual variability of circulating levels of ethinyl estradiol and progestins. Contraception 78: 4–9.
26. You L, Zhu X, Shrubsole MJ, Fan H, Chen J, et al. (2011) Renal function, Bisphenol A, and Alkylphenols: Results from the National Health and Nutrition Examination Survey (NHANES 2003–2006). Environ Health Perspect 119: 527–533.
27. Krieter DH, Canaud B, Lemke HD, Rodriguez A, Morgenroth A, et al. (2013) Bisphenol A in chronic kidney disease. Artif Organs 37: 283–290.
28. Vandenberg LN, Welshons WV, Vom Saal FS, Toutain PL, Myers JP (2014b) Should oral gavage be abandoned in toxicity testing of endocrine disruptors? Environ Health 13: 46.
29. EFSA (2008) Toxicokinetics of Bisphenol A - Scientific Opinion of the Panel on Food additives, Flavourings, Processing aids and Materials in Contact with Food (AFC). European Food Safety Authority July, 2008. http://www.efsa.europa.eu/EFSA/efsa_locale-1178620753812_1211902017492.htm. Accessed September 2, 2014.
30. FDA (2008a) Food and Drug Administration draft assessment of bisphenol A for use in Food contact applications, August 14, 2008. http://www.fda.gov/food/ingredientspackaginglabeling/foodadditivesingredients/ucm166145.htm. watAccessed August 6, 2014.
31. Patterson TA, Twaddle NC, Roegge CS, Callicott RJ, Fisher JW, et al. (2013) Concurrent determination of bisphenol A pharmacokinetics in maternal and fetal rhesus monkeys. Toxicol Appl Pharmacol 267: 41–48.
32. Vandenberg LN, Hauser R, Marcus M, Olea N, Welshons WV (2007) Human exposure to bisphenol A (BPA). Reproductive Toxicology 24: 139–177.
33. Gayrard V, Lacroix MA, Collet SH, Viguié C, Bousquet-Melou A, et al. (2013) Interpreting Bbsphenol A absorption in the canine oral cavity. Environ Health Perspect 121: A323–A324.
34. Rochester JR (2013) Bisphenol A and human health: A review of the literature. Reprod Toxicol 42: 132–155.
35. Lang IA, Galloway TS, Scarlett A, Henley WE, Depledge M, et al. (2008) Association of urinary bisphenol A concentration with medical disorders and laboratory abnormalities in adults. JAMA 300: 1303–1310.
36. Melzer D, Osborne NJ, Henley WE, Cipelli R, Young A, et al. (2012) Urinary bisphenol a concentration and risk of future coronary artery disease in apparently healthy men and women. Circulation 125: 1482–1490.
37. Trasande L (2014) Further limiting bisphenol a in food uses could provide health and economic benefits. Health Aff (Millwood) 33: 316–323.
38. Ehrlich S, Calafat AM, Humblet O, Smith T, Hauser R (2014) Handling of thermal receipts as a source of exposure to bisphenol A. JAMA 311: 859–860.
39. Braun JM, Kalkbrenner AE, Calafat AM, Bernert JT, Ye X, et al. (2011) Variability and predictors of urinary bisphenol A concentrations during pregnancy. Environ Health Perspect 119: 131–137.
40. Zalko D, Jacques C, Duplan H, Bruel S, Perdu E (2011) Viable skin efficiently absorbs and metabolizes bisphenol A. Chemosphere 82: 424–430.
41. Vanderford BJ, Drewes JE, Eaton A, Guo YC, Haghani A, et al. (2014) Results of an Interlaboratory Comparison of Analytical Methods for Contaminants of Emerging Concern in Water. Anal Chem 86: 774–782.
42. Volkel W, Colnot T, Csanady GA, Filser JG, Dekant W (2002) Metabolism and kinetics of bisphenol a in humans at low doses following oral administration. Chem Res Toxicol 15: 1281–1287.
43. Churchwell MI, Camacho L, Vanlandingham MM, Twaddle NC, Sepehr E, et al. (2014) Comparison of life-stage-dependent internal dosimetry for bisphenol A, ethinyl estradiol, a reference estrogen, and endogenous estradiol to test an estrogenic mode of action in Sprague Dawley rats. Toxicol Sci 139: 4–20.
44. Ye X, Zhou X, Hennings R, Kramer J, Calafat AM (2013) Potential external contamination with bisphenol A and other ubiquitous organic environmental chemicals during biomonitoring analysis: an elusive laboratory challenge. Environ Health Perspect 121: 283–286.
45. Vinas R, Watson CS (2013) Bisphenol S disrupts estradiol-induced nongenomic signaling in a rat pituitary cell line: effects on cell functions. Environ Health Perspect 121: 352–358.
46. Welshons WV, Nagel SC, vom Saal FS (2006) Large effects from small exposures. III. Endocrine mechanisms mediating effects of bisphenol A at levels of human exposure. Endocrinol 147: S56–S69.
47. Liao C, Liu F, Alomirah H, Loi VD, Mohd MA, et al. (2012) Bisphenol S in Urine from the United States and Seven Asian Countries: Occurrence and Human Exposures. Environ Sci Technol 46: 6860–6866.
48. EnvironmentCanada (2008) Screening Assessment for The Challenge Phenol, 4,4′ -(1-methylethylidene) bis- (Bisphenol A) Chemical Abstracts Service Registry Number 80-05-7. Environment Canada and Health Canada, Ottawa, October 2008.
49. Liao C, Kannan K (2012b) High levels of bisphenol a in paper currencies from several countries, and implications for dermal exposure. Environ Sci Technol 45: 6761–6768.

11

Label-Free LC-MS^e in Tissue and Serum Reveals Protein Networks Underlying Differences between Benign and Malignant Serous Ovarian Tumors

Wouter Wegdam[1]*, Carmen A. Argmann[2], Gertjan Kramer[3], Johannes P. Vissers[4], Marrije R. Buist[1], Gemma G. Kenter[1], Johannes M. F. G. Aerts[3], Danielle Meijer[1], Perry D. Moerland[5]

1 Department of Gynecology, Academic Medical Center, University of Amsterdam, Amsterdam, the Netherlands, **2** Department of Genetics and Genomic Sciences, Icahn Institute for Genomics and Multiscale Biology, Icahn School of Medicine at Mount Sinai, New York, New York, United States of America, **3** Clinical Proteomics Group, Department of Medical Biochemistry, Academic Medical Center, University of Amsterdam, Amsterdam, the Netherlands, **4** Waters Corporation MS Technologies Center, Manchester, United Kingdom, **5** Bioinformatics Laboratory, Department of Clinical Epidemiology, Biostatistics and Bioinformatics, Academic Medical Center, University of Amsterdam, Amsterdam, the Netherlands

Abstract

Purpose: To identify proteins and (molecular/biological) pathways associated with differences between benign and malignant epithelial ovarian tumors.

Experimental Procedures: Serum of six patients with a serous adenocarcinoma of the ovary was collected before treatment, with a control group consisting of six matched patients with a serous cystadenoma. In addition to the serum, homogeneous regions of cells exhibiting uniform histology were isolated from benign and cancerous tissue by laser microdissection. We subsequently employed label-free liquid chromatography tandem mass spectrometry (LC-MS^e) to identify proteins in these serum and tissues samples. Analyses of differential expression between samples were performed using Bioconductor packages and in-house scripts in the statistical software package R. Hierarchical clustering and pathway enrichment analyses were performed, as well as network enrichment and interactome analysis using MetaCore.

Results: In total, we identified 20 and 71 proteins that were significantly differentially expressed between benign and malignant serum and tissue samples, respectively. The differentially expressed protein sets in serum and tissue largely differed with only 2 proteins in common. MetaCore network analysis, however inferred GCR-alpha and Sp1 as common transcriptional regulators. Interactome analysis highlighted 14-3-3 zeta/delta, 14-3-3 beta/alpha, Alpha-actinin 4, HSP60, and PCBP1 as critical proteins in the tumor proteome signature based on their relative overconnectivity. The data have been deposited to the ProteomeXchange with identifier PXD001084.

Discussion: Our analysis identified proteins with both novel and previously known associations to ovarian cancer biology. Despite the small overlap between differentially expressed protein sets in serum and tissue, APOA1 and Serotransferrin were significantly lower expressed in both serum and cancer tissue samples, suggesting a tissue-derived effect in serum. Pathway and subsequent interactome analysis also highlighted common regulators in serum and tissue samples, suggesting a yet unknown role for PCBP1 in ovarian cancer pathophysiology.

Editor: Rossella Rota, Ospedale Pediatrico Bambino Gesu', Italy

Funding: The study was funded by the Academic Medical Center, University of Amsterdam. Co-author Johannes P. Vissers is employed by Waters Corporation (MS Technologies Center, Manchester, United Kingdom). Waters Corporation provided support in the form of salary for author Johannes P. Vissers. The specific role of this author is articulated in the 'author contributions' section. Both funders, Academic Medical Center and Waters Corporation, had no role in study design, data collection and analysis, decision to publish, or preparation of the manuscript.

Competing Interests: Johannes P. Vissers is employed by Waters Corporation. The methods described in the manuscript make use of the following Waters Corporation marketed products: a nanoAcquity system, a Synapt G2 MS mass spectrometer, ProteinLynx GlobalSERVER (PLGS) v2.5, Mass Prep Quantitation standard, and RapiGest SF.

* Email: W.Wegdam@amc.uva.nl

Introduction

Epithelial ovarian cancer is the leading cause of gynecologic cancer deaths in the Western world [1]. Approximately 70% of epithelial ovarian cancers are detected at an advanced stage. Although about 80% of the patients have complete remission of the disease after treatment with extensive debulking surgery and chemotherapy, the recurrence rate is very high. Currently, there are no curative treatment options for patients with recurrent disease and the 5-year survival rate is less than 30% [1]. In order to improve upon this poor survival rate many studies have tried to identify more sensitive early detection markers and methods for discriminating between different pelvic masses [2,3]. A large number of these studies used various mass-spectrometric methods to search for new markers in patient material such as serum [4]. The OVA1 test, which has been approved by the Food and Drug Administration (FDA) in 2009, was one of the first multimarker diagnostic tests that resulted from this type of research [5]. However, when Moore et al. [6] evaluated several of these biomarkers alone and in combination with CA 125 in prediagnostically collected sera from women in the Prostate, Lung, Colorectal and Ovarian Cancer Screening trial the addition of these biomarkers to CA125 did not improve sensitivity for preclinical diagnosis. Other strategies involve a combination of known serum biomarkers such as Human Epididymal secretory protein 4 (HE4) and CA125 in a discriminatory algorithm such as ROMA (Risk of Ovarian Malignancy Algorithm) [7]. Most of the biomarkers being investigated or used in the clinic today are serum-based proteins, which are logical targets both for use as biomarkers for screening and diagnosis, as well as potential drug targets. However, most of the recently found biomarkers in serum or plasma are acute phase proteins that are not specific for one type of cancer or disease [8]. In fact, only a few FDA approved cancer markers in current clinical use are tumor-derived proteins (e.g., prostate-specific antigen, carcinoembryonic antigen), and are present in serum at very low concentrations (1-10 ng/mL) only [9]. In this study we have tried to overcome the problematic aspecific aspects of blood-based protein markers by aiming to identify proteins differentially expressed between tumor tissue samples of patients with a serous adenocarcinoma of the ovaries versus a benign serous tumor. In tumor tissue the potential marker proteins are present at much higher concentrations, which could facilitate protein identification. By comparing the protein content of tumor tissue with that of serum samples, we aimed to detect or infer reliable tumor-produced serum biomarkers. Directly studying tumor tissue, even though it enhances the probability of finding tumor-derived markers, is challenging nevertheless. Accurate analysis of tumors is often hampered by within-tumor heterogeneity, for example due to the presence of contaminating stroma cells, necrosis or infiltrating lymphocytes [10]. Laser microdissection minimizes this problem via the rapid and reliable isolation of a specific cell population or type from a tissue section under direct microscopic visualization [11,12].

Using laser microdissection we obtained homogenous tumor samples that were subsequently measured with a mass spectrometric approach called LC-MS^e. LC-MS^e differs from traditional data-dependent acquisition (DDA) modes in that all precursor and fragment ions are measured by alternating the collision energy between a low (precursor ions) and elevated (fragment ions) profile without selection of ions. Thus LC-MS^e is able to identify and quantify more peptides in complex samples using a single dimension reversed phase ultra-high pressure liquid chromatography (UPLC) separation, than DDA on quadrupole time-of-flight instruments (QTOF) [13,14].

The primary objective of the present study was to identify differentially expressed proteins in tissue and serum, comparing benign and malignant serous ovarian tumors. After initial protein identification we performed extensive pathway and network analyses in order to find differences in the underlying protein pathways associated with benign and malignant ovarian tumors.

Experimental Procedures

Patients and Ethics Statement

After written informed consent was obtained, serum and tissue samples were prospectively collected from patients admitted at the Academic Medical Center (AMC) for treatment of an ovarian tumor. The study was performed in agreement with the Helsinki Declaration and approved by the Ethical Committee at the Academic Medical Center, University of Amsterdam. For serum analysis, we included 6 patients that were newly diagnosed with non-familial invasive serous epithelial ovarian carcinoma, stage IIIB or higher based on FIGO (Fédération Internationale de Gynécologie Obstétrique) criteria, and 6 patients with benign serous cystadenomas. For 4 of the 6 patients with benign disease and 3 of the 6 with a malignant tumor, also tissue was available. To increase sample size for the tissue comparison, we included two additional patients with benign disease and two additional patients with a malignant tumor. Both in serum and tissue, the two groups were matched for age, body mass index (BMI), menopausal status and sample-storage duration. Clinicopathological data are listed in Table 1. All samples were collected using a strict protocol. Blood was collected from all patients by the same operator, at least two hours after the patient's last meal, and left to clot for 30 minutes. After centrifugation (at 1750×g) serum was immediately frozen and stored at -80°C. Samples used for these experiments were only thawed once.

Laser microdissection and protein isolation

During surgery tumor tissue was collected, snap frozen in liquid nitrogen, and stored at −80°C within 30 minutes of surgery. From these samples 10 µm cryostat sections were prepared. One section was stained with hematoxylin and examined microscopically in order to detect tissue areas of interest for microdissection. Corresponding consecutive tissue sections were mounted on a microscope slide coated with a membrane (polyethylene naphtalate (PEN) Zeiss/Palm, Bernried, Germany) and stored at −80°C. Comparison of stained and unstained tissue sections revealed that hematoxylin staining had no influence on the quantitative protein measurements and identification using LC-MS^e.

Tissue areas were cut using a Veritas Microdissection System (Arcturus Molecular Devices, CA, USA), as described earlier [15]. Slides were stained for 1 minute with hematoxylin. Dissected cancer samples contained at least 90% cancer cells (Figure 1). Using microdissection, the samples from benign cystadenomas were enriched for 75%–90% epithelial cells.

We obtained 100,000 cells from each sample. Cells were denatured in 20 µl 0,1% RapiGest detergent solution (Waters Corp., Milford, MA) and heated at 80°C for 15 minutes. After centrifugation at 1750×g for 10 min, the supernatants were collected. Several tests were performed to determine optimal lysis conditions. Protein concentrations were measured using a Bicinchoninic Acid (BCA) solution (Sigma-Aldrich Chemie GmbH, Schnelldorf, Germany) and 4% CuSO4. The average protein concentration obtained from 100.000 cells was 1 mg/ml.

Sample preparation for LC-MS analysis

Serum samples were diluted in 50 mM ammoniumhydrogencarbonate (Fluka), 1% RapiGest SF (Waters Corp., Milford, MA) to ~10 µg/µl total protein concentration. Laser dissected tissue samples were lysed in 50 mM ammoniumhydrogencarbonate, 0.1% RapiGest SF, prior to protein determination by BCA-assay (Thermo-Scientific) according to the manufacturer's protocol. Subsequently serum samples were denatured at 80°C for 15 min and tissue samples at 95°C for 10 min prior to reduction of

Table 1. Patients characteristics.

	Serum		Tissue	
	Malignant	*Benign*	*Malignant*	*Benign*
Patients	6	6	5	6
Age (mean, SD)	53 (16.5)	57 (7.2)	51 (15.2)	56 (9.8)
BMI (mean, SD)	25 (4.9)	25 (5.1)	23 (3.3)	26 (4.8)
Pre-menopausal	3	1	2	2
Post-menopausal	3	5	3	4
CA125 kU/L (median, range)	6946 (113–14100)	12 (7–26)	2651 (113–7737)	70 (7–376)
Differentiation grade				
2	1		1	
3	5		4	
Figo Stage				
III	5		5	
IV	1			

Clinicopathological characteristics of the patient groups. SD: standard deviation.

disulfide bridges 5 mM dithiorthreitol at 60°C for 30 min. Free sulfhydryl groups were alkylated by addition of 15 mM iodoacetamide and incubation at ambient temperature for 30 min. in the dark. Samples were digested overnight by addition of 0.3 activity units/μg total protein content of sequencing grade modified trypsin (Promega, Madison WI) and incubation overnight at 37°C. Following digestion the acid-labile detergent was hydrolyzed by incubation in the presence of 0.5% trifluoroaceticacid (Biosolve, the Netherlands) at 37°C for 45 min and removal of immiscible debris by centrifugation at 20.000×g for 10 min, collecting the supernatant. Prior to analyses, serum digest samples were diluted with aqueous 0.1% formic acid solution (Biosolve, the Netherlands) to ~0.5 μg/μl total protein concentration. Subsequently both serum digest and tissue digest samples were mixed 1:1 with a Mass Prep Quantitation standard (Waters, Milford MA) for quantitation purposes (mix with either 100 fmol/μl Enolase or Alcohol dehydrogenase 1 from *S. cerevisiae* for tissue samples or 250 fmol/μl ClpB from *Escherichia coli* for serum samples).

LC-MS analysis

0.5 μg of total protein was loaded onto a Nano-Acquity system (Waters Corporation) equipped with a Bridged Ethyl Hybrid C18 1.7 μm, 15-cm×150-μm analytical reversed phase column (Waters Corporation) and operated at a column flow rate of 1 μl/min. All samples were measured in triplicate. Apart from the column dimension and flow rate, all other gradient conditions were as detailed earlier [14]. Analysis of tryptic peptides was performed using a Synapt G2 quadrupole time of flight mass spectrometer (Waters Corporation, Manchester, UK) with the operating and experimental conditions as previously described [14]. Accurate mass precursor and fragment ion LC-MS data were collected in data-independent MS^e mode of acquisition. This method alternates the energy applied to the collision cell of the mass spectrometer between a low and elevated energy state [16,17]. Briefly, the low energy portion of the obtained data sets is typically used for quantification of the proteins, whereas the combined low and elevated energy information are utilized for identification purposes. In both modes of acquisition, mass spectral information was obtained from *m/z* 50 to 1990 at a resolving power of at least 10,000 full width half maximum.

Data processing and protein identification

Continuum LC-MS^e data were processed and searched using ProteinLynx Globalserver version 2.5 (PLGS 2.5, Waters Corporation). Protein identifications were obtained with the embedded ion accounting algorithm [18] of the software and searching the

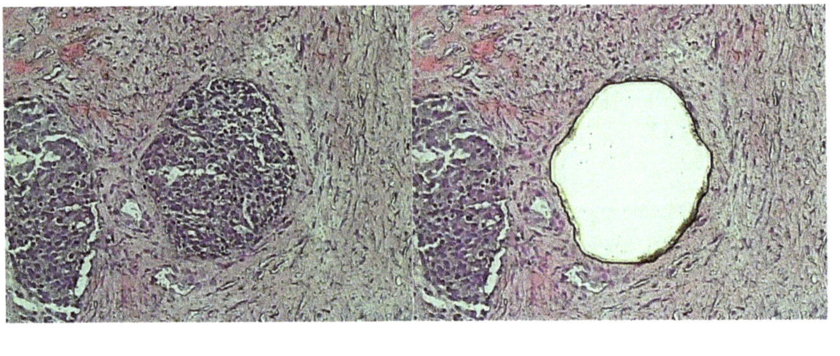

Figure 1. Laser capture microdissection of tumor tissue. A 10 μm hematoxylin stained cryostat section of a serous adenocarcinoma of the ovaries. The picture on the left is prior to microdissection, on right the same slide after microdissection is shown.

human SwissProt entries of the UniProt database (release 13.2) that was modified to include N-terminal processing of proteins using the protein maturation device software [19] and to which enolase and alcohol dehydrogenase 1 of *S. cerevisiae* or ClpB from *Escherichia coli* were appended as the internal standard to provide the ability to address technical variation and to accommodate concentration determinations [13]. The search tolerances were set to automatic, typically 10 ppm for precursor and 25 ppm for product ions, cysteine carbamidomethylation specified as a fixed modification and N-terminal acetylation, deamidation of asparagine and glutamine and oxidation of methionine as variable modifications. Estimation of false positive identification rates was performed by searches in a shuffled version of the UniProt human protein database generated in PGLS 2.5. Robust criteria were applied for quantification, including the identification of minimally three and seven product ion matches per peptide and protein, respectively. In addition, at least two peptides per protein had to be identified and the identification had to occur in at least two independent patient serum or tissue samples. Protein false positive identification rate, taking into account the criteria mentioned above, was less than one percent. Label free quantitation of proteins was based on the sum of the signal intensities of the three most abundant peptides of a protein, divided by the sum of the signal intensities of the three most abundant peptides of the internal standard, times the amount in fmol of standard injected on the column. This gives an estimation of the molar amount of each protein injected on the column. PLGS 2.5 determines the molar amount (the amount in ng is determined using the molecular weight in the database) for each protein based on the ratio of its three most abundant peptides (HI3) determined in each individual experiment [13]. These measured amounts were used for proteins that met the criteria for identification indicated above in order to calculate the average concentration of each protein in g/L using the dilution factor of the samples. Protein identity and quantitative data were exported as a comma separated value file for further statistical and pathway analysis. The mass spectrometry proteomics data have been deposited to the ProteomeXchange consortium (http://proteomecentral.proteomexchange.org) [20] via the PRIDE partner repository with the dataset identifier PXD001084. A list of filenames deposited in ProteomeXchange and their corresponding sample annotation can be found in the supporting information section (Table S1, worksheet 'Filenames').

Statistical analyses

Statistical analyses were performed using Bioconductor packages and in-house scripts in the statistical software package R [21]. Serum and tissue data were analyzed separately. Missing values in the raw quantitative data were imputed with the minimum value measured for the sample in which the missing value occurred. Data were scale normalized to the same mean intensity across samples; resulting values were then log2-transformed with an offset of 1 in order to stabilize their variance. The array Quality Metrics R package was used to assess whether all MS samples were of good quality. The tissue samples were measured in two separate batches; quality control clearly showed the presence of a pronounced batch effect in the normalized data. Tissue data were made comparable across batches by fitting a linear model, including both batches and regular conditions, and removing the component due to the batch effects (function 'removeBatchEffect' from the R package limma). After normalization and batch correction (tissue study), the technical replicate samples for each patient were highly similar. A more detailed description of the quality control analysis is given in Text S1. The technical replicates of the batch corrected data were averaged and resulting data was used for hierarchical clustering analyses. For benign tissue sample 4 only two technical replicates were used for data analyses due to technical problems with the third measurement.

For each identified protein a linear model was fit on the normalized data containing the two conditions (benign and malignant) as explanatory variable; for the tissue study a batch factor was also included in the linear model. A consensus between-replicate correlation was estimated for the technical replicates (function 'duplicateCorrelation' from the R package limma) and included in the linear model fit. Differentially expressed proteins between benign and malignant tumors were detected using a moderated t-test. P-values were adjusted for multiple-testing using the Benjamini-Hochberg false discovery rate [22]. Proteins were considered to be significantly differentially expressed between the two conditions with an adjusted p-value<0.05, and a fold change ≤ -1.4 or ≥ 1.4. Moreover, the protein had to be present before imputation in at least 50% of the samples in at least one of the two conditions.

Hierarchical clustering and enrichment analyses

Two-dimensional clustering (Pearson correlation, average linkage) was performed on protein expression values using the function 'heatmap.2' from the R package gplots [23]. The Cytoscape plugin "ClueGO" v2.0.2 was used for protein set enrichment analysis by uploading the list of proteins with their UniProt IDs and using a custom background reference set consisting of all proteins detected in the experiment. [24,25]. For exploratory pathway enrichment analyses a less stringent cutoff, using an unadjusted p-value less than 0.05 was used. Lists of serum or tumor proteins differentially expressed between malignant and benign cases were submitted for protein set enrichment analysis according to the gene ontology (GO) biological process domain. Within ClueGO we used the 'compare lists' feature and compared protein set enrichment (one-sided hypergeometric test) for the differentially expressed serum and tumor proteomes simultaneously. The edges of the resulting ClueGO network are based on kappa statistics and reflect the relationships between the GO terms (network nodes) based on the similarity of their associated proteins.

Protein accession numbers and their corresponding fold changes were imported into the web-based integrative software MetaCore (v 6.8 build 30387; Thomson Reuters, St. Joseph, MI) for network analysis [26]. MetaCore analysis was used for network enrichment and interactome analysis using the differentially expressed proteins (unadjusted p-value<0.05) in either the serum or tissue samples of benign versus malignant samples with the background reference set consisting of all proteins detected in the experiment. Relative connectivity of proteins inside a set (intra-connectivity) and between a set and the global interactome (inter-connectivity) were calculated using MetaCore protein interaction database. A ranking of importance was given by using a "knowledge-based" analysis that considers the differentially expressed proteins in the context of their known interactors in complex protein and molecular networks.

Results

Hierarchical clustering of serum and tissue proteome

In total, we identified 84 proteins in serum and 209 in tissue, which were present in at least 50% of the samples in at least one of the conditions (benign or malignant) (Table S1). Of those proteins 20 and 71 were significantly differentially expressed between benign and malignant disease in serum and tissue samples, respectively (Figure 2). Only 16 proteins were detected in both

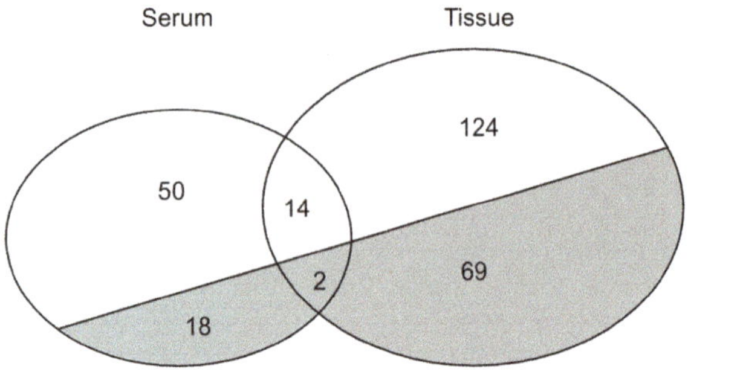

Figure 2. Venn diagram of the detected proteins. We detected a total of 84 proteins in serum and 209 in tissue, present in at least 50% of the samples in at least one of the conditions (benign or malignant). The grey area represents the proteins with an adjusted p-value of <0.05 when comparing benign with malignant.

serum and tissue samples (highlighted in yellow in Table S1). Of these, only two proteins had an adjusted p-value of <0.05, Apolipoprotein A-I and Serotransferrin.

Hierarchical cluster analysis was used to group serum and tumor samples according to the similarity of their expression profiles. Clustering the 84 and 209 proteins detected in serum and tumor samples respectively, could perfectly separate the benign and the malignant tumors (Figure 3). This illustrates that malignancy was the strongest signal in this dataset and that the benign and malignant samples constitute well-defined groups that could reveal differences in underlying biology between the processes leading to malignancy. This result also supported our methodology in which we minimized heterogeneity by going through detailed patient and sample selection and by micro-dissecting the tumor tissue.

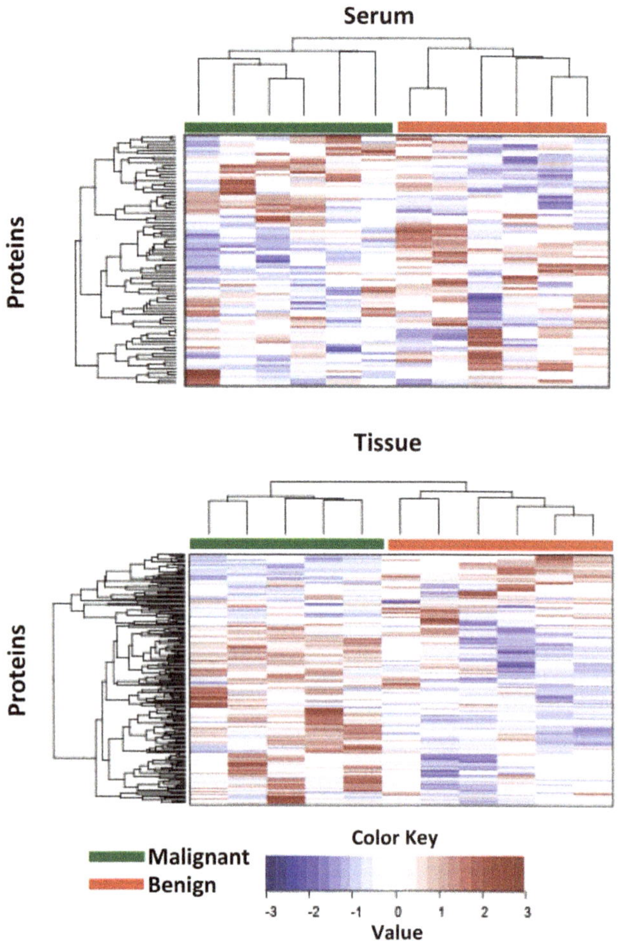

Figure 3. Unsupervised hierarchical clustering. Unsupervised hierarchical clustering was performed of the 84 and 209 proteins detected in serum and tumor tissue samples, respectively. The key color bar indicates standardized protein expression levels (dark red indicates relatively higher expression; dark blue indicates relatively lower expression).

Biological functions and networks enriched in serum and tumor signatures between malignant and benign samples

To explore and compare the biological processes that contribute to changes of the serum and tumor proteome during ovarian cancer development, a protein set biological enrichment analysis was performed on the differentially expressed protein signatures derived from the serum and tissue comparisons. The serum proteome signature was significantly enriched in categories associated with immune function and lipoprotein metabolism. In contrast, the tumor proteome signature was significantly enriched in categories associated with glucose metabolism and the unfolded protein response (Figure 4; Bonferroni corrected p-value<0.05). Interestingly, there is little overlap in the biological processes enriched in serum and tissue signatures. The proteins associated with these protein sets and the relevant statistics are summarized in Table S2.

Key transcriptional regulatory networks in ovarian cancer

We subjected the lists of differentially expressed serum and tissue proteins to the transcriptional regulation network algorithm in MetaCore. This was used to infer potentially important transcription factors in the carcinogenic process. Summaries of the top scoring transcriptional regulatory networks and the key associated transcription factors in respectively serum and tissue are shown in Table S3. The most significant transcriptional regulatory network in serum was GCR-alpha (glucocorticoid receptor alpha) signaling. Eleven proteins that are upstream or downstream of GCR-alpha signaling were found differentially expressed in the serum of patients with a serous adenocarcinoma of the ovaries compared to patients with a serous cystadenoma. The pathways linked to GCR-alpha signaling may explain regulation of the acute inflammatory response that was seen altered in the cancer patients. In the tumor tissue, GCR-alpha was also highlighted in the top scoring transcriptional networks although associated with pathways related to cellular localization and protein folding (Table S3). Figure 5A summarizes, which proteins in our dataset are potentially regulated by GCR-alpha. Interestingly, despite the limited overlap in terms of differentially expressed proteins (Figure 2) and significantly enriched biological processes (Figure 4), two GCR-alpha target proteins, ApoA-1 and Serotransferrin, were present in the signatures of both the serum and the tumor proteome (Figure 5A). These results suggest that the serum cancer proteome could be used to detect changes in GCR-alpha tumor associated processes.

Sp1 was associated with the third top scoring transcriptional network in tumor tissue (Table S3) after the well-known cancer-related transcription factor c-Myc and also CREB-1 that was recently found to be associated with OVCA cell line platinum sensitivity and overall survival [27]. Sp1 was also associated with the top scoring transcriptional networks in the cancerous serum

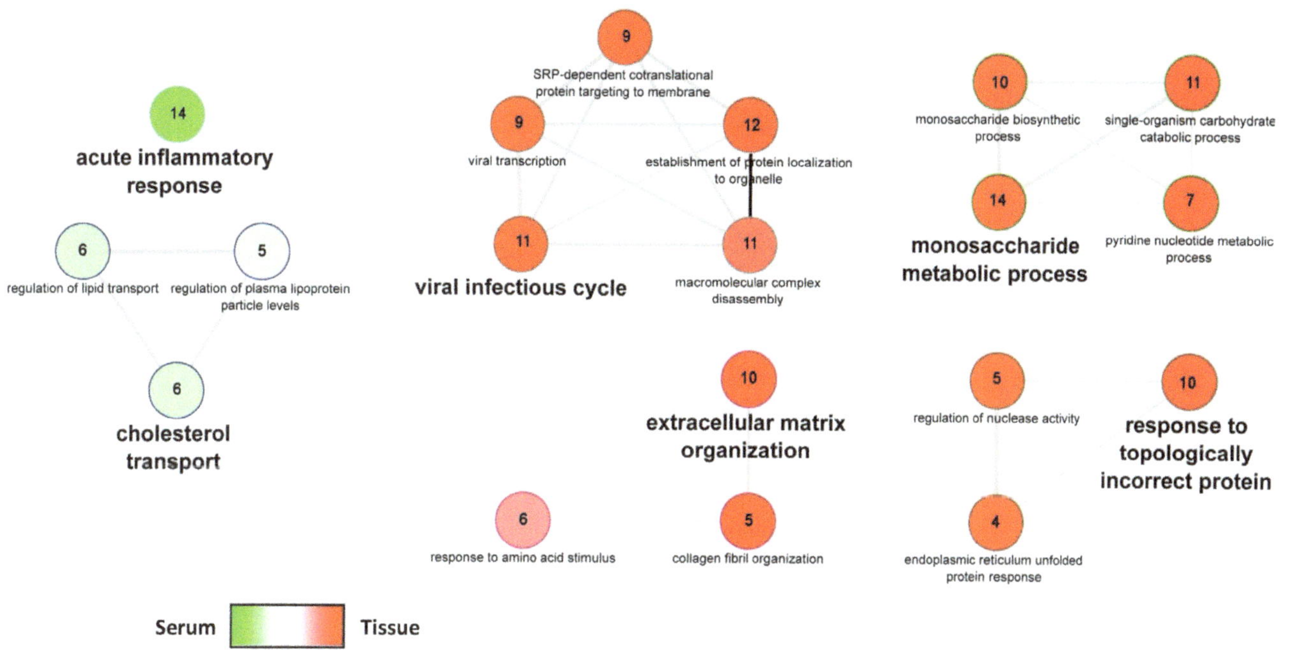

Figure 4. Protein set enrichment analysis using the Cytoscape plugin 'ClueGO'. In the network, only significantly enriched categories (p-value<0.05, Bonferroni corrected) are shown. The node color represents the commonality of members of either the differentially expressed serum or tumor proteome list. Dark red highlights categories that are specific to the tissue proteome signature while dark green represents biological processes that are specific to the serum proteome signature. The number of proteins associated with each GO category are indicated within the corresponding node. The edges of the resulting ClueGO network are based on kappa statistics and reflect the relationships between the GO terms (network nodes) based on the similarity of their associated proteins. The complete results and relevant statistics are summarized in Table S2.

signature. In total, 32 proteins associated with the Sp1 transcriptional pathway were differentially expressed between benign and malignant tissue samples (Figure 5B). Biological processes associated with Sp1 included several pathways related to lipid metabolism such as regulation of cholesterol and sterol transport, and acute-phase response and response to endogenous stimulus. This suggests that this transcriptional regulator might be an important contributor to the metabolic reprogramming that occurs within the tumor as highlighted by our ontology analysis (Figure 4).

Overlap between candidate key-regulatory transcription factors in serum and tumor tissue as highlighted by the transcriptional regulatory network analysis was far greater than at the individual protein level. Nine of the top-20 significantly associated transcription factors in serum were also found in the top-20 of tumor tissue, among them well known cancer-associated transcription factors such as p53 and c-Jun.

Key proteins differentially expressed between benign and malignant ovarian tumors

In an attempt to move beyond transcriptional regulation and find other regulatory proteins that are statistically significantly "overconnected" within our proteomics signatures, we subjected the list of differentially expressed proteins in ovarian tumor samples to "interactome analysis by protein function". This helps in prioritizing potentially relevant individual proteins or hubs. Table 2 summarizes the results of the interactome analysis. Only five proteins were found to be significantly over-connected in the tumor proteome signature namely, PCBP1, 14-3-3 zeta, 14-3-3 beta, alpha actinin-4, and HSP60 (CH60/HSPD-1). These proteins were significantly upregulated in malignant tumors and have all been linked to cancer previously and all but one, PCBP1, specifically to ovarian cancer.

To further investigate the role of PCBP1 in ovarian cancer, we retrieved the transcriptional profiles of an independent ovarian cancer dataset containing 30 tumors of low malignant potential and 60 serous ovarian cancer tumor samples [28] available at Gene Expression Omnibus (http://www.ncbi.nlm.nih.gov/geo/; accession no. GSE12172). Compared to low malignant potential tumors, there was a significant increase in PCBP1 gene expression in malignant ovarian tumors (Figure 6). Furthermore, OncoPrints from the cBioportal for Cancer Genomics (http://www.cbioportal.org) showed that about 10% of all serous malignant ovarian tumors had an altered PCBP1 mRNA expression (data not shown) [29]. The combined observations of elevated protein expression of PCBP1, with the computational analysis highlighting over-representation of PCBP1 protein interactions in this study, as well as the elevated gene expression in a microarray dataset, are suggestive of a role of PCBP1 in ovarian tumor biology, a previously unreported finding.

Discussion

In order to identify proteins and pathways underlying the differences between benign and malignant ovarian tumors, we performed a comparative proteomic analysis of ovarian tumor tissue and serum, from a limited number of patients using a combination of LC-MS^e label-free mass-spectrometry and extensive bioinformatics analyses. Our control group consisted of patients with a benign ovarian tumor instead of healthy women. Therefore, the proteins differentially expressed in our study are more likely to be ovarian tumor-specific instead of reflecting a more general response to disease. We further enhanced robustness

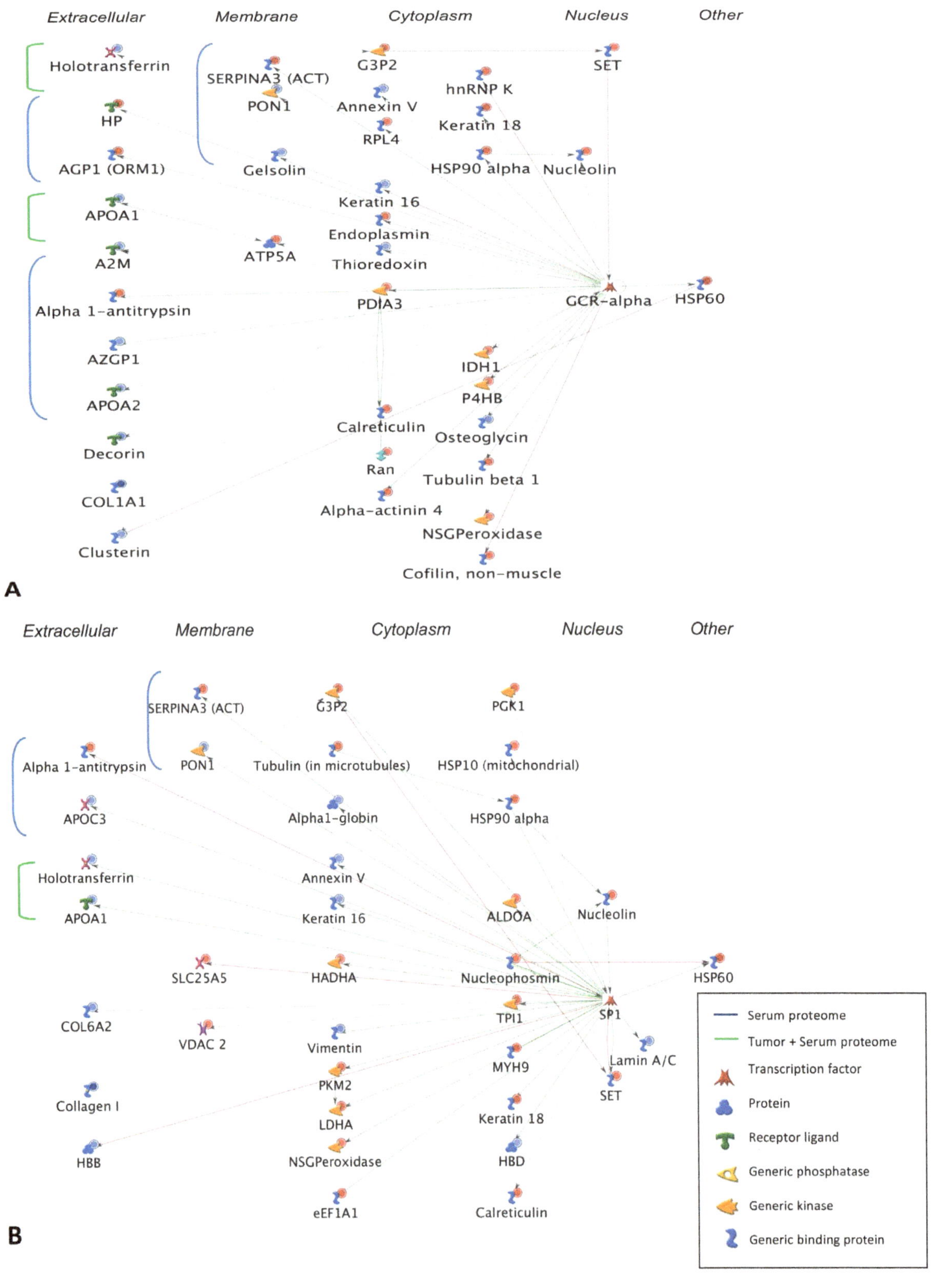

Figure 5. Proteins in the serum and tumor datasets that are potentially associated with GCR-alpha (A) and SP1 (B) pathways. The proteins marked in blue were found in the serum dataset, those marked in green in both tumor and serum. Unmarked proteins are specific for the tumor signature (except GCR-alpha and SP1). Proteins are ordered according to their position within the cell (extracellular, membrane bound, cytoplasmic or nucleic). Individual proteins are represented as nodes, the different shapes of the nodes represent the functional class of the proteins. The arrowheads indicate the direction of the interaction, the color of the lines between nodes describes activation (green), inhibition (red), and unspecified (black) interactions. The small circles on top of the protein symbols indicate up-regulation (red) or down-regulation (blue).

Table 2. Interactions by protein function.

Protein	Actual	n	R	N	Expected	Ratio	p-value	z-score
PCBP-1	11	108	13	296	4.743	2.319	0.000402	3.68
Alpha-actinin 4	14	108	19	296	6.932	2.019	0.000754	3.476
HSP60	17	108	27	296	9.851	1.726	0.003122	2.993
14-3-3 beta/alpha	34	108	56	296	20.43	1.664	3.71E-05	4.176
14-3-3 zeta/delta	55	108	97	296	35.39	1.554	5.33E-07	5.035

Interactions by protein function based on the connectivity with the tumor tissue signatures and with proteins from the human proteome MetaCore database. The proteins were considered over-connected when the number of observed interactions exceeded the number of expected interactions. Actual: number of network objects in the signature which interact with the chosen object; n: number of network objects in the signature; R: number of network objects in the background list which interact with the chosen object; N: total number of protein-based objects in the background list; Expected: mean of hypergeometric distribution. Ratio: connectivity ratio (Actual/Expected); z-score: (Actual-Expected)/(standard deviation); p-value: probability to have the value of Actual or higher (lower for negative z-score) by chance under null hypothesis of no over- or under-connectivity.

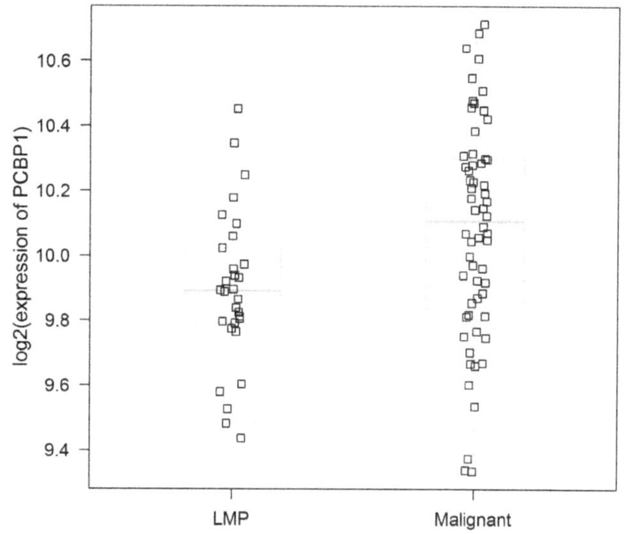

Figure 6. PCBP1 expression in serous ovarian cancer. Expression of PCBP1 (probeset 208620_at) in serous tumors of low malignant potential (LMP) versus malignant serous ovarian tumors [28]. PCBP1 was significantly up-regulated ($p = 0.003$, Welch's t-test) in malignant tumors. Squares represent the individual samples used in the microarray experiment. Boxplots are overlaid with the lower and upper ends of a box indicating the 25th and 75th percentiles, respectively. The solid black line inside a box indicates the median.

of our results by using well matched patient groups and by reducing within-tumor heterogeneity via the use of laser micro-dissected tumor tissue lysates. In addition we used strict experimental protocols, extensive quality control and state-of-the-art bioinformatics analyses to control for false positive results.

Our study revealed a large number of changes in protein expression in serum and tissue from patients suffering from benign and malignant ovarian tumors. Some proteins were already known to play a role in ovarian cancer, others are new candidates, which may provide new insights into the etiology of the disease or act as potential new disease markers. For a large subset of proteins identified in this study, literature searches confirmed their role in ovarian cancer. For example, Dieplinger et. al. also measured decreased plasma concentrations of Afamin and APOA4 in patients with ovarian cancer, with APOA4 adding independent diagnostic information to CA125 and age for differentiating ovarian cancer from benign and healthy samples [30]. The observed reduction in serum of PON1, that usually mediates enzymatic protection against oxidative stress, may lead to increasing DNA damage and consequently to malignant transformation. It has been suggested before, that SNPs reducing PON1 activity may be associated with an increased risk of epithelial ovarian cancer [31]. In addition, we found a significant decrease of APOA1 in serum of ovarian cancer patients as has been shown before in various studies [32,33] and in tissue. To our knowledge this significant decrease in tumor tissue samples has not been described yet. The altered serum signature, which is also enriched for other proteins involved in cholesterol and lipid metabolism, suggests that an alteration of these pathways may be beneficial for the cancer cells.

Although substantial efforts have been devoted to detect new serum biomarkers for ovarian cancer, we are the first to describe proteomic analysis in both serum and tissue. This approach may lead to detection of serum proteins directly derived from the tumor, which can give new insights in the pathways active in benign and malignant disease. Only 16 proteins were identified in both serum and tissue, however, with only Apolipoprotein A-I and Serotransferrin being significantly differentially expressed in both. This limited overlap is probably due to the fact that we only detect abundant proteins in both serum and tissue and that abundant tissue proteins have a different concentration in serum and vice versa. Some of the detected proteins are also compartment specific, and therefore only detectable in serum or tissue.

In order to see whether there might be similarities in significantly enriched processes or altered transcription factors within the serum and tissue datasets we performed enrichment analyses using MetaCore. This analysis revealed that 9 out of the top-20 transcription factors associated with key transcriptional regulatory networks in serum were also found in the top-20 of tumor tissue. These results indicate that although the detected proteins only overlap to a limited extent between the 2 datasets, the detected tumor cancer proteome is reflected by the serum proteome at the molecular subnetwork level. This approach may provide another strategy for biomarker discovery.

Amongst others Sp1 and GCR-alpha were detected as potential key transcription factors of the key transcriptional regulatory networks underlying the proteomic signatures in both tissue and serum. The protein encoded by the Sp1 gene is a zinc finger transcription factor that binds to GC-rich motifs of many promoters. It is involved in many cellular processes, including cell differentiation, cell growth, apoptosis, immune response, response to DNA damage, and chromatin remodeling [34]. Post-translational modifications such as phosphorylation, acetylation, glycosylation, and proteolytic processing significantly affect the activity of this protein, which can be an activator or a repressor. Sp1 has been suggested to be responsible for many features of ovarian cancer cells like oncogenic transformation and epithelial to mesenchymal transition for example through activation of KLF8 [35]. Expression of Sp1 is frequently increased in human epithelial ovarian cancers and inhibitors of Sp1-dependent transcription both in vitro and in tumor xenografts have been suggested as interesting candidates for treatment [36].

Receptors for glucocorticoids, like GCR-alpha, are present in tumor cells of almost 90% of ovarian cancer cells and mRNA of GCR-alpha was detected in a wide range of ovarian cancer cell lines [37]. In vitro studies suggests that glucocorticoids may have an adverse effect on outcome in several cancers, including ovarian [38]. However, other investigators have reported favorable effects of GCs in vitro [39]. A study in GCR-positive patients gave no evidence that GCR expression had any prognostic value nor was there any evidence of poorer survival in a small subset of GCR-positive patients who received GC treatment [40]. A recent study has discovered a role for the glucocorticoid receptor within the SLIT glycoprotein ligand and their ROBO receptor pathway. This pathway plays a fundamental role in mammalian development by promoting apoptosis and repulsing aberrant cell migration. SLIT/ROBO expression could be increased by reducing the expression of the glucocorticoid receptor using siRNA. Their findings indicate that in the post-ovulatory phase a role of cortisol may be to temporarily inhibit SLIT/ROBO expression to facilitate regeneration of the ovarian surface epithelium. Therefore this pathway may be a target to develop strategies to manipulate the SLIT/ROBO system in ovarian cancer [41].

Interactome analysis revealed 5 proteins that were significantly overconnected in our tumor tissue signature, meaning they had more connections within the tumor signature than expected by chance and thus are potentially highly relevant in tumor pathophysiology. Two of those, 14-3-3 beta/alpha and 14-3-3 zeta/delta, are members of the 14-3-3 protein family which have been described in previous studies to promote cell survival through suppression of apoptosis [42]. Due to its upregulation in a variety of human tumors and its involvement in cancer progression and treatment resistance, 14-3-3 zeta is currently undergoing extensive investigation as a novel therapeutic target [43].

The other overconnected proteins were actinin-4, HSP60, and PCBP1. Actinin-4 is an isoform of non-muscular-actinin, which enhances cell motility by bundling the actin cytoskeleton [44]. Implications of actinin-4 have been demonstrated in some human malignancies including ovarian cancer. Yamamoto *et al.* have demonstrated high actinin-4 protein expression in 57% of the primary ovarian carcinomas [45,46]. High expression was associated with serous histology, high histological grade, and poor patient outcome.

Heat shock proteins (HSPs), like HSP60, are important players in protein homeostasis and cell and tissue physiology, as well as in protection against stressors [47]. HSPs intervene not only in protein folding, refolding, trafficking and degradation but also in the regulation of cell growth and differentiation, apoptosis and cell-to-cell crosstalk, inflammation, and tissue repair [47,48]. The importance of HSPs has come into focus in the past few years because it has been realized that they can be pathogenic factors in a variety of conditions. Among these pathologies there are various forms of cancer, in which the proteins are normal but work in favor of the tumor rather than protect the patient [49]. In these conditions, HSPs enhance tumor cell survival and growth by inhibiting apoptosis and the anti-tumor immune response, or by promoting neoangiogenesis [50]. In our study, several of the HSPs had altered expression. Besides the overconnected HSP60, six HSP family members were found to be upregulated in the malignant tissue samples, further highlighting their importance in ovarian cancer biology.

The fifth overconnected protein, PCBP1, was originally discovered as an RNA-binding protein, which participates in mRNA processing at multiple steps. Subsequent studies showed that PCBP1 possesses multiple functions in transcription, splicing, and translation. The protein is capable of switching among its various functions depending upon its state of phosphorylation as well as its cellular localization, and can therefore act as a corepressor and a coactivator in response to different environmental signals [51]. In the cBioPortal database, almost all neighboring genes connected to PCBP1 have altered expression in more than 20% of the serous ovarian cancer samples (data not shown) providing further evidence of a critical role for PCBP1 in the pathophysiological processes underlying malignant ovarian tumors. Importantly, we further implicated PCBP1 within ovarian tumor biology by the fact that the network built in MetaCore using the 5 overconnected proteins as seed notes and their nearest neighbors, generated a network highly interconnecting all 5 seed nodes. The results of this network analysis also revealed an interesting connection to the androgen receptor-signaling pathway (Figure 7). As PCBP1 has been previously found to regulate the androgen receptor in androgen-responsive cells, like the prostate cancer LNCaP cells [52], this connection might be underlying the function of PCBP1 in ovarian tumor biology as well. Overall this network analysis, which attempts to reconstruct the biological mechanism underlying the proteomics profile, provides further mechanistic insights for future validation as well as potential targets of intervention.

In summary, by quantifying protein expression in serum and tissue we found proteins differentially expressed between benign and malignant samples. These included proteins previously identified to play a role in ovarian cancer, but also candidates

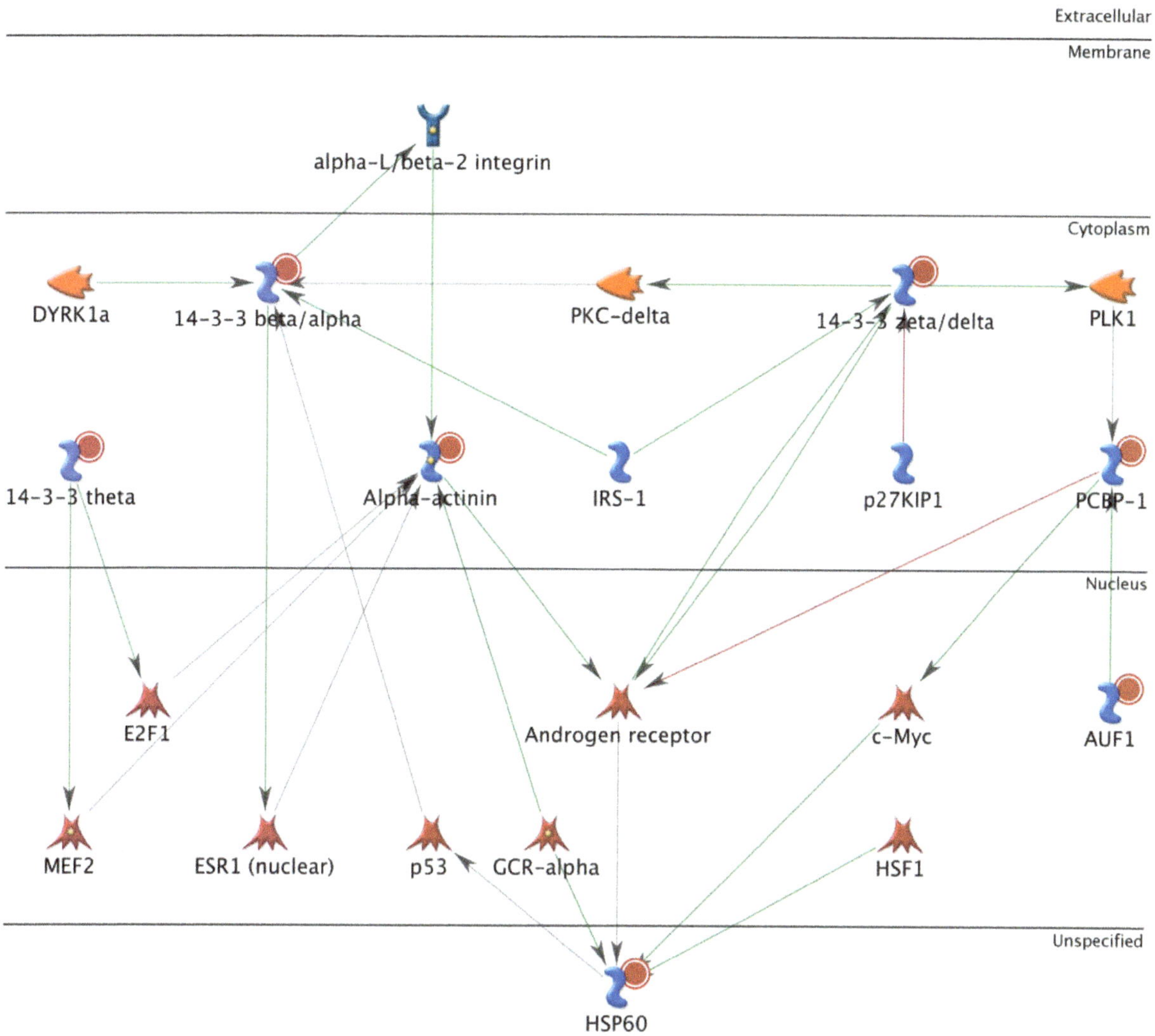

Figure 7. Interactions between overconnected proteins in tumor tissue. A network built in MetaCore using the 5 overconnected proteins, PCBP-1, Alpha-actinin 4, HSP60, 14-3-3 beta/alpha and 14-3-3 zeta/delta as seed nodes yielded a highly interconnected network amongst the seed nodes and implicated a role for androgen receptor signaling.

that had not been implicated in the disease process before. We observed not only a significant decrease in serum APOAI and Serotransferrin, as previously reported, but provide evidence for decreased expression in the tumor site as well. Although the serum and tissue signatures had only 16 proteins in common, we highlighted common transcription factors potentially relevant for changes in both the serum and tumor proteome through in-silico analyses. Important roles are suggested for GCR-alpha and Sp1. In addition, our results implicate an as yet unknown role for PCBP1 in ovarian cancer. We hypothesize that the protein network including PCBP1 contributes to the malignant properties of ovarian tumors, possibly through regulation of the androgen receptor. Further experiments are warranted to unravel the precise mechanism of PCBP1 in ovarian cancer.

Supporting Information

Table S1 List of proteins identified in serum and tissue of ovarian cancer vs. benign patients. List of file names as reported in ProteomeXchange with the corresponding sample annotation in worksheet named 'Filenames'. List of all the measured samples with a complete list of protein identifications in worksheet named 'Raw data' together with separate worksheets containing the filtered data named 'Serum (filtered)' and 'Tissue (filtered)'. Detailed information on the annotation of the proteins and the outcome of the differential expression analysis is provided.

Table S2 Protein set enrichment analysis using the Cytoscape plugin "ClueGO". The proteins associated with significant GO categories are displayed as well as the p-value associated with the GO term. The first four categories are mostly specific to the serum proteome signature while the other categories represent biological processes that are mainly specific to the tissue proteome signature.

Table S3 Serum and tissue transcriptional regulation network list. The column 'GO processes' states the different biological processes associated with the network. The total number of objects in the network is indicated in the 'Total nodes' column. The p-values represent the probability of intersection between the experimental signature and the prebuilt content in MetaCore. The column 'zScore' gives the level of saturation of the networks taking into account the size of the database, the number of objects in the subnetwork and the number of objects in the signature used to construct the network. The higher the z-score the more saturated a subnetwork is. The transcriptional regulation networks are ranked according to p-value.

Text S1 Batch effect and batch correction for the tissue samples.

Acknowledgments

The Department of Pathology of the Academic Medical Center is kindly acknowledged for their assistance with the laser microdissection experiments. Dr. Richard R. Sprenger for initial technical support of the project.

Author Contributions

Conceived and designed the experiments: WW DM PDM MRB JMFGA GGK. Performed the experiments: WW DM GGK. Analyzed the data: PDM CAA WW DM. Contributed reagents/materials/analysis tools: JMFGA. Wrote the paper: WW DM CAA PDM. Provided technical support during the mass-spectrometry measurements, but did not have any additional role in the study design, data collection and analysis, decision to publish, or preparation of the manuscript: JPV.

References

1. Jemal A, Siegel R, Xu J, Ward E (2010) Cancer statistics, 2010. CA Cancer J Clin 60: 277–300.
2. Zhang Z, Bast RC, Yu Y, Li J, Sokoll LJ, et al. (2004) Three biomarkers identified from serum proteomic analysis for the detection of early stage ovarian cancer. Cancer Res 64: 5882–5890.
3. Rai AJ, Zhang Z, Rosenzweig J, Shih I-MI, Pham T, et al. (2002) Proteomic approaches to tumor marker discovery. ArchPatholLab Med 126: 1518–1526.
4. Skates SJ, Horick N, Yu Y, Xu F-J, Berchuck A, et al. (2004) Preoperative sensitivity and specificity for early-stage ovarian cancer when combining cancer antigen CA-125II, CA 15-3, CA 72-4, and macrophage colony-stimulating factor using mixtures of multivariate normal distributions. J Clin Oncol 22: 4059–4066.
5. Ueland FR, Desimone CP, Seamon LG, Miller RA, Goodrich S, et al. (2011) Effectiveness of a multivariate index assay in the preoperative assessment of ovarian tumors. Obstet Gynecol 117: 1289–1297.
6. Moore LE, Pfeiffer RM, Zhang Z, Lu KH, Fung ET, et al. (2012) Proteomic biomarkers in combination with CA 125 for detection of epithelial ovarian cancer using prediagnostic serum samples from the Prostate, Lung, Colorectal, and Ovarian (PLCO) Cancer Screening Trial. Cancer 118: 91–100.
7. Moore RG, Jabre-Raughley M, Brown AK, Robison KM, Miller MC, et al. (2010) Comparison of a novel multiple marker assay vs the Risk of Malignancy Index for the prediction of epithelial ovarian cancer in patients with a pelvic mass. Am J Obstet Gynecol 203: 228.e1–6.
8. Füzéry AK, Levin J, Chan MM, Chan DW (2013) Translation of proteomic biomarkers into FDA approved cancer diagnostics: issues and challenges. Clin Proteomics 10: 13.
9. Ludwig JA, Weinstein JN (2005) Biomarkers in cancer staging, prognosis and treatment selection. Nat Rev Cancer 5: 845–856.
10. Xu BJ (2010) Combining laser capture microdissection and proteomics: methodologies and clinical applications. Proteomics Clin Appl 4: 116–123.
11. Espina V, Wulfkuhle JD, Calvert VS, VanMeter A, Zhou W, et al. (2006) Laser-capture microdissection. Nat Protoc 1: 586–603.
12. Lawrie LC, Curran S (2005) Laser capture microdissection and colorectal cancer proteomics. Methods Mol Biol 293: 245–253.
13. Silva JC, Gorenstein M V, Li G-Z, Vissers JPC, Geromanos SJ (2006) Absolute quantification of proteins by LCMSE: a virtue of parallel MS acquisition. Mol Cell Proteomics 5: 144–156.
14. Vissers JPC, Langridge JI, Aerts JMFG (2007) Analysis and quantification of diagnostic serum markers and protein signatures for Gaucher disease. Mol Cell Proteomics 6: 755–766.
15. Wegdam W, Moerland PD, Meijer D, de Jong SM, Hoefsloot HCJ, et al. (2012) A critical assessment of SELDI-TOF-MS for biomarker discovery in serum and tissue of patients with an ovarian mass. Proteome Sci 10: 45.
16. Geromanos SJ, Vissers JPC, Silva JC, Dorschel CA, Li G-Z, et al. (2009) The detection, correlation, and comparison of peptide precursor and product ions from data independent LC-MS with data dependant LC-MS/MS. Proteomics 9: 1683–1695.
17. Silva JC, Denny R, Dorschel CA, Gorenstein M, Kass IJ, et al. (2005) Quantitative proteomic analysis by accurate mass retention time pairs. Anal Chem 77: 2187–2200.
18. Li G-Z, Vissers JPC, Silva JC, Golick D, Gorenstein M V, et al. (2009) Database searching and accounting of multiplexed precursor and product ion spectra from the data independent analysis of simple and complex peptide mixtures. Proteomics 9: 1696–1719.
19. Martens L, Vandekerckhove J, Gevaert K (2005) DBToolkit: processing protein databases for peptide-centric proteomics. Bioinformatics 21: 3584–3585.
20. Vizcaíno JA, Deutsch EW, Wang R, Csordas A, Reisinger F, et al. (2014) ProteomeXchange provides globally coordinated proteomics data submission and dissemination. Nat Biotechnol 32: 223–226.
21. Gentleman RC, Carey VJ, Bates DM, Bolstad B, Dettling M, et al. (2004) Bioconductor: open software development for computational biology and bioinformatics. Genome Biol 5: R80.
22. Benjamini Y, Hochberg Y (1995) Controlling the false discovery rate: a practical and powerful approach to multiple testing. J R Stat Soc Series B: 289–300.
23. Warnes GR, Bolker B, Bonebakker L, Gentleman R, Huber W, et al. (2013) Various R programming tools for plotting data. Available: http://cran.r-project.org/web/packages/gplots/gplots.pdf.
24. Bindea G, Mlecnik B, Hackl H, Charoentong P, Tosolini M, et al. (2009) ClueGO: a Cytoscape plug-in to decipher functionally grouped gene ontology and pathway annotation networks. Bioinformatics 25: 1091–1093.
25. Smoot ME, Ono K, Ruscheinski J, Wang P-L, Ideker T (2011) Cytoscape 2.8: new features for data integration and network visualization. Bioinformatics 27: 431–432.
26. Bessarabova M, Ishkin A, JeBailey L, Nikolskaya T, Nikolsky Y (2012) Knowledge-based analysis of proteomics data. BMC Bioinformatics 13 Suppl 1: S13.
27. Bicaku E, Xiong Y, Marchion DC, Chon HS, Stickles XB, et al. (2012) In vitro analysis of ovarian cancer response to cisplatin, carboplatin, and paclitaxel identifies common pathways that are also associated with overall patient survival. Br J Cancer 106: 1967–1975.
28. Anglesio MS, Arnold JM, George J, Tinker A V, Tothill R, et al. (2008) Mutation of ERBB2 provides a novel alternative mechanism for the ubiquitous activation of RAS-MAPK in ovarian serous low malignant potential tumors. Mol Cancer Res 6: 1678–1690.
29. Cerami E, Gao J, Dogrusoz U, Gross BE, Sumer SO, et al. (2012) The cBio cancer genomics portal: an open platform for exploring multidimensional cancer genomics data. Cancer Discov 2: 401–404.
30. Dieplinger H, Ankerst DP, Burges A, Lenhard M, Lingenhel A, et al. (2009) Afamin and apolipoprotein A-IV: novel protein markers for ovarian cancer. Cancer Epidemiol Biomarkers Prev 18: 1127–1133.
31. Lurie G, Wilkens LR, Thompson PJ, McDuffie KE, Carney ME, et al. (2008) Genetic polymorphisms in the Paraoxonase 1 gene and risk of ovarian epithelial carcinoma. Cancer Epidemiol Biomarkers Prev 17: 2070–2077.
32. Melvin JC, Seth D, Holmberg L, Garmo H, Hammar N, et al. (2012) Lipid profiles and risk of breast and ovarian cancer in the Swedish AMORIS study. Cancer Epidemiol Biomarkers Prev 21: 1381–1384.
33. Clarke CH, Yip C, Badgwell D, Fung ET, Coombes KR, et al. (2011) Proteomic biomarkers apolipoprotein A1, truncated transthyretin and connective tissue activating protein III enhance the sensitivity of CA125 for detecting early stage epithelial ovarian cancer. Gynecol Oncol 122: 548–553.
34. Li L, Davie JR (2010) The role of Sp1 and Sp3 in normal and cancer cell biology. Ann Anat 192: 275–283.
35. Wang X, Urvalek AM, Liu J, Zhao J (2008) Activation of KLF8 transcription by focal adhesion kinase in human ovarian epithelial and cancer cells. J Biol Chem 283: 13934–13942.
36. Previdi S, Malek A, Albertini V, Riva C, Capella C, et al. (2010) Inhibition of Sp1-dependent transcription and antitumor activity of the new aureolic acid analogues mithramycin SDK and SK in human ovarian cancer xenografts. Gynecol Oncol 118: 182–188.
37. Gubbay O, Guo W, Rae MT, Niven D, Langdon SP, et al. (2005) Inflammation-associated gene expression is altered between normal human ovarian surface epithelial cells and cell lines derived from ovarian adenocarcinomas. Br J Cancer 92: 1927–1933.
38. Runnebaum IB, Brüning A (2005) Glucocorticoids inhibit cell death in ovarian cancer and up-regulate caspase inhibitor cIAP2. Clin Cancer Res 11: 6325–6332.
39. Yano A, Fujii Y, Iwai A, Kageyama Y, Kihara K (2006) Glucocorticoids suppress tumor angiogenesis and in vivo growth of prostate cancer cells. Clin Cancer Res 12: 3003–3009.
40. Woenckhaus J, Franke FE, Hackethal A, Von Georgi R, Münstedt K (2006) Glucocorticosteroid receptors in ovarian carcinomas. Oncol Rep 15: 1137–1140.
41. Dickinson RE, Fegan KS, Ren X, Hillier SG, Duncan WC (2011) Glucocorticoid regulation of SLIT/ROBO tumour suppressor genes in the ovarian surface epithelium and ovarian cancer cells. PLoS One 6: e27792.

42. Zhao J, Meyerkord CL, Du Y, Khuri FR, Fu H (2011) 14-3-3 proteins as potential therapeutic targets. Semin Cell Dev Biol 22: 705–712.
43. He Y, Wu X, Liu X, Yan G, Xu C (2010) LC-MS/MS analysis of ovarian cancer metastasis-related proteins using a nude mouse model: 14-3-3 zeta as a candidate biomarker. J Proteome Res 9: 6180–6190.
44. Honda K, Yamada T, Endo R, Ino Y, Gotoh M, et al. (1998) Actinin-4, a novel actin-bundling protein associated with cell motility and cancer invasion. J Cell Biol 140: 1383–1393.
45. Yamamoto S, Tsuda H, Honda K, Kita T, Takano M, et al. (2007) Actinin-4 expression in ovarian cancer: a novel prognostic indicator independent of clinical stage and histological type. Mod Pathol 20: 1278–1285.
46. Yamamoto S, Tsuda H, Honda K, Onozato K, Takano M, et al. (2009) Actinin-4 gene amplification in ovarian cancer: a candidate oncogene associated with poor patient prognosis and tumor chemoresistance. Mod Pathol 22: 499–507.
47. Macario AJL, Conway de Macario E (2005) Sick chaperones, cellular stress, and disease. N Engl J Med 353: 1489–1501.
48. Ciocca DR, Calderwood SK (2005) Heat shock proteins in cancer: diagnostic, prognostic, predictive, and treatment implications. Cell Stress Chaperones 10: 86–103.
49. Cappello F, Marino Gammazza A, Palumbo Piccionello A, Campanella C, Pace A, et al. (2014) Hsp60 chaperonopathies and chaperonotherapy: targets and agents. Expert Opin Ther Targets 18: 185–208.
50. Barazi HO, Zhou L, Templeton NS, Krutzsch HC, Roberts DD (2002) Identification of heat shock protein 60 as a molecular mediator of alpha 3 beta 1 integrin activation. Cancer Res 62: 1541–1548.
51. O'Malley BW, Kumar R (2009) Nuclear receptor coregulators in cancer biology. Cancer Res 69: 8217–8222.
52. Cloke B, Shah K, Kaneda H, Lavery S, Trew G, et al. (2010) The poly(c)-binding protein-1 regulates expression of the androgen receptor. Endocrinology 151: 3954–3964.

12

Metabolomics as a Tool for Discovery of Biomarkers of Autism Spectrum Disorder in the Blood Plasma of Children

Paul R. West[1]*, David G. Amaral[2], Preeti Bais[3], Alan M. Smith[1], Laura A. Egnash[1], Mark E. Ross[1], Jessica A. Palmer[1], Burr R. Fontaine[1], Kevin R. Conard[1], Blythe A. Corbett[4], Gabriela G. Cezar[1¤], Elizabeth L. R. Donley[1], Robert E. Burrier[1]

1 Stemina Biomarker Discovery, Madison, Wisconsin, United States of America, **2** The M.I.N.D. Institute and Department of Psychiatry and Behavioral Sciences, University of California Davis, Davis, California, United States of America, **3** The Jackson Laboratory for Genomic medicine, University of Connecticut Health Center, Farmington, Connecticut, United States of America, **4** Department of Psychiatry, Psychology and Kennedy Center, Vanderbilt University, Nashville, Tennessee, United States of America

Abstract

Background: The diagnosis of autism spectrum disorder (ASD) at the earliest age possible is important for initiating optimally effective intervention. In the United States the average age of diagnosis is 4 years. Identifying metabolic biomarker signatures of ASD from blood samples offers an opportunity for development of diagnostic tests for detection of ASD at an early age.

Objectives: To discover metabolic features present in plasma samples that can discriminate children with ASD from typically developing (TD) children. The ultimate goal is to identify and develop blood-based ASD biomarkers that can be validated in larger clinical trials and deployed to guide individualized therapy and treatment.

Methods: Blood plasma was obtained from children aged 4 to 6, 52 with ASD and 30 age-matched TD children. Samples were analyzed using 5 mass spectrometry-based methods designed to orthogonally measure a broad range of metabolites. Univariate, multivariate and machine learning methods were used to develop models to rank the importance of features that could distinguish ASD from TD.

Results: A set of 179 statistically significant features resulting from univariate analysis were used for multivariate modeling. Subsets of these features properly classified the ASD and TD samples in the 61-sample training set with average accuracies of 84% and 86%, and with a maximum accuracy of 81% in an independent 21-sample validation set.

Conclusions: This analysis of blood plasma metabolites resulted in the discovery of biomarkers that may be valuable in the diagnosis of young children with ASD. The results will form the basis for additional discovery and validation research for 1) determining biomarkers to develop diagnostic tests to detect ASD earlier and improve patient outcomes, 2) gaining new insight into the biochemical mechanisms of various subtypes of ASD 3) identifying biomolecular targets for new modes of therapy, and 4) providing the basis for individualized treatment recommendations.

Editor: Subhabrata Sanyal, Biogen Idec, United States of America

Funding: Stemina funded this study. The funder provided support in the form of salaries for authors (PRW, LAE, AMS, MER, JAP, BRF, KRC, GGC, ELRD, and REB), but did not have any additional role in the study design, data collection and analysis, decision to publish, or preparation of the manuscript.

Competing Interests: All authors except Blythe Corbett have, within the past five years, received salary from, and/or hold stocks or stock options in, Stemina Biomarker Discovery, which as a company may gain or lose financially from the publication of this manuscript. PRW, LAE, AMS, MER, JAP, BRF, KRC, GGC, ELRD and REB are employees of Stemina, whose company funded this study and holds, or is currently, applying for patents relating to the content of the manuscript as follows: BIOMARKERS OF AUTISM SPECTRUM DISORDER; PCT App No. PCT/US2014/045397 and METABOLIC BIOMARKERS OF AUTISM; PCT Application No. PCT/US2011/034654. There are no further patents, products in development, or marketed products to declare.

* Email: pwest@stemina.com

¤ Current address: Pfizer Inc., São Paulo, Brazil

Introduction

Autism spectrum disorder (ASD) is a lifelong neurodevelopmental disorder characterized by social deficits, impaired verbal and nonverbal communication and repetitive movements or circumscribed interests [1]. About 1 in 68 children has been identified with autism spectrum disorder (ASD) according to estimates from CDC's Autism and Developmental Disabilities Monitoring (ADDM) Network. The current process for a clinical diagnosis includes establishing a developmental history and assessments of speech, language, intellectual abilities, and educational or vocational attainment. In practice, these methods lead to a diagnosis at an average age of 4 years [2] in the United States. It is recognized that establishing personalized therapy for children with ASD at the earliest age possible improves outcomes including a higher level of cognitive and social function and improved communication as well as decreased financial and emotional burden on families [3,4]. Development of blood-based diagnostic tests to aid in the assessment of risk for a diagnosis of ASD at an early age would facilitate implementing intensive behavioral therapy at the earliest age possible.

The etiology of the vast majority of cases of ASD are unknown and their genetics have proven to be incredibly complex [5,6]. There is now widespread appreciation that there will be many causes of ASD with varying combinations of genetic and environmental risk factors at play. Numerous studies have attempted to identify the causes of the disorder by studying transcriptomics and genomics, leading to the identification of multiple genes associated with ASD [6,7]. There are currently hundreds of observable genetic variants that account for about 20% of the cases of autism. These data are currently most useful in understanding the intra-familial genetics of autism. For this reason, clinical tests based on genomic measures often include genetic counseling to assess the chance of disease occurrence or recurrence within a family [8,9]. Prediction accuracies of ASD risk based on genomic approaches range from 56% to 70% depending largely on the population of patients assessed. Separate analyses of at least one of the genomic studies by Skafidas *et al.* has questioned whether the results have been confounded by biases due to ancestral origins [10,11]. An additional limitation of genomic studies is that the results of environmental influences on the child and/or mother are not discernible. Metabolomics is sensitive to biochemical changes caused by even subtle environmental influences and therefore can complement genomic approaches by addressing some of these factors that may be closer to phenotype.

Given the complexities of the genetic environment of ASD, metabolomic profiling may provide an alternative path to developing early diagnostic tests. Previous metabolic studies of ASD have used biological matrices such as cells, organelles, urine and blood, and have implicated a wide range of metabolites including fatty acids, sterols, intermediary metabolites, phospholipids, and molecules associated with oxidative stress [12–16]. Two recent reports highlight the potential use of metabolomic analysis of urine to identify signatures of ASD. One study used 1H-NMR methods and showed changes in metabolites associated with the tryptophan/nicotinic acid metabolic pathway, sulphur and amino acid pathways, as well as microbial metabolites implicating the involvement of microbial metabolism in the etiology of ASD [16]. Ming *et al.* used a combination of liquid- and gas-chromatography based mass spectrometry methods to identify changes in a number of amino acids and antioxidants such as carnosine, as well as confirming the changes associated with altered gut microbiomes [17].

Measurement of metabolites offers an excellent opportunity to identify differences in small molecule abundance that may have the ability to characterize some forms of ASD. High resolution mass spectrometry (HRMS) is not only a very sensitive detection method for small molecule metabolites, it also provides accurate mass data that aids in metabolite identification through molecular formulae determination [18]. HRMS offers an additional distinct advantage in the ability to distinguish between compounds with the same nominal mass (isobaric compounds), providing enhanced chemical formula and structure information [19]. Unfortunately there is not one universal chromatographic mass spectrometric technique capable of detecting all of the metabolites in blood. To identify novel potential biomarkers associated with ASD, it is necessary to facilitate broad metabolite detection coverage. Toward this goal, we applied an orthogonal approach to chromatographic separation, mass spectral ionization and detection [20]. The current study employed multiple chromatographic mass spectrometric metabolomic methods including gas chromatography-mass spectrometry (GC-MS) and liquid chromatography-high resolution mass spectrometry (LC-HRMS) to discover a wide range of metabolites in blood plasma samples that were able to differentiate TD individuals from those with ASD. Subsequently, tandem mass spectrometry (MS-MS) experiments were employed to aid in structural confirmation of the metabolites discovered by LC-HRMS.

The aim of the study was to perform a broad evaluation of small molecules in blood plasma to discover metabolites that may lead to biomarkers associated with ASD. Univariate, multivariate and machine learning methods were employed to discover metabolites or groups of metabolites exhibiting statistically significant abundance differences that can be used as biomarkers to distinguish children with ASD from TD individuals.

Materials and Methods

Subject Samples

The experimental subjects were initially recruited through the UC Davis M.I.N.D. Institute Clinic, Regional Centers, referrals from clinicians, area school districts and community support groups such as Families for Early Autism Treatment (FEAT). Subjects were limited to an age range of 4–6 years. Typically developing participants were recruited from area school districts and community centers. All facets of this study were approved by the University of California at Davis Institutional Review Board (IRB). Written informed consent was obtained from the parent or guardian of each participant and data were analyzed without personal information identifiers then subjects completed diagnostic and psychological measures. Study participants with ASD were enrolled under inclusion criteria consisting of a diagnosis of autism spectrum disorder based on the DSM-IV criteria determined by an experienced neuropsychologist (BAC), which was further corroborated by the following measures using research reliable clinicians: the Autism Diagnostic Observation Schedule-Generic (ADOS-G) provides observation of a child's communication, reciprocal social interaction, and stereotyped behavior including an algorithm with cutoffs for autism and autism spectrum disorder; the Autism Diagnostic Interview-Revised (ADI-R) is a comprehensive, semi-structured parent interview that assesses a child's developmental history and relevant ASD characteristic behaviors and generates a diagnostic algorithm for children with ASD. Based on the DSM-IV criteria [21], only children with strictly defined autistic disorder were enrolled whereas children with pervasive developmental disorder-not otherwise specified (PDD-NOS) or Asperger Syndrome were excluded from the study. The Social Communication Questionnaire (SCQ) was used as a screening tool to ensure the absence of symptoms of ASD in the TD children. The patients recruited for this study were primarily Caucasian and the ages were similar between groups. However, the participants with autism had lower IQ scores than the TD subjects [22,23].

The exclusion criteria for all subjects included the presence of Fragile X or other serious neurological (e.g., seizures), psychiatric (e.g., bipolar disorder) or known medical conditions such as autoimmune disease and inflammatory bowel diseases/celiac disease. All subjects were screened via parental interview for current and past physical illness. Children with known endocrine, cardiovascular, pulmonary, and liver or kidney disease were excluded from enrollment in the study. Dietary restriction for participation in the study was not required with the exception of an overnight fast. Participation in the study required two clinical visits for behavioral assessment and blood draws. After application of exclusion criteria, the final study group consisted of 104 children, 69 with ASD and 35 in the TD group.

Samples were collected on Thursday morning visits to the M.I.N.D. Institute over a period of 13 months. Blood was drawn into a 9.6 mL EDTA Vaccutainer tube by an experienced pediatric phlebotomist between the hours of 8 and 10 AM following an overnight fast. Tubes were immediately inverted 6–8 times to assure mixing with the anticoagulant and placed on ice. Immediately after plasma separation and aliquoting, samples were sent on the morning of the draw via courier with a barcode label, wrapped tube cap with a strip of parafilm; bubble wrapped then set in a biohazard bag which was placed inside a carrier between coolant packs. Samples were stored at −80°C.

Samples from 103 of the 104 children were sent to Stemina for metabolomic analyses on dry ice… Upon receipt, 5 samples were removed after visual inspection and observation of overt hemolysis and the remaining 98 samples were analyzed by mass spectrometry. Quality checks of the raw mass spectrometric data from the 98 samples were performed, resulting in removing data from 16 patient samples that did not contain MS data from all 5 methods from further analysis. The final 82 samples used in these studies originated from 52 children with ASD and 30 children in the TD group. The children were chosen so that the age and gender distributions were similar across the groups. There was no statistical difference in age between ASD cases and the TD children for the current study (Welch's t-test $p = 0.25$) (see Table 1).

Regarding patient medication, 18 out of 52 of the subjects with ASD in this study were taking medications which included Risperidone (5), Sertraline (3), Aripiprazole (2), antihistamines (2), antivirals (2), antifungals (2), and various other less frequent drugs. Three of the 30 typical subjects were taking medications, which included methylphenidate (1), albuterol (1) and loratadine (1). Ten of the 52 ASD subjects were on a gluten and/or casein-free (GFCF) diet. Importantly, blood draws were administered prior to eating and any morning administration of any medication.

Sample Preparation for LC-MS

Plasma samples were split into 50 µl aliquots and stored at −80°C prior to metabolite extraction. Samples were kept on ice during these procedures. Samples were randomized into three batches for the LC-HRMS analysis such that diagnosis, IQ, age and ethnicity were equally distributed in each batch. Small molecules were extracted from 50 µL plasma aliquots using 450 µL of 8:1 methanol: water solution at −20°C [24]. The extraction solution also contained internal standards. The samples were agitated for 10 minutes at 2–8°C then centrifuged at 18,400×G for 20 minutes at 4°C to remove the precipitate. The supernatant was transferred to a fresh tube and the centrifugation step was repeated to remove any residual precipitate. After the final centrifugation, 450 µL of supernatant was transferred to a fresh tube then evaporated to dryness in a SpeedVac, then resolublized in 45 µL of a 50:50 mixture of 0.1% formic acid in acetonitrile: 0.1% formic acid, also containing internal standards. This solution was then transferred to a high performance liquid chromatograph (HPLC) autosampler injection vial for LC-HRMS analysis.

Mass Spectrometry

Both targeted GC-MS as well as untargeted LC-HRMS were employed for better metabolome coverage. Four untargeted LC-HRMS methods were used including C8 or HILIC chromatography coupled to electrospray ionization in both positive and negative ion polarities, resulting in 4 separate data acquisitions per sample. For each methodology and condition, only a single sample aliquot was assessed, due to limited material availability.. LC-HRMS methods were developed and tested prior to the evaluation of the clinical patient samples to optimize the breadth of coverage of small molecule metabolites.

Liquid Chromatography High Resolution Mass Spectrometry

LC-HRMS was performed using an Agilent G6540 Quadrupole Time of Flight (QTOF) system consisting of an Agilent 1290 HPLC coupled to a high resolution (QTOF) mass spectrometer. Electrospray ionization (ESI) in both positive and negative ion modes was employed using a dual ESI source under high-resolution exact mass conditions. 2 µL of sample was injected. A Waters Acquity ultra high performance liquid chromatography (UPLC) BEH Amide column with dimensions 2.1×150 mm, 1.7 µM particle size was used for Hydrophilic Interaction Liquid Chromatography (HILIC), and maintained at 40°C. Data was acquired for each sample for 29 minutes at a flow rate of 0.5 mL/minute using a solvent gradient with 0.1% formic acid in water and 0.1% formic acid in acetonitrile. An Agilent Zorbax Eclipse Plus C8 2.1×100 mm, 1.8 µM particle size column was used for C8 chromatography and data was acquired for each sample for

Table 1. Patient demographic information.

Demographic		TD	ASD	Overall
Group Size		30	52	82
Sex (male %)		86.67	78.85	81.7
	Range	4.17–6.92	4–6.92	4–6.92
Age (Years)	Average	5.6	5.37	5.46
	Std. Dev.	0.95	0.81	0.87
	Range	88–137	40–110	40–137
IQ	Average	114.3	67.48	80
	Std. Dev.	10.78	17.69	27.47

50 minutes at a flow rate of 0.5 mL/minute using a gradient with 0.1% formic acid in water and 0.1% formic acid in acetonitrile and maintained at 40°C.

Gas Chromatography - Mass Spectrometry

GC-MS analyses were performed at the West Coast Metabolomics Center at UC Davis as described in [25]. GC-MS data was acquired using an Agilent 6890 gas chromatograph coupled to a LECO Pegasus IV TOF mass spectrometer. Metabolite identification was done by comparing sample data to a database of over 1,000 compounds identified by GC-MS that includes mass spectra, retention indices, structures and links to external metabolic databases.

Metabolite chemical structure confirmation by LC-HRMS-MS

The chemical structures of key metabolites were further confirmed using tandem mass spectrometry (LC-HRMS-MS) methods with chromatographic conditions identical to those used for their discovery. LC-HRMS-MS analyses were performed on an Agilent QTOF mass spectrometer for patient samples and/or, reference blood samples with collision energy conditions optimized to obtain the highest quality product ion spectra. The resulting product ion spectra were then compared to MS-MS spectra available in public spectral databases such as METLIN [26], MassBank [27] and Stemina's own SteminaMetDB database.

Data Analysis

LC-HRMS Data preprocessing. Raw mass spectral data and were initially examined for quality criteria established during method development such as abundance thresholds, retention time and peak shape consistency for total ion chromatograms, and extracted ion chromatograms for internal standards and markers. Data files exhibiting chromatograms that failed these quality criteria were removed from further analysis. A portion of these were retested, depending on the nature of the QC failure. Raw data were converted to open source mzData files [28]. Peak picking and feature creation were performed using XCMS [29] and then deviations in retention times were corrected using the obiwarp algorithm [30] based on a non-linear clustering approach to align the LC-HRMS data. Mass features were generated using the XCMS density based grouping algorithm. Missing features were integrated based on retention time and mass range of a feature bin using iterative peak filling. A "mass feature" (also abbreviated here as "feature") is a moiety detected by the mass spectrometer that is defined by 2 properties 1) the detected mass-to-charge ratio (*m/z*) and 2) the chromatographic retention time.

A series of data filters were then employed to remove features exhibiting low abundance levels, those resulting from background noise, ions with non-biological mass defects, and known contaminants from subsequent data analyses. To reduce LC-HRMS batch variations in feature detection, the abundance values were then normalized by sample to the experiment-wide median area of spiked-in internal reference standards. The integrated areas of the normalized mass features from the GC-MS and LC-HRMS platforms were combined into a single dataset. There were 4572 features for the training set of samples that passed preprocessing filters.

Training and Independent Validation Sets. The 82 patient samples (52 ASD and 30 TD samples) were split into two sets, (1) a training set of 61 samples (39 ASD and 22 TD) for identification of statistically significant features and classification modeling and (2) a 21-sample independent validation set (13 ASD and 8 TD) used to evaluate performance of the classification models. This was accomplished by randomizing the samples using the diagnosis, patient IQ, and gender in these training and validations sets so that each set contained a similar proportion of factors used in randomization. The validation sample set was withheld from the univariate filtering and model development process to act as an independent external sample set to evaluate model performance. Detailed patient demographics for the samples in the training and validation sets are provided in Table S4.

Univariate Filtering of Mass Features. T-tests were used to reduce the overall feature set, the potential for over-fitting, and increase the biological interpretability of the predictive signature [31]. The integrated areas of mass features normalized to internal standards (IS) from the GC-MS and LC-HRMS platforms were combined into a single dataset. The 4572 features passing the preprocessing filters for the training set of samples were further filtered using Welch T-tests under the null hypothesis that no difference in mean integrated areas of a mass feature is present between the experimental classes, and the alternative hypothesis that there is a difference in mean integrated areas between ASD and TD training set samples to identify differential features. For each feature that exhibited a statistically significant change with an uncorrected p-value <0.05, its extracted ion chromatogram (EIC) was reviewed for consistency of integration across samples, peak shape, and a minimum peak height requirement of >3000. Features passing this EIC quality review process were then utilized in the classification modeling. False discovery rates (FDRs) were calculated using the Benjamini Hochberg method of p-value correction [32].

Classification Modeling. Model development was performed with two primary goals: 1) to robustly rank the importance of metabolites in discriminating ASD using a VIP (Variable Importance in the Projection) score index and 2) to identify the minimum set of predictive metabolites needed to reach the highest levels of differentiation of the ASD and TD experimental classes. The final models were created by training a Partial Least Squares Discriminant Analysis (PLS-DA) or Support Vector Machine (SVM) classifier using the entire 61-sample training set. The modeling techniques PLS-DA as well as SVM with a linear kernel [33,34] were both utilized to demonstrate that the molecular signature can be predictive using multiple approaches. PLS and SVM classification models were created using the R package Classification and Regression Training "caret" version 5.17–7 [35]. Receiver operator Curve (ROC) analysis was performed using the R package ROCR version 1.0–5 [36].

A nested cross validation (CV) approach (Figure 1) was used to meet the first objective of model development - a robust measure of feature VIP scores. The 179 features from the 61 sample training set were analyzed using 100 resamples with an 80:20 split to weight the importance of each of the 179 statistically significant features. The tuning loop utilized 10-fold cross validation to tune model parameters (cost parameter C for SVM and the number of components for PLS-DA). The recursive feature elimination loop was used to identify the best performing feature subset from each iteration using steps of 20 features. The results from the 100 resamples were used to estimate model performance and create a robust biomarker VIP score index to rank the importance of each of the 179 features in classification of ASD from TD individuals.

Feature VIP robustness was measured by resampling the training set 100 times using an 80:20 split into 49-sample CV training and 12-sample CV test sets. VIP scores were calculated for each of the 100 resamples and the most informative features at each resample were identified by backwards recursive feature

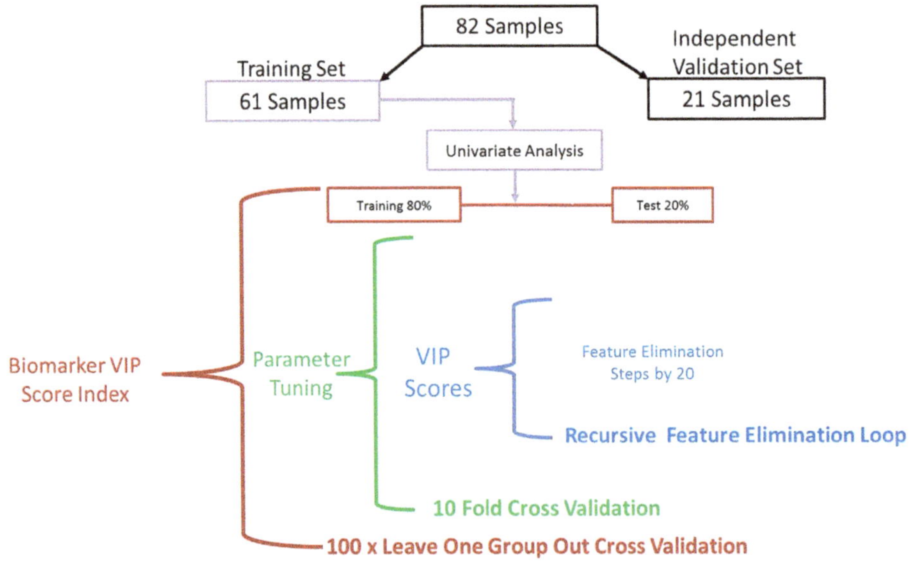

Figure 1. Classification modeling process. A three-layer nested cross-validation approach was applied using both PLS-DA and SVM modeling methods to determine significant features capable of classifying children with ASD from TD children. The 179 features of the training set were analyzed using a leave-one-group-out cross-validation loop as described. The results from this cross-validation process were used to estimate model performance and create a robust feature VIP score index to rank the ASD vs TD classification importance of each of the 179 features. These feature ranks were used to evaluate the performance of the molecular signature using an independent validation set.

elimination (in 20-feature steps) using the Area Under the ROC Curve (AUC). The most informative set of features was then used to predict each CV test set. The VIP scores were averaged across the 100 resamples to create the VIP index for each feature. The classification performance metrics of the CV test sets were averaged across resamples to understand potential future performance.

The second objective of the classification modeling approach was to identify the minimum number of features with the highest level of classification accuracy. This objective was met using feature subsets based on the ordered VIP score index and evaluating the subset performance in the validation set of samples. The classification models were created using the entire 61 sample training set and by stepping through features. The feature stepping process utilized the 20 top VIP features then added the next 20 highest weighted features until all 179 features were evaluated.

Performance metrics (Accuracy, Sensitivity, Specificity, and ROC analysis) were determined based on the prediction of the 21 sample independent validation set for assessment of the molecular signature at each feature subset bin size (Table S3). Accuracy is defined as the proportion of correctly classified participants and is calculated by dividing the number of correctly classified participants by the total number of participants in a sample set. Specificity is the proportion of correctly classified TD individuals out of all TD participants in a sample set. Sensitivity is the proportion of correctly classified ASD individuals out of all participants with ASD in a sample set. The top 179 features were also compared for rank between SVM and PLS modeling methods (Figure 2).

Feature Metabolite Annotations. Metabolite annotation (assignment of putative chemical structures) was carried out for each feature. Annotation was accomplished by comparing *m/z* value of each mass feature to the *m/z* value of common ESI adducts contained in public chemical databases and/or Stemina's internal metabolite database. All mass features that were annotated with chemical identities in that the measured exact mass was consistent (within 20 ppm relative mass error) with one or more chemical structures. These annotations were considered to be putative until the chemical structure of the feature was further confirmed by LC-HRMS-MS.

The molecular formulae of the mass features with putative annotations were then input into the "Find by Formula" (FBF) algorithm in the Agilent Technologies MassHunter Qualitative Analysis software which tests whether the mass spectra for a given feature is a reasonable match with the proposed formula. In most cases, the annotations for any feature with a median FBF score of less than 70, a retention time difference greater than 35 seconds or which was present in less than 50% of the data files was not included for further analysis due to lack of confidence in the formula assignment of the annotation.

Features from the GC-MS analysis were identified as described by [25]. This procedure used comparison of the sample data to spectra of metabolite reference standards that had been previously acquired by the same identical GC-MS method. Therefore, the data analysis and confirmation of the metabolite chemical structures was performed by a simple comparison of the acquired patient sample data to the database. GC-MS data also contained peaks that remained unidentified and showed statistically significant changes depending on sample class.

Results

The use of multiple orthogonal analytical methods provided a broad coverage of the metabolome and each method contributed mass features to the model for classification of the children with ASD from the TD controls. Each analytical method was assessed for the unique features it provided. The HILIC LC-HRMS method resulted in the highest number of distinctive mass features in the models, followed by C8 LC-HRMS then GC-MS. Univariate analysis filtering was performed on the 4572 features that passed the preprocessing filters. About 60% of the LC-HRMS features were putatively annotated with a chemical structure and

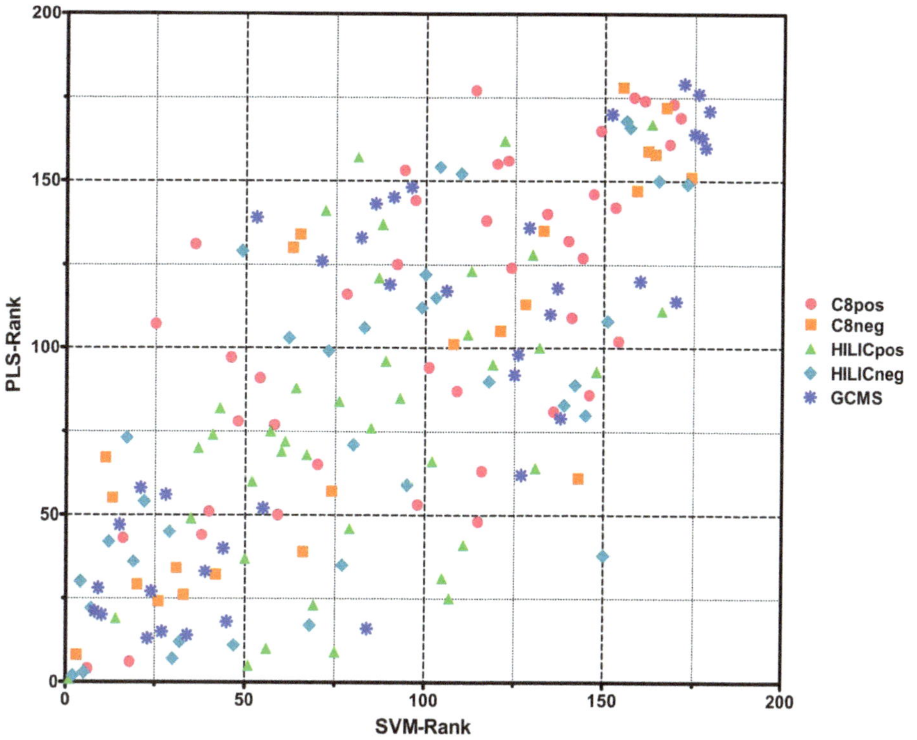

Figure 2. Feature Importance Rankings. The top 179 features were compared for rank between SVM and PLS modeling methods. The lowest rank scores represent the most important features.

8% (503) of the annotated features passed the FBF procedural criteria. Approximately 36% (142) of the targeted GC-MS features were confirmed metabolites. A breakdown of these results is contained in Table 2.

Data across the 61-sample training set from all analytical platforms were used to identify and robustly rank the features that could be utilized to discriminate plasma samples from children with ASD from samples from TD children. The univariate analysis filtering, as described in the methods, resulted in 389 statistically significant features. Following feature QC, 210 features were removed from the analysis due to poor quality EICs, leaving 179 features that were included in classification modeling. The 179 features comprised 3% of the LC-HRMS and 8% of the GC-MS preprocessed set of features and are shown in Table S1.

Training Set Model Performance

SVM and PLS classification methods were used to discriminate between samples from children with ASD and TD children using the 179 selected features as variables and each feature's contribution toward classification was evaluated for future biomarker development efforts. Based on the best performing model from each of the 100 nested CV resampling iterations, ROC plots were generated for the average of the 100 resamples to understand performance of each modeling method (SVM and PLS-DA). Both SVM and PLS modeling methods indicated that a metabolic signature could be detected that could classify children with ASD from TD individuals (Table S2). For the 61-sample training set, the average ASD prediction accuracy of the SVM model was 0.86, with AUC values of 0.95 (95% CI 0.94–0.96). The PLS model gave an average prediction accuracy of 0.84 with AUC values of 0.92 (95% CI 0.91–0.94). To confirm that the model classification accuracies were not random results, the modeling process was repeated with random permutations of the diagnosis class labels. These results showed near random classification, with AUC values of 0.52 (95% CI 0.48–0.57) and 0.52 (95% CI 0.49–0.56) for SVM and PLS, respectively, indicating that the 179 features did not discriminate the classes by chance (Figure 3).

Anticipating that blood tests for ASD may be more efficient and less expensive if they measure an optimally lower number of metabolites, the classification modeling paradigm also included a feature number optimization in each model, based on the highest resulting AUC. The feature sets were evaluated using feature subsets based on the ordered VIP scores of individual features to identify the minimum number of features that maximized performance for each modeling method (Table S2). These data together indicate that not all of the features contributed equally to the models and that the number of features could be reduced by removing those that contributed less while still retaining model accuracy and robustness. As a result, the entire set of 179 features was not required for optimal model performance for either of the modeling methods (Figure 3). The results from the model training process indicated that SVM models that were trained using an 80 feature set exhibited the best combined classification performance metrics (when compared to PLS and other SVM results) with an average accuracy of 90%, an average sensitivity of 92%, an average specificity of 87%, and an average AUC of 0.95 (Table S2).

Validation Set Model Performance

Different subsets of features, created based on the weighted VIP scores, were evaluated independently of the outer cross-validation loop using the 21-sample independent validation set. The 80-feature SVM model described above had a classification predic-

Table 2. A breakdown of the numbers of features resulting from filtering and annotation processes, based on molecular formula.

Platform	Raw Features	Annotated Features	Unique Formula within a Platform	Features Passing Preprocessing Filters	Features Passing Univariate Filter
HILIC +	3207	1985	146	1527	40
HILIC−	1865	1061	140	950	35
C8+	3062	1902	140	1096	42
C8−	1568	847	77	514	23
GC-MS	485	178*	142*	485	39
Total	**10187**	**5795**	**645**	**4572**	**179**

This table also helps to illustrate the orthogonality and contribution of each of the 5 analytical platforms. Molecular formulae are being used here only to approximate the method orthogonality, since any given molecular formula may be associated with multiple chemical structures. *These annotations were confirmed in the GCMS platform and the formula were confirmed by using the KEGG database instead of the FBF procedure used in the 4 LCMS platforms.

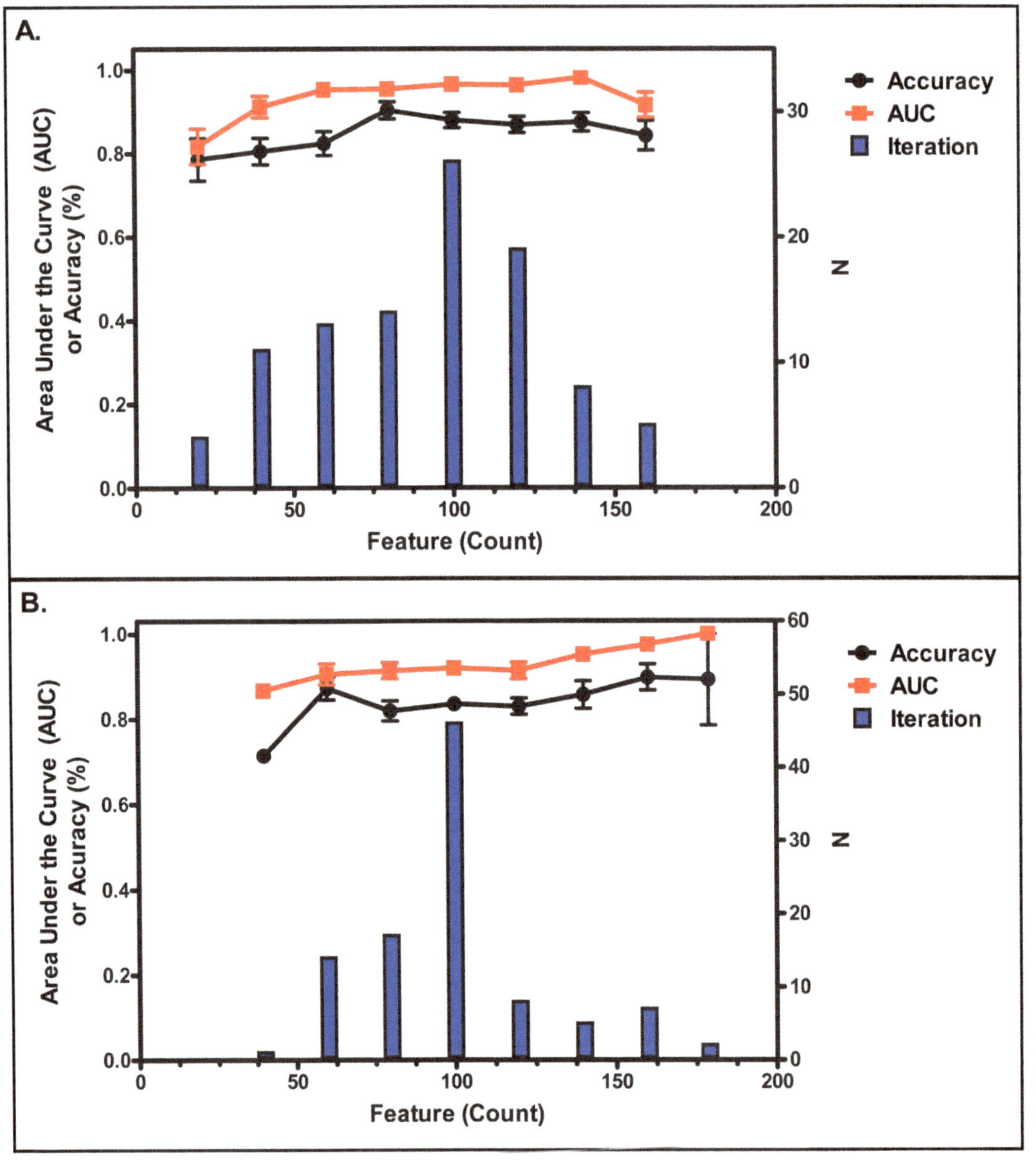

Figure 3. Performance of the SVM and PLS models. Average AUC and accuracy of the (a) SVM and (b) PLS models containing different numbers of features. The bar graphs show the number of optimal models which were derived from recursive feature elimination process that was included in the resampling process for the indicated number of features.

tion accuracy of 81%, a sensitivity of 85%, a specificity of 75% and an AUC of 84% (Figure 4, red line; Table 3). The best performing PLS model, comprised of 160 variables, had an accuracy of 81%, a sensitivity of 92%, a specificity of 63% and an AUC of 0.81% (Figure 4, blue line; Table 3). Detailed results are shown in Table S3. The results suggest that at least 40 features are needed to reach an accuracy of 70% and that a range of 80 to 160 features had the best performance with this independent validation sample set as well as the training set of samples.

Confirmation of Metabolite Chemical Structures

The chemical identities of the 7 LC-MS mass features that were confirmed by LC-HRMS-MS are shown in Table 4. Included in the metabolites confirmed by LC-HRMS-MS or targeted GC-MS was homocitrulline, which was decreased in ASD patients. Other metabolites showing significant up or down regulation in our study include: aspartate, glutamate, DHEAS, citric acid, succinic acid, methylhexa-, tetra- and hepta-decanoic acids, isoleucine, glutaric acid, 3-aminoisobutyric acid and creatinine. These are listed in Table 4 and represent a variety of molecular classes including amino acids, organic acids, sterols, and fatty acids.

Discussion

Our metabolomic approach was not biased toward possible biochemical pathways other than by the separation and detection limits of the analytical methods used. We used robust VIP scores and recursive feature elimination to estimate that between 80 and 160 mass features are required to produce an optimal predictive signature in this set of patients. The predictive signatures in this study are the result of modeling a 62-patient training set, then applying those models to predict a 21-patient validation set. This approach has resulted in the discovery of a biochemically diverse set of metabolites that might be useful in distinguishing individuals at risk for ASD. It is difficult to determine how generalizable these predictive signatures will be in the broader population, given the small sample size. Larger studies need to be performed in order to assess and refine a signature into a clinical diagnostic. Several of the metabolites identified so far in these signatures point to biological mechanisms that have been previously identified as having a role in the etiology of ASD. Our signatures will most likely represent a portion of the metabolic changes that will be critical in the diagnosis of ASD through metabolic end points.

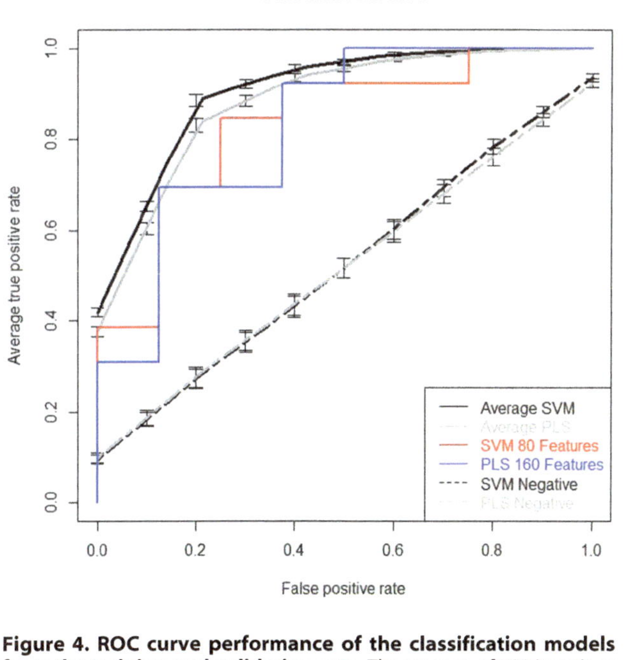

Figure 4. ROC curve performance of the classification models from the training and validation sets. The average of 100 iterations of the classifier for the best performing feature sets following recursive feature elimination comparing ASD vs. TD samples (Black and Grey Lines). The blue (PLS) and red (SVM) lines are ROC curves of the best performing validation feature subsets. Vertical bars represent the standard error of the mean.

Identification of metabolites previously associated with ASD

Examples of metabolites showing significant up or down regulation in the current study that have been previously associated with autism include:

- Tricarboxylic acid cycle associated molecules including citric acid (decreased) and succinic acid (increased) were found to be significantly altered in the ASD participants. Elevations in urinary succinate [16,17] and decreased urinary citrate [37] in children with autism have been previously reported.
- Fatty acids have previously been observed to be decreased in the plasma of children with ASD, similar to our observations for methylhexa-, tetra- and hepta-decanoic acids [12]. Links between saturated fatty acid metabolism and oxidative stress have been reported in erythrocytes in children with ASD [38].
- 3-aminoisobutyric acid was increased in samples from participants with ASD. This is also consistent with previous findings [39].
- Creatinine was decreased in children with ASD and is consistent with the findings of Whitely *et al,* who observed similar changes in urinary creatinine in children diagnosed with PDD [40].

Evidence for a role in mitochondrial dysfunction in ASD

The goal of this study was to evaluate biomarkers in blood. When metabolism is disrupted, active transporters and tissue specific differences in metabolism can cause different levels of the same metabolites in different biological compartments (plasma, urine, CSF, etc.). When discussing individual metabolites in the context of autism, it is important to recognize that autism is a systemic disease that affects other organ systems besides the brain. For example, serotonin levels have been reported to be elevated in blood in some patients with autism, and other evidence suggests that intracerebral serotonergic activity is decreased in ASD. Serotonin does not cross the blood brain barrier, and the brain has different enzymes for serotonin synthesis than peripheral tissues [41].

Many of the confirmed metabolites that are associated with ASD are relevant to aspects of mitochondrial biology. Mitochondrial disease or dysfunction may be a risk factor for autism [42]. In addition, several other observed metabolites are associated with other processes already proposed to be involved in ASD including oxidative stress [43] and energy production [44].

- Aspartate and glutamate levels in blood were significantly elevated in ASD, as has been observed in previous studies [45,46]. Mutations in the aspartate/glutamate mitochondrial transporter, SLC25A12, have been previously associated with ASD [47]. This transporter is an important component of the malate/aspartate shuttle, a crucial system supporting oxidative

Table 3. Classifier performance metrics based on predictions on the independent 21-sample validation set, showing the feature sets with the highest accuracy.

Model	Feature No.	Accuracy	Sensitivity	Specificity	AUC
SVM	80	0.81	0.85	0.75	0.84
PLS	160	0.81	0.92	0.63	0.81

Feature No. corresponds to the number of the ordered, ranked VIP features that were evaluated. Table S3 shows the results for all feature sets.

phosphorylation, adenosine triphosphate production, and key metabolites for the urea cycle [47].

- DHEAS, the predominant plasma sterol, was increased in children with ASD. DHEA is known to affect mitochondrial energy production through inhibition of enzymes associated with the respiratory chain [48] with variable findings in children with ASD [49,50].
- The branched chain amino acid isoleucine was reduced in samples from children with ASD versus TD children as observed by others [51]. Possible molecular mechanisms would include mutation in the branched chain amino acid kinase dehydrogenase (BCKD-kinase), a mitochondrial enzyme [52] as well as amino acids in energy metabolism [53].
- Glutaric acid levels were elevated in children with ASD. Increased urinary glutaric acid occurs in a variety of neuronal deficiencies such as glutaryl-CoA dehydrogenase (GCDH) deficiency. A significant portion of the glutaric acid metabolism takes place in the mitochondria [54].

The potential relationship of the gut microbiome with ASD

This potential connection between the gut microbiome and ASD is also receiving considerable attention [55]. Metabolomic studies of urine from individuals with ASD have identified molecules associated with the microbiome such as dimethylamine, hippuric acid and phenylacetylglutamine [16,17]. We observed decreased plasma levels of p-hydroxyphenyllactate, a metabolite associated with bifidobacteria and lactobacilli that is known to serve as an antioxidant both in the circulation and tissues [56]. We have yet to identify other microbiome related metabolites.

Novel metabolic alterations in ASD

We identified novel statistically significant changes in some metabolites that had not been previously reported in other metabolomics profiling as well as identifying novel changes in metabolites that had never before been associated with ASD. Significant changes in the levels of aspartate, citrate, creatinine, DHEA-S, hydroxyphenyllactate, indoleacetate, isoleucine, glutamate and glutarate between ASD and TD individuals were identified in this study compared to previous metabolomics studies of urine metabolites where changes in these metabolites were not significant [17]. These differences could be related to transport and accumulation of metabolites in the urine compared to the blood, differences in the study populations, or application different LC-MS and GC-MS methodology allowing better detection of these metabolites in this study.

We also identified a new, previously undescribed potential ASD biomarker, homocitrulline. This metabolite was decreased in ASD patients and had the highest rank of all features in both SVM and PLS classification models. Homocitrulline is a poorly understood molecule which is known to be formed inside the mitochondria from lysine and carbamoyl phosphate. The decreased homocitrulline levels in the blood suggests that homocitrulline metabolism in the brain may also be disrupted, Homocitrulline levels are increased in urine and blood in patients with ornithine translocase (SLC25A15) deficiency which diverts carbamyl phosphate to react with lysine. These patients can exhibit behavioral abnormalities similar to ASD such as developmental delay, ataxia, spasticity, learning disabilities, cognitive deficits and/or unexplained seizures [57]. Rats treated with intracerebroventricular administration of homocitrulline are also observed to have disrupted brain redox status and energy metabolism [58,59]. These observations suggest that elevated brain levels of homocitrulline are deleterious; however additional studies are needed to define the brain levels of homocitrulline and the potential role in the development of ASD.

Summary

The current study profiled metabolites in blood plasma using metabolomics methods to evaluate the possibility that differences in the metabolite abundances might provide a metabolic signature that could prove useful in distinguishing individuals at high risk for developing ASD. The cohort of subjects enrolled in this study was carefully assembled to reflect a diagnosis of ASD by strict research criteria. Beyond careful clinical diagnosis, great pains were taken to ensure that fasting blood collection was obtained at the same time for all study participants and that complicating factors such as illness were minimized. We consider the current work as a proof of concept that there are predictive metabolic signatures which can be used to distinguish ASD and TD individuals.

Two independent statistical classification methods (PLS and SVM) were employed to determine the most influential metabolites and mass features that could be used to discriminate between ASD and TD individuals. Both classification modeling methods yielded relatively similar results with respect to maximum prediction accuracy of about 81% as evaluated by an independent 21-sample validation sample set. This was followed by recursive feature elimination to establish the minimal numbers of features needed for a predictive model. Interestingly, several of the key features for classification, such as homocitrulline, were common between the two methods indicating their importance in the development of future blood based diagnostics. It is clear that access to a larger sample set will be required to further validate and confirm the annotations of the key features. Metabolomics determines changes in small molecule metabolites that are reactants and products of endogenous biochemical processes as well as small molecules derived from diet, the gut microbiome and contact with the environment. Perturbations in their abundance can result not only from genomic and proteomic influences, but from environmental and epigenetic influences as well. A metabolomic approach may therefore provide enhanced predictive results by keying in on common, end stage metabolites rather than on specific genomic or proteomic determinants.

Table 4. Confirmed metabolites.

Analytical Platform	Metabolite	Feature ID	HMDB ID [61]	Fold Change (ASD/TD)	p-value (ASD vs. TD)	FDR	SVM Rank	PLS Rank
HILICpos	homocitrulline	M190T512	HMDB00679	0.67	<0.001	0.059	1	1
C8neg	2-hydroxyvaleric acid	M117T127	HMDB01863	0.80	0.0289	0.53	33	26
HILICpos	cystine	M241T774	HMDB00192	0.91	0.0277	0.532	87	121
GCMS	aspartic acid	GCMS_aspartic.acid	HMDB00191	1.33	<0.001	0.086	34	14
HILICpos	isoleucine	M132T248	HMDB00172	0.76	0.0351	0.541	60	69
HILICpos	creatinine	M114T262	HMDB00562	0.88	0.0471	0.576	57	75
GCMS	serine	GCMS_serine	HMDB00187	1.16	0.00275	0.267	137	118
HILICneg	4-hydroxyphenyllactic acid	M181T66	HMDB00755	0.84	0.0344	0.541	47	11
GC-MS	citric acid	GCMS_citric.acid	HMDB00094	0.91	0.0492	0.580	84	16
GC-MS	glutamic acid	GCMS_glutamic.acid	HMDB00148	1.28	0.00144	0.188	15	47
GC-MS	lactic acid	GCMS_indol.3.lactate	HMDB00671	0.87	0.0181	0.457	55	52
C8neg	DHEA sulfate	M367T736	HMDB01032	2.55	0.00152	0.188	11	67
GC-MS	glutaric acid	GCMS_glutaric.acid	HMDB00661	1.36	0.00492	0.322	27	15
GC-MS	5-hydroxynorvaline	GCMS_X5. Hydroxy norvaline.NIST	HMDB31658	1.27	0.0457	0.576	177	163
GC-MS	heptadecanoic acid	GCMS_heptadecanoic.acid.NIST	HMDB02259	0.81	0.0270	0.527	135	110
GC-MS	5-aminovaleric acid lactam	GCMS_X5.aminovaleric.acid.lactame	HMDB11749	2.43	0.00211	0.22	127	62
GC-MS	succinic acid	GCMS_succinic.acid	HMDB00254	1.11	0.0457	0.576	175	164
GC-MS	myristic acid	GCMS_myristic.acid	HMDB00806	0.76	0.00892	0.371	24	27
GC-MS	2-hydroxyvaleric acid	GCMS_X2.hydroxyvaleric.acid	HMDB01863	1.41	0.0406	0.564	179	171
GC-MS	methylhexadecanoic acid	GCMS_methylhexadecanoic.acid	NA	0.82	0.0399	0.564	160	120
GC-MS	3-aminoisobutyric acid	GCMS_X3.aminoisobutyric.acid	HMDB02166	1.19	0.0473	0.576	176	176

Statistically significant metabolites from the 61-sample training set with chemical structures confirmed by LC-HRMS-MS or GC-MS.

Limitations

While the patient population was very well characterized, represented all severity levels of ASD and the blood samples were taken in a very systematic fashion, the total number of subjects (ASD = 52; TD = 30) was not large enough to definitively create a model for prediction of ASD or characterize metabolic differences that may be more highly associated with ASD subtypes.

Due to the small sample size, analysis of the data with respect to medication, sex, special diet, race, ethnicity or other potential confounding covariates was not conclusive. These are important considerations which require a larger sample size to address properly. A much larger study is currently in progress. Randomization methods were implemented to help prevent biasing the results based on any single covariate. The 4 misclassified patients in the 80 feature SVM model in the validation test set were Caucasian male and females whereas the Hispanic, Asian, and other ethnicity were predicted correctly.

Strong evidence of hemolysis, based on visual observation, was observed in 5 samples from ASD children. These samples were excluded from analysis Hemolysis can be a result of poor medical condition, but can also result from suboptimal blood collection and handling. However, Yin et. al. found that if EDTA tubes were placed on ice immediately, as was done in this protocol, the metabolome was very stable. Therefore, it remains possible, but unlikely, that minor hemolysis may confound the data by effecting some of the metabolite fold changes that were observed [60].

Conclusions

This initial study provides proof of concept to further pursue development of metabolic biomarkers of ASD. We have demonstrated that a profile of altered metabolites in the blood plasma from a well-curated sample set from clinically diagnosed children with ASD and TD individuals between 4 and 6 years of age, can be detected by a combination of several MS-based metabolomic analyses. Statistical models developed from the derived metabolic data distinguished children with ASD from TD individuals with better than 80% accuracy in both the 61-sample training set and the 21 sample validation set.

The broad metabolite profiling methods developed here can also be employed to discover a wide variety of additional metabolites, leading to the determination of biochemical pathways and mechanisms that are involved in the etiologies of ASD, and advancing the understanding of autism in broader patient populations, eventually leading to new modes of therapy. Given the pronounced clinical and co-morbid features of ASD, it is possible that metabolic profiling of individual patients may enable individualized therapeutic approaches for improved outcomes.

Future Endeavors

Further research is currently being carried out in much larger and younger patient populations to confirm these results, discover and confirm additional diagnostic metabolites and determine which are the most robust for evaluating ASD risk. We are also comparing metabolite profiles in clinically defined subtypes of ASD to determine whether predictive accuracy can be increased through better phenotyping of the ASD population. Analysis and consequential stratification will be performed based on covariables such as medication, sex, special diet, race, ethnicity, onset and co-morbid features such as gastrointestinal distress or seizure disorders may lead to a more accurate set of diagnostic metabolic profiles.

Supporting Information

Table S1 Metabolic features used in the classification models. A table of all 179 model features.

Table S2 Results from the cross-validation (CV) training sets.

Table S3 Classifier performance metrics based on predictions on the independent 21-sample validation set.

Table S4 Patient gender and ethnicity.

Table S5 Complete Feature Data. All mass feature data used for modelling.

Acknowledgments

The authors thank Agilent Technologies for providing instrumentation, software and assistance.

Author Contributions

Conceived and designed the experiments: PRW DGA PB AS JAP GC ELRD REB. Performed the experiments: PRW LE MR KC. Analyzed the data: PRW LE AS KC BF PB. Wrote the paper: PRW DGA PB LE AS BF BAC JAP ELRD REB.

References

1. American Psychiatric Association (2013) Desk Reference to the Diagnostic Criteria from DSM-5. 5th ed. Washington, D.C.: American Psychiatric Association.
2. Centers for Disease Control and Prevention (2014) Prevalence of autism spectrum disorder among children aged 8 years - autism and developmental disabilities monitoring network, 11 sites, United States, 2010. MMWR Surveill Summ 63: 1–21. Available: http://www.ncbi.nlm.nih.gov/pubmed/24670961.
3. Dawson G, Rogers S, Munson J, Smith M, Winter J, et al. (2010) Randomized, controlled trial of an intervention for toddlers with autism: the Early Start Denver Model. Pediatrics 125: e17–23. Available: http://www.ncbi.nlm.nih.gov/pubmed/19948568. Accessed 12 August 2013.
4. Ganz ML (2007) The lifetime distribution of the incremental societal costs of autism. Arch Pediatr Adolesc Med 161: 343–349. Available: http://www.ncbi.nlm.nih.gov/pubmed/17404130.
5. State MW, Šestan N (2012) Neuroscience. The emerging biology of autism spectrum disorders. Science 337: 1301–1303. Available: http://www.ncbi.nlm.nih.gov/pubmed/22984058. Accessed 27 February 2013.
6. Berg JM, Geschwind DH (2012) Autism genetics: searching for specificity and convergence. Genome Biol 13: 247. Available: http://www.pubmedcentral.nih.gov/articlerender.fcgi?artid=3491377&tool=pmcentrez&rendertype=abstract.
7. Huguet G, Ey E, Bourgeron T (2013) The genetic landscapes of autism spectrum disorders. Annu Rev Genomics Hum Genet 14: 191–213. Available: http://www.ncbi.nlm.nih.gov/pubmed/23875794. Accessed 11 December 2013.
8. Bucan M, Abrahams BS, Wang K, Glessner JT, Herman EI, et al. (2009) Genome-wide analyses of exonic copy number variants in a family-based study point to novel autism susceptibility genes. PLoS Genet 5: e1000536. Available: http://www.pubmedcentral.nih.gov/articlerender.fcgi?artid=2695001&tool=pmcentrez&rendertype=abstract. Accessed 7 August 2013.
9. Wang K, Zhang H, Ma D, Bucan M, Glessner JT, et al. (2009) Common genetic variants on 5p14.1 associate with autism spectrum disorders. Nature 459: 528–533. Available: http://www.pubmedcentral.nih.gov/articlerender.fcgi?artid=2943511&tool=pmcentrez&rendertype=abstract. Accessed 9 August 2013.
10. Belgard TG, Jankovic I, Lowe JK, Geschwind DH (2014) Population structure confounds autism genetic classifier. Mol Psychiatry 19: 405–407. doi: 10.1038/mp.2013.34.
11. Skafidas E, Testa R, Zantomio D, Chana G, Everall IP, et al. (2012) Predicting the diagnosis of autism spectrum disorder using gene pathway analysis. Mol Psychiatry in press. Available: http://www.ncbi.nlm.nih.gov/pubmed/22965006. Accessed 24 October 2012.

12. El-Ansary AK, Bacha AG Ben, Al-Ayahdi LY (2011) Plasma fatty acids as diagnostic markers in autistic patients from Saudi Arabia. Lipids Health Dis 10: 62. Available: http://www.pubmedcentral.nih.gov/articlerender.fcgi?artid=3107800&tool=pmcentrez&rendertype=abstract. Accessed 6 August 2013.
13. James SJ, Melnyk S, Fuchs G, Reid T, Jernigan S, et al. (2009) Efficacy of methylcobalamin and folinic acid treatment on glutathione redox status in children with autism 1–3. Am J Clin Nutr 89: 425–430.
14. Lee RWY, Tierney E (2011) Hypothesis: the role of sterols in autism spectrum disorder. Autism Res Treat 2011: 653570. Available: http://www.pubmedcentral.nih.gov/articlerender.fcgi?artid=3420784&tool=pmcentrez&rendertype=abstract. Accessed 23 August 2013.
15. Damodaran LPM, Arumugam G (2011) Urinary oxidative stress markers in children with autism. Redox Rep 16: 216–222. Available: http://www.ncbi.nlm.nih.gov/pubmed/22005342. Accessed 23 August 2013.
16. Yap IKS, Angley M, Veselkov K a, Holmes E, Lindon JC, et al. (2010) Urinary metabolic phenotyping differentiates children with autism from their unaffected siblings and age-matched controls. J Proteome Res 9: 2996–3004. Available: http://www.ncbi.nlm.nih.gov/pubmed/20337404.
17. Ming X, Stein TP, Barnes V, Rhodes N, Guo L (2012) Metabolic perturbance in autism spectrum disorders: a metabolomics study. J Proteome Res 11: 5856–5862. Available: http://www.ncbi.nlm.nih.gov/pubmed/23106572.
18. Dunn WB, Bailey NJC, Johnson HE (2005) Measuring the metabolome: current analytical technologies. Analyst 130: 606–625. Available: http://www.ncbi.nlm.nih.gov/pubmed/15852128. Accessed 19 August 2013.
19. Gross ML (1994) Accurate masses for structure confirmation. J Am Soc Mass Spectrom 5: 57. Available: http://link.springer.com/10.1016/1044-0305(94)85036-4.
20. Bruce SJ, Jonsson P, Antti H, Cloarec O, Trygg J, et al. (2008) Evaluation of a protocol for metabolic profiling studies on human blood plasma by combined ultra-performance liquid chromatography/mass spectrometry: From extraction to data analysis. Anal Biochem 372: 237–249. Available: http://www.ncbi.nlm.nih.gov/pubmed/17964273. Accessed 12 August 2013.
21. American Psychiatric Association (2000) Desk Reference to the Diagnostic Criteria from DSM IV. 4th ed. Washington, D.C.: American Psychiatric Association.
22. Corbett BA, Kantor AB, Schulman H, Walker WL, Lit L, et al. (2007) A proteomic study of serum from children with autism showing differential expression of apolipoproteins and complement proteins. Mol Psychiatry 12: 292–306. Available: http://www.ncbi.nlm.nih.gov/pubmed/17189958. Accessed 14 January 2013.
23. Ashwood P, Corbett BA, Kantor A, Schulman H, Van de Water J, et al. (2011) In search of cellular immunophenotypes in the blood of children with autism. PLoS One 6: e19299. Available: http://www.pubmedcentral.nih.gov/articlerender.fcgi?artid=3087757&tool=pmcentrez&rendertype=abstract. Accessed 21 January 2013.
24. Jiye A, Trygg J, Gullberg J, Johansson AI, Jonsson P, et al. (2005) Extraction and GC/MS analysis of the human blood plasma metabolome. Anal Chem 77: 8086–8094. Available: http://www.ncbi.nlm.nih.gov/pubmed/16351159.
25. Fiehn O, Wohlgemuth G, Scholz M, Kind T, Lee DY, et al. (2008) Quality control for plant metabolomics: reporting MSI-compliant studies. Plant J 53: 691–704. doi: 10.1111/j.1365-313X.2007.03387.x.
26. Smith CA, O'Maille G, Want EJ, Qin C, Trauger S a, et al. (2005) METLIN: a metabolite mass spectral database. Ther Drug Monit 27: 747–751. Available: http://www.ncbi.nlm.nih.gov/pubmed/16404815.
27. Horai H, Arita M, Kanaya S, Nihei Y, Ikeda T, et al. (2010) MassBank: a public repository for sharing mass spectral data for life sciences. J Mass Spectrom 45: 703–714. Available: http://www.ncbi.nlm.nih.gov/pubmed/20623627. Accessed 23 August 2013.
28. Orchard S, Montechi-Palazzi L, Deutsch EW, Binz P-A, Jones AR, et al. (2007) Five years of progress in the Standardization of Proteomics Data 4th Annual Spring Workshop of the HUPO-Proteomics Standards Initiative April 23-25, 2007 Ecole Nationale Supérieure (ENS), Lyon, France. Proteomics 7: 3436–3440. Available: http://www.ncbi.nlm.nih.gov/pubmed/17907277. Accessed 1 May 2014.
29. Smith CA, Want EJ, O'Maille G, Abagyan R, Siuzdak G (2006) XCMS: processing mass spectrometry data for metabolite profiling using nonlinear peak alignment, matching, and identification. Anal Chem 78: 779–787. Available: http://www.ncbi.nlm.nih.gov/pubmed/16448051.
30. Prince JT, Marcotte EM (2006) Chromatographic alignment of ESI-LC-MS proteomics data sets by ordered bijective interpolated warping. Anal Chem 78: 6140–6152. Available: http://www.ncbi.nlm.nih.gov/pubmed/16944896.
31. Haury A-C, Gestraud P, Vert J-P (2011) The influence of feature selection methods on accuracy, stability and interpretability of molecular signatures. PLoS One 6: e28210. Available: http://www.ncbi.nlm.nih.gov/pubmed/22205940. Accessed 1 May 2014.
32. Benjamini Y, Hochberg Y (1995) Controlling the false discovery rate: a practical and powerful approach to multiple testing. J R Stat Soc Ser B 57: 289–300.
33. Wold H (1985) Partial least squares. In: Kotz S, Johnson NL, editors. Encyclopedia of statistical sciences. New York: Wiley, Vol. 6. pp. 581–591.
34. Cortes C, Vapnik V (1995) Support-vector networks. Mach Learn 20: 273–297. Available: http://link.springer.com/article/10.1007/BF00994018. Accessed 1 May 2014.
35. Kuhn M (2008) Building predictive models in R using the caret package. J Stat Softw 28: 1–26.
36. Sing T, Sander O, Beerenwinkel N, Lengauer T (2005) ROCR: visualizing classifier performance in R. Bioinformatics 21: 3940–3941. Available: http://www.ncbi.nlm.nih.gov/pubmed/16096348. Accessed 29 April 2014.
37. Frye RE, Melnyk S, Macfabe DF (2013) Unique acyl-carnitine profiles are potential biomarkers for acquired mitochondrial disease in autism spectrum disorder. Transl Psychiatry 3: e220. Available: http://www.pubmedcentral.nih.gov/articlerender.fcgi?artid=3566723&tool=pmcentrez&rendertype=abstract. Accessed 9 January 2014.
38. Ghezzo A, Visconti P, Abruzzo PM, Bolotta A, Ferreri C, et al. (2013) Oxidative Stress and Erythrocyte Membrane Alterations in Children with Autism: Correlation with Clinical Features. PLoS One 8: e66418. Available: http://www.pubmedcentral.nih.gov/articlerender.fcgi?artid=3686873&tool=pmcentrez&rendertype=abstract. Accessed 7 August 2013.
39. Adams JB, Audhya T, McDonough-Means S, Rubin RA, Quig D, et al. (2011) Nutritional and metabolic status of children with autism vs. neurotypical children, and the association with autism severity. Nutr Metab (Lond) 8: 34. Available: http://www.pubmedcentral.nih.gov/articlerender.fcgi?artid=3135510&tool=pmcentrez&rendertype=abstract.
40. Whiteley P, Waring R, Williams L, Klovrza L, Nolan F, et al. (2006) Spot urinary creatinine excretion in pervasive developmental disorders. Pediatr Int 48: 292–297. Available: http://www.ncbi.nlm.nih.gov/pubmed/16732798. Accessed 22 July 2013.
41. Whitaker-Azmitia PM (2005) Behavioral and cellular consequences of increasing serotonergic activity during brain development: a role in autism? Int J Dev Neurosci 23: 75–83. Available: http://www.ncbi.nlm.nih.gov/pubmed/15730889. Accessed 12 November 2013.
42. Marazziti D, Baroni S, Picchetti M, Landi P, Silvestri S, et al. (2012) Psychiatric disorders and mitochondrial dysfunctions. Eur Rev Med Pharmacol Sci 16: 270–275. Available: http://www.ncbi.nlm.nih.gov/pubmed/22428481.
43. Rossignol DA, Frye RE (2012) A review of research trends in physiological abnormalities in autism spectrum disorders: immune dysregulation, inflammation, oxidative stress, mitochondrial dysfunction and environmental toxicant exposures. Mol Psychiatry 17: 389–401. Available: http://www.pubmedcentral.nih.gov/articlerender.fcgi?artid=3317062&tool=pmcentrez&rendertype=abstract. Accessed 5 February 2013.
44. Blaylock RL (2009) A possible central mechanism in autism spectrum disorders, part 2: immunoexcitotoxicity. Altern Ther Health Med 15: 60–67. Available: http://www.ncbi.nlm.nih.gov/pubmed/19161050.
45. Shinohe A, Hashimoto K, Nakamura K, Tsujii M, Iwata Y, et al. (2006) Increased serum levels of glutamate in adult patients with autism. Prog Neuropsychopharmacol Biol Psychiatry 30: 1472–1477. Available: http://www.ncbi.nlm.nih.gov/pubmed/16863675. Accessed 15 July 2013.
46. Moreno-Fuenmayor H, Borjas L, Arrieta A, Valera V, Socorro-Candanoza L (1996) Plasma excitatory amino acids in autism. Invest Clin 37: 113–128.
47. Napolioni V, Persico AM, Porcelli V, Palmieri L (2011) The mitochondrial aspartate/glutamate carrier AGC1 and calcium homeostasis: physiological links and abnormalities in autism. Mol Neurobiol 44: 83–92.
48. Safiulina D, Peet N, Seppet E, Zharkovsky A, Kaasik A (2006) Dehydroepiandrosterone inhibits complex I of the mitochondrial respiratory chain and is neurotoxic in vitro and in vivo at high concentrations. Toxicol Sci 93: 348–356. Available: http://www.ncbi.nlm.nih.gov/pubmed/16849397. Accessed 9 January 2014.
49. Strous RD, Golubchik P, Maayan R, Mozes T, Tuati-Werner D, et al. (2005) Lowered DHEA-S plasma levels in adult individuals with autistic disorder. Eur Neuropsychopharmacol 15: 305–309. Available: http://www.ncbi.nlm.nih.gov/pubmed/15820420. Accessed 23 August 2013.
50. Tordjman S, Anderson GM, McBride PA, Hertzig ME, Snow ME, et al. (1995) Plasma androgens in autism. J Autism Dev Disord 25: 295–304. Available: http://www.ncbi.nlm.nih.gov/pubmed/7559294.
51. Arnold GL, Hyman SL, Mooney RA, Kirby RS (2003) Plasma amino acids profiles in children with autism: potential risk of nutritional deficiencies. J Autism Dev Disord 33: 449–454. Available: http://www.ncbi.nlm.nih.gov/pubmed/12959424.
52. Novarino G, El-Fishawy P, Kayserili H, Meguid N a, Scott EM, et al. (2012) Mutations in BCKD-kinase lead to a potentially treatable form of autism with epilepsy. Science 338: 394–397. Available: http://www.ncbi.nlm.nih.gov/pubmed/22956686. Accessed 24 October 2012.
53. Valerio A, D'Antona G, Nisoli E (2011) Branched-chain amino acids, mitochondrial biogenesis, and healthspan: an evolutionary perspective. Aging (Albany NY) 3: 464–478. Available: http://www.pubmedcentral.nih.gov/articlerender.fcgi?artid=3156598&tool=pmcentrez&rendertype=abstract.
54. Müller E, Kölker S (2004) Reduction of lysine intake while avoiding malnutrition–major goals and major problems in dietary treatment of glutaryl-CoA dehydrogenase deficiency. J Inherit Metab Dis 27: 903–910. Available: http://www.ncbi.nlm.nih.gov/pubmed/15505398.
55. Mulle JG, Sharp WG, Cubells JF (2013) The gut microbiome: a new frontier in autism research. Curr Psychiatry Rep 15: 337. Available: http://www.ncbi.nlm.nih.gov/pubmed/23307560. Accessed 7 August 2013.
56. Beloborodova N, Bairamov I, Olenin A, Shubina V, Teplova V, et al. (2012) Effect of phenolic acids of microbial origin on production of reactive oxygen species in mitochondria and neutrophils. J Biomed Sci 19: 89. Available: http://www.pubmedcentral.nih.gov/articlerender.fcgi?artid=3503878&tool=pmcentrez&rendertype=abstract. Accessed 6 August 2013.

57. Palmieri F (2004) The mitochondrial transporter family (SLC25): physiological and pathological implications. Pflugers Arch 447: 689–709.
58. Viegas CM, Busanello ENB, Tonin AM, de Moura AP, Grings M, et al. (2011) Dual mechanism of brain damage induced in vivo by the major metabolites accumulating in hyperornithinemia-hyperammonemia-homocitrullinuria syndrome. Brain Res 1369: 235–244. Available: http://www.ncbi.nlm.nih.gov/pubmed/21059345. Accessed 26 August 2014.
59. Sokoro A a H, Lepage J, Antonishyn N, McDonald R, Rockman-Greenberg C, et al. (2010) Diagnosis and high incidence of hyperornithinemia-hyperammonemia-homocitrullinemia (HHH) syndrome in northern Saskatchewan. J Inherit Metab Dis 33 Suppl 3: S275–81. Available: http://www.ncbi.nlm.nih.gov/pubmed/20574716. Accessed 26 August 2014.
60. Yin P, Peter A, Franken H, Zhao X, Neukamm SS, et al. (2013) Preanalytical aspects and sample quality assessment in metabolomics studies of human blood. Clin Chem 59: 833–845. Available: http://www.ncbi.nlm.nih.gov/pubmed/23386698. Accessed 18 August 2014.
61. Kanehisa M (1997) A database for post-genome analysis. Trends Genet 13: 375–376.

13

Biospecimen Long-Chain N-3 PUFA and Risk of Colorectal Cancer

Bo Yang[1,2], Feng-Lei Wang[1], Xiao-Li Ren[3], Duo Li[1]*

1 Department of Food Science and Nutrition, Zhejiang University, Hangzhou, China, **2** Department of Preventive Medicine, Wenzhou Medical University, Wenzhou, China, **3** Medical Laboratory Animal Center, Wenzhou Medical University, Wenzhou, China

Abstract

Background: Several prospective cohort and case-control studies reported the inconsistent association between biospecimen composition of C20 and C22 long-chain (LC) n-3 polyunsaturated fatty acid (PUFA) and colorectal cancer (CRC) risk. The aim of the present study was to investigate the association of biospecimen LC n-3 PUFA with CRC risk based on prospective cohort and case-control studies.

Methods and Results: Cochrane Library, PubMed, and EMBASE database were searched up to February 2014 for eligible studies. Risk ratios (RRs) or odds ratios (ORs) from prospective and case-control studies were combined using a random-effects model in the highest vs. lowest categorical analysis. Nonlinear dose-response relationships were assessed using restricted cubic spline regression models. Difference in tissue composition of LC n-3 PUFA between cases and noncases was analyzed as standardized mean difference (SMD). Three prospective cohort studies and 8 case-control studies were included in the present study, comprising 60,627 participants (1,499 CRC cases and 59,128 noncases). Higher biospecimen LC n-3 PUFA was significantly associated with a lower risk of CRC in case-control (pooled OR: 0.76; 95% CI: 0.59, 0.97; $I^2 = 10.00\%$) and prospective cohort studies (pooled RR: 0.70; 95% CI: 0.55, 0.88; $I^2 = 0.00\%$), respectively. A significant dose-response association was found of biospecimen C20:5n-3 (P for nonlinearity $= 0.02$) and C22:6n-3 (P for trend $= 0.01$) with CRC risk, respectively. Subjects without CRC have significantly higher biospecimen compositions of C20:5n-3 (SMD: 0.27; 95%: 0.13, 0.41), C22:6n-3 (SMD: 0.23; 95%: 0.11, 0.34) and total LC n-3 PUFA (SMD: 0.22; 95% CI: 0.07, 0.37) compared with those with CRC.

Conclusions: The present evidence suggests human tissue compositions of LC n-3 PUFA may be an independent predictive factor for CRC risk, especially C20:5n-3 and C22:6n-3. This needs to be confirmed with more large-scale prospective cohort studies.

Editor: Antonio Moschetta, IRCCS Istituto Oncologico Giovanni Paolo II, Italy

Funding: This was an independent study; the study subsidies of postgraduate students were paid from grants from the National Natural Science Foundation of China (No: 81273054) and the PhD Programs Foundation of Ministry of Education of China (No: 20120101110107). The funders had no role in study design, data collection and analysis, decision to publish, or preparation of the manuscript.

Competing Interests: The authors have declared that no competing interests exist.

* Email: duoli@zju.edu.cn

Introduction

Colorectal cancer (CRC) is the most frequently diagnosed, and has a higher incidence or mortality in both women and men in developed countries than in developing countries [1–3]. Dietary factors were postulated to play an important role in the prevention of CRC [4]. Data from human studies suggested that dietary fatty acids, as subtypes of fat in most foods, were closely associated with the development of CRC [5,6]. Recently, a meta-analysis of 13 prospective cohort studies [7] assessed the impact of total dietary fat on the risk of CRC, and indicated that dietary polyunsaturated fatty acid (PUFA) was not associated with the increased risk of CRC. One of the explains was that the true associations might be modified by the different effects of PUFA (omega-3 and omega-6) on the development of CRC. Seafood-derived long-chain (LC) omega-3 polyunsaturated fatty acid (n-3 PUFA), including C20:5n-3, C22:5n-3 and C22:6n-3, is suggested to reduce the risk of CRC in many epidemiological studies [8,9]. However, dietary data from meta-analyses of prospective cohort studies provided an insufficient evidence of protective effects of dietary LC n-3 PUFA on CRC risk [10,11], which may be due to inaccuracy in dietary assessment and an insufficient amount or variety of intake. Taking into account the difficulty in measuring dietary fatty acids accurately, more comprehensive attentions should be paid to a biomarker as a helpful tool that has been used to reflect intake closely to act as objective indices of true dietary intake. The most common biomarkers for dietary intake of LC n-3 PUFA from marine food or fish oil are C20:5n-3 and C22:6n-3, which can be determined in a variety of human biospecimens such as blood (serum/plasma/erythrocytes), adipose tissue (AT) and hair.

Accumulating evidences from in vitro and in vivo studies [12–14] indicate that LC n-3 PUFA as constituents of membrane phospholipids can work through several actions to protect against the initiation and early stages of CRC, including activating protein kinase C, enhancing CRC cell apoptosis, reducing inflammation and decreasing fecal bile acids as well as neutral sterol excretion. Nevertheless, results from prospective and case-control studies revealed inconsistent associations of human tissue LC n-3 PUFA with CRC risk. Most of case-control studies [15–17] reported that tissue composition of LC n-3 PUFA was inversely associated with CRC risk, whereas prospective cohort studies showed inverse [18] or null associations [19,20] between tissue LC n-3 PUFA and CRC risk. Tissue compositions of LC n-3 PUFA were reported to be significantly lower in subjects with CRC (cases) compared with control subjects without CRC (noncases) in some case-control studies [21,22], whereas inconsistent results were reported in other case-control studies [16,17,23–25].

The aim of the present study was to examine the relationship between LC n-3 PUFA compositions in human biospecimens and CRC risk based on prospective cohort and case-control studies. Additionally, the differences in biospecimens (plasma/serum/erythrocytes/whole blood/AT) compositions of LC n-3 PUFA between cases and noncases were also investigated based on case-control studies. We therefore conducted a meta-analysis to clarify the role of tissue compositions of LC n-3 PUFA in the etiology of CRC.

Methods

Literature research

We identified prospective and case-control studies which reported the association between LC n-3 PUFA composition in biospecimen and CRC risk from PubMed, EMBASE and Cochrane Library database up to February 2014. Search strategy was ("Fatty Acids, omega-3" AND "Colorectal Neoplasms") for PubMed, ("Colorectal tumor" AND "omega 3 fatty acid") for EMBASE and ("Fatty Acids, Omega-3" AND "Colorectal Neoplasms") for Cochrane Library databases. We also searched systematic reviews from the above-mentioned database, and check the reference lists to identify studies that might have been missed. We followed MOOSE guidelines of observational studies [26] for conducting and reporting meta-analyses (Checklist S1).

Eligibility criteria

To examine the associations of human biospecimen LC n-3 PUFA with risk of CRC, the inclusion criteria were: 1) Participants: Any aged adults from the same population; 2) Exposure: LC n-3 PUFA compositions in human biospecimen (serum/plasma/whole blood/erythrocytes/AT); 3) Outcomes: evaluating CRC incidence as outcome variable and providing risk ratio (RR) or odds ratio (OR) with the corresponding 95% confidence interval (CI) of CRC for all categories of LC n-3 PUFA compositions; 4) Study design: prospective studies (cohort, nested case-control and case-cohort study) and case-control study.

To investigate the differences in human biospecimens LC n-3 PUFA compositions between cases and noncases, the inclusion criteria were: 1) Participants: both the cases and noncases in each study were from the same population; 2) Outcomes: human biospecimen compositions of C22:6n-3, C22:5n-3, C20:5n-3 or total LC n-3 PUFA in cases and noncases; 3) Study design: case-control study.

Definition of exposure

In the present meta-analysis, biospecimen LC n-3 PUFA composition was defined as the sum of C22:6n-3, C22:5n-3, C20:5n-3 compositions in human biospecimens (serum/plasma/whole blood/erythrocytes/AT). Blood LC n-3 PUFA composition was defined as the sum of C22:6n-3, C22:5n-3, C20:5n-3 compositions in human blood (plasma/serum/erythrocytes/whole blood).

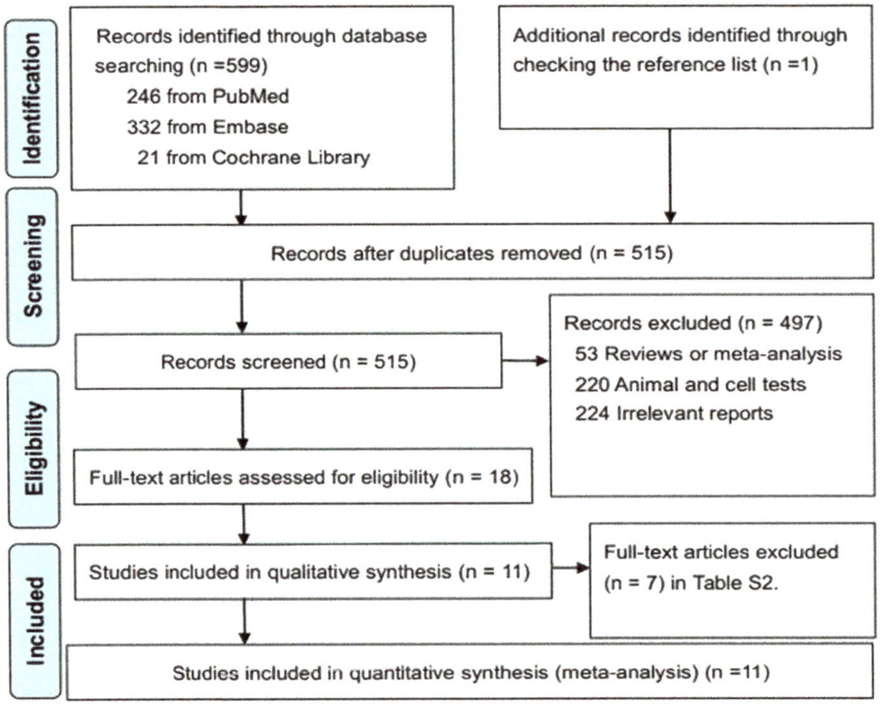

Figure 1. PRISMA Flow Diagram for included prospective cohort and case-control studies.

Table 1. Characteristics of included prospective and case-control studies in the meta-analysis of association between biospecimen long-chain n-3 PUFA and the risk of colorectal cancer.

Author (year)	Design (Nation)	Population (case/participants)	Gender (Age)	Exposure of interest: Measurement	Exposure of interest: Range (H vs. L)	Outcomes RR/OR (95%CI)	Covariates adjusted
Cottet (2013)	Cohort (France)	Subjects from E3N-EPIC cohort (328/19934)	F 40–65 y	Erythrocyte GLC (% tFC)	EPA:>1.18 vs. <0.89	0.88 (0.62–1.25)	BMI, physical activity, energy intake, alcohol consumption, smoking, educational level, menopausal status, and family history
					DHA:>7.21 vs. <6.10	0.83 (0.57–1.22)	
Pot (2008)	Case-control (Netherlands)	Subjects from the POLIEP study (498/861)	Both 18–75 y	Serum GLC (% tFC)	EPA:>1.00 vs. <0.70	0.79 (0.55–1.15)	Family history, BMI, indication for endoscopy, physical activity, smoking regular use of drugs, hormone replacement therapy, diet change due to gastrointestinal complaints, and daily intake of energy, alcohol, fat, fiber, red meat, vegetables and legumes and cholesterol.
					DHA:>0.60 vs. <0.50	0.71 (0.49–1.02)	
Ghadimi (2008)	Case-control (Japan)	Subjects form study on dietary, lifestyle factors and colon cancer (203/382)	F and M 35–75 y	Serum GLC (% tFC)	**F**:		Age, BMI, history of CRC, history of diabetes; smoking, alcohol consumption, vigorous exercise and season of data collection.
					EPA:>10.48 vs. <5.50	0.62 (0.22–1.80)	
					DPA:>1.80 vs. <1.00	1.60 (0.35–7.31)	
					DHA:>20.2 vs. <13.8	0.43 (0.14–1.38)	
					LC n-3:>32.8 vs. <21.3	0.54 (0.19–1.54)	
					M:		
					EPA:>9.50 vs. <5.70	1.22 (0.48–3.54)	
					DPA:>1.70 vs. <1.10	0.40 (0.15–1.09)	
					DHA:>19.2 vs. <14.2	2.30 (0.675–7.35)	
					LC n-3:>29.5 vs. <21.8	0.86 (0.28–2.21)	
Hall (2007)	Cohort (USA)	Subjects from the primary prevention of cancer and CVD disease (178/14916)	M 40–84 y	Whole blood GLC (% tFC)	EPA: 2.21–4.07 vs. 0.89–1.55	0.60 (0.29–1.23)	BMI, multivitamin use, history of diabetes, useof drugs, vigorous exercise, alcohol intake, and quartile of red meat intake.
					DHA: 2.83–6.22 vs. 0.69–1.87	0.69 (0.39–1.23)	
					LC n-3: 6.06–11.41 vs. 2.43–4.43	0.60 (0.32–1.11)	

Table 1. Cont.

Author (year)	Design (Nation)	Population (case/participants)	Gender (Age)	Exposure of interest		Outcomes RR/OR (95%CI)	Covariates adjusted
				Measurement	Range (H vs. L)		
Kuriki (2006)	Case-control (Japan)	Subjects form Hospital-based Epidemiologic Research Program; (74/295)	Both 20–80 y	EM; GLC (% tFC)	EPA:>1.70 vs. <1.18	0.69 (0.32–1.50)	BMI, habitual exercise, drinking and smoking status, green-yellow vegetable intake, and family history.
					DPA:>1.50 vs. <1.24	0.83 (0.34–2.05)	
					DHA:>6.10 vs. <5.06	0.36 (0.14–0.93)	
Kojima (2005)	Cohort (Japan)	Subjects from Collaborative Cohort Study for the Evaluation of Cancer Risk (JACC Study); 169/23863;	F and M 20–81y	Serum; GLC (% tFC)	**F**:		Family history, BMI, education, smoking and alcohol drinking, green leafy vegetable intake, and physical exercise
					F-EPA:>3.33 vs. <1.73	0.83 (0.39–1.80)	
					DPA:>0.94 vs. <0.66	0.64 (0.30–1.39)	
					DHA:>5.92 vs. <4.20	0.80 (0.33–1.93)	
					M:		
					EPA:>3.84 vs. <1.91	0.44 (0.18–1.08)	
					DPA:>1.02 vs. <0.68	0.30 (0.11–0.80)	
					DHA:>6.25 vs. <4.23	0.23 (0.07–0.76)	
Busstra (2003)	Case-control (Netherlands)	Subjects from colorectal adenomas study; 52/109;	Both <75 y	Adipose; GLC (% tFC)	LC n-3:>0.27 vs. <0.20	0.30 (0.10–1.10)	Age, family background, energy intake and gender

Abbreviations: H: the highest category; L: the lowest category; F: females; M: males; GLC: Gas liquid chromatography; tFC: total fatty acid; EPA: eicosapentaenoic acid (C20: 5n-3); DPA: docosapentaenoic acid (C22: 5n-3); DHA: docosahexaenoic acid (C22: 6n-3); LC n-3: long-chain n-3 polyunsaturated fatty acid (C20: 5n-3+C22: 5n-3+C22: 6n-3).

Table 2. Characteristics of included case-control studies in the mea-analysis of different long-chain n-3 PUFA compositions between subjects with and without colorectal cancer.

Author (year)	Design (Nation)	Gender (F or M)	Mean age (years)	No. of subjects		Biospecimen LC n-3 PUFA compositions (% total fatty acids)			
				Cases	Controls	Biospecimen	Subtypes	Case vs. Control (Mean ±SD)	P^a value
Okuno (2013)	Case-control (Japan)	Both	60.5	41	61	Plasma	C20:5n-3	2.27±1.14 vs 3.04±1.65	0.006
						Plasma	C22:5n-3	0.99±0.26 vs1.00±0.22	0.80
						Plasma	C22:6n-3	7.63±1.43 vs 7.84±1.59	0.49
						Erythrocyte	C20:5n-3	1.86±0.71 vs 2.23±0.85	0.02
						Erythrocyte	C22:5n-3	2.11±0.30 vs 2.12±0.27	0.93
						Erythrocyte	C22:6n-3	7.81±0.90 vs 7.90±1.06	0.64
						Adipose	C20:5n-3	0.12±0.19 vs 0.10±0.07	0.62
						Adipose	C22:5n-3	0.28±0.18 vs 0.25±0.22	0.37
						Adipose	C22:6n-3	0.58±0.32 vs 0.66±0.39	0.28
Giuliani (2013)	Case-control (Italy)	Both	60.0	52	50	Adipose	C20:5n-3	0.02 ± 0.03 vs 0.02±0.03	NS
						Adipose	C22:5n-3	0.16±0.10 vs 0.15±0.12	NS
						Adipose	C22:6n-3	0.16±0.12 vs 0.14±0.12	NS
Pot (2008)	Case-control (Netherlands)	Both	46.5	363	498	Serum	C22:5n-3	0.80±0.50 vs 0.80±0.60	NS
						Serum	C22:6n-3	0.60±0.30 vs 0.60±0.30	NS
Ghadimi (2008)	Case-control (Japan)	F	58.0	55	112	Serum	C20:5n-3	0.24±0.13 vs 0.27±0.15	0.12
						Serum	C22:5n-3	0.07±0.03 vs 0.05±0.04	0.001
						Serum	C22:6n-3	0.48±0.16 vs 0.56±0.31	0.02
						Serum	LC n-3	0.79±0.27 vs 0.88±0.54	0.18
		M	60.0	148	67	Serum	C20:5n-3	0.24±0.10 vs 0.26±0.12	0.220.
						Serum	22:5n-3	0.07±0.04 vs 0.06±0.05	001
						Serum	C22:6n-3	0.50±0.25 vs 0.57±0.20	0.06
						Serum	LC n-3	0.80±0.34 vs 0.89±0.37	0.53
Kuriki (2006)	Case-control (Japan)	Both	50.0	74	221	Erythrocyte	C20:5n-3	1.40±0.50 vs 1.50±0.60	NS
						Erythrocyte	C22:5n-3	1.40±0.40 vs 1.40±0.30	NS
						Erythrocyte	C22:6n-3	5.30±1.00 vs 5.50±1.30	NS
						Erythrocyte	LC n-3	8.10±1.60 vs 8.40±2.00	NS
Busstra (2003)	Case-control (Netherlands)	F	46.5	52	57	Adipose	LC n-3	1.10±0.09 vs 1.14±0.10	NS
Baro (1998)	Case-control (Spain)	Both	58.5	17	29	Plasma	C20:5n-3	0.96±0.19 vs 0.79±0.21	NS
						Plasma	C22:5n-3	0.70±0.05 vs 0.65±0.09	NS
						Plasma	C22:6n-3	3.02±0.18 vs 2.91±0.28	NS
						Erythrocyte	C22:6n-3	6.25±0.20 vs 6.34±0.33	NS
Fernandez-Banares (1996)	Case-control (Spain)	Both	62.0	22	12	Plasma	C20:5n-3	0.46± 0.03 vs 0.70±0.07	0.001

Table 2. Cont.

Author (year)	Design (Nation)	Gender (F or M)	Mean age (years)	No. of subjects		Biospecimen LC n-3 PUFA compositions (% total fatty acids)			
				Cases	Controls	Biospecimen	Subtypes	Case vs. Control (Mean ±SD)	P^a value
						Plasma	C22:5n-3	0.58± 0.06 vs 0.47±0.05	NS
						Plasma	C22:6n-3	3.42± 0.19 vs 3.45±0.15	NS

Abbreviations: F: females; M: males; NO.: Number; NS: no significance; LC n-3: long-chain n-3 polyunsaturated fatty acid (C20: 5n-3+C22: 5n-3+C22: 6n-3).
[a]P value for different LC n-3 PUFA compositions between cases and controls.

Data extraction

Data extraction was finished independently and performed twice by two reviewers (XLR and FLW), and disagreements were reconciled by consensus. The following data were extracted form each original study: participant characteristics (e.g., nationality, age, gender and number of participants), biospecimen LC n-3 composition as exposure of interest (e.g., measurement method, exposure source, and exposure range), biospecimen compositions of C22:6n-3, C22:5n-3, C20:5n-3 and total LC n-3 PUFA in cases and noncases, adjusted covariates and RR (OR) including 95% CI for all categories of LC n-3 PUFA composition. Our search was restricted to human studies, and we did not contact authors for the detailed information of primary studies and unpublished studies.

Statistic analysis

We conducted two types of meta-analysis. Firstly, we performed a meta-analysis for the highest category vs. lowest. Multivariate adjusted RR (OR) for the highest vs lowest category to assess the association of biospecimen LC n-3 with CRC risk from each original study was firstly transformed to their logarithm (logRR or logOR), and the corresponding 95% CIs were used to calculate corresponding standard errors (selogRR or selogOR). Summary RR (SRR) including corresponding 95% CI as the summary risk estimate for all prospective and case-control studies was estimated using a random-effects model [27], which considers both within-study and between-study variability. The second meta-analysis was that the differences in biospecimen compositions of C22:6n-3, C22:5n-3, C20:5n-3 and total LC n-3 compositions between cases and noncases were also analyzed as standardized mean difference (SMD) by pooling the data from case-control studies, respectively. Heterogeneity among studies was assessed with the Q test and I^2 statistic. I^2 statistic describes the proportion of total variation attributable to between-study heterogeneity as opposed to random error or chance. We defined the low, moderate and high degrees of heterogeneity by I^2 values of 25%, 50% and 75% as cut-off points [28], and considered an I^2 value greater than 50% as indicative of heterogeneity according to Cochrane Handbook. In the presence of substantial heterogeneity, stratified analysis was conducted to identify the possible sources of heterogeneity by study design (case-control and prospective study), different regions (Asia and West (Europe and USA)), gender (women and men) and biospecimen types (blood and adipose tissue). Meta-regression with restricted maximum likelihood (REML) estimation was conducted to assess the potentially important covariates exerting substantial impact on between-study heterogeneity. Sensitivity analysis was performed to evaluate possible influence of individual study with potential bias on overall risk. Publication bias was quantitatively examined by Begg's test and Egger's regression test [29].

Furthermore, the dose-response association of biospecimen LC n-3 PUFA with CRC risk was performed in the present study. Original studies with 3 or more categories were included in the dose-response analysis. Midpoint of upper and lower boundaries was taken as the dose of the quantile if the study only reported the range; if the highest quantile was open-ended, its dose was regarded as 1.2-fold the highest boundary [30]; if the lowest quantile or reference category was open-ended, the midpoint of lowest boundary and zero was taken as the dose of lowest quantile. A nonlinear (curvilinear) trend was tested by using a 2-stage random-effects dose-response meta-analysis [31,32]. The compositionof LC n-3 PUFA in biospecimen was modeled by using restricted cubic splines with 3 knots (2 spline transformations) at percentiles (25%, 50%, and 75%) of the distribution [33]. A P-value for nonlinearity was calculated by testing the null hypothesis that the coefficient of the second spline is equal to zero [34]. In the

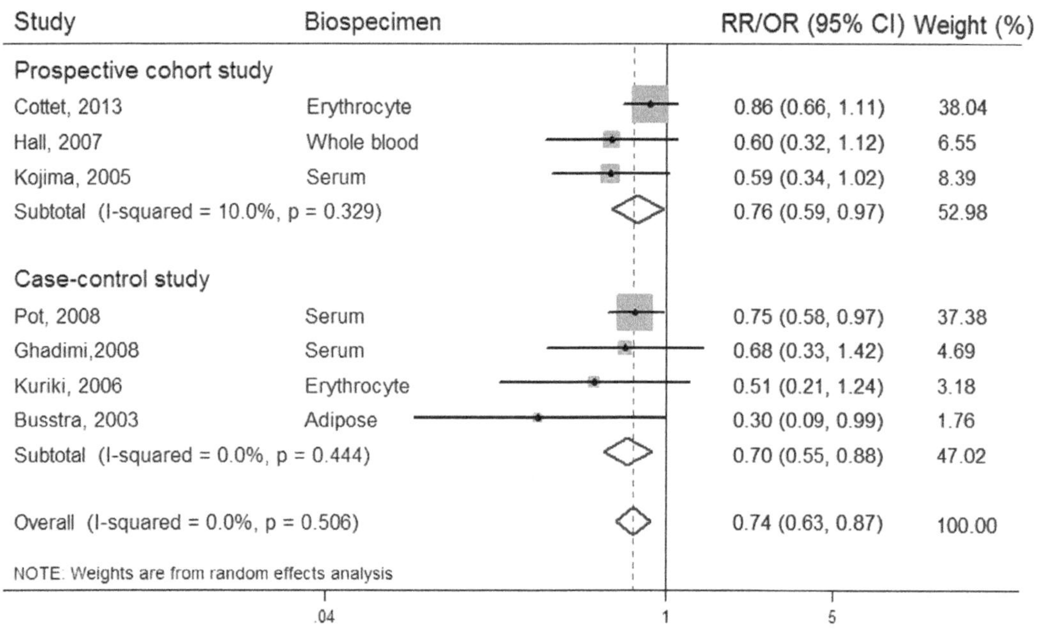

Figure 2. Forest plot corresponding to the random-effects meta-analysis quantifying the relationship between LC n-3 PUFA composition and CRC risk for the highest vs. lowest category. Relative risks (RRs) or odds ratios (ORs) compared the highest vs. lowest category of biospecimen LC n-3 PUFA composition and were grouped by study designs. The size of the gray box representing each risk estimate was proportional to the weight that the risk estimate contributed to the summary risk estimate. The diamonds denoted summary risk estimate.

presence of substantial linear trends (P-value for nonlinearity >0.05), a linear dose-response analysis [32] was conducted to examine the association between every 1% increment of LC n-3 PUFA composition in biospecimens and the risk of CRC. Statistical analyses of the combined data were performed by STATA version 11.0 (Stata CORP, College Station, TX). P-value less than 0.05 were considered statistically significant in the present study.

Results

Study characteristics

We identified 599 potential studies from electronic search, and 515 studies were left after removing duplicates. Eleven relevant studies were eligible for the present study after full text review (Figure 1; Table S1). A total of 1,499 CRC cases among 60,627 participants were included in the present study, separately from 3 prospective cohort [18–20] and 8 case-control studies [15–17,21–25]. Of the 3 cohort studies, 2 studies were conducted in West (Europe [19] and USA [20]), and 1 study was conducted in Japan [18]. Of the 8 case-control studies, 5 studies were conducted in Europe [15,16,22,24,25], and 3 studies were conducted in Japan [17,21,23]. Of the 11 included studies, 6 studies assessed serum (plasma) biomarker of LC n-3 composition [15,18,20,21,23–25], 4 studies assessed RBC biomarker [17,19,21,24], 1 study [20] assessed whole blood biomarker and 3 studies assessed AT biomarker [16,21,22]. LC n-3 PUFA compositions in biospecimens were quantified by gas liquid chromatography (GLC), and measurement unit was percentage of total fatty acids (% tFC) except for 1 study (mg/dL) [23]. Two studies separately provided data of males (M) and females (F) [18,23], 1 study only provided data of females [19], and 1 study only provided data of males [20]. For the analysis on association between biospecimen LC n-3 PUFA and CRC risk, the characteristics of included 3 prospective cohort and 4 case-control studies were summarized in Table 1.

For the analysis of different biospecimen LC n-3 PUFA compositions between subjects with CRC (cases) and control subjects without CRC (noncases), the characteristics of included 8 case-control studies were summarized in Table 2.

Highest vs lowest category

Overall, 3 prospective cohort [18–20] and 4 case-control studies [15–17,23] were eligible for the meta-analysis on the association of LC n-3 PUFA composition in biospecimens with CRC risk, comprising 60,360 participants. A significantly inverse association between biospecimens LC n-3 PUFA and CRC risk was observed in 60,360 participants (summary RR = 0.74; 95% CI: 0.63, 0.87), with no between-study heterogeneity ($I^2 = 0.00\%$) (Figure 2). Biospecimen C20:5n-3 and C22:6n-3 were both inversely associated with the risk of CRC, and the summary RR was 0.78 (95% CI: 0.64, 0.96; $I^2 = 0.00\%$) and 0.68 (95% CI: 0.54, 0.84; $I^2 = 0.00\%$), respectively (Table 3). However, no significant association was found of biospecimen C22:5n-3 with CRC risk in 15,593 participants from 1 prospective and case-control studies (summary OR = 0.80; 95% CI: 0.42, 1.52; $I^2 = 47.60\%$).

In stratified analysis (Table 3), there was no evidence that the estimated summary RR differed significantly by sex (P for meta-regression = 0.14). We further focused on the difference in pooled association estimate between prospective cohort and case-control study. In 3 cohort studies, biospecimen C20:5n-3, C22:6n-3 and LC n-3 PUFA was all significantly associated with the lower risk of CRC, and the pooled RR was 0.77 (95% CI: 0.58, 1.00; $I^2 = 0.00\%$), 0.76 (95% CI: 0.56, 1.01; $I^2 = 0.00\%$), and 0.76 (95% CI: 0.59, 0.97; $I^2 = 10.00\%$), respectively. However, only one prospective cohort study separately reported an association between serum C22:5n-3 and CRC risk in Japan males and females [18], and the pooled RR is 0.47 (95% CI: 0.23, 0.97; $I^2 = 28.60\%$). In 4 case-control studies, higher biospecimen LC n-3 composition was also significantly associated with a lower risk of CRC (pooled OR = 0.70; 95% CI: 0.55, 0.88; $I^2 = 0.00\%$),

Table 3. Subgroup analysis for association between biospecimen long-chain n-3 PUFA and risk of colorectal cancer.

Factors stratified	C20:5n-3					C22:6n-3					LC n-3 PUFA				
	N^a	SRR (95% CI)	Heterogeneity		P^c	N	SRR (95% CI)	Heterogeneity		P	N	SRR (95% CI)	Heterogeneity		P
			I^2 (%)	P^b				I^2 (%)	P				I^2 (%)	P	
Overall analysis	6	0.78 (0.64, 0.96)	0.00	0.89		6	0.68 (0.54, 0.84)	0.00	0.42		7	0.74 (0.63, 0.87)	0.00	0.50	
Study design					0.93					0.37					0.63
PC	3	0.77 (0.58, 1.00)	0.00	0.49		3	0.76 (0.56, 1.01)	0.00	0.30		3	0.76 (0.59, 0.97)	10.00	0.33	
CC	3	0.79 (0.58, 1.05)	0.00	0.89		3	0.55 (0.36, 0.85)	30.60	0.00		4	0.70 (0.55, 0.88)	0.00	0.45	
Regions					0.65					0.10					0.30
West (USA and Europe)	4	0.81 (0.63, 1.02)	0.00	0.64		3	0.75 (0.59, 0.96)	0.00	0.80		4	0.76 (0.61, 0.93)	19.70	0.29	
Asia	2	0.72 (0.48, 1.07)	0.00	0.77		3	0.34 (0.13, 0.85)	43.00	0.17		3	0.60 (0.40, 0.89)	0.00	0.88	
Gender					0.42					0.24					0.14
Female	3	0.85 (0.62, 1.15)	0.00	0.82		2	0.78 (0.56, 1.09)	0.00	0.56		3	0.83 (0.66, 1.05)	0.00	0.70	
Male	3	0.65 (0.19,1.11)	13.00	0.32		5	0.47 (0.26, 0.88)	33.00	0.22		3	0.53 (0.33, 0.84)	13.70	0.32	
Biospecimens					0.68					0.58					0.73
Serum	3	0.77 (0.57, 1.02)	0.00	0.57		3	0.63 (0.45, 0.86)	0.00	0.38		3	0.71 (0.57, 0.89)	0.00	0.73	
Erythrocytes	2	0.80 (0.60, 1.06)	0.00	0.74		2	0.70 (0.48, 1.01)	23.50	0.27		2	0.79 (0.55, 1.15)	17.80	0.27	
Whole blood	1	0.80 (0.60, 1.06)	.	.		1	0.69 (0.39, 1.23)	.	.		1	0.60 (0.32, 1.12)	.	.	

Abbreviations: LC n-3: long-chain n-3 polyunsaturated fatty acid (C20: 5n-3+C22: 5n-3+C22: 6n-3); SRR: summary risk ratio; PC: prospective cohort study; CC: case-control study.
[a]*N*, number of included studies.
[b]*P* value for heterogeneity within subgroup.
[c]*P* value for heterogeneity between subgroups with meta-regression analysis.

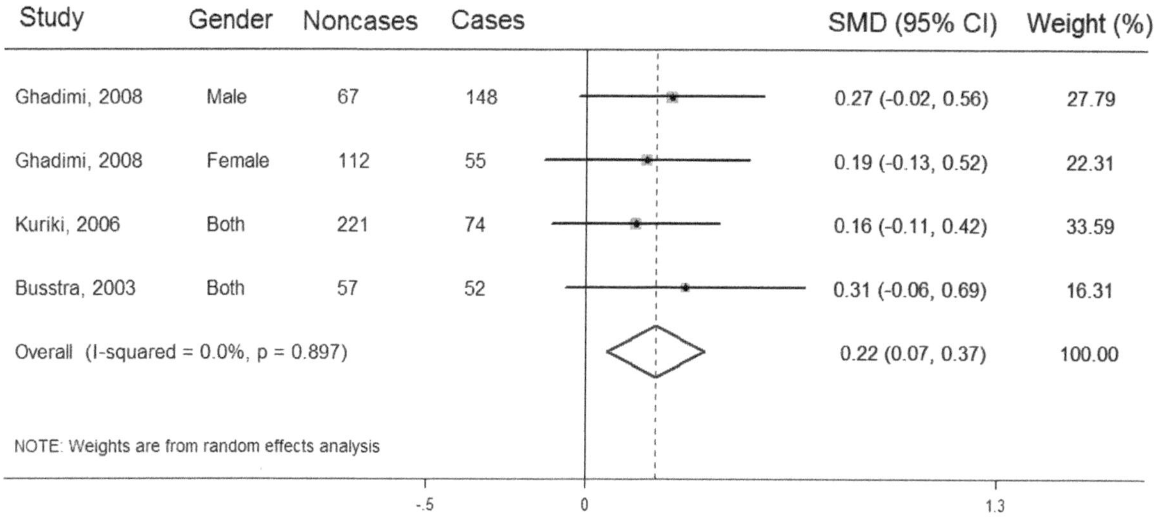

Figure 3. Forest plot corresponding to the random-effects meta-analysis analysis on difference in biospecimen compositions of LC n-3 PUFA between cases and noncases. Case-control studies are referred to by first author, year of publication, gender and biospecimen types. The combined standardized mean difference (SMD) was achieved using random-effects model. Grey square represents SMD in each study, with square size reflecting the study-specific weight and the 95% CI represented by horizontal bars. SMD from individual study were pooled by random effect model. The diamond indicates summary SMD.

especially biospecimen C22:6n-3 (pooled OR = 0.55; 95% CI: 0.36, 0.85; I^2 = 30.60%), whereas biospecimen C20:5n-3 exhibited no significant association (pooled OR = 0.79; 95% CI: 0.58, 1.05; I^2 = 0.00%). There were 2 case-control studies reported the association of biospecimen C22:5n-3 with CRC risk [17,23], and the pooled OR is 1.25 (95% CI: 0.65, 2.41; I^2 = 0.00%). However, the results of the meta-regression did not show the significant difference between the two study designs. No evidence of significant difference was found between other subgroups with meta-regression (Table 3).

In a sensitivity analysis, we sequentially omitted 1 study at a time and reanalyzed the remaining data. We found that exclusion of any individual study did not substantially change the overall association. In publication bias analysis, there was also no indication of publication bias as suggested by visual inspection of Begg's funnel plot (*P* for bias = 0.452) and Egger's regression test (*P* for bias = 0.175).

Difference in LC n-3 PUFA compositions between cases and noncases

There were 4 case-control studies eligible for the analysis of different biospecimen total LC n-3 PUFA composition between cases and noncases [15–17,23]. Compared with 329 cases, 457 noncases have a significantly higher LC n-3 PUFA composition in biospecimens (SMD: 0.22; 95% CI: 0.07, 0.37), with no between-study heterogeneity (I^2 = 0.00%) (Figure 3). Similarly, there were 7 case-control studies eligible for analyses on different biospecimen C20:5n-3 and C22:6n-3 composition between cases and noncases [15,17,21–25], respectively. Compared with 623 CRC cases, 1315 noncases have significantly higher biospecimen C20:5n-3 (SMD: 0.27; 95% CI: 0.13, 0.41; I^2 = 36.20%) and C22:6n-3 composition (SMD: 0.23; 95% CI: 0.11, 0.34; I^2 = 0.00%) (Table 4). However, no significant difference was found in biospecimen C22:5n-3 composition between 587 cases and 817 noncases from 6 case-control studies (SMD: −0.08; 95% CI: −0.22, 0.06; I^2 = 17.60%) (Table 4).

Stratified analysis indicated that there was a significantly higher blood C20:5n-3 and C22:6n-3 compositions in noncases compared with cases, whereas adipose tissue C20:5n-3 and C22:6n-3 compositions exhibited no significant difference between cases and noncases (Table 4). Results from meta-regression only showed a significant difference in C20:5n-3 composition between the two biospecimens (*P* value = 0.05). Furthermore, biospecimen compositions of C20:5n-3 and C22:6n-3 were both significantly higher in Asian noncases compared with cases, whereas no significant difference was observed in Western noncases compared with cases. There was no significant difference between the two populations with meta-regression (Table 4).

Dose-response analysis

Four eligible studies were available to evaluate the dose-response association of biospecimen LC n-3 PUFA with CRC risk [16,17,20,23], and there was a significantly nonlinear trend in 15,593 participants (*P* for nonlinearity = 0.01; *P* for trend = 0.01) (Figure 4D). Six eligible studies were available to evaluate the dose-response analysis on relationship of biospecimen C20:5n-3 and C22:6n-3 with CRC risk in 60,291 participants [15,17–20,23], respectively (Figure 4 A and C). A significantly nonlinear dose-response association was observed between biospecimen C20:5n-3 and CRC risk (*P* for nonlinearity = 0.021; *P* for trend = 0.001). The nonlinear association between biospecimen C22:6n-3 and CRC risk was not significant (*P* for nonlinearity = 0.10), but the overall association in the linear dose-response model was significant (*P* for trend = 0.012), with a 1% increment of biospecimen C22:6n-3 composition associated with 5% reduced risk of CRC (pooled RR = 0.95; 95% CI: 0.92, 0.98; I^2 = 15.00%). Likewise, three relevant studies were available to evaluate the dose-response relationship between biospecimen C22:5n-3 and CRC risk [17,18,23], but no significant nonlinear and linear trend was observed in 24,540 individuals, respectively (*P* for nonlinearity = 0.10; *P* for trend = 0.38) (Figure 4B).

Discussion

To our knowledge, this is the first meta-analysis evaluating an association between biospecimen LC n-3 PUFA and CRC risk.

Table 4. Subgroup analysis for different biospecimen long-chain n-3 PUFA compositions between subjects with and without CRC.

Factors stratified	C20:5n-3					C22:5n-3					C22:6n-3				
	N^a	SMD (95% CI)	Heterogeneity		P^c	N	SMD (95% CI)	Heterogeneity		P	N	SMD (95% CI)	Heterogeneity		P
			I^2 (%)	P^b				I^2 (%)	P				I^2 (%)	P	
Overall analysis	7	0.27 (0.13, 0.41)	36.20	0.18		6	−0.08 (−0.22, 0.06)	17.60	0.17		7	0.23 (0.11, 0.34)	0.00	0.38	
Region					0.74					0.12					0.45
West	4	0.29 (−0.10, 0.67)	56.00	0.07		3	−0.33 (−0.64, 0.00)	0.00	0.43		4	0.30 (−0.06, 0.67)	51.00	0.08	
East	3	0.24 (0.08, 0.40)	27.90	0.23		3	−0.02 (−0.16, 0.11)	0.00	0.44		3	0.24 (0.11, 0.38)	0.00	0.94	
Gender					0.90					0.22					0.25
Female	1	0.22 (−0.10, 0.55)	.	.		1	−0.28 (−0.61, 0.04)	.	.		1	0.29 (−0.04, 0.61)	.	.	
Male	1	0.34 (0.14, 0.55)	.	.		1	0.05 (−0.15, 0.25)	.	.		1	0.37 (0.21, 0.52)	.	.	
Both	5	0.26 (0.05, 0.46)	50.10	0.05		5	−0.03 (−0.28, 0.05)	12.60	0.33		5	0.18 (0.03, 0.33)	10.80	0.34	
Biospecimens					0.05					0.54					0.55
Blood	5	0.30 (0.15, 0.44)	17.60	0.27		4	−0.04 (−0.20, 0.11)	26.70	0.12		5	0.24 (0.10, 0.40)	18.0	0.25	
Adipose	2	−0.07 (−0.35, 0.20)	0.00	0.59		2	−0.02 (−0.35, 0.30)	28.10	0.24		2	0.19 (−0.09, 0.47)	0.00	0.84	

Abbreviations: CRC, colorectal cancer; *N*: number of included case-control studies; PC: prospective cohort study; CC: case-control study; SMD: standard mean difference compared with colorectal cancer subjects.
[a] *N*, number of included studies.
[b] *P* value for heterogeneity within each subgroup.
[c] *P* value for heterogeneity between subgroups with meta-regression analysis.

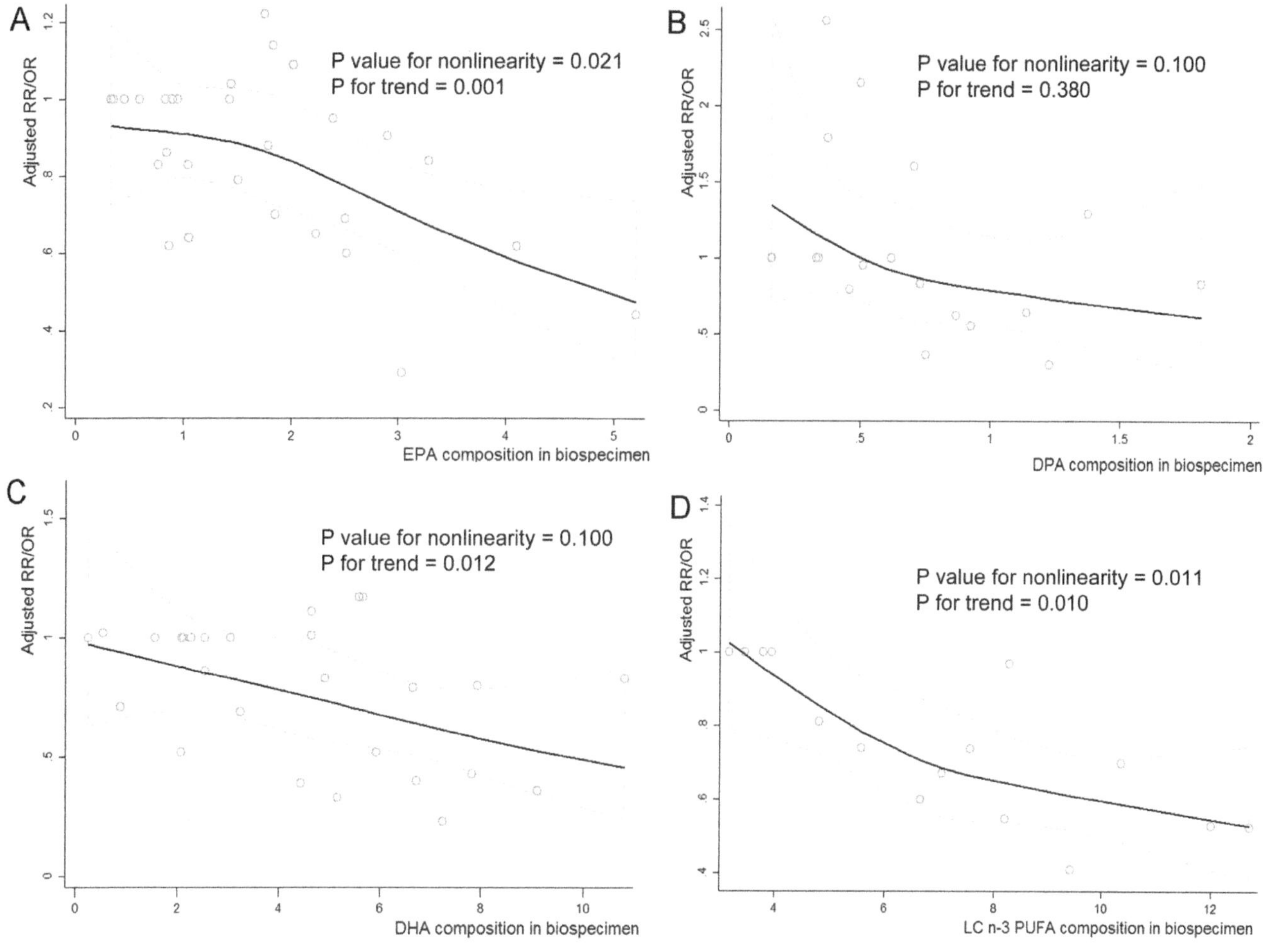

Figure 4. Nonlinear dose-response trend analysis assessed by restricted cubic spline model with three knots. Adjusted ORs (RRs) from all category of biospecimen C20:5n-3, C22:5n-3, C22:6n-3 and total LC n-3 PUFA in each study were separately represented by the small gray circle in the figure A, B, C and D, and corresponding nonlinear dose-response relationship was represented by the black solid line shown in figure A, B, C, and D by using restricted cubic splines functional model with three knots at percentiles 25%, 50%, and 75% of the distribution, respectively.

Overall, our findings suggested that biospecimen composition of LC n-3 PUFA was inversely associated with CRC risk, especially C20:5n-3 and C22:6n-3. Tissue compositions of C20:5n-3, C22:6n-3 and total LC n-3 PUFA were all significantly lower in CRC subjects compared with controls without CRC.

There are several hypothesized mechanisms explaining the possible protective role of tissue LC n-3 PUFA in the etiology of CRC carcinogenesis. The lower composition of LC n-3 PUFA in cases was observed in the present study, suggesting that the characteristic LC n-3 PUFA composition in biospecimen may be involved in the mechanism of CRC progression. Firstly, LC n-3 PUFA existing in biomembrane phospholipids has been found to be involved in the regulation of downstream receptor activity, cell proliferation and apoptosis process by alternation of the fluidity, structure and/or function of lipid rafts or caveolae located in cell surface [13,35,36]. In addition, LC n-3 PUFA, especially C20:5n-3, can may modulate cyclooxygenases (COX) activity, leading to the reduction of n-6 family derived 2-series PG (e.g., PGE_2) with promoting tumor growth effects [37] in favor of n-3 family derived 3-series PG (e.g., PGE_3) with suppressive effects in several cell types including CRC cells [38,39]. Lastly, LC n-3 PUFA may have an antineoplastic effect through alteration in the cellular redox state and increased oxidative stress. The evidence from experimental studies indicated that the oxidative stress and colonocyte apoptosis induced by the fermentation product short-chain fatty acid butyrate might be potentiated by both intrinsic and extrinsic apoptosis pathways medicated by C22:6n-3 [36,40].

In subgroup analyses by study design for the highest category vs lowest, the pooled association estimates of LC n-3 PUFA including the specific subtypes were all significant in prospective cohort studies, although the pooled estimate of C20:5n-3 and C22:5n-3 from case-control studies did not reach statistical significance. Prospective cohort studies greatly decreased the possibility of recall bias and selection biases, which are always inherent in retrospective case-control studies, in view of exposure information was collected before suffering from the disease. Thus, prospective cohort designs are warranted to elucidate causal relationships. In addition, the difference in the number and types of the potential covariates adjusted in multivariable statistic models probably resulted in the discrepant results between cohort and case-control studies. Therefore, we cannot exclude the possibility that the true associations might be distorted in case-control studies adjusting for few confounding factors. For the stratified analysis of LC n-3 PUFA composition between cases and noncases by biospecimen types, blood (serum/plasma/erythrocytes) compositions of LC n-3 PUFA revealed that a statistically significant difference between cases and noncases, but not AT. The heterogeneity between the two biospecimens may be partially explained by different metabolic characteristics of these human biospecimens (serum/plasma/erythrocyte/AT) as biomarkers. Plasma (serum) biomarker represents a combination of triacylglycerol, cholesterol esters and phospholipids found in lipoproteins, and reflects dietary intakes of the past few hours or days [41]. Determination of LC n-3 PUFA composition in erythrocytes provides a biomarker for over several weeks, considering that the half-life of erythrocytes is 120 days [42]. Conversely, AT biomarker represents mostly triacylglycerol, and reflects long-term dietary intake of fatty acids, mainly because of its slow turnover and lack of response to acute diseases. However, given that concentrations of PUFA are very low in AT [43], this tissue does not seem to be a perfect biomarker of LC n-3 PUFA. Furthermore, although biospecimen compositions of fatty acids were mainly determined by GLC in these observational studies, all measurement steps may be accomplished by different methodological procedures, chemicals, and equipments. Hence, the difference between blood and AT biomarker of LC n-3 PUFA may be partly attributed to no agreed standard procedures.

Several strengths could be highlighted in our study. Firstly, our present study showed a characteristic biospecimen compositions of LC n-3 PUFA associated with CRC risk, and further analyzed the difference in the compositions of biospecimen LC n-3 PUFA between CRC cases and noncases. In addition, a biomarker as an indicator of some biological state or condition can closely reflect an integrated measurement of diet over time, thus recall bias might not occur in case-control studies. Finally, no evidence of potential publication bias was observed in the present study, though publication bias could be of concern because small studies with null results tend not to be published. In addition, there are also several potential limitations in the present study. Firstly, meta-analyses of observational studies are susceptible to inherent biases (e.g., report biases and unknown residual confoundings), which might have affected the summarized results. Secondly, selection bias might be unavoidable, due to inclusion of case-control studies with regards to elucidating causal relationships. Thirdly, data on association of tissue biomarker with colon or rectal cancer risk was not provided by the original studies, respectively. Given that therapeutic strategy for colon cancer and rectal cancer may differ [2,44], future epidemiological studies should further investigate whether LC n-3 PUFA in human tissues could be beneficial for colon or rectal cancer, respectively. Fourthly, the limited numbers of cohort studies included in this meta-analysis might diminish the statistical power to detect the association between biospecimen LC n-3 PUFA and CRC risk. Therefore, care must be exercised in the extrapolation of our findings to larger populations of CRC individuals.

In conclusion, this meta-analysis provided a sufficient evidence that human biospecimen LC n-3 composition was inversely associated with the risk of CRC, especially C20:5n-3 and C22:6n-3. Populations without CRC have higher tissue compositions of C20:5n-3, C22:6n-3 and total LC n-3 PUFA than those with CRC. These evidences have important public health implications for CRC prevention. LC n-3 PUFA profile in human tissues may be an independent predictive factor for CRC risk. Future epidemiological studies should focus on whether the risk of colon or rectal cancer could be modified by increasing LC n-3 PUFA composition in human tissues, respectively. Nevertheless, the protective effect of human tissue LC n-3 PUFA on CRC risk needs to be replicated by further large-scale prospective studies.

Supporting Information

Checklist S1 MOOSE Checklist of the Present Meta-Analysis.

Table S1 Observational studies Excluded from Meta-Analysis.

Author Contributions

Wrote the paper: BY DL. Study conception and design: DL BY. Acquisition of data: FLW XLR. Analysis and interpretation of data: BY FLW.

References

1. Butler LM, Wang R, Koh WP, Yu MC (2008) Prospective study of dietary patterns and colorectal cancer among Singapore Chinese. Br J Cancer 99: 1511–1516.
2. Cai F, Dupertuis YM, Pichard C (2012) Role of polyunsaturated fatty acids and lipid peroxidation on colorectal cancer risk and treatments. Curr Opin Clin Nutr Metab Care 15: 99–106.
3. Ji BT, Devesa SS, Chow WH, Jin F, Gao YT (1998) Colorectal cancer incidence trends by subsite in urban Shanghai, 1972–1994. Cancer Epidemiol Biomarkers Prev 7: 661–666.
4. Penkov A, Popov B (2011) Diet and colorectal cancer. Annals of Nutrition and Metabolism 58: 375–376.
5. Zhong X, Fang YJ, Pan ZZ, Li B, Wang L, et al. (2013) Dietary fat, fatty acid intakes and colorectal cancer risk in Chinese adults: A case-control study. European Journal of Cancer Prevention 22: 438–447.
6. Murff HJ, Shrubsole MJ, Cai Q, Smalley WE, Dai Q, et al. (2012) Dietary intake of PUFAs and colorectal polyp risk. Am J Clin Nutr 95: 703–712.
7. Liu L, Zhuang W, Wang RQ, Mukherjee R, Xiao SM, et al. (2011) Is dietary fat associated with the risk of colorectal cancer? A meta-analysis of 13 prospective cohort studies. Eur J Nutr 50: 173–184.
8. Song M, Chan AT, Fuchs CS, Ogino S, Hu FB, et al. (2014) Dietary intake of fish, omega-3 and omega-6 fatty acids and risk of colorectal cancer: A prospective study in U.S. men and women. Int J Cancer.
9. Pham NM, Mizoue T, Tanaka K, Tsuji I, Tamakoshi A, et al. (2013) Fish consumption and colorectal cancer risk: an evaluation based on a systematic review of epidemiologic evidence among the Japanese population. Jpn J Clin Oncol 43: 935–941.
10. Shen XJ, Zhou JD, Dong JY, Ding WQ, Wu JC (2012) Dietary intake of n-3 fatty acids and colorectal cancer risk: A meta-analysis of data from 489000 individuals. British Journal of Nutrition 108: 1550–1556.
11. Geelen A, Schouten JM, Kamphuis C, Stam BE, Burema J, et al. (2007) Fish consumption, n-3 fatty acids, and colorectal cancer: A meta-analysis of prospective cohort studies. American Journal of Epidemiology 166: 1116–1125.
12. Yang T, Fang S, Zhang HX, Xu LX, Zhang ZQ, et al. (2013) N-3 PUFAs have antiproliferative and apoptotic effects on human colorectal cancer stem-like cells in vitro. J Nutr Biochem 24: 744–753.
13. Turk HF, Chapkin RS (2013) Membrane lipid raft organization is uniquely modified by n-3 polyunsaturated fatty acids. Prostaglandins Leukot Essent Fatty Acids 88: 43–47.
14. Kansal S, Bhatnagar A, Agnihotri N (2014) Fish oil suppresses cell growth and metastatic potential by regulating PTEN and NF-kappaB signaling in colorectal cancer. PLoS One 9: e84627.
15. Pot GK, Geelen A, van Heijningen EM, Siezen CL, van Kranen HJ, et al. (2008) Opposing associations of serum n-3 and n-6 polyunsaturated fatty acids with colorectal adenoma risk: an endoscopy-based case-control study. Int J Cancer 123: 1974–1977.
16. Busstra MC, Siezen CLE, Grubben MJAL, Van Kranen HJ, Nagengast FM, et al. (2003) Tissue levels of fish fatty acids and risk of colorectal adenomas: A case-control study (Netherlands). Cancer Causes and Control 14: 269–276.
17. Kuriki K, Wakai K, Hirose K, Matsuo K, Ito H, et al. (2006) Risk of colorectal cancer is linked to erythrocyte compositions of fatty acids as biomarkers for dietary intakes of fish, fat, and fatty acids. Cancer Epidemiol Biomarkers Prev 15: 1791–1798.
18. Kojima M, Wakai K, Tokudome S, Suzuki K, Tamakoshi K, et al. (2005) Serum levels of polyunsaturated fatty acids and risk of colorectal cancer: A prospective study. American Journal of Epidemiology 161: 462–471.
19. Cottet V, Collin M, Gross AS, Boutron-Ruault MC, Morois S, et al. (2013) Erythrocyte membrane phospholipid fatty acid concentrations and risk of colorectal adenomas: a case-control nested in the French E3N-EPIC cohort study. Cancer Epidemiol Biomarkers Prev 22: 1417–1427.

20. Hall MN, Campos H, Li H, Sesso HD, Stampfer MJ, et al. (2007) Blood levels of long-chain polyunsaturated fatty acids, aspirin, and the risk of colorectal cancer. Cancer Epidemiol Biomarkers Prev 16: 314–321.
21. Okuno M, Hamazaki K, Ogura T, Kitade H, Matsuura T, et al. (2013) Abnormalities in fatty acids in plasma, erythrocytes and adipose tissue in Japanese patients with colorectal cancer. In Vivo 27: 203–210.
22. Giuliani A, Ferrara F, Scimo M, Angelico F, Olivieri L, et al. (2013) Adipose tissue fatty acid composition and colon cancer: a case-control study. Eur J Nutr.
23. Ghadimi R, Kuriki K, Tsuge S, Takeda E, Imaeda N, et al. (2008) Serum concentrations of fatty acids and colorectal adenoma risk: a case-control study in Japan. Asian Pac J Cancer Prev 9: 111–118.
24. Baro L, Hermoso JC, Nunez MC, Jimenez-Rios JA, Gil A (1998) Abnormalities in plasma and red blood cell fatty acid profiles of patients with colorectal cancer. Br J Cancer 77: 1978–1983.
25. Fernandez-Banares F, Esteve M, Navarro E, Cabre E, Boix J, et al. (1996) Changes of the mucosal n3 and n6 fatty acid status occur early in the colorectal adenoma-carcinoma sequence. Gut 38: 254–259.
26. Stroup DF, Berlin JA, Morton SC, Olkin I, Williamson GD, et al. (2000) Meta-analysis of observational studies in epidemiology: a proposal for reporting. Meta-analysis Of Observational Studies in Epidemiology (MOOSE) group. JAMA 283: 2008–2012.
27. DerSimonian R, Laird N (1986) Meta-analysis in clinical trials. Control Clin Trials 7: 177–188.
28. Higgins JP, Thompson SG, Deeks JJ, Altman DG (2003) Measuring inconsistency in meta-analyses. BMJ 327: 557–560.
29. Egger M, Davey Smith G, Schneider M, Minder C (1997) Bias in meta-analysis detected by a simple, graphical test. BMJ 315: 629–634.
30. Liu Q, Cook NR, Bergström A, Hsieh CC (2009) A two-stage hierarchical regression model for meta-analysis of epidemiologic nonlinear dose–response data. Computational Statistics & Data Analysis 53: 4157–4167.
31. Jackson D, White IR, Thompson SG (2010) Extending DerSimonian and Laird's methodology to perform multivariate random effects meta-analyses. Stat Med 29: 1282–1297.
32. Orsini N, Bellocco R, Greenland S (2006) Generalized least squares for trend estimation of summarized dose-response data. Stata Journal 6: 40–57.
33. Harrell FE Jr, Lee KL, Pollock BG (1988) Regression models in clinical studies: determining relationships between predictors and response. J Natl Cancer Inst 80: 1198–1202.
34. Orsini N, Li R, Wolk A, Khudyakov P, Spiegelman D (2012) Meta-analysis for linear and nonlinear dose-response relations: examples, an evaluation of approximations, and software. Am J Epidemiol 175: 66–73.
35. Rogers KR, Kikawa KD, Mouradian M, Hernandez K, McKinnon KM, et al. (2010) Docosahexaenoic acid alters epidermal growth factor receptor-related signaling by disrupting its lipid raft association. Carcinogenesis 31: 1523–1530.
36. Hull MA (2011) Omega-3 polyunsaturated fatty acids. Best Pract Res Clin Gastroenterol 25: 547–554.
37. Hawcroft G, Loadman PM, Belluzzi A, Hull MA (2010) Effect of eicosapentaenoic acid on E-type prostaglandin synthesis and EP4 receptor signaling in human colorectal cancer cells. Neoplasia 12: 618–627.
38. Hopkins GJ, Kennedy TG, Carroll KK (1981) Polyunsaturated fatty acids as promoters of mammary carcinogenesis induced in Sprague-Dawley rats by 7,12-dimethylbenz[a]anthracene. J Natl Cancer Inst 66: 517–522.
39. Poole EM, Bigler J, Whitton J, Sibert JG, Kulmacz RJ, et al. (2007) Genetic variability in prostaglandin synthesis, fish intake and risk of colorectal polyps. Carcinogenesis 28: 1259–1263.
40. Kolar SS, Barhoumi R, Callaway ES, Fan YY, Wang N, et al. (2007) Synergy between docosahexaenoic acid and butyrate elicits p53-independent apoptosis via mitochondrial Ca(2+) accumulation in colonocytes. Am J Physiol Gastrointest Liver Physiol 293: G935–943.
41. Kohlmeier L (1995) Future of dietary exposure assessment. Am J Clin Nutr 61: 702S–709S.
42. Theret N, Bard JM, Nuttens MC, Lecerf JM, Delbart C, et al. (1993) The relationship between the phospholipid fatty acid composition of red blood cells, plasma lipids, and apolipoproteins. Metabolism 42: 562–568.
43. Hirsch J, Farquhar JW, Ahrens EH Jr, Peterson ML, Stoffel W (1960) Studies of adipose tissue in man. A microtechnic for sampling and analysis. Am J Clin Nutr 8: 499–511.
44. Cockbain AJ, Toogood GJ, Hull MA (2012) Omega-3 polyunsaturated fatty acids for the treatment and prevention of colorectal cancer. Gut 61: 135–149.

14

Integrated Exon Level Expression Analysis of Driver Genes Explain Their Role in Colorectal Cancer

Mohammad Azhar Aziz[1]*, Sathish Periyasamy[2], Zeyad Al Yousef[3], Ibrahim AlAbdulkarim[1], Majed Al Otaibi[1], Abdulaziz Alfahed[1], Glowi Alasiri[1]

1 Medical Genomics, King Abdullah International Medical Research Center, Riyadh, Saudi Arabia, **2** Bioinformatics, King Abdullah International Medical Research Center, Riyadh, Saudi Arabia, **3** Surgery, National Guard Health Affairs, Riyadh, Saudi Arabia

Abstract

Integrated analysis of genomic and transcriptomic level changes holds promise for a better understanding of colorectal cancer (CRC) biology. There is a pertinent need to explain the functional effect of genome level changes by integrating the information at the transcript level. Using high resolution cytogenetics array, we had earlier identified driver genes by 'Genomic Identification of Significant Targets In Cancer (GISTIC)' analysis of paired tumour-normal samples from colorectal cancer patients. In this study, we analyze these driver genes at three levels using exon array data – gene, exon and network. Gene level analysis revealed a small subset to experience differential expression. These results were reinforced by carrying out separate differential expression analyses (SAM and LIMMA). ATP8B1 was found to be the novel gene associated with CRC that shows changes at cytogenetic, gene and exon levels. Splice index of 29 exons corresponding to 13 genes was found to be significantly altered in tumour samples. Driver genes were used to construct regulatory networks for tumour and normal groups. There were rearrangements in transcription factor genes suggesting the presence of regulatory switching. The regulatory pattern of AHR gene was found to have the most significant alteration. Our results integrate data with focus on driver genes resulting in highly enriched novel molecules that need further studies to establish their role in CRC.

Editor: Osman El-Maarri, University of Bonn, Institut of experimental hematology and transfusion medicine, Germany

Funding: This study was funded by King Abdullah International Medical Research Center through research grant RC10/083 awarded to MAA. The funders had no role in study design, data collection and analysis, decision to publish, or preparation of the manuscript.

Competing Interests: The authors have declared that no competing interests exist.

* Email: azharbiotech@yahoo.com

Introduction

There is a wealth of information at omics level that associates cytogenetics and gene expression changes leading to colorectal cancer (CRC). The integration of gene expression and copy number (CN) data to identify DNA CN alterations that induce changes in the expression levels of the associated genes is a common task in cancer studies [1–3]. The central dogma of molecular biology has thus been addressed at two important levels. There have been many reports providing evidence of changes at the genome level in the form of copy number aberration [4], single nucleotide polymorphisms, loss of heterozygosity that attempt to understand the molecular events associated with colorectal cancer. These somatic or hereditary changes have different mechanism of contributing to initiation and progression of CRC. Loss and gain of crucial chromosomal regions leading to deletion or amplification of cancer related genes has been very well established. The functional significance of these molecular events has been measured using different tools and algorithms. Genes targeted by somatic copy-number alterations (SCNAs), in particular, play central roles in oncogenesis and cancer therapy [5]. Several tools have been made available to assess the potential of genes that get affected by SCNAs in causing colorectal cancer. 'Genomic Identification of Significant Targets in Cancer' (GISTIC) tool has successfully been used in identifying 'driver SCNAs' based on the frequency and amplitude of observed events [6,7]. The second aspect of changes happening in tumour cells is at the transcription level. Differential expression analysis has been carried out to find out important genes playing a role in causing colorectal cancer. There could be several mechanisms by which the SCNA affected genes exert their effect at functional level. Amplifications and deletions in the genomic region are reflected in the transcript levels and could be detected by carrying out expression microarray based studies. By employing exon arrays, we gain extra dimension of the events happening at the exon level, which may lead to alternative splicing resulting in different gene isoforms. Alternative splicing is a crucial step in the generation of protein diversity and its misregulation is observed in many human cancer types [8].

The quest to explore the relationship between copy number changes and the expression level of affected genes/exons has received limited success owing to a number of reasons [9]. Technological improvements in the array design for cytogenetics as well as transcriptomics have improved the accuracy and precision of the data generated. Combining this with better analytical techniques and algorithms, possibilities of finding target genes responsible for causing colorectal cancer has further increased.

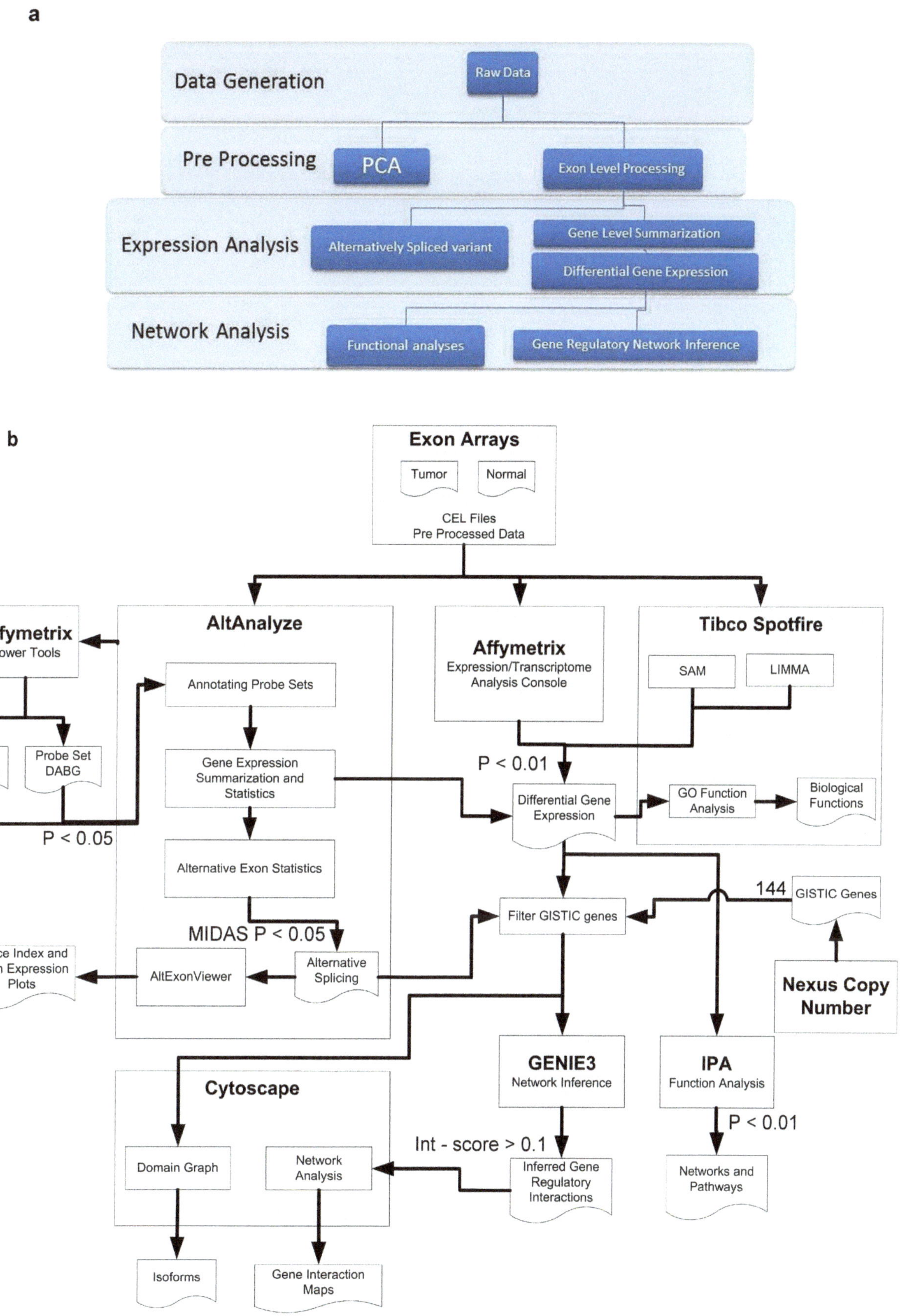
a
Data Generation
Raw Data
Pre Processing
PCA
Exon Level Processing
Expression Analysis
Alternatively Spliced variant
Gene Level Summarization
Differential Gene Expression
Network Analysis
Functional analyses
Gene Regulatory Network Inference
b
Exon Arrays
Tumor
Normal
CEL Files
Pre Processed Data
Affymetrix
Power Tools
Probe Set Expression
Probe Set DABG
P < 0.05
AltAnalyze
Annotating Probe Sets
Gene Expression Summarization and Statistics
Alternative Exon Statistics
MIDAS P < 0.05
Alternative Splicing
AltExonViewer
Splice Index and Exon Expression Plots
Affymetrix
Expression/Transcriptome Analysis Console
Tibco Spotfire
SAM
LIMMA
P < 0.01
Differential Gene Expression
GO Function Analysis
Biological Functions
144
GISTIC Genes
Nexus Copy Number
Filter GISTIC genes
GENIE3
Network Inference
IPA
Function Analysis
P < 0.01
Networks and Pathways
Int - score > 0.1
Inferred Gene Regulatory Interactions
Cytoscape
Domain Graph
Network Analysis
Isoforms
Gene Interaction Maps

Figure 1. Flow diagram for Analysis Strategy. A)The entire analyses is categorized into fours stages from 'Data Generation' to 'Network Analyses'. B) Analysis strategy using different programs is displayed in this diagram. There are three components of the analysis – Gene, Exon and Network handled by different programs. Gene level analyses are conducted using 'Affymetrix, Expression/Transcriptome analysis console' and 'Tibco Spotfire'. Exon level analysis is carried out by 'AltAnalyze' and 'Affymetrix power tools'. Network analyses employed 'GENIE3', 'IPA' and 'Cytoscape'. 'Nexus Copy Number' is a program used in earlier studies to eventually generate a list of 144 driver genes.

Past few decades have seen a quest for finding novel genes that can serve as therapeutic targets or biomarkers. However, genes or proteins do not function alone but interact with each other to form networks or pathways so as to carry out biological functions [10]. Network-based approaches to finding biomarkers more closely represent *in vivo* molecular biology where a perturbation in one gene may affect many downstream genes. Cancer has thus been rightly addressed as a systems biology disease [11] as opposed to diseases caused by changes in few genes or mutations. Reconstructing gene regulatory networks in healthy and diseased tissues is therefore critical to understanding cancer phenotypes and devising effective therapeutics [12].

With the availability of tools and techniques to capture the molecular changes happening at different stages of the central dogma with increased precision and accuracy, we are yet to develop an integrated comprehensive picture that could help us in finding better targets for colorectal cancer. In the present study, we aim to integrate the information from the cytogenetic analysis with the exon level expression data using paired normal-tumour samples from colorectal cancer patients. A set of driver genes suggested by GISTIC analysis (termed as 'driver genes' from now onwards) were queried at gene, exon and network level. Both DNA and RNA for cytogenetics and transcriptomic studies, respectively, were extracted from the same tissue in a single workflow to minimize variation. This study provides evidence for

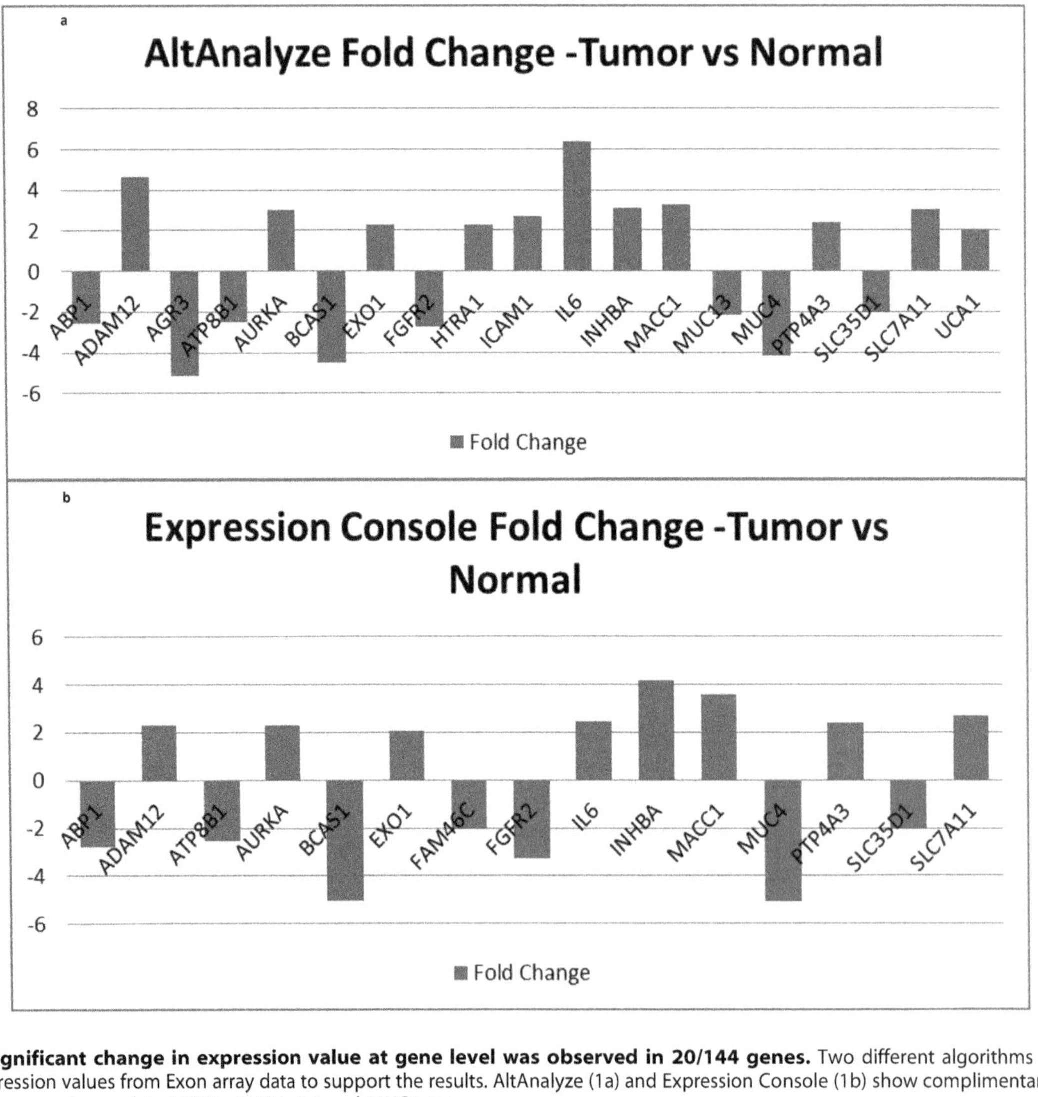

Figure 2. Significant change in expression value at gene level was observed in 20/144 genes. Two different algorithms were used to measure expression values from Exon array data to support the results. AltAnalyze (1a) and Expression Console (1b) show complimentary results with maximum changes observed in BCAS1, INHBA, IL6 and MUC4 genes.

Table 1. Driver Genes from GISTIC analysis showing more than two fold change in expression value as calculated by two different programs – AltAnalyze and Expression Console.

Gene Symbol	GISTIC score	AltAnalyze	Expression Console
BCAS1[a,b]	5.323	−4.50771	−5.02
AURKA[a,b]	4.772	3.044088	2.31
ATP8B1[a]	2.326	−2.49709	−2.55
IL6[a,b]	2	6.353318	2.45
INHBA[a,c]	1.944	3.071911	4.18
PTP4A3[a,b,c]	1.892	2.366951	2.41
ABP1[a,b]	1.859	−2.54991	−2.78
AGR3	1.772	−5.12325	N/A
MACC1	1.772	3.272925	3.57
UCA1	1.155	2.058481	N/A
FGFR2[a,b]	0.892	−2.72455	−3.28
ADAM12[a,b]	0.871	4.646741	2.33
MUC13	0.704	−2.15979	N/A
MUC4[a,b,c]	0.66	−4.18466	−5.06
SLC7A11[a]	0.637	3.051363	2.72
ICAM1	0.532	2.655218	N/A
EXO1	0.405	2.268313	2.05
FAM46C[a]	0.271	−1.7528	−2.03
HTRA1	0.231	2.301062	N/A
SLC35D1[a]	0.217	−2.0238	−2.06

N/A = No annotation for these genes were found in the analysis program.
[a]Genes found to be differentially expressed in SAM/LIMMA analyses. CLDN7 and LOX genes were additional driver genes that were differentially expressed.
[b]Genes found to have high splice index values.
[c]Genes found to be eligible as biomarkers for colorectal cancer.

explaining different possible mechanisms by which SCNA affected driver genes can exert their functional effect. A subset of driver genes were found to show gene level changes in expression. Most of these genes also indicated the exon level changes resulting in the formation of different isoforms. Network of GISTIC genes showed a clear shift in the transcription factors (TF) regulation. ATP8B1 gene was found to have novel association with colorectal cancer at cytogenetic, gene and exon level.

Materials and Methods

The study is approved by the ethics committee and Institutional Review Board (IRB) of King Abdullah International medical Research Center after due review process of the ethical aspects of the proposal. The necessary procedural and ethical consent forms were signed by each patient prior to sample collection.

Sample collection and RNA extraction

Sample collection was done as described previously [13]. The type and stage of all patient samples are provided in Table S1. The study was approved by institutional review board after the due process. Patients were consented and the records maintained in an approved manner. RNA was extracted from the same piece of

Table 2. Differentially regulated genes found to have incoherent expression levels and genomic changes.

Gene	Genomic level	Gene level (AA, EC)	Network level
ABP1	Gain 53.33, Loss 13.33	−2.55, −2.78	TF in Normal = CTCFL TF Tumour = Unknown
AGR3	Gain 60, Loss 0	−5.12	TF in Normal =SMAD2 TF Tumour = Unknown
BCAS1	Gain 80, Loss 0	−4.5, −5	TF in Normal =SMAD4 TF Tumour = Unknown
HTRA1	Gain 6.7, Loss 26.7	2.3	TF in Normal =CTCFL TF Tumour =AHR

AA = Fold change value as calculated by AltAnalyze program.
EC = Fold change value as calculated by Expression Console program.
TF = Transcription Factor. Unknown is the TF that is not found in the driver genes.

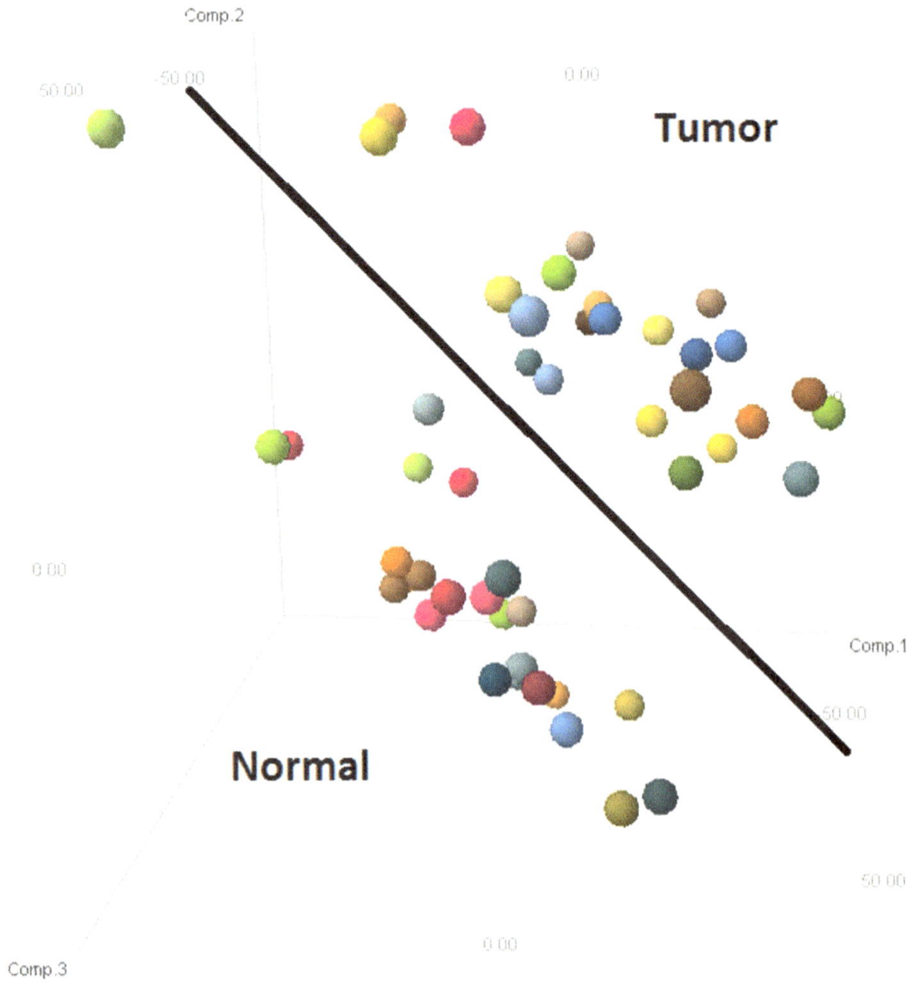

Figure 3. Principal Component Analysis of Exon array data from 32 patients. 60 samples from 32 patients were subjected to PCA and the outliers were removed. 4 normal and 7 tumour samples were removed from the final analysis.

tissue that was used to extract DNA for cytogenetic studies in a single workflow. Maceherey Nagel trio prep kit (Germany) was used to extract DNA and RNA in the same protocol. Quality and quantity was checked using Nanodrop (Thermo Fisher Scientific, USA).

Exon microarray

GeneChip Human Exon 1.0 ST Arrays along with WT Terminal Labelling and Controls Kit and Hybridization, Wash, and Stain Kit were obtained from Affymetrix USA. Ambion WT Expression Kit was obtained by Ambion, USA. 31 Tumour and 29 normal samples from 32 patients were processed. The data was extracted using Expression Console software from Affymetrix, USA. Quality control was carried out using Principal Component Analysis (PCA) and Integromics biomarker suite (TIBCO spotfire). All the data is deposited in GEO database with an accession number GSE50421.

Data Analysis

Before carrying out any gene/exon level analysis, principal component analysis (PCA) was done to identify outliers. Data from 4 normal samples and 7 tumour samples was subsequently removed.

Data analysis specifically with driver genes

Gene level analysis. For checking expression levels of 144 driver gene list generated by GISTIC analysis (13), we employed two different softwares – Expression console and AltAnalyze [14]. Two different softwares were used to confirm our results using independent methods. Signal estimates were derived from the CEL files of 60 samples (29 normal and 31 tumour) using Robust Multi-Array Average (RMA) for normalizing the data. The core exon-level probe sets were used to summarize the gene expression levels.

The same list of 144 driver genes with expression values calculated using 'Altanalyze' was used for inference based (GENIE3) pathway/network analysis.

Exon level expression analysis. Altanalyze program was used to evaluate alternative splicing in driver genes. The raw data was filtered to remove probe sets that were considered to be non-expressed. A splicing score for filtered exons was calculated using splicing index method and exon/intron/splicing annotation were

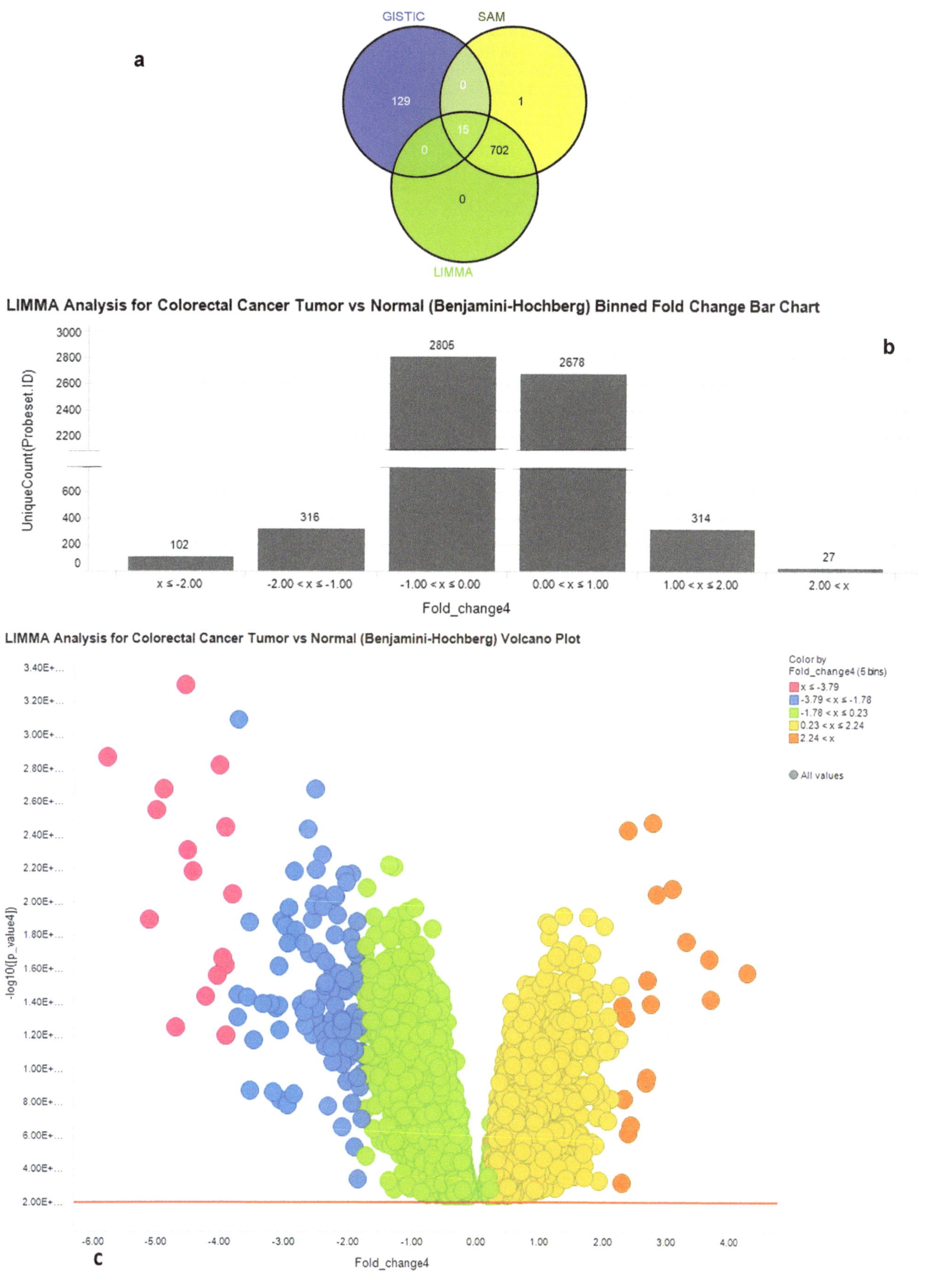
a
GISTIC
SAM
LIMMA
129
0
1
15
0
702
0
LIMMA Analysis for Colorectal Cancer Tumor vs Normal (Benjamini-Hochberg) Binned Fold Change Bar Chart
b
UniqueCount(Probeset.ID)
3000
2800
2600
2400
2200
600
400
200
0
102
316
2805
2678
314
27
x ≤ -2.00
-2.00 < x ≤ -1.00
-1.00 < x ≤ 0.00
0.00 < x ≤ 1.00
1.00 < x ≤ 2.00
2.00 < x
Fold_change4
LIMMA Analysis for Colorectal Cancer Tumor vs Normal (Benjamini-Hochberg) Volcano Plot
-log10([p_value4])
3.40E+...
3.20E+...
3.00E+...
2.80E+...
2.60E+...
2.40E+...
2.20E+...
2.00E+...
1.80E+...
1.60E+...
1.40E+...
1.20E+...
1.00E+...
8.00E+...
6.00E+...
4.00E+...
2.00E+...
Color by
Fold_change4 (5 bins)
x ≤ -3.79
-3.79 < x ≤ -1.78
-1.78 < x ≤ 0.23
0.23 < x ≤ 2.24
2.24 < x
All values
-6.00
-5.00
-4.00
-3.00
-2.00
-1.00
0.00
1.00
2.00
3.00
4.00
c
Fold_change4

Figure 4. Differential Expression analysis of genes yielded genes common with GISTIC analysis. (a) Venn diagram of common genes among GISTIC, SAM and LIMMA analyses. All genes were annotated and compared using IPA 'compare' function. 43 genes from Integromics analyses were not mapped by IPA.15 genes are common among all three analyses. (b) Binned fold change bar chart of LIMMA analysis. Total 6242 genes were having adjusted p-value <0.01 of which 759 showed significant fold change (<−1 or>1). (c) Volcano plot showing highly significant genes (pink = downregulated, orange = upregulated) in terms of p- value and fold change.

assigned to these results. A splice index p-value cut-off of <0.05 was used to filter alternative exon results. AltExonViewer – a component of Altanalyze and DomainGraph - a Cytoscape plugin were used to visualize splice index values and alternatively spliced exons. The splicing index (SI) value was calculated as described in [15]. Briefly, SI is $\log_2$ ratio of normalized intensities of tumour and normal samples. In our analysis 'sample 1' in the numerator was normal and 'sample 2' in the denominator was tumour.

Causal network analysis. For network analysis, knowledge and inference based approaches were used. For inference based approaches, GENIE3 [16,17] was used to generate gene regulatory networks for tumour and normal samples. To generate the network, driver genes were classified as TF genes and target genes. Although 1000 interactions were inferred for each of the group, an interaction score>0.1 was chosen as a cut-off value. Using this information the regulatory networks were independently inferred for tumour and normal samples using Cytoscape.

Data analysis with entire probeset

Integromics Biomarker Discovery Suite. In order to find differentially expressed genes in our dataset, without any prior bias, data from CEL files was analyzed using the Integromics software (TIBCO Spotfire, USA) pipeline for affymetrix exon 1.0 ST arrays. Quantile normalization was done after removing the outliers using PCA. Both Significance Analysis of Microarrays (SAM) and Linear Models for MicroArray data (LIMMA) analyses was carried out with a cut-off of 0.01 for adjusted p-value and fold change of>1 or <−1. Two different yet complimentary methodologies were used to make our results more confident. Gene ontology enrichment was carried out on a list of 760 differentially expressed genes obtained from LIMMA analysis.

Ingenuity pathway Analysis. List of 760 genes from SAM/LIMMA analysis done using Integromics was used to perform 'core' and 'biomarker' analyses. Core analysis was done as described before [13]. For biomarker analysis following filters were used: Consider only molecules where (species = Human) AND (tissues/cell lines = KM-12 OR HCT-116 OR RKO OR Colon Cancer Cell Lines not otherwise specified OR COLO205 OR HT29 OR HCC-2998 OR HCT-15 OR SW-480 OR Other Colon Cancer Cell Lines OR Tissues and Primary Cells not otherwise specified OR SW-620) AND (diseases = Cancer) AND ((biomarker applications = All Biomarker Applications) AND (biomarker diseases = colon cancer OR colon carcinoma OR colon neoplasm OR colorectal adenoma OR colorectal cancer OR colorectal carcinoma)).

Results

The analysis strategy leading to following results is illustrated in Figure 1a&b.

A small subset of genes identified by GISTIC show a significant change in expression level. We studied expression patterns of driver genes at gene level using AltAnalyze and Expression Console softwares. These analyses produced complimentary results and yielded a list of 20 genes that were found to have a significant fold change of greater than 2 and a p-value < 0.01 [Table 1]. 9 genes experienced a down regulation. BCAS1 with highest GISTIC score of 5.323 was among the most significantly downregulated genes. 11 genes showed an upregulation with IL6 and INHBA showing the highest fold change [Figure 2a (AltAnalyze), 2b (Expression Console)]. Fold change values of all 144 driver genes are given in Table S2.

Three significantly down regulated genes (BCAS1, ABP1 and AGR3) were found in amplified regions of the genome whereas upregulated HTRA1 was found mostly in regions of loss. These genes experienced a change in their transcription factor in tumour and normal samples [Table 2].

Differential expression analysis using tumour-normal paired sample data of exon arrays from 32 patients was carried out. After removing outliers using PCA [Figure 3], 25 normal and 24 tumour samples were found suitable for further analyses. We employed non-parametric (SAM) and parametric (LIMMA) methods and found complimentary results. 6242 genes were differentially expressed with adjusted p-value of <0.01. 760 genes were found to be differentially regulated (fold change>1or <−1) of which 15 genes were common with driver genes from GISTIC analysis [Figure 4a-c and Figure S1]. BCAS1, AURKA, ATP8B1, IL6 and INHBA were the differentially regulated genes found to be among the top scorers in list of driver genes.

Significant changes in isoform expression is exhibited by genes identified by GISTIC analysis. Exon level analysis of 144 driver genes was carried out. 29 exons belonging to 13 genes were shown to have significant changes in isoform expression as reflected in their splice index scores [Table 3]. While exons E25-1 of MUC4 and E3-2 of PTP4A3 showed high negative SI values, exons E2-2 of IL6 and E21-2 of ADAM12 showed high positive SI values. Negative SI values indicate exons are enriched in tumour samples and are skipped or repressed in normal samples and vice versa for positive SI values. For MUC4 gene, exons E25-1, E2-2, E2-1, I4-6 and I3-6 recorded negative SI values and exon E8-1 recorded a positive SI value. Exons E2-2 and E4-3 of IL6 recorded positive SI values. [Figure 5 ai-ii & bi-ii and figure S2]. Exons in MYLK and ANK3 showed significant change in splicing pattern but did not show a significant fold change in gene expression value. Microarray Detection of Alternative Splicing (MiDAS) p-value range of 0.01–0.04 was observed in the filtered results.

Causal Network analysis displays switch in transcription factors in tumor samples. Causal Network analysis displays switch in transcription factors in tumour samples. The most significant influence of TF genes in tumour and normal samples was reflected in the alteration in number of directed edges [Table 4]. CHAF1A, AHR, PRPF4B, ZNF200, SMAD2, RUVBL1, SMAD4, TSHZ1, CTCFL and CEBPE were among the top influencers. The regulatory hierarchy between these groups changed with respect to TFs. While RUVBL1 transformed into a master regulator in tumours, TSHZ1 has lost its capacity to master regulate other genes in tumours [Figure 6a]. Significant rearrangement in modularity is also observed between these two groups. More target genes function as modules in tumours as

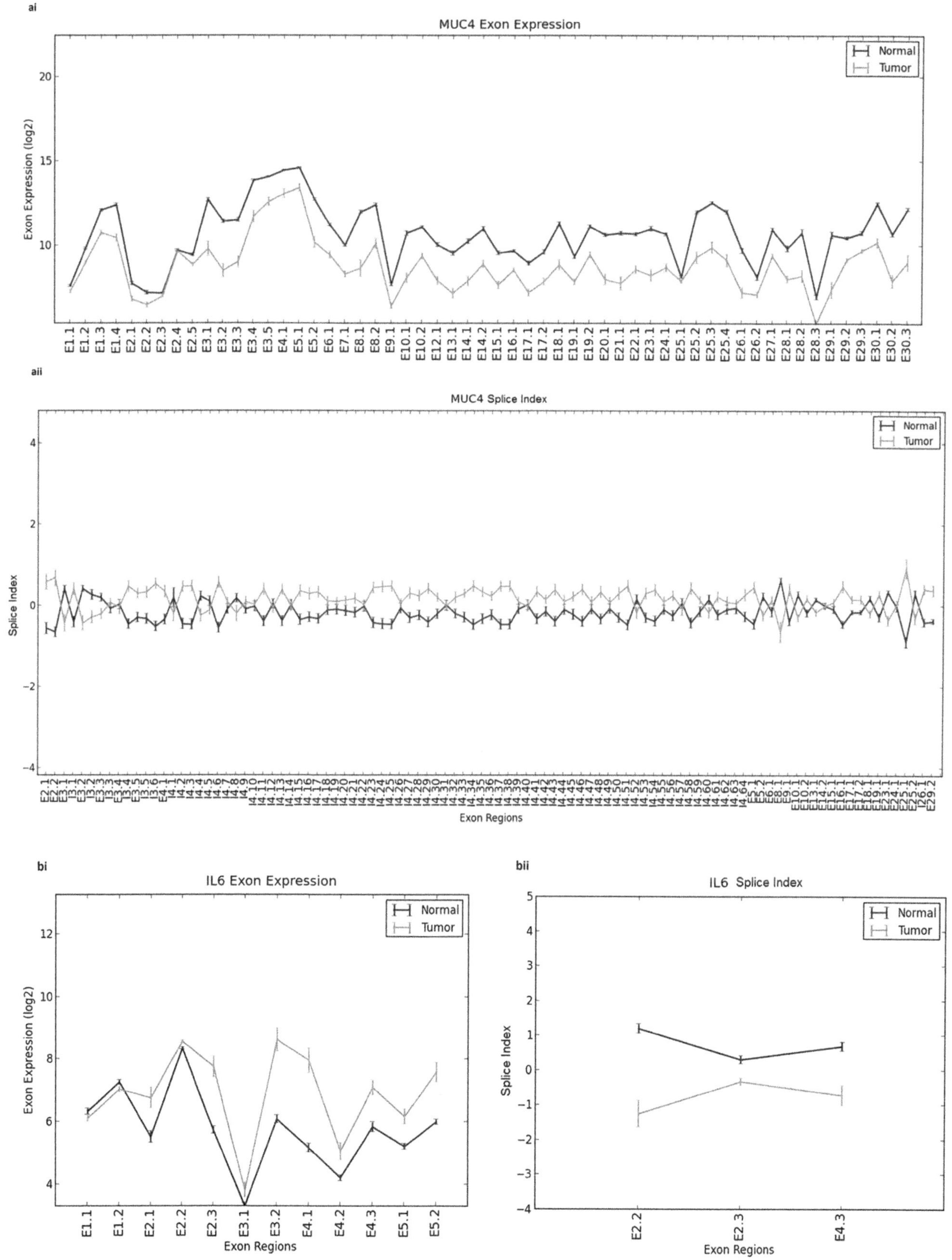
ai
MUC4 Exon Expression
Exon Expression (log2)
Normal
Tumor
aii
MUC4 Splice Index
Splice Index
Exon Regions
Normal
Tumor
bi
IL6 Exon Expression
Exon Expression (log2)
Exon Regions
Normal
Tumor
bii
IL6 Splice Index
Splice Index
Exon Regions
Normal
Tumor

Figure 5. Differential Expression at exon level was observed in thirteen GISTIC genes. Exon expression (i) and splice index (ii) values were mapped for both tumour and normal samples for twenty nine exons affecting thirteen genes. Exon 25-1 of MUC4 gene (a) shows highest negative splice index value (a ii) whereas exon 2-2 of IL6 (b) showed highest value of 2.44 (b ii). Exon expression and splice index values for rest 27 exons are provided as supplementary figure 1.

observed in modules regulated by AHR, CHAF1A and PRPF4B. Further, there is significant regulatory crosstalk among the genes in the normal group [Figure 6b]. While the tumours have lost the scale-free properties in its regulatory interaction, normal group exhibit approximate scale-free out degree distributions, signifying the potential of TF to regulate host of target genes. The tumours do not show this type of regulation which indicate unidirectional feed forward regulatory mode.

Functional analysis of differentially expressed genes confirms their role in colorectal cancer and reveal important pathways and biomarkers. Gene Ontology enrichment of 760 differentially expressed genes obtained from SAM/LIMMA analyses showed cell division, mitosis and cell adhesion to be the most significant biological processes affected [figure S3]. Ingenuity pathway analysis of 760 genes showed cancer and gastrointestinal disease among the top functions followed by cellular movement growth and proliferation [Figure 7a]. NF-kB signalling, cell cycle G_2/M DNA damage checkpoint regulation, colorectal cancer metastasis were among the top scoring pathways followed by agranulocyte adhesion [figure 7b]. TGFB1 was among the top upstream regulators. Network analysis suggests MYC, MMP and IL6 genes as important nodes [Fig 7c-e]. Biomarker analysis reveals 28 molecules relevant for colorectal cancer [Table 5]. INHBA, CLDN7 and MUC4 were eligible as biomarkers and are common with GISTIC, SAM and LIMMA analyses results.

Table 3. Significant changes in exon level expression of driver genes.

Probeset	GeneID	Exon ID	Regulation Call	SI	SI p-value	MiDAS p-value
2712254	MUC4	E25-1	Upregulated	−1.80873	2.79E-08	0.021609
3118824	PTP4A3	E3-2	Upregulated	−1.61711	9.95E-12	0.012046
2712381	MUC4	E2-2	Upregulated	−1.3477	7.19E-07	0.026458
3310161	FGFR2	E11-1	Upregulated	−1.29699	4.55E-08	0.023093
3310118	FGFR2	E29-1	Upregulated	−1.27723	1.86E-09	0.01652
3910391	BCAS1	E4-3	Upregulated	−1.25187	3.35E-07	0.021612
3031671	ABP1	E11-1	Upregulated	−1.24918	1.22E-10	0.014292
3310159	FGFR2	E12-1	Upregulated	−1.17574	2.50E-07	0.026414
2712382	MUC4	E2-1	Upregulated	−1.15152	1.33E-05	0.037457
3290897	ANK3	E60-1	Upregulated	−1.14825	1.19E-04	0.041986
2712354	MUC4	I4-6	Upregulated	−1.12743	3.39E-07	0.028327
2712361	MUC4	I3-6	Upregulated	−1.05374	8.25E-07	0.03115
3290925	ANK3	E53-5	Upregulated	−1.05177	2.60E-05	0.040567
3268341	HTRA1	E1-8	Downregulated	1.007325	5.53E-10	0.016611
3310147	FGFR2	E17-1	Downregulated	1.086154	2.78E-06	0.031111
3268338	HTRA1	E1-5	Downregulated	1.086203	3.38E-11	0.013645
2388253	EXO1	E18-1	Downregulated	1.08806	3.11E-05	0.044937
3311901	ADAM12	E10-1	Downregulated	1.089706	1.70E-09	0.018986
3910807	AURKA	E1-2	Downregulated	1.105387	2.78E-07	0.026314
3820445	ICAM1	E3-3	Downregulated	1.222886	3.84E-07	0.027735
2712282	MUC4	E8-1	Downregulated	1.267574	1.63E-05	0.039593
2692532	MYLK	E13-1	Downregulated	1.273764	4.27E-07	0.030277
3268334	HTRA1	E1-1	Downregulated	1.288045	1.63E-12	0.011119
3310142	FGFR2	E20-1	Downregulated	1.403702	1.07E-09	0.015743
3268335	HTRA1	E1-2	Downregulated	1.404729	1.43E-12	0.011016
2992599	IL6	E4-3	Downregulated	1.406659	4.60E-05	0.044146
3311894	ADAM12	E11-1	Downregulated	1.420516	1.99E-10	0.016023
3311853	ADAM12	E21-2	Downregulated	2.016734	1.96E-09	0.018149
2992593	IL6	E2-2	Downregulated	2.448861	1.85E-07	0.027456

List of 29 exons corresponding to 13 genes are listed along with their respective splice index and MiDAS p values.
Probeset IDs are according to Affymetrix database
SI = Splice Index
MiDAS = Microarray Detection of Alternative Splicing

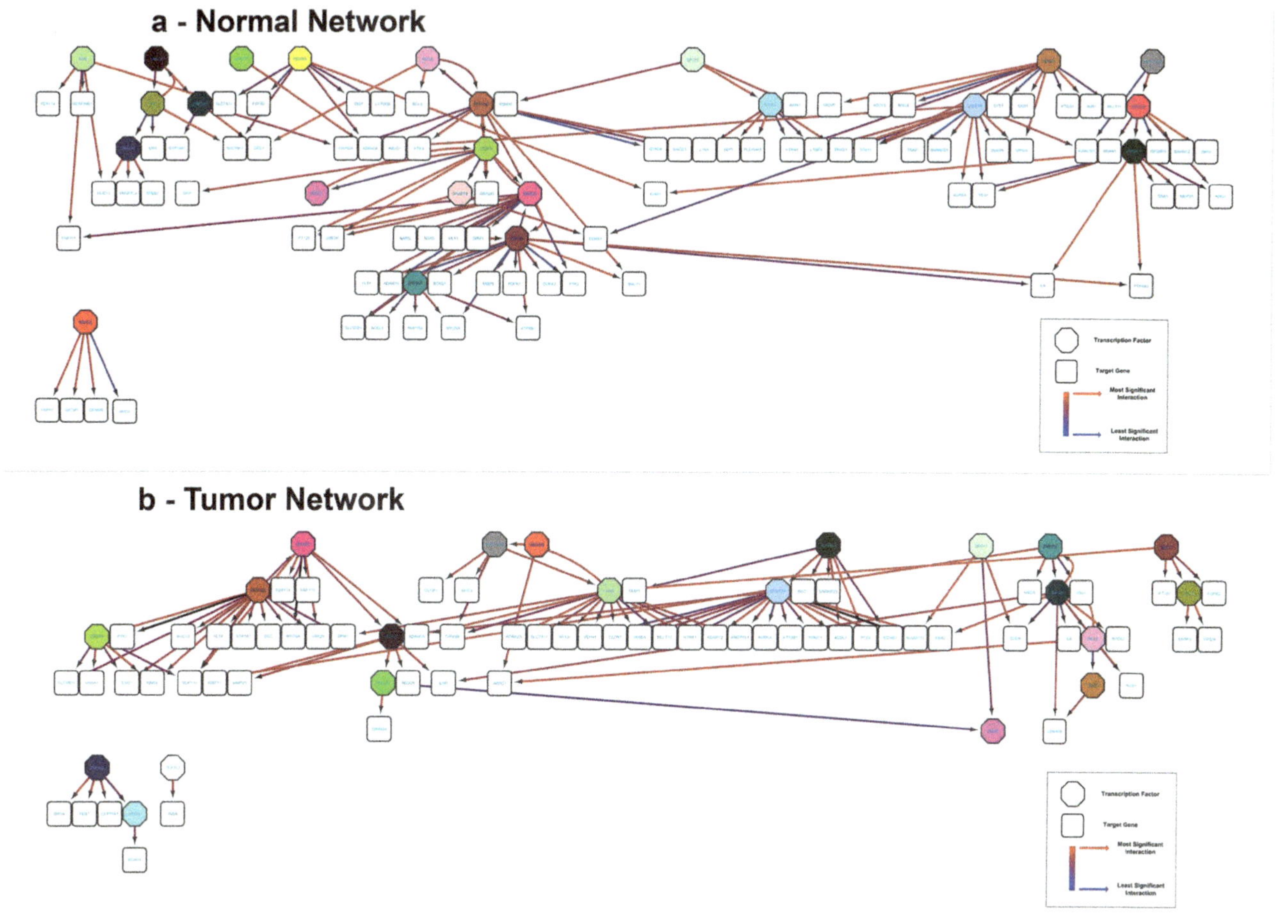

Figure 6. Gene Regulatory Network Inference diagram for Tumor and Normal Groups. A hierarchical network topology is used to visualize the degrees of interaction between transcription factor genes and target genes. (a) The inferred network for tumour group showing RUVBL1 as master regulator. (b) The inferred network for normal group showing TSHZ1as master regulator.

Discussion

In this study we attempt to understand the transcription level changes in driver genes affected by SCNAs in colorectal cancer. We queried these genes from three perspectives using gene/exon/network level analysis tools. Our integrated analysis at genomic/transcriptomic levels resulted in finding genes of high priority that can be experimentally studied to establish their role in colorectal cancer. Functional significance of differentially expressed genes confirmed the outcome of our analyses.

Due to the unavailability of high resolution cytogenetic arrays large size of chromosomal regions were implicated in causing colorectal cancer through copy number changes. The commercial SNP genotyping arrays focus on variants that are present in 5% or more of the population and feature a limited number of CNV probes. Therefore, sub microscopic structural variants are poorly captured by available SNP genotyping arrays that were designed to evaluate SNPs. The recent introduction of the Affymetrix CytoScan HD Array (CNV-targeted array), which is based on the validated Genome-Wide Human SNP Array 6.0 and contains more than 2.6 million markers for copy number variants and approximately 750,000 SNPs, has enabled the detection of copy number aberrations with high resolution across the genome [18]. Data from this platform was used to obtain the list of driver genes which could thus be considered to be most precise and accurate. Earlier, results from different groups often lead to a high level of discordance with an overlap of <5% in some cases. GISTIC analysis was able to address this issue and differentiate between passenger and driver mutations with a high level of precision and accuracy [6]. The correlation between expression and CN data is very complex [19] and is very much affected by the type of platform used for generating the data as well as the analysis strategies. Our analysis strategy aimed at reducing the confounding factors. We extracted DNA/RNA from the same piece of tissue in a single protocol [20]. We used matched paired tumour-normal control which is arguably the best way to do a comparative study [21]. Several approaches have been employed for cancer gene prioritization by integrative analysis [22,23]. We employed a modified two-step approach by filtering the cancer genes using GISTIC and then carried out exon expression analysis.

Gene Level. The effect of chromosomal changes is not always direct. Global amplification at genomic level would result into higher level expression of selected genes [9]. Our gene level analysis showed only 20 of 144 driver genes to experience significant change at transcription level. 5 of these genes were

Table 4. Transcription factor genes showing significant change in their effect as represented by the change in number of outbound and inbound edges in tumour and normal samples.

Transcription Factor	In bound edges (Normal, Tumour)	Out bound edges (Normal, Tumour)
CHAF1A	*1,1*	*16,12*
AHR	*0,2*	*5,14*
PRPF4B	*2,1*	*11,14*
ZNF200	*1,2*	*3,9*
SMAD2	*3,1*	*13,8*
RUVBL1	*1,0*	*8,7*
CEBPE	*2,1*	*7,5*
SMAD7	1,2	2,5
HIST1H1B	0,1	2,4
MLL3	1,1	3,4
SMAD4	*2,0*	*14,4*
ZNF217	1,1	6,4
ZNF442	1,0	3,4
SPO11	0,0	3,3
NHLH2	0,1	1,2
TP53	1,1	4,2
CTCFL	*1,1*	*6,1*
SMAD3	0,0	4,1
TCF7L2	1,0	6,1
TSHZ1	*0,1*	*12,1*

listed among the top scoring driver genes. Our results correlate focal amplifications with increased expression levels and have been reported earlier using array CGH (aCGH) for FGFR2, GNAS and AURKA genes [24]. With an average amplicon size of 4.56 Mb, it could be misleading to report all affected genes/non-coding regions to be associated with CRC. FAM46C, EGFR2 and IL6 genes from our analysis have also been listed in the updated cancer gene census [5,25]. BCAS1 gene that scored the highest in the GISTIC analysis was earlier reported to undergo alternative splicing and downregulation [26] which is consistent with our results. Upregulation of human SLC7A11 mRNA in stromal fibroblast cells from liver metastases is associated with metastatic colorectal cancer in human [27]. PTP4A3 reported to be significantly upregulated in this study has recently been implicated in colon tumorigenesis [28]. ATP8B1 is the gene that has not yet been reported to have any association with colorectal cancer and would be an important molecule for further studies.

Our differential expression analysis of tumour and normal exon array datasets using two independent tools (SAM and LIMMA) showed an overlap of 15 genes with the driver genes. Analysis of> 44,000 probes resulting in differentially expressed genes provide an unbiased approach and lends further confidence in the list of overlapping genes. Both LIMMA and SAM approaches generated same results at the functional level as evidenced by Ingenuity Pathway Analysis (IPA).

ABP1, AGR3 and BCAS1 showed downregulation despite amplification at the genome level. This is supported by earlier studies for BCAS1in MCF7 cell line [29]. We observed that the influence of SMAD4 transcription factor was lost in tumour cells and may be responsible for this observation. Similar changes in transcription factors was observed for two other genes indicating the switching behaviour as discussed below.

Exon Level. Exon level analysis for measuring gene expression changes is challenging but rewarding. Even the improved algorithms have limitations in providing absolute quantification of the transcript levels. Earlier methods have found exon level data to be more informative about the nature and level of transcripts [30]. Now with the knowledge that more than 90% of all genes undergo alternative splicing to produce more than one transcript for a gene, the potential of exon level data is being realized more than ever [31–33]. Gene centric approach for carrying out integrated analysis using aCGH and exon array data has yielded more of confirmatory results and lack the use of full potential of whole genome arrays [34]. FGFR2 gene was shown to be amplified and upregulated which is misleading due to the truncated form of FGFR2. Wt FGFR2 gene was not measured and hence could not be compared with our study [34].

Exon level studies in colorectal cancer have been few and carry several limitations in terms of data analysis. Many of these studies compared tumour and normal from different sources [35]. Our results show a subset of differentially expressed genes to experience change in splicing pattern. 29 exons belonging to 13 genes showed significant splice index (SI) and MiDAS p-values. Both the values are strong indicators to measure alternative splicing. MUC4 is very well known to undergo alternative splicing and cause cancer [36] but the alternative splicing of IL6 is novel in association with CRC. ADAM12 that scored a high SI value has been implicated earlier in lung cancer [37]. 5 genes (ACTN1, CALD1, SLC3A2,

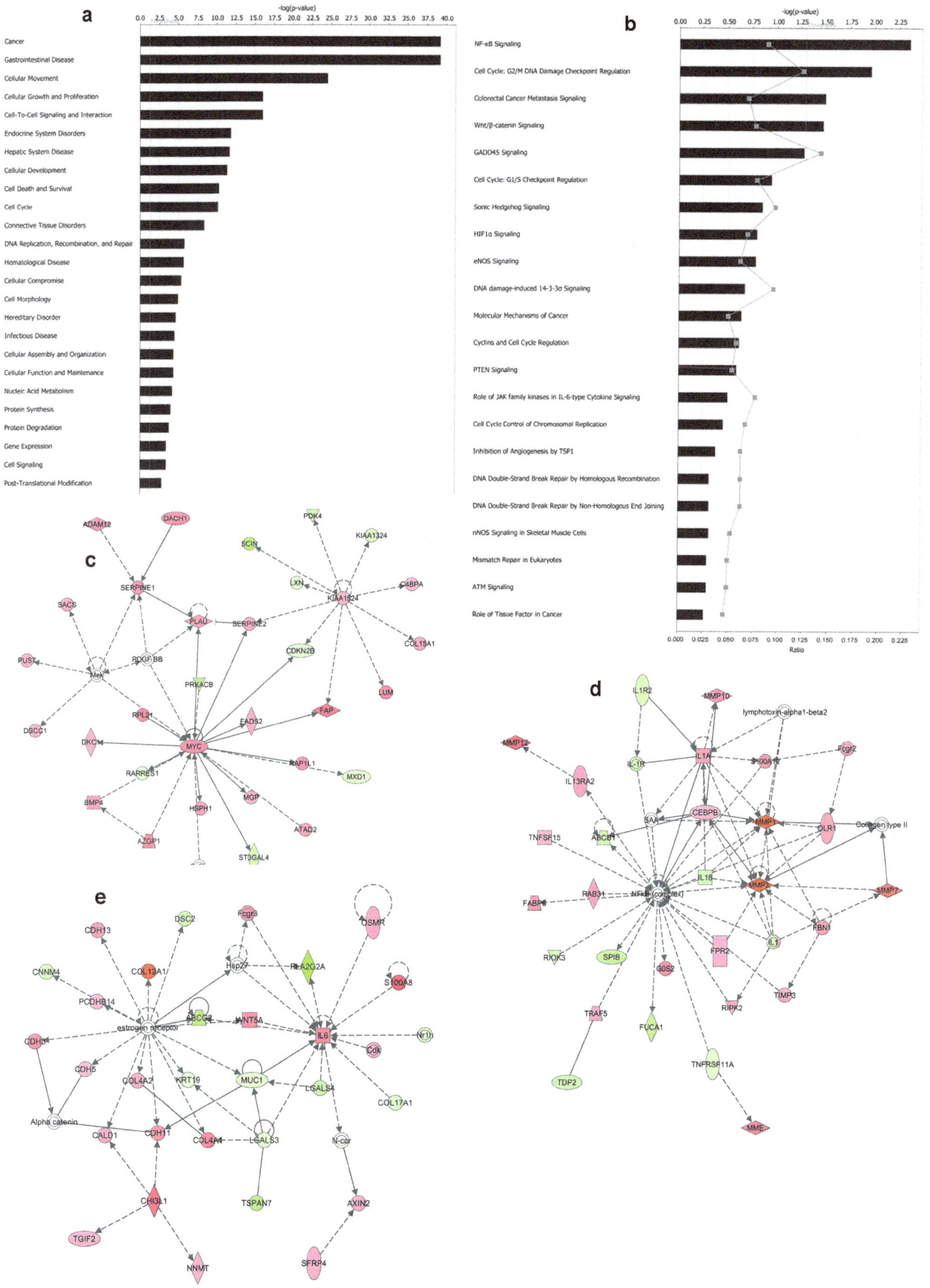
a
-log(p-value)
0.0 2.5 5.0 7.5 10.0 12.5 15.0 17.5 20.0 22.5 25.0 27.5 30.0 32.5 35.0 37.5 40.0
Cancer
Gastrointestinal Disease
Cellular Movement
Cellular Growth and Proliferation
Cell-To-Cell Signaling and Interaction
Endocrine System Disorders
Hepatic System Disease
Cellular Development
Cell Death and Survival
Cell Cycle
Connective Tissue Disorders
DNA Replication, Recombination, and Repair
Hematological Disease
Cellular Compromise
Cell Morphology
Hereditary Disorder
Infectious Disease
Cellular Assembly and Organization
Cellular Function and Maintenance
Nucleic Acid Metabolism
Protein Synthesis
Protein Degradation
Gene Expression
Cell Signaling
Post-Translational Modification
b
-log(p-value)
0.00 0.25 0.50 0.75 1.00 1.25 1.50 1.75 2.00 2.25
NF-κB Signaling
Cell Cycle: G2/M DNA Damage Checkpoint Regulation
Colorectal Cancer Metastasis Signaling
Wnt/β-catenin Signaling
GADD45 Signaling
Cell Cycle: G1/S Checkpoint Regulation
Sonic Hedgehog Signaling
HIF1α Signaling
eNOS Signaling
DNA damage-induced 14-3-3σ Signaling
Molecular Mechanisms of Cancer
Cyclins and Cell Cycle Regulation
PTEN Signaling
Role of JAK family kinases in IL-6-type Cytokine Signaling
Cell Cycle Control of Chromosomal Replication
Inhibition of Angiogenesis by TSP1
DNA Double-Strand Break Repair by Homologous Recombination
DNA Double-Strand Break Repair by Non-Homologous End Joining
nNOS Signaling in Skeletal Muscle Cells
Mismatch Repair in Eukaryotes
ATM Signaling
Role of Tissue Factor in Cancer
0.000 0.025 0.050 0.075 0.100 0.125 0.150 0.175 0.200 0.225
Ratio
c
ADAM12
DACH1
PDK4
KIAA1324
SCIN
LXN
C4BPA
SERPINE1
KIAA1524
SACS
PLAU
SERPINE2
COL15A1
PDGF BB
CDKN2B
PUS7
Mek
PRKACB
LUM
FAP
RPL21
FADS2
DSCC1
DKC1
MYC
RAP1L1
MXD1
RARRES1
BMP4
MGP
HSPH1
ATAD2
AZGP1
ST3GAL4
d
IL1R2
MMP10
lymphotoxin-alpha1-beta2
MMP12
Fcgr2
IL1A
IL-1R
S100A12
IL13RA2
CEBPB
SAA
MMP1
OLR1
Collagen type II
TNFSF15
ABCB1
IL18
RAB31
NFkB (complex)
MMP3
MMP7
FABP6
FBN1
FPR2
IL1
RIOK3
SPIB
G0S2
TIMP3
RIPK2
TRAF5
FUCA1
TNFRSF11A
TDP2
MME
e
CDH13
DSC2
Fcgr3
OSMR
CNNM4
COL12A1
Hsp27
PLA2G2A
S100A8
PCDHB14
ABCG2
WNT5A
estrogen receptor
IL6
Nr1h
CDH3
Cdk
CDH5
COL4A2
KRT19
MUC1
LGALS4
COL17A1
Alpha catenin
CALD1
CDH11
COL4A1
LGALS3
N-cor
CHI3L1
TSPAN7
AXIN2
TGIF2
NNMT
SFRP4

Figure 7. Core Analysis of Differentially Expressed Genes using IPA. Core analysis using IPA was carried out using set of 760 genes that were differentially expressed in tumour samples. Important biological functions (a) pathways (b) and networks (c-e) were revealed by this analysis.

CTTN and FN1) reported earlier as differentially spliced [38] have been found in the our study as well which used a different analysis strategy.

ANK3 is known to use alternative transcription start sites in colorectal cancer [8] and could also be the mechanism for other gene MYLK for which we did not see a significant change in gene level expression.

Network Level. Pathways analysis has been used to measure the relevance of the genes affected by CNAs by creating networks among them [1]. However, these networks are limited in their useful interpretation owing to the absence of directionality. Our causal network analysis provides more useful information on the genes involved in these networks. We observed a significant difference in the number of target genes between tumour and normal. In case of genes found in the amplified region but were downregulated we observed a loss of the transcription factor regulation, whereas in the upregulated gene found in the deleted region there was a switch in the transcription factor. From the list of driver genes we chose the transcription factors and studied their change in behaviour in tumour samples. AHR has been established as a tumour suppressor gene in colon and other cancers [39]. This study further explains the enhanced role of AHR by the increased number of outbound (target) genes in tumour. Our study provides evidence that TSHZ1 loses its role as master regulator in normal cells while RUVBL1 assumes that role. These provide interesting opportunities for mechanistic studies of network/pathways affected in CRC. It has been envisaged through integrated studies that many different genomic alterations potentially dys-regulate the same pathways in complex diseases [40]. Further studies of the regulatory level changes in this study will be able to establish this concept in CRC.

Functional role of the differentially expressed genes and the identification of MYC, MMP and IL6 as important nodes in the affected networks provide leads that need to be validated to

Table 5. Biomarker molecules among the differentially expressed genes.

Symbol	Fold Change	p-value	Location	Type(s)
ANGPT2	2.055	6.89E-14	Extracellular Space	growth factor
CD34	1.104	4.27E-10	Plasma Membrane	other
CD44	1.256	9.28E-14	Plasma Membrane	enzyme
CDH13	1.338	4.13E-11	Plasma Membrane	other
CLDN7	−1.030	1.81E-09	Plasma Membrane	other
CXCL10	1.073	8.50E-03	Extracellular Space	cytokine
EREG	1.352	2.39E-05	Extracellular Space	growth factor
GDF15	1.191	6.33E-06	Extracellular Space	growth factor
IGF2	1.398	3.85E-04	Extracellular Space	growth factor
IL8	3.641	2.55E-17	Extracellular Space	cytokine
INHBA	2.225	1.71E-12	Extracellular Space	growth factor
KRT20	−2.032	4.90E-12	Cytoplasm	other
MET	1.049	1.87E-07	Plasma Membrane	kinase
MKI67	1.015	1.58E-10	Nucleus	other
MMP2	1.764	2.31E-09	Extracellular Space	peptidase
MUC1	−1.070	1.65E-05	Plasma Membrane	transcription regulator
MUC4	−2.264	3.71E-11	Extracellular Space	growth factor
OSMR	1.166	4.95E-07	Plasma Membrane	transmembrane receptor
PDCD4	−1.572	9.64E-13	Nucleus	other
PDGFRB	1.090	1.47E-10	Plasma Membrane	kinase
PDPN	1.136	5.95E-11	Plasma Membrane	transporter
PTGS2	2.303	5.99E-09	Cytoplasm	enzyme
PTP4A3	1.132	2.47E-12	Plasma Membrane	phosphatase
SERPINE1	1.418	4.29E-09	Extracellular Space	other
SPP1	2.648	6.37E-10	Extracellular Space	cytokine
TIMP1	1.938	9.22E-13	Extracellular Space	other
TNS4	1.486	3.15E-07	Cytoplasm	other
TSPAN8	−1.031	2.83E-09	Plasma Membrane	other

Fold change and p-values were calculated using Integromics biomarker suite.

establish their association with CRC. Biomarkers, especially MUC4 will be an important molecule to study mechanistically and establish their use in clinical studies. This study provides wealth of analyzed data and an enriched list of genes that can serve as potential clues to understand the biology of colorectal cancer.

Supporting Information

Figure S1 Significance of Microarray analysis. SAM analysis was performed using Integromics biomarker discovery suites on all samples. The results were complimentary to LIMMA analysis as reflected in the number of differentially expressed genes.

Figure S2 Splice index and exon expression plots for remaining 11 genes. Splice index and exon expression values of all 13 genes that were found significant among the driver genes were plotted. Comparison of 'Normal' and 'Tumor' samples is depicted to observe the change in splice index as well the expression pattern at exon level.

Figure S3 Biological processes enrichment chart for differentially expressed genes. This bar plot shows the differentially expressed genes (as obtained from Integromics) are enriched in three functions viz., cell division, mitosis and cell adhesion.

Table S1 Types and stages of all the patient samples used in the study.

Table S2 Fold change values of all 144 GISTIC genes as calculated by AltAnalyze Program.

Acknowledgments

The help extended by Drs. Balwi and Hussein in providing facilities for conducting experiments and analyses is acknowledged.

Author Contributions

Conceived and designed the experiments: MAA. Performed the experiments: MAO AA GA. Analyzed the data: MAA SP. Contributed reagents/materials/analysis tools: ZAY IA. Wrote the paper: MAA.

References

1. Fan B, Dachrut S, Coral H, Yuen ST, Chu KM, et al. (2012) Integration of DNA copy number alterations and transcriptional expression analysis in human gastric cancer. PLoS One 7: e29824.
2. Lu T-P, Lai L-C, Tsai M-H, Chen P-C, Hsu C-P, et al. (2011) Integrated Analyses of Copy Number Variations and Gene Expression in Lung Adenocarcinoma. PLoS One 6: e24829.
3. Louhimo R, Lepikhova T, Monni O, Hautaniemi S (2012) Comparative analysis of algorithms for integration of copy number and expression data. Nat Methods 9: 351–355.
4. Yoshida T, Kobayashi T, Itoda M, Muto T, Miyaguchi K, et al. (2010) Clinical omics analysis of colorectal cancer incorporating copy number aberrations and gene expression data. Cancer Inform 9: 147–161.
5. Santarius T, Shipley J, Brewer D, Stratton MR, Cooper CS (2010) A census of amplified and overexpressed human cancer genes. Nat Rev Cancer 10: 59–64.
6. Beroukhim R, Getz G, Nghiemphu L, Barretina J, Hsueh T, et al. (2007) Assessing the significance of chromosomal aberrations in cancer: methodology and application to glioma. Proc Natl Acad Sci U S A 104: 20007–20012.
7. Mermel C, Schumacher S, Hill B, Meyerson M, Beroukhim R, et al. (2011) GISTIC2.0 facilitates sensitive and confident localization of the targets of focal somatic copy-number alteration in human cancers. Genome Biology 12: R41.
8. Thorsen K, Mansilla F, Schepeler T, Øster B, Rasmussen MH, et al. (2011) Alternative Splicing of SLC39A14 in Colorectal Cancer is Regulated by the Wnt Pathway. Molecular & Cellular Proteomics 10.
9. Platzer P, Upender MB, Wilson K, Willis J, Lutterbaugh J, et al. (2002) Silence of chromosomal amplifications in colon cancer. Cancer Res 62: 1134–1138.
10. Wen Z, Liu ZP, Liu Z, Zhang Y, Chen L (2013) An integrated approach to identify causal network modules of complex diseases with application to colorectal cancer. J Am Med Inform Assoc 20: 659–667.
11. Hornberg JJ, Bruggeman FJ, Westerhoff HV, Lankelma J (2006) Cancer: A Systems Biology disease. Biosystems 83: 81–90.
12. Madhamshettiwar P, Maetschke S, Davis M, Reverter A, Ragan M (2012) Gene regulatory network inference: evaluation and application to ovarian cancer allows the prioritization of drug targets. Genome Med 4: 1–16.
13. Hisham ElDai SP, Al Qarni S, Al Rodayyan M, Mustafa S, Deeb A, et al. (2013) Novel Genes Associated with Colorectal Cancer Are Revealed By High Resolution Cytogenetic Analysis in a Patient Specific Manner. PLOS ONE 8: e76251.
14. Emig D, Salomonis N, Baumbach J, Lengauer T, Conklin BR, et al. (2010) AltAnalyze and DomainGraph: analyzing and visualizing exon expression data. Nucleic Acids Res 38: W755–W762.
15. Srinivasan K, Shiue L, Hayes JD, Centers R, Fitzwater S, et al. (2005) Detection and measurement of alternative splicing using splicing-sensitive microarrays. Methods 37: 345–359.
16. Marbach D, Costello JC, Kuffner R, Vega NM, Prill RJ, et al. (2012) Wisdom of crowds for robust gene network inference. Nat Meth 9: 796–804.
17. Huynh-Thu VA, Irrthum A, Wehenkel L and Geurts P (2010) Inferring Regulatory Networks from Expression Data Using Tree-Based Methods. PLoS ONE 5: e12776.
18. Chen W, Yuan L, Cai Y, Chen X, Chi Y, et al. (2013) Identification of chromosomal copy number variations and novel candidate loci in hereditary nonpolyposis colorectal cancer with mismatch repair proficiency. Genomics 102: 27–34.
19. Tsafrir D, Bacolod M, Selvanayagam Z, Tsafrir I, Shia J, et al. (2006) Relationship of gene expression and chromosomal abnormalities in colorectal cancer. Cancer Res 66: 2129–2137.
20. Mathieson W, Thomas GA (2013) Simultaneously extracting DNA, RNA, and protein using kits: is sample quantity or quality prejudiced? Anal Biochem 433: 10–18.
21. Mojica W and Hawthorn L (2010) Normal colon epithelium: a dataset for the analysis of gene expression and alternative splicing events in colon disease. BMC Genomics 11: 5.
22. Lahti L, Schafer M, Klein HU, Bicciato S, Dugas M (2013) Cancer gene prioritization by integrative analysis of mRNA expression and DNA copy number data: a comparative review. Brief Bioinform 14: 27–35.
23. Bisognin A, Pizzini S, Perilli L, Esposito G, Mocellin S, et al. (2013) An integrative framework identifies alternative splicing events in colorectal cancer development. Mol Oncol.
24. Camps J, Nguyen QT, Padilla-Nash HM, Knutsen T, McNeil NE, et al. (2009) Integrative genomics reveals mechanisms of copy number alterations responsible for transcriptional deregulation in colorectal cancer. Genes Chromosomes Cancer 48: 1002–1017.
25. Futreal PA, Coin L, Marshall M, Down T, Hubbard T, et al. (2004) A census of human cancer genes. Nat Rev Cancer 4: 177–183.
26. Correa RG, de Carvalho AF, Pinheiro NA, Simpson AJ, de Souza SJ (2000) NABC1 (BCAS1): alternative splicing and downregulation in colorectal tumors. Genomics 65: 299–302.
27. Nakagawa H, Liyanarachchi S, Davuluri RV, Auer H, Martin EW Jr, et al. (2004) Role of cancer-associated stromal fibroblasts in metastatic colon cancer to the liver and their expression profiles. Oncogene 23: 7366–7377.
28. Zimmerman MW, Homanics GE, Lazo JS (2013) Targeted Deletion of the Metastasis-Associated Phosphatase *Ptp4a3* (PRL-3) Suppresses Murine Colon Cancer. PLoS One 8: e58300.
29. Collins C, Rommens JM, Kowbel D, Godfrey T, Tanner M, et al. (1998) Positional cloning of ZNF217 and NABC1: Genes amplified at 20q13.2 and overexpressed in breast carcinoma. Proceedings of the National Academy of Sciences 95: 8703–8708.
30. Bemmo A, Benovoy D, Kwan T, Gaffney DJ, Jensen RV, et al. (2008) Gene expression and isoform variation analysis using Affymetrix Exon Arrays. BMC Genomics 9: 529.
31. Consiglio A, Carella M, De Caro G, Delle Foglie G, Giovannelli C, et al. (2012) BEAT: Bioinformatics Exon Array Tool to store, analyze and visualize Affymetrix GeneChip Human Exon Array data from disease experiments. BMC Bioinformatics 13 Suppl 4: S21.
32. Pan Q, Shai O, Lee LJ, Frey BJ, Blencowe BJ (2008) Deep surveying of alternative splicing complexity in the human transcriptome by high-throughput sequencing. Nat Genet 40: 1413–1415.
33. Wang ET, Sandberg R, Luo S, Khrebtukova I, Zhang L, et al. (2008) Alternative isoform regulation in human tissue transcriptomes. Nature 456: 470–476.
34. Furuta K, Arao T, Sakai K, Kimura H, Nagai T, et al. (2012) Integrated analysis of whole genome exon array and array-comparative genomic hybridization in gastric and colorectal cancer cells. Cancer Sci 103: 221–227.

35. Piepoli A, Palmieri O, Maglietta R, Panza A, Cattaneo E, et al. (2012) The expression of leucine-rich repeat gene family members in colorectal cancer. Exp Biol Med (Maywood) 237: 1123–1128.
36. Singh AP, Chaturvedi P, Batra SK (2007) Emerging roles of MUC4 in cancer: a novel target for diagnosis and therapy. Cancer Res 67: 433–436.
37. Xi L, Feber A, Gupta V, Wu M, Bergemann AD, et al. (2008) Whole genome exon arrays identify differential expression of alternatively spliced, cancer-related genes in lung cancer. Nucleic Acids Res 36: 6535–6547.
38. Gardina PJ, Clark TA, Shimada B, Staples MK, Yang Q, et al. (2006) Alternative splicing and differential gene expression in colon cancer detected by a whole genome exon array. BMC Genomics 7: 325.
39. Zudaire E, Cuesta N, Murty V, Woodson K, Adams L, et al. (2008) The aryl hydrocarbon receptor repressor is a putative tumor suppressor gene in multiple human cancers. The Journal of Clinical Investigation 118: 640–650.
40. Kim YA, Wuchty S, Przytycka TM (2011) Identifying causal genes and dysregulated pathways in complex diseases. PLoS Comput Biol 7: e1001095.

15

Calcium-Sensing Receptor-Mediated Osteogenic and Early-Stage Neurogenic Differentiation in Umbilical Cord Matrix Mesenchymal Stem Cells from a Large Animal Model

Nicola Antonio Martino[1]*, Stephan Joel Reshkin[2], Elena Ciani[2], Maria Elena Dell'Aquila[1¤]

1 Department of Emergency and Organ Transplantation (DETO) – Section of Veterinary Clinics and Animal Productions, University of Bari Aldo Moro, Valenzano, Bari, Italy,
2 Department of Biosciences, Biotechnologies and Biopharmaceutics (DBBB), University Campus "Ernesto Quagliariello" University of Bari Aldo Moro, Bari, Italy

Abstract

Background: Umbilical cord matrix mesenchymal stem cells (UCM-MSCs) present a wide range of potential therapeutical applications. The extracellular calcium-sensing receptor (CaSR) regulates physiological and pathological processes. We investigated, in a large animal model, the involvement of CaSR in triggering osteogenic and neurogenic differentiation of two size-sieved UCM-MSC lines, by using AMG641, a novel potent research calcimimetic acting as CaSR agonist.

Methodology/Principal Findings: Large (>8μm in diameter) and small (<8μm) equine UCM-MSC lines were cultured in medium with high calcium (Ca^{2+}) concentration ($[Ca^{2+}]_o$; 2.87 mM) and dose-response effects of AMG641 (0.01 to 3μM) on cell proliferation were evaluated. Both cell lines were then cultured in osteogenic or neurogenic differentiation medium containing: 1) low $[Ca^{2+}]_o$ (0.37 mM); 2) high $[Ca^{2+}]_o$ (2.87 mM); 3) AMG641 (0.05, 0.1 or 1 μM) with high $[Ca^{2+}]_o$ and 4) the CaSR antagonist NPS2390 (10 mM for 30 min) followed by incubation with AMG641 in high $[Ca^{2+}]_o$. Expression of osteogenic or neurogenic differentiation biomarkers was compared among groups. In both cell lines, AMG641 dose-dependently increased cell proliferation (up to $P<0.001$). Osteogenic molecular markers expression was differentially regulated by AMG641, with stimulatory (OPN up-regulation) in large or inhibitory (RUNX2 and OPN down-regulation) effects in small cells, respectively. AMG641 significantly increased alkaline phosphatase activity and calcium phosphate deposition in both cell lines. Following treatment with AMG641 during osteogenic differentiation, in both cell lines CaSR expression was inversely related to that of osteogenic markers and inhibition of CaSR by NPS2390 blocked AMG641-dependent responses. Early-stage neurogenic differentiation was promoted/triggered by AMG641 in both cell lines, as Nestin and CaSR mRNA transcription up-regulation were observed.

Conclusions/Significance: Calcium- and AMG641-induced CaSR stimulation promoted *in vitro* proliferation and osteogenic and early-stage neurogenic differentiation of UCM-MSCs. CaSR activation may play a fundamental role in selecting specific differentiation checkpoints of these two differentiation routes, as related to cell commitment status.

Editor: Shree Ram Singh, National Cancer Institute, United States of America

Funding: The study was supported by ONEV MIUR PONa3_00134 – n.254/R&C 18/05/2011. The authors received AMG641 from ERA-Amgen (Amgen Inc., Thousand Oaks, California, United States of America; Research Program Agreement n ° 2011568566). The funders had no role in study design, data collection and analysis, decision to publish, or preparation of the manuscript.

Competing Interests: ERA-Amgen provided AMG641 for this study. (Amgen Inc., Thousand Oaks, California, United States of America; Research Program Agreement n ° 2011568566).

* Email: nicmartino@libero.it

¤ Current address: Department of Biosciences, Biotechnologies and Biopharmaceutics (DBBB), University Campus "Ernesto Quagliariello" University of Bari Aldo Moro, Bari, Italy

Introduction

Recent developments in stem cell biology research area have revealed that umbilical cord matrix (UCM, also known as Wharton's jelly) is a pivotal source of "young" mesenchymal stem cells (MSCs) considered as much more proliferative, immunosuppressive and even more therapeutically active than those from adult tissue sources [1]. Several groups reported success in isolating and establishing MSCs cultures from UCM in human [2–8] as well as in large animal models, such as horses [9–16], pigs [17,18], and dogs [19–22].

The equine UCM (eUCM) is a well known source of MSCs that can be easily isolated, cryogenically preserved and *in vitro*-differentiated into adipocytes, chondrocytes, osteoblasts and in cells with a morphology typical of neurons with axon- and dendrite-like processes [9-12]. Moreover, eUCM-MSCs show expression of embryonic markers (Oct-4, SSEA-4, c-Myc), specific MSCs markers (CD44, CD90, CD105, and CD146) and lack expression of HLA-ABC, HLA1AG, and MHC II [12]. The low immunogenicity makes eUCM-MSCs ideal for cell therapy and regenerative medicine applications, both for species-specific purposes in equine medicine and as a large animal model of pre-clinical trials. The horse is of particular interest in the orthopaedic field, as bone, tendon and ligament diseases have a significant impact on equine industry. Also, enhancing research programs in this species could establish a particularly suitable animal model useful for pre-clinical trials in humans. Infact, current laboratory practices in equine regenerative medicine mirror those in the human field. Morever, the translational use of autologous and allogeneic MSCs for patient therapy far exceeds what is currently permitted in human medicine [23]. To date, stem cell therapy in equine orthopaedic diseases, a relatively new research area, has been based mainly on the use of bone marrow (BM-MSCs; [24,25]), adipose tissue (Ad-MSCs; [26]), amnion-derived (AM-MSCs; [24]) and umbilical cord blood (UCB-MSCs; [27]). The use of stem cells in equine neurological diseases/ neuropathies is still in a planning stage. The use of UCM-MSCs, due to their particularly advantageous features, such as ease of sourcing, high *in vitro* expandability and differentiation ability, immune-evasion and immune-regulation capacities, high homing ability, limited constraints due to ethical issues, low tumorigenicity, and even tumoricidal ability [1,6,28,29] could allow significant improvements of clinical therapeutical applications.

An important procedural aspect of stem cell-based therapies is the control of proliferation and differentiation and extracellular calcium ion (Ca^{2+}) is known as a potent mediator of the balance between proliferation and differentiation in a number of different cell types [30,31]. The extracellular calcium-sensing receptor (CaSR) is a G protein–coupled receptor able to bind extracellular Ca^{2+} ions [32], firstly identified in bovine parathyroid cells by Brown et al., [33], and subsequently involved in the regulation of whole-body Ca^{2+} metabolism [30].

In this context, a large body of evidence supports a role of CaSR in cell proliferation [31,34–41]. Indeed, a recent study from our unit reported the CaSR is expressed in eUCM-MSCs and is functionally active since calcium and the selective CaSR agonist NPS R-467 stimulate cell growth/proliferation in these cell lines, an effect which is reversed by the CaSR antagonist NPS2390 [13]. On the other hand, limited information is available on the role of CaSR in cell differentiation. Indeed, studies reported to date investigate its involvement in differentiation of specific lineages, such as osteoblasts [42,43], osteoclasts [44], perinatal sympathetic neurons [45], epidermal initiation sites in mouse developing embryos and epidermic tissues [46] and preadipocytes [47] whereas only few studies reported its role in driving/regulating differentiation of embryonic [48] or fetal-derived stem cells ([49], for amniotic fluid-derived stem cells). No studies are reported to date on CaSR role in UCM-MSC differentiation.

Investigating whether CaSR affects ostegenic and neurogenic differentiation potency of UCM-derived MSCs by means of its selective agonists could contribute to elucidate differentiation mechanisms and to optimize differentiation protocols and the development of novel (even *in utero* and/or neonatal) targeted therapies in both bone diseases and neurodegenerative disorders. The aim of the present study was to investigate, in the horse as a large animal model, the involvement of CaSR on osteogenic and neurogenic differentiation potency of size-sieved UCM-MSC lines, by testing the *in vitro* effects of AMG641, a novel research calcimimetic acting as a CaSR agonist.

Materials and Methods

Chemicals

AMG641 (chemical name: (1R)-N- ((6-(methyloxy)-4′-(trifluoromethyl)-3-biphenylyl)methyl)-1-phenylethanamine;) was provided by Amgen Inc. (Thousand Oaks, California, USA; Research Program Agreement n° 2011568566). NPS2390

(Quinoxaline-2-carboxilic acid adamantan-1-ylamide) was purchased by Sigma (N4786), Milan Italy. NPS R-467 ((R)-N-(3-phenylpropyl)-a-methyl-3-methoxybenzylamide hydrochloride) was a kind gift of Dr. R. Caroppo (Dept. Biosciences, Biotechnologies and Biopharmaceutics, University of Bari, Italy)

Cell lines isolation and stemness molecular charaterization

The study was carried out on two homogeneous subpopulations of equine UCM-MSCs (eUCM-MSCs) [12,13]. Cells were isolated from perivascular Wharton's jelly by using a multi-dishes plate with transwell inserts of 8 µm pores [12]. Therefore, we have referred to the cells as size-sieved stem cells separated by their dimension, one larger than 8µm (namely, large cell line) and the other smaller than 8µm in diameter (namely, small cell line). The two cell lines were molecularly characterized and found as expressing CaSR at mRNA and protein level [13], pluripotency-specific antigens (OCT-4 and c-Myc), MSC markers (CD105, CD44, CD29 and CD166) and showing weak expression of antigens TRA-1-60 and SSEA-4 and lack of expression of the hematopoietic markers CD34, CD14 and MHC-II [12]. As well, in these cell lines, cell growth significantly increased in presence of high $[Ca^{2+}]_o$, (2.87 mM $CaCl_2$), as previously reported [13].

Culture conditions

Cells were cultured at 38.5°C in a humidified atmosphere (95%) under 5% CO_2 in standard expansion medium, consisting of Dulbecco's Modified Eagle's Medium - High Glucose (DMEM) (Sigma D-5546) supplemented with 10% Fetal Calf Serum (FCS) (Sigma F3018), 100 U/ml penicillin, 100 µg/ml streptomycin, 0.25 µg/ml amphoterycin solution (Sigma A-5955), 2 mM L-glutamine (Sigma G-7513) and 10 ng/ml Epidermal Growth Factor (EGF; Sigma E-9644).

Cell freezing

Standard medium supplemented with 10% (v/v) FCS and 10% (v/v) dimethyl sulfoxide (DMSO, Sigma D-5879) was used to cryopreserve cells in cryotubes that were stored at −80°C and then transferred to cryogenic containers with liquid nitrogen until molecular analysis.

Osteogenic and neurogenic differentiation induction

Osteogenic and neurogenic *in vitro* differentiation potential was induced as previously reported [21,50]. Cells at P3 were seeded at a density of 3000 cells /cm^2 in six-well plates and were cultured until they reached approximately 80–90% confluence. For differentiation of MSCs into osteogenic lineage, cells were cultured for 21 days in medium consisting of HG-DMEM, supplemented with 10% FCS (Sigma), 100 U/ ml penicillin, 100µg/ml streptomycin, 0.25µg/ml amphotericin B, 2 mM L-glutamine, 10 mM beta-glycerophosphate, 0.1 µM dexamethasone and 250 µM ascorbic acid. Neurogenic induction was performed by culturing cells for 24 h in pre-induction medium consisting of HG-DMEM, 20% FCS and 1 mM beta-mercaptoethanol, with neural induction then performed by switching to a medium composed of DMEM plus 2% FCS, 2% dimethylsulphoxide (DMSO) and

200 mM butylated hydroxyanisole for 3 days. Non-induced control cells (negative controls) were cultured for the same length of time in standard medium (HG-DMEM supplemented with 10% FCS, 100 U/ ml penicillin, 100 µg/ml streptomycin, 0.25µg/ml amphotericin B, 2 mM L-glutamine).

Osteogenic differentiation assessment

Osteogenesis was assessed by alkaline phosphatase (ALP) assay [51] and von Kossa staining [50] and by evaluating the relative abundance of the transcripts of two osteogenic differentiation markers, such as Runt-related transcription factor 2 (RUNX2) and Osteopontin (OPN). Briefly, ALP activity, a typical osteoblast marker, was assessed by using the Alkaline Phosphatase Kit (Sigma Aldrich), a commercial kit based on naphthol AS-BI and fast red violet LB [51]. After treatments in the conditions described below (Experiment 2), cells were fixed with a citrate-acetone-formaldehyde fixative for 30 sec at room temperature. After being rinsed with distilled water, cells were incubated for 15 min in dark with alkaline-dye mixture (NaNO2, FRV-Alkaline Solution, Naphthol AS-BI Alkaline Solution) and washed with distilled water. Cells were counterstained with hematoxylin solution, washed in tap water and evaluated under light microscopy. For von Kossa staining, cells were washed with PBS and then fixed with 10% formalin for 1 h at room temperature. The formalin was removed and cells were washed with distilled water. A 5% (w/v) silver nitrate solution was added and cells were exposed to UV light for 20 min. Reaction was stopped by using a 5% sodium thiosulphate solution for 2 min. Cells were washed with distilled water. Calcium phosphate deposits stained black [50].

Neurogenic differentiation assessment

Neurogenic differentiation was assessed by conventional Nissl staining, beta III tubulin immunostaining and by evaluating the relative abundance of the transcripts of the two neurogenic differentiation markers, Glial Fibrillary Acidic Protein (GFAP) and Nestin. Briefly, for Nissl staining, cells were washed with PBS and then fixed with 10% formalin for 15 min at room temperature. The formalin was removed and cells were washed with distilled water and incubated in a 0.1% cresyl violet solution for 20 min. Cells were washed with distilled water and observed under light microscopy for the evaluation of Nissl bodies [50]. For beta III tubulin, a specific neuronal marker, cells were seeded on cover glass slides at the density of 1000 cell/cm^2. After treatments in the conditions described below (Experiment 2), cells were permeabilized with 0.03% Triton X-100 for 15 min at room temperature and then incubated for 10 min in 1% (w/v) Bovine Serum Albumin (BSA) in PBS (PBS-BSA). After that, cells were incubated overnight at room temperature with a 1:1000 dilution of a primary rabbit polyclonal antibody against the beta III tubulin (ab18207; Abcam, Cambridge, UK) in PBS-BSA. Cells incubated overnight in PBS-BSA were used as negative (no primary antibody) controls. At the end of incubation, cells were washed in PBS-BSA and incubated for 2 h at room temperature with a fluorescein isothiocyanate (FITC)- conjugated goat anti-rabbit IgG-secondary antibody (ab6717, Abcam) diluted 1:500 in PBS-BSA. After washing, cells were fixed in 2% para-formaldehyde solution in PBS, mounted on slides and observed under oil immersion (630x magnification) with a C1/TE2000-U Nikon confocal laser-scanning microscope, equipped with an Argon Ions 488 laser and an 495–519 (B2-A) nm excitation/emission filter.

Total RNA extraction

The RNeasy kit (QIAGEN, Milan, Italy) was used to extract total RNA. After thawing, cells were washed in PBS and then disrupted in Lysis Buffer RLT and homogenized at room temperature. A 70% ethanol solution was then added to the lysate, creating conditions that promoted selective binding of RNA to the RNeasy membrane. The lysate was transferred to an RNeasy spin column and centrifuged for 15 sec at 10000 rpm. The column was washed twice with washing buffer and finally, the total RNA was eluted in 30 µl of RNase-free water and stored at −80°C. The total amount of RNA of each sample was measured using the BioPhotometer plus (Eppendorf, Milan, Italy).

Reverse Transcription PCR

The High Capacity cDNA Reverse Transcription kit (4368814, LifeTechnologies, Monza, Italy) was used to convert RNA to cDNA. After thawing, 1 µg of total RNA of each sample was added to 2 µL 10X RT Buffer, 0.8 µL 25X dNTP Mix, 2 µL RT Random Primers, 1 µL M-MLV Reverse Transcriptase, 1 µLRNase Inhibitor and nuclease-free water for a total volume of 20 µl and then, the solution was mixed gently and centrifuged briefly. Reaction tubes were incubated at 10°C for 10 min, then at 37°C for 120 min and finally at 85°C for 5 min. cDNA was stored at −20°C until Real Time PCR analysis.

Real Time PCR

Real Time PCR was performed by using Real Time TaqMan technology and analyzed on automated "StepOne System" (Applied Biosystem, Monza, Italy). All TaqMan equine primers and probes were purchased from Life Technologies. Life Technologies inventored gene assays were adopted for Hypoxanthine phosphoribosyltransferase 1 (HPRT1; Ec03470219_m1) used as endogenous control, GFAP (Ec03470056_m1) and RUNX2 (Ec03469741_m1). For the equine CaSR, OPN and Nestin genes, primers and probes were specifically designed in the present study across an exon-exon junction, using Primer Express 3.0 software (Applied Biosystem) based on NCBI *Equus caballus* available nucleotidic sequences. The oligonucleotide sequences of the above Real Time PCR primers and probes are shown in Table 1. The TaqMan MGB (minor groove-binder) hybridization probe was labeled with a reporter dye (6-carboxy-fluorescein, FAM) on the 5′ nucleotide and a quenching dye with NFQ (non fluorescent quencher) on the 3′ nucleotide where MGB hyper-stabilized duplexes with complementary DNA. Samples were run in duplicates on Microamp fast optical 48-well reaction plate (Life Technologies) where twenty-microliters reactions for each well contained: 10 µL TaqMan gene expression Master Mix 2X (Life Technologies), 1µL 800 nM Primers and 250 nM Probe, 1–4 µL cDNA and RNase Free H_2O. Cycling parameters were: 2 min at 50°C, 10 min at 95°C followed by 40 cycles of 15 s at 95°C and 1 min at 60°C. Data were collected by using the StepOne Software (Applied Biosystem, Monza, Italy) and relative quantification was performed by using comparative method after determining the Ct (threshold cycle) values for the reference endogenous control (HPRT1) and the target gene in each sample sets, according to the $2^{-\Delta\Delta Ct}$ method as described by the manufacturer. Changes in mRNA expression levels were calculated after normalization to HPRT1. The program calculates the ΔCt and the ΔΔCt with the formulas below: ΔCt = Ct_Mean(HPRT1) – Ct_Mean(target gene); ΔΔCt = ΔCt – ΔCt_Mean, so that the gene expression level $= 2^{-\Delta\Delta Ct}$. Changes in gene expression were reported as percentage changes relative to controls.

Table 1. Oligonucleotide sequences used for Real Time-PCR analysis.

Markers	Forward Primer 5′→ 3′	Reverse Primer 5′→ 3′	Probe 5′→ 3′
Calcium-Sensing Receptor (CaSR)	CTTGGCAGGTCCTGAAGCA	TGGTTGTTATACCCCCTGGTC	CTACGGCACCTCAAC
Osteopontin (OPN)	CGCAGATCTGAAGACCAGTATCCT	TTGCTTTCCACAGGTGATGTG	TGCTACGGAAGAGGAC
Nestin (Nes)	ACTGAGAAGTTCCAGCTGGC	GGACATCTTGAGGTGTGCCA	GGGCCTGCAGAGCCAGATCGCCCAGG

Experimental Design

Experiment 1: Effects of AMG641 on *in vitro* proliferation of size-sieved eUCM-MSCs

To evaluate the optimal concentration of the calcimimetic, large and small eUCM-MSCs cells were seeded in six well plates and cultured in the standard medium supplemented with rising concentrations of AMG641 (0.01, 0.05, 0.1, 0.5, 1 and 3 μM) in presence of 2.5 mM $CaCl_2$. Calcium concentration was selected on the basis of a previous study from our unit [13] in which 2.5 mM $CaCl_2$ was considered as CaSR EC_{50} in both cell lines. External Ca^{2+} concentration ($[Ca^{2+}]_o$) in the present study, as in our previous study by Martino et al., [13] was actually either 0.37 (low $[Ca^{2+}]_o$) or 2.37 mMCa^{2+} (high $[Ca^{2+}]_o$). Infact, standard medium was supplemented with 10% FCS and, since average $[Ca^{2+}]_o$ in FCS was around 1.6 mg/dL, thus 3.7 mM [52], $[Ca^{2+}]_o$ in our standard medium (10% FCS) was around 0.37 mM. When additional 2.5 mMCa^{2+} was included, final $[Ca^{2+}]_o$ was 2.87 mM (0.37+2.5 = 2.87 mM). Control cells were cultured in medium with additional 2.5 mM $CaCl_2$ in the absence of AMG641. Negative controls were referred to cells cultured in medium with low calcium concentration (0.37 mM $CaCl_2$) whereas positive controls were referred to values observed in cells cultured in high calcium concentration and in presence of 3 μM NPS R-467. For DT calculation, cells were seeded, at the density of 1000 cell/cm^2. The DT data were calculated by using the following formula: CD = ln(Nf/Ni)/ln2 and DT = CT/CD, where DT is the cell-doubling time, CD is the cell-doubling number, CT is the cell culture time, Nf is the final number of cells and Ni the initial number of cells. Cells of each well were detached by using 0.05% trypsin/0.02% EDTA in PBS and were counted, by dilution (1:1) in Trypan blue, with Burker's counting chamber. Cell counts were performed on days 4th after the beginning of the treatments. Data were expressed as mean ± standard deviation of values obtained in three replicates. The Student's t-test was used to evaluate statistical significances and values with $P<0.05$ were considered as statistically different.

Experiment 2: Effects of AMG641 on osteogenic and neurogenic differentiation potential of eUCM-MSCs

Based on the results of experiment 1, three concentrations of AMG641 (0.05, 0.1 and 1 μM AMG641), that were shown to significantly stimulate cell proliferation, were selected to test its effects on osteogenic (experiment 2a) and neurogenic (experiment 2b) differentiation potential of eUCM-MSCs.

Cells were cultured in following conditions: 1) control (CTRL): osteogenic or neurogenic differentiation medium, as described above; 2) high external calcium (2.5 mM $CaCl_2$): differentiation medium +2.5 mM $CaCl_2$; 3) agonist (2.5 mM $CaCl_2$+ AMG641): differentiation medium plus 2.5 mM$CaCl_2$ and AMG641 (0.05 or 0.1 or 1 μM); 4) antagonist/agonist (2.5 mM $CaCl_2$ + NPS2390 + AMG641): standard differentiation medium plus 2.5 mM $CaCl_2$ and 1 μM AMG641. In these samples, before CaSR agonist addition, cells were preincubated for 30 min with 10 mM NPS2390. In both cell lines, after 14 days in vitro culture under osteogenic differentiation induction conditions, ALP activity was analyzed and, after 21 days, von Kossa staining was performed and CaSR and osteogenic differentiation markers mRNA expression levels were evaluated. As well, in both cell lines, after 4 days of neurogenic differentiation treatments, Nissl staining and beta III tubulin immunostaining were performed and CaSR and neurogenic differentiation markers mRNA expression levels were evaluated. The Student's t-test was used to evaluate the statistical significance of the results. Within each differentiation lineage, differentiation biomarkers relative expression in the four above mentioned treatments groups (CTRL, high calcium, agonist and antagonist/agonist) were compared. ALP activity, extracellular matrix mineralization (calcium deposits), Nissl bodies formation and beta III tubulin immunostaining were quantified by densitometric analysis using Adobe Photoshop. For each experimental condition, areas of constant size were measured. Staining intensity was evaluated by recording: 1) the total stained area, 2) the number of stained spots and 3) the mean spot area. Data (mean ± standard deviation of values obtained in three replicates) were expressed as number of pixels. The Student's t-test was used to evaluate statistical significances and values with $P<0.05$ were considered as statistically different.

Results

Experiment 1: AMG641 stimulates *in vitro* proliferation of eUCM-MSCs

In both cell lines, the proliferation rate was significantly increased upon AMG641 treatment and the effects of this compound were very similar between the two cell lines. In detail, in the large cell line, AMG641 significantly reduced DT values compared with controls ($P<0.01$ in cells treated with the two lowest AMG641 concentrations, i.e. 0.01 and 0.05μM AMG641; $P<0.001$ in cells treated with the four remaining higher AMG641 concentrations, i.e. 0.1, 0.5, 1 and 3 μM AMG641; Fig. 1, Panel A). Likewise, in the small cell line, AMG641 significantly reduced DT values compared with controls ($P<0.05$ in cells treated with the two lowest AMG641 concentrations; $P<0.001$ in cells treated with the remaining higher AMG641 concentrations; Fig. 1, Panel B). In both cell lines, DT values in cells cultured in medium with low calcium concentration (negative controls, CTRL) were significantly higher than that of cell cultured in high calcium ($P<0.05$). As well, in both cell types, DT values of cells cultured in presence of 3 μM NPS R-467 (positive controls) were significantly higher that those of 0.1 to 3 μM AMG641-treated cells ($P<0.001$ in both large and small cells), indicating a more sustained action of AMG641 than NPS R-467. In both cell lines, treatment with AMG641 had no effect on cell viability (Fig. 2; Panel A and Panel B), indicating non toxic effect of this compound on these cell lines.

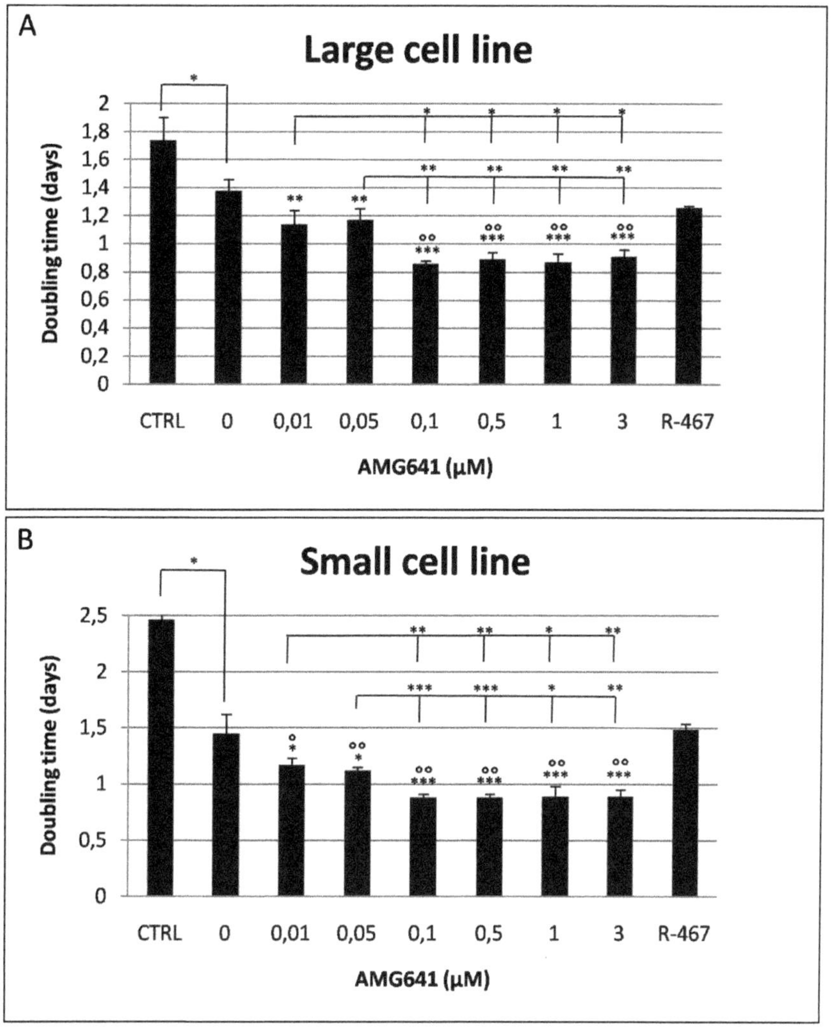

Figure 1. Effects of the calcimimetic AMG641 on *in vitro* proliferation of size-sieved eUCM-MSC lines. Cells were plated in 6-wells plates and treated as described in materials and methods. The effects of increasing doses of AMG641 in presence of 2.5 mM extracellular Ca^{2+} on the large (Panel A) and the small (Panel B) eUCM-MSC cell line are shown. In both cell lines, AMG641 significantly increased cell proliferation, expressed as significantly reduced doubling time (DT) values. DT values in cells cultured in medium with low calcium concentration (negative controls, CTRL) were significantly higher than those of cell cultured in high calcium (0 μM AMG641). DT values of cells cultured in presence of NPS R-467 (3μM, positive controls) were significantly higher that those of AMG641-treated cells. Data are mean ± standard deviation of values obtained in three replicates. Student's t-test: comparisons AMG641-treated cells vs controls (low and high calcium) and among used AMG641 concentrations: *$P<0.05$; **$P<0.01$; ***$P<0.001$; comparisons AMG641- vs NPS R-467-treated cells: $^{\circ}P<0.01$; $^{\circ\circ}P<0.001$.

Experiment 2a: CaSR activation promotes osteogenic differentiation of eUCM-MSCs

Effects of AMG641 on bone-like cell morphology and histochemical features. As a first approach to evaluate the effects of higher Ca^{2+} on AMG641 action on osteogenic differentiation potency of eUCM-MSCs lines, cell morphology, cytochemical and histochemical characteristics were analyzed. Cells were evaluated at P3. In both cell lines, ALP positivity was found in cells induced to differentiate through the osteogenic lineage with significantly higher proportions of ALP+ cells after treatment with high $[Ca^{2+}]_o$ plus AMG641 compared with high $[Ca^{2+}]_o$ alone ($P<0.05$ and $P<0.01$ for the large and the small cell lines, respectively). As well, in both cell lines, the CaSR antagonist NPS2390 reversed the stimulatory effect of AMG641 ($P<0.01$; Fig. 3, panel A, B). ALP quantification analysis confirmed these observations, as significantly higher ALP activity was found in AMG641-treated cells compared with high $[Ca^{2+}]_o$ alone controls ($P<0.05$) and this effect was reversed by addition of NPS2390 ($P<0.05$; Fig. 3, panel C, D). Figures 4 and 5 show representative photomicrographs of ALP and von Kossa stained cells in both large and small cell lines, respectively. Clearly evident ALP positivity and conspicuous mineralized extracellular matrix deposition by von Kossa staining with no apparent differences among those cultured in presence of low (Fig. 4 A, F) or high $[Ca^{2+}]_o$ (Fig. 4 B, G) or high $[Ca^{2+}]_o$ plus AMG641 (Fig. 4 C, H) were observed. Instead, in cells pre-incubated with the CaSR antagonist NPS2390 and subsequently treated with AMG641, reduced proportion of ALP+ cells and reduced amount of calcium phosphate deposits were observed (Fig. 4 D, I). Non-induced negative control cell lines showed neither ALP positivity nor relevant calcium phosphate deposits after von Kossa staining (Fig. 4 E, L). These observations can be similarly referred to the large, as well as to the small cell line (Fig. 5 A to L). Quantification

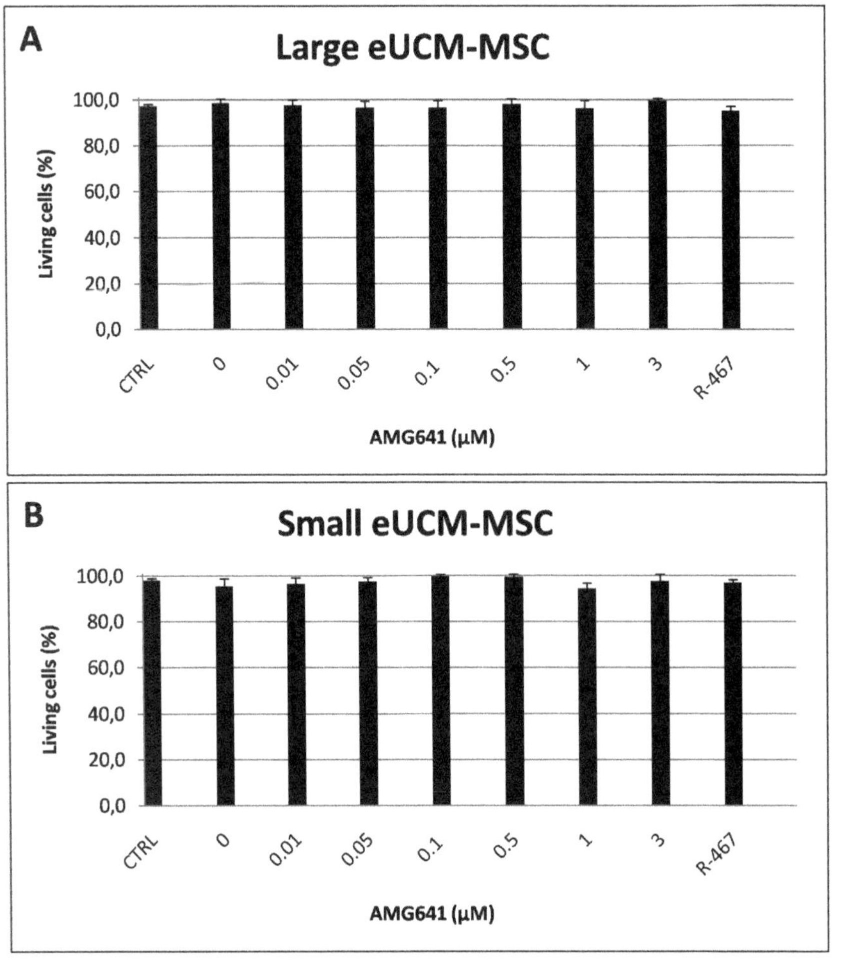

Figure 2. Effects of the calcimimetic AMG641 on cell viability of size-sieved eUCM-MSC lines. Cell viability is expressed as percentage of living (unstained) cells after Trypan blue staining. The effects of increasing doses of AMG641 in presence of 2.5 mM extracellular Ca^{2+} on the large (Panel A) and the small (Panel B) eUCM-MSC cell line are shown. Cell viability remained at high values, indicating non toxic effects of AMG641 on these cell lines. As in Figure 1, values in cells cultured in medium with low calcium concentration are referred as negative controls (CTRL) and values observed in cells cultured in presence of 3 µM NPS R-467 are referred as positive controls (R-467). Data are mean ± standard deviation of values obtained in three replicates. Student's t-test: NS.

analysis of von Kossa stained specimens allowed to observe that cells induced to osteogenic differentiation showed significantly higher mineralization level in response to CaSR activation by the calcimimetic AMG641 (comparison 1 µM AMG641-treated cells vs high high $[Ca^{2+}]_o$ control: $P<0.05$ in large cells, Fig. 6, Panel A; $P<0.001$ in small cells, Fig. 6, Panel B). The addition of the CaSR antagonist NPS2390 significantly reversed the agonists effects ($P< 0.001$ in both large and small cells).

Effects of high $[Ca^{2+}]_o$ on CaSR and osteogenic biomarkers expression. Elevating $[Ca^{2+}]_o$ in culture medium during osteogenic differentiation significantly increased the relative abundance of osteogenic differentiation biomarkers compared with that observed in standard differentiation conditions (CTRL). In the large cell line, additional Ca^{2+} up-regulated Osteopontin (OPN, $P<0.05$) and CaSR ($P<0.05$) mRNA expression even if it had no effect on relative expression of the Runt-related transcription factor, RUNX2 (Fig. 7, Panel A) whereas in the small cell line, high $[Ca^{2+}]_o$ significantly increased both OPN and RUNX2 transcripts level ($P<0.001$ and $P<0.01$, respectively; Fig. 7, Panel B) but it had no effects on CaSR expression.

Effects of AMG641 on CaSR and osteogenic biomarkers expression. The addition of AMG641 in presence of high $[Ca^{2+}]_o$ during osteogenic differentiation induced opposite effects in the two cell lines. In the large cell line, AMG641 increased OPN transcription ($P<0.05$ and $P<0.01$ with 0.1 and 1 µM AMG641, respectively) and had no effect on RUNX2 expression (Fig. 8, Panel A) while, conversely, in the small cell line, AMG641 significantly down-regulated OPN ($P<0.05$, $P<0.01$ and $P<0.05$ in cells stimulated with 0.05, 0.1 and 1 µM AMG641, respectively) and RUNX2 transcription ($P<0.05$ in cells treated with 0.1 µM AMG641) (Fig. 8, Panel B). Interestingly, CaSR transcription was found to be inversely related to the expression of osteogenic markers. In fact, it was significantly down-regulated in the large cell line ($P<0.01$ at 0.05 and 0.1 µM AMG641), but markedly up-regulated in the small cell line, with a clear dose-response effect ($P<0.05$, $P<0.01$ and $P<0.0001$, at 0.05, 0.1 and 1 µM AMG641, respectively). In both cell lines, the addition of NPS2390 reversed the effects of the CaSR agonist AMG641 on OPN mRNA levels, with significant down-regulation in large cells ($P<0.01$) and up-regulation in small cells ($P<0.001$) whereas it had no effects on RUNX2 mRNA levels. In both cell lines, NPS2390

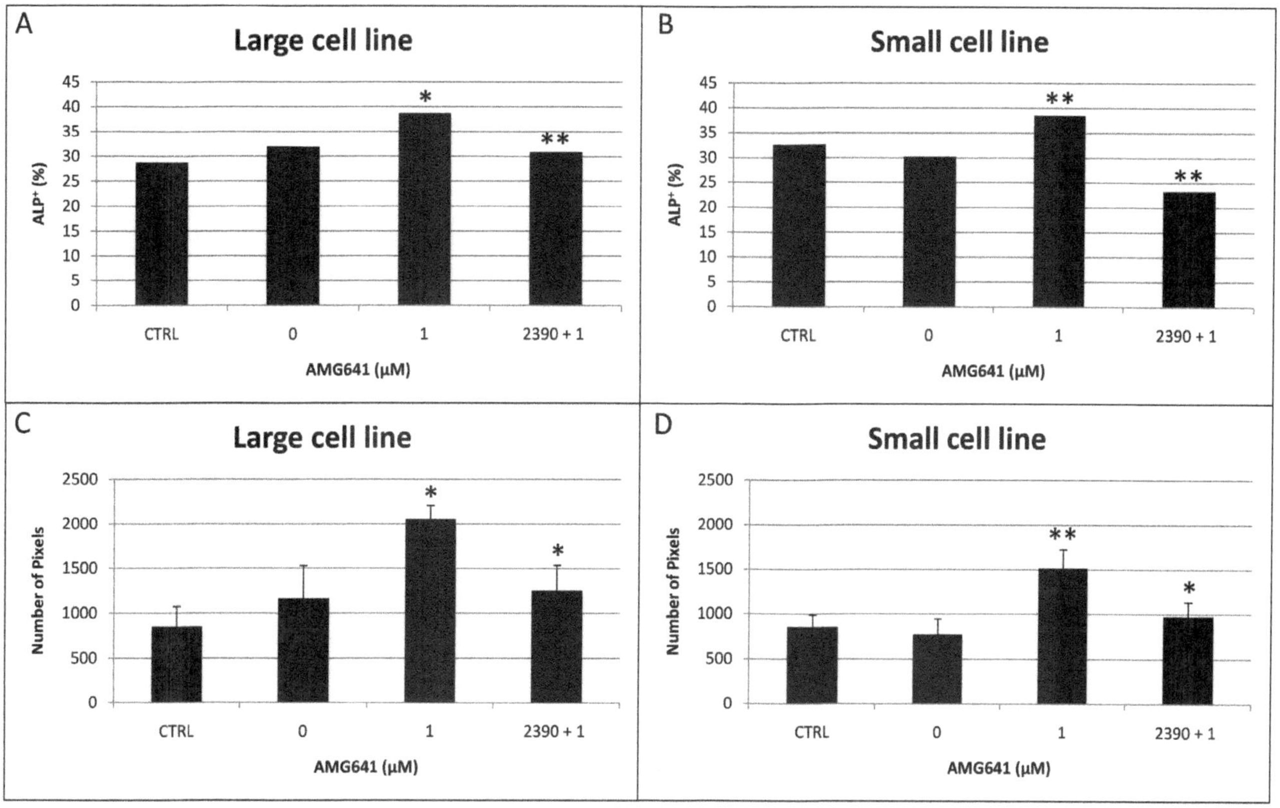

Figure 3. Effects of calcium and the calcimimetic AMG641 on osteogenic differentiation efficiency of size-sieved eUCM-MSC lines, as assessed by ALP activity. Panel A: percentages of ALP+ cells in the large and small cell lines observed after treatments, as described in M&M, Experiment 2: (CTRL) control cells differentiated *in vitro* in presence of low $[Ca^{2+}]_o$; (0) cells differentiated *in vitro* in presence of high $[Ca^{2+}]_o$; (1) AMG641-treated cells (treated with 1 μM AMG641 in presence of of high $[Ca^{2+}]_o$); (NPS2390+1) NPS2390/AMG641-treated cells (cells pre-incubated for 10 min in 10 mM NPS2390 and then cultured in 1 μM AMG641in presence of of high $[Ca^{2+}]_o$). A minimum of 500 cells per experimental condition was counted. In both cell lines, the addition of AMG641 significantly increased the proportion of ALP+ cells (1 vs 0: $P<0.05$ and $P<0.01$ for large and small cell lines, respectively). As well, in both cell lines, the CaSR antagonist reversed the stimulatory effect of AMG641 on ALP activity ($P<0.01$). Panel B: Quantification analysis was performed by measuring the total stained area normalized on the number of counted cells. Data are expressed as number of pixels. Significantly higher ALP activity was found after AMG641 treatment (1 vs 0: $P<0.05$) and significantly lower ALP activity was found after antagonist treatment compared with AMG641 (NPS2390+1 vs 1: $P<0.05$). Non-induced controls (non induced to differentiate in vitro) showed 0 value in both cell lines and in both panels, as ALP positivity was not observed at all in these samples (data not shown).

was not able to reverse the effect of AMG641 on CaSR relative abundance.

Experiment 2b: CaSR activation promotes neurogenic differentiation of eUCM-MSCs

Effects of AMG641 on neuron-like cell morphology. The effects of AMG641 in presence of additional Ca^{2+} on neurogenic differentiation potency of eUCM-MSC lines, were assessed by cell morphology and cytochemical characteristics. Cells were evaluated at P3. Cells directed toward neurogenic differentiation showed diffused discrete granular bodies after Nissl staining, with no apparent differences among those cultured in presence of low (Fig. 4 M) or high $[Ca^{2+}]_o$ (Fig. 4 N) or high $[Ca^{2+}]_o$ plus AMG641 (Fig. 4 O) or in cells pre-incubated with the CaSR antagonist NPS2390 and subsequently treated with AMG641 (Fig. 4 P). A low percentage of cells (around 1%) became more elongated and showed neuronal-like morphology, as they displayed beta III tubulin immunopositivity throughout the cell body, the axon and dendritic-like extensions (Fig. 4 R,S,T,U). Non-induced negative controls showed neither Nissl nor beta III tubulin labeling (Fig. 4 Q, V). These observations can be similarly referred to the small cell line (Fig. 5 M to V). In both cell lines, densitometric analysis for Nissl bodies quantification did not show statistically significant differences among groups (Fig.6, Panel C and Panel D). Densitometric analysis of beta III tubulin labeled cells did not reveal statistical differences among groups (data not shown).

Effects of high $[Ca^{2+}]_o$ on CaSR and neurogenic biomarkers expression. In both cell lines, additional Ca^{2+} up-regulated Nestin ($P<0.05$ in the large cell line, Fig. 7, Panel C; $P<0.01$ in the small cell line, Fig. 7, Panel D) and CaSR ($P<0.05$ in both cell lines) mRNA expression whereas the GFAP transcript was never detected in any examined culture condition.

Effects of AMG641 on CaSR and neurogenic biomarkers expression. The addition of AMG641 during neurogenic differentiation induced similar effects in the two cell lines. In detail, in both cell lines, it significantly increased Nestin mRNA level when added at 1 μM ($P<0.05$; Fig. 8 Panels C and D). The GFAP transcript was never detected in both cell lines, either cultured with or without AMG641. As well, in both cell lines, the treatment with AMG641 significantly increased the CaSR transcript level ($P<0.05$ and $P<0.001$ at 0.05 and 1 μM AMG641 respectively in the large cell line; Fig. 8, Panel C and $P<0.05$ an $P<0.001$ at 0.05 and 0.1 μM AMG641, respectively in

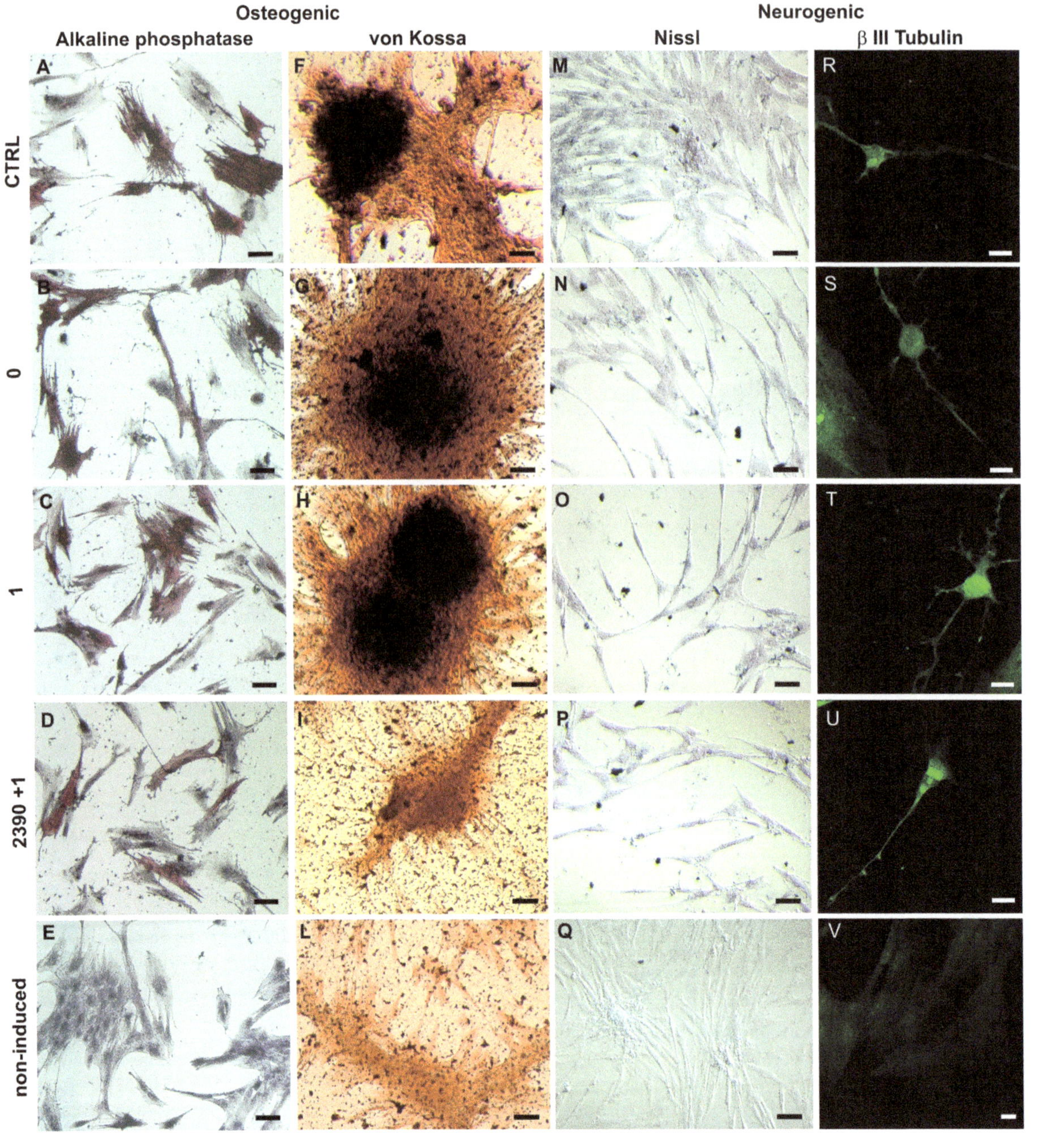

Figure 4. Bone-like and neuron-like morphology, cytochemical and histochemical features of AMG641-treated large eUCM-MSCs as evaluated by ALP activity, von Kossa and Nissl stainings and beta III tubulin immunodetection. Photomicrographs representative of the morphological appearance of the large eUCM-MSC line induced to differentiate *in vitro* toward osteogenic (1st and 2nd column) or neurogenic (3rd and 4th column) lineages in presence of 1μM AMG641 and observed after ALP activity assay, von Kossa and Nissl stainings, and beta III tubulin immunostaining. (A, F, M, R) control cells differentiated *in vitro* in presence of low $[Ca^{2+}]_o$; (B, G, N, S) cells differentiated *in vitro* in presence of high $[Ca^{2+}]_o$; (C, H, O, T) AMG641-treated cells (treated with 1 μM AMG641 in presence of of high $[Ca^{2+}]_o$); (D, I, P, U) NPS2390/AMG641-treated cells (cells pre-incubated for 10 min in 10 mM NPS2390 and then cultured in 1 μM AMG641in presence of of high $[Ca^{2+}]_o$); (E, L, Q, V) non-induced controls. Osteogenic differentiation was evidenced by increased ALP activity observed after 14 days *in vitro* culture and by the formation of mineralized matrix as shown by von Kossa staining after 21 days *in vitro* culture. No apparent differences can be seen for ALP activity and for the presence of mineral deposits after treatment with high $[Ca^{2+}]_o$ (B, G) or with AMG641 in high $[Ca^{2+}]_o$ (C, H) compared with controls (CTRL: A, F). ALP positivity and amount of calcium phosphate deposits appear to be reduced in antagonist/agonist-treated cells (D, I) compared with those treated with the CaSR agonist AMG641 (C, H). Neurogenic differentiation was evidenced by the presence of Nissl bodies and beta III tubulin positivity, as observed after 4 days *in vitro* culture. All cells directed toward neurogenic differentiation showed diffused discrete granular bodies after Nissl staining with no apparent differences among those cultured in presence of low (M) or high $[Ca^{2+}]_o$ (N) or high $[Ca^{2+}]_o$ plus AMG641 (O) or in cells pre-incubated with the CaSR antagonist NPS2390 and subsequently treated with AMG641 (P). Some cells showed neuron-like appearance and pancytoplasmic beta III tubulin immunopositivity in all induced conditions (R,S,T, U) with no apparent differences among treatments. Non-induced control cells were unstained for osteogenic (E, L) and neurogenic (Q, V) markers. Black scale bars indicate 10 μm; white scale bars indicate 5 μm.

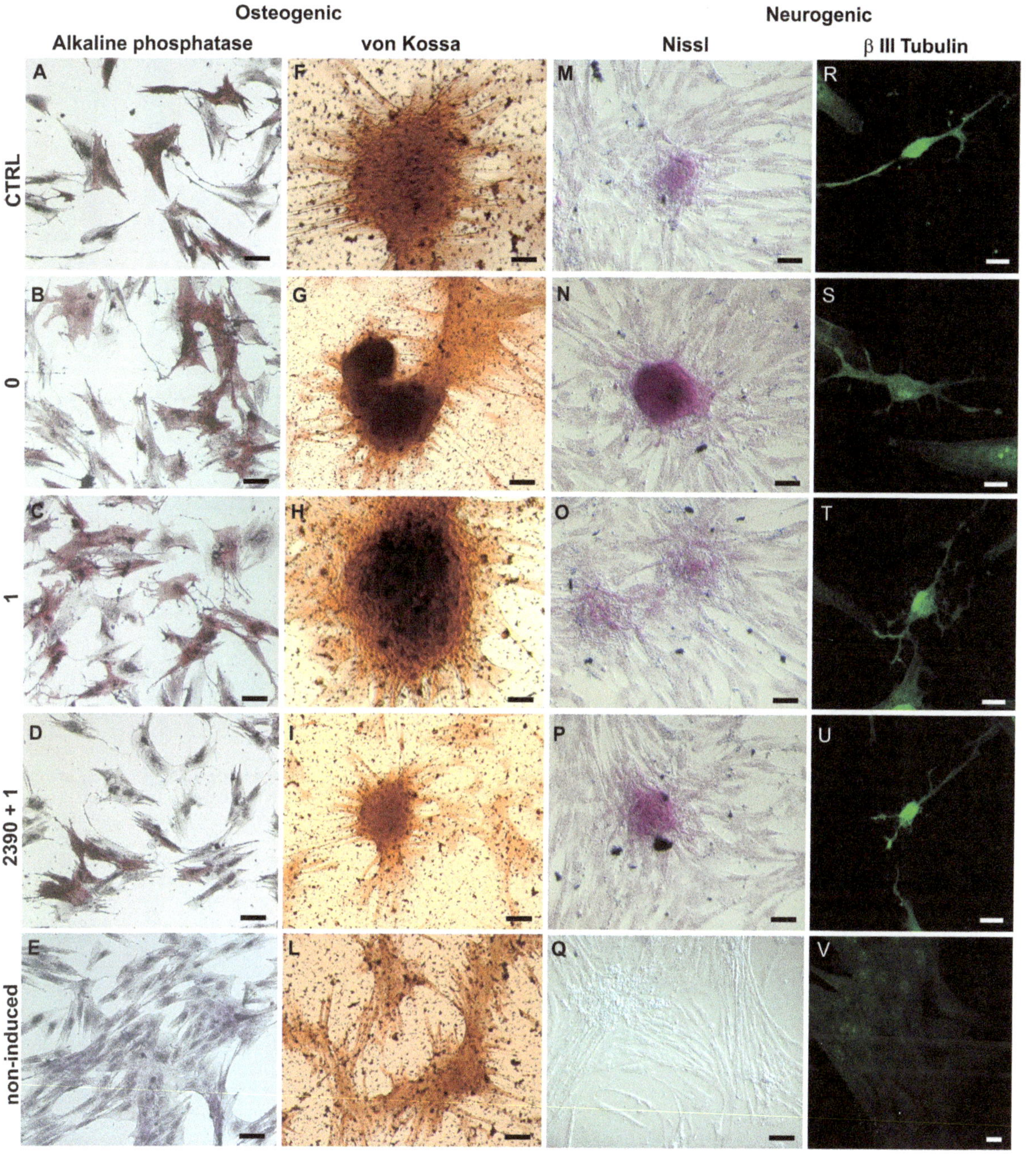

Figure 5. Bone-like and neuron-like morphology, cytochemical and histochemical features of AMG641-treated small eUCM-MSCs as evaluated by ALP activity, von Kossa and Nissl stainings and beta III tubulin immunodetection. Photomicrographs representative of morphological appearance of the small eUCM-MSC line induced to differentiate *in vitro* toward osteogenic (1st and 2nd column) or neurogenic (3rd and 4th column) lineages in presence of 1μM AMG641 and observed after ALP activity assay, von Kossa and Nissl stainings, and beta III tubulin immunostaining. As in Figure 4, control cells differentiated *in vitro* in the presence of low $[Ca^{2+}]_o$ (A, F, M, R), cells differentiated *in vitro* in the presence of high $[Ca^{2+}]_o$ (B, G, N, S), AMG641-treated cells (treated with 1 μM AMG641 in the presence of high $[Ca^{2+}]_o$) (C, H, O, T), NPS2390/AMG641-treated cells (cells pre-incubated for 10 min in 10 mM NPS2390 and then cultured in 1 μM AMG641in the presence of high $[Ca^{2+}]_o$) (D, I, P, U) and non-induced controls (E, L, Q, V) are shown. As in the large cells, no apparent differences can be seen for ALP activity and for the presence of mineral deposits after treatment with high $[Ca^{2+}]_o$ (B, G) or with AMG641 in high $[Ca^{2+}]_o$ (C, H) compared with controls (CTRL: A, F). Even in small cells, ALP positivity and the amount of calcium phosphate deposits appears to be significantly reduced in antagonist/agonist-treated cells (D, I) compared with those treated with the CaSR agonist AMG641 (C, H). All cells directed toward neurogenic differentiation showed discrete granular bodies after Nissl staining no apparent differences among those cultured in presence of low (M) or high $[Ca^{2+}]_o$ (N) or high $[Ca^{2+}]_o$ plus AMG641 (O) or in cells pre-incubated with the CaSR antagonist NPS2390 and subsequently treated with AMG641 (P) can be seen. Some cells showed neuron-like appearance as they displayed beta III tubulin immunopositivity throughout the cell body, the axon and dendritic-like extensions with no apparent differences among treatments. Non-induced control cells were unstained for osteogenic (E, L) and neurogenic (Q, V) markers. Black scale bars indicate 10 μm; white scale bars indicate 5 μm.

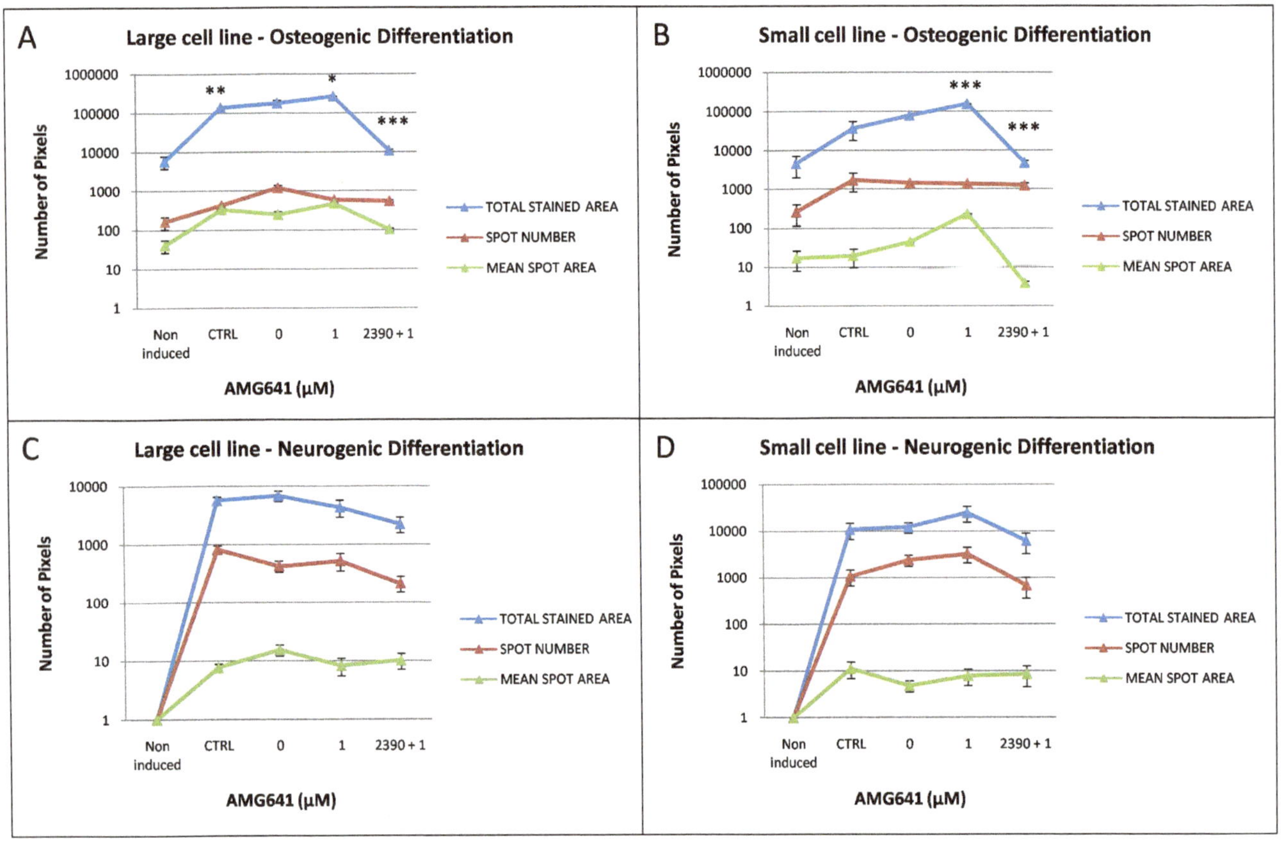

Figure 6. Effects of calcium and the calcimimetic AMG641 on osteogenic and neurogenic differentiation efficiency of size-sieved eUCM-MSC lines, as assessed by quantification of extracellular matrix mineralization and Nissl bodies formation. Densitometric analysis was performed in large and small cells after von Kossa (Panel A and B) and Nissl staining (Panel C and D). For each experimental condition, areas of constant size were measured. Staining intensity was evaluated by recording: 1) the total stained area, 2) the number of stained spots and 3) the mean spot area. Data (mean ± standard deviation of values obtained in three replicates) are expressed as number of pixels. Cells induced to osteogenic differentiation showed higher mineralization levels in response to CaSR activation by the calcimimetic AMG641 (large and small cells). The addition of the CaSR antagonist NPS2390 reversed the agonists effects. In both cell lines, no statistical differences were noticed among treatments for Nissl staining intensity values. Student's t-test: comparisons AMG641-treated cells vs controls (low and high calcium) and among used AMG641 concentrations: *P<0.05; **P<0.01; ***P<0.001.

the small cell line; Fig. 8, Panel D). No repeatable reverse effects were obtained upon NPS2390 addition.

Discussion

The proliferation study was performed with the aim to preliminary testing *in vitro* AMG641 activity on equine fetal adnexa-derived size-sieved UCM-MSCs. A dose-response effect of AMG641 on the proliferation rate of eUCM-MSCs was observed. AMG641 in presence of high $[Ca^{2+}]_o$ significantly increased cell proliferation in both large and small eUCM-MSCs lines. To the best of our knowledge, this is the first study on the effects of AMG641 on cell proliferation of *in vitro* cultured cell lines and, more specifically, in fetal-adnexa derived mesenchymal stem cell lines. AMG641 is a research calcimimetic mainly reported to date in studies on calcium homeostasis disorders [54–57]. Recent studies reported its effect as selective activator of CaSR [55,58–61]. Only one study has been reported to date, on the effects of AMG641 on *in vivo* cell proliferation [58] and reduced or unchanged proliferation rates were observed in cells obtained from parathyroid tissues of five-sixth nephrectomized rats, after the application of a long or short term *in vivo* administration protocol of AMG641, respectively. Our data cannot be easily compared with those of the study by Mendoza et al., [58], due to different *in vivo* versus *in vitro* adopted experimental approaches. Moreover, AMG641 has been reported as having different effects attending to cell types [60]. Further comparisons can be performed with previous studies reporting the effects of other selective CaSR agonists on the proliferation of fetal-adnexa derived MSCs. Our group reported that NPS R-467 stimulates cell proliferation in the same cell lines, eUCM-MSCs [13]. Interestingly, the stimulatory effect of AMG641 on cell proliferation was evident even at the very low tested concentrations (0.01 μM) whereas higher concentrations of NPS R-467 (3μM; [13,38]) or its precursor NPS R-568 (0.3–1 μM; [35]) were reported in previous studies. The stimulatory effect of NPS R-467 was confirmed in the present proliferation study, as it was used as positive control. This finding could be considered of high importance for the use of this novel potent calcimimetic as a component of media for fetal-derived MSC cultures, in protocols aimed to obtain enough cells for downstream purposes of cell therapy applications.

Given that it was previously demonstrated that physiological changes in $[Ca^{2+}]_o$ control, via CaSR, the fate of progenitor cells of specific lineages (such as osteogenic, neurogenic, adipogenic and epidermic lineages: see Introduction for references) toward their specific differentiation routes, after testing the dose-response effect

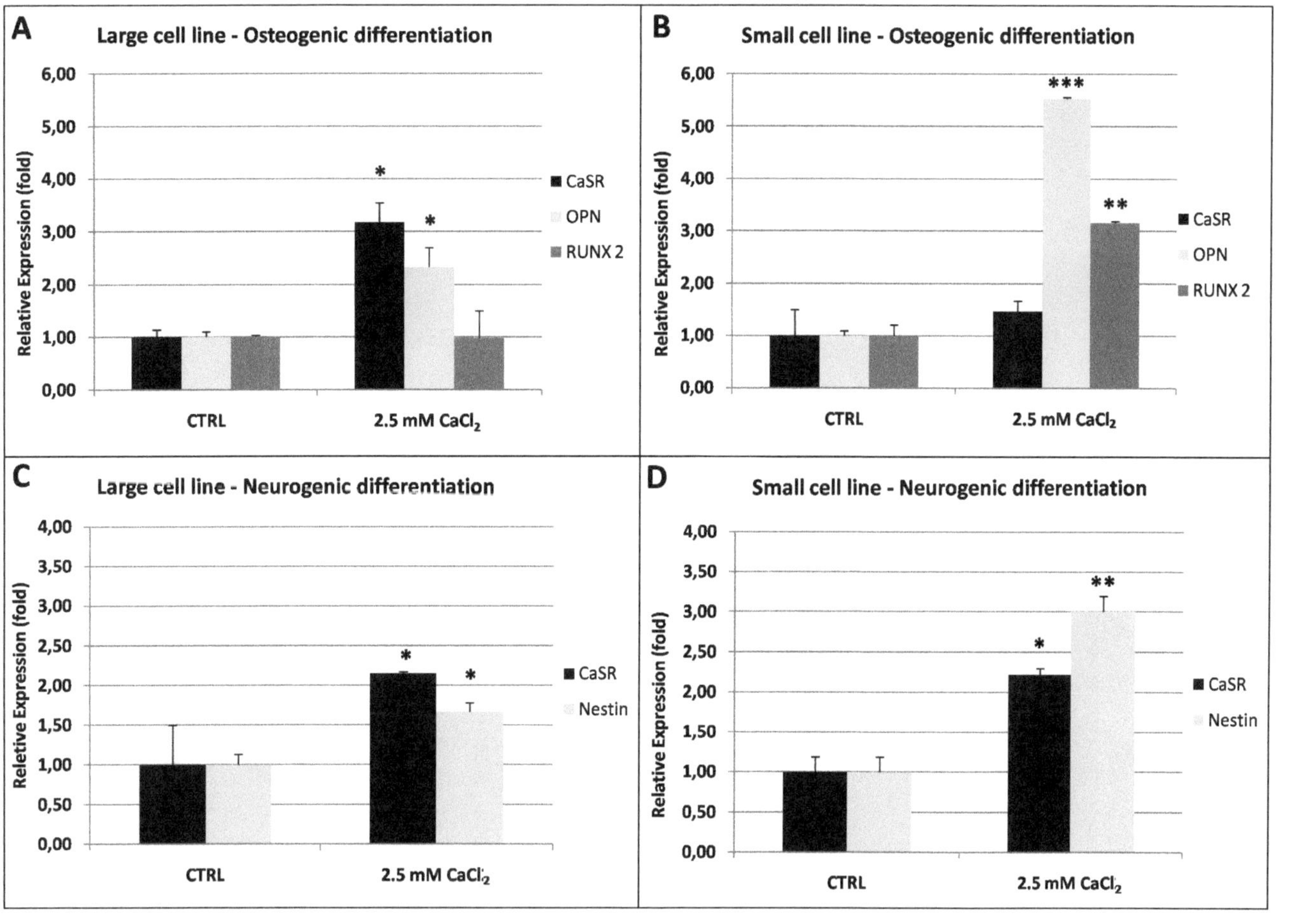

Figure 7. Relative abundance of CaSR and specific osteogenic and neurogenic differentiation biomarkers in eUCM-MSCs upon Ca^{2+}-induced CaSR stimulation. Panels A, B: Quantitative Real Time RT-PCR analysis of CaSR, OPN and RUNX2 transcripts in high $[Ca^{2+}]_o$-treated equine UCM-MSCs (2.5 mM $CaCl_2$) versus low $[Ca^{2+}]_o$ controls (CTRL). In the large cell line, additional Ca^{2+} up-regulated CaSR ($P<0.05$) and OPN ($P<0.05$) mRNA expression even if it had no effect on RUNX2 (Panel A). In the small cell line, high $[Ca^{2+}]_o$ significantly increased both OPN and RUNX2 transcripts level ($P<0.001$ and $P<0.01$, respectively; Panel B) but it had no effects on CaSR expression. Panels C, D: Quantitative Real Time RT-PCR analysis of CaSR, Nestin and GFAP transcripts in high $[Ca^{2+}]_o$-treated equine UCM-MSCs (2.5 mM $CaCl_2$) versus low $[Ca^{2+}]_o$controls (CTRL). In both cell lines, additional Ca^{2+} up-regulated Nestin ($P<0.05$ in the large cell line, Panel C; $P<0.01$ in the small cell line, Panel D) and CaSR ($P<0.05$) mRNA expression whereas the GFAP transcript was not detected. For each sample, average Ct data (mean±SD of three independent experiments in duplicate) were normalized relatively to the abundance of HPRT1 mRNA (endogenous control) and normalized values were compared between groups. Student's t-Test; $^{*}P<0.05$; $^{**}P<0.01$; $^{***}P<0.001$.

of AMG641 on cell proliferation, we wanted to test the effects of this potent research calcimimetic on the differentiation potency of fetal mesenchymal stem cell populations, such as UCM-MSCs, considered as less committed and having wider stemness bounderies than progenitor cells of specific lineages.

In UCM-MSCs, we showed that keeping elevated $[Ca^{2+}]_o$ in culture medium during osteogenic differentiation induced over-expression of bone differentiation-related genes. The observed cell responses had different extent in the two examined cell lines. In detail, in the large cell line, high $[Ca^{2+}]_o$ up-regulated OPN mRNA expression, whereas in the small cell line it increased both OPN and RUNX2 mRNA levels. These results may be interpreted in light of different roles played by these osteogenic biomarkers. Indeed, RUNX2 (also known as Core binding factor alfa 1, Cbfa 1) is the master osteoblast transcription factor responsible for osteoblast differentiation and mineralization whereas OPN is a major osteoblast organic matrix protein downstream of RUNX2 [42]. Thus, it could be possible that in the small cell line (less committed), high $[Ca^{2+}]_o$ was able to up-regulate the master gene RUNX2 and, consequently, its downstream gene OPN. Whereas, in the large cell line (more committed), high $[Ca^{2+}]_o$ was only able to stimulate OPN expression. These findings are in part in agreement with studies published meanwhile our study was performed [49,62]. In human bone marrow mesenchymal stromal cells cultured *in vitro*, elevated $[Ca^{2+}]_o$ was reported to induce over-expression of genes coding for bone-related extracellular matrix proteins, such as OPN, Osteocalcin and bone sialoprotein but it had no effects on RUNX2 [62]. In the same study, the authors reported evidences demonstrating that the signaling pathway between extracellular $Ca^{2+}$and bone morphogenetic protein 2 (BMP-2), a protein essential to maintain bone homeostasis and having a prominent role in fracture healing, involves type L voltage-dependent Ca^{2+}channels (L-VDCC) rather/more than CaSR. A subsequent study strengthen the role of CaSR in supporting osteogenic differentiation, as it demonstrated that extracellular calcium promotes osteogenic differentiation in human periodontal ligament stem/progenitor cells and that CaSR and L-VDCC appear

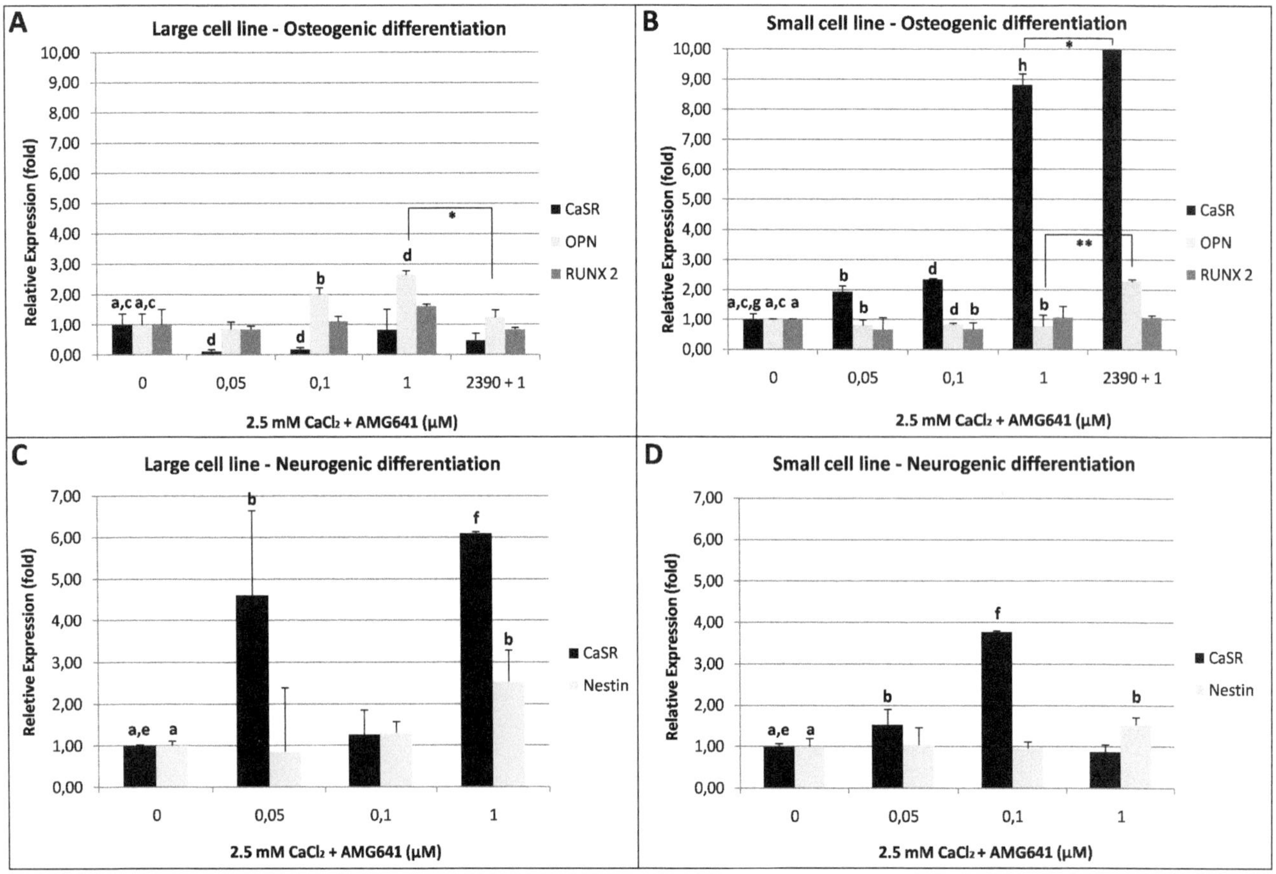

Figure 8. Relative abundance of CaSR and specific osteogenic and neurogenic differentiation biomarkers in eUCM-MSCs upon calcimimetic AMG641-induced CaSR stimulation. Panels A, B: Quantitative Real Time RT-PCR analysis of CaSR, OPN and RUNX2 transcripts inhigh $[Ca^{2+}]_o$ and (0.05, 0.1 or 1 µM) calcimimetic AMG641-treated equine UCM-MSCs (2.5 mM $CaCl_2$+AMG641) or cells pre-incubated with the CaSR antagonist NPS2390 (2.5 mM $CaCl_2$+NPS2390+AMG641) versus cells cultured in high $[Ca^{2+}]_o$ (2.5 mM $CaCl_2$) alone (indicated as 0 µM AMG641). In the large cell line, AMG641 increased OPN transcription ($P<0.05$ and $P<0.01$ with 0.1 and 1 µM AMG641, respectively) and had no effect on RUNX2 expression (Panel A). In the small cell line, AMG641 significantly down-regulated OPN ($P<0.05$, $P<0.01$ and $P<0.05$ respectively in cells stimulated with 0.05, 0.1 and 1 µM AMG641) and RUNX2 transcription ($P<0.05$ in cells treated with 0.1 µM AMG641) (Panel B). Upon AMG641 addition, CaSR expression was significantly down-regulated in the large cell line ($P<0.01$ at 0.05 and 0.1 µM AMG641), but markedly up-regulated (up to approximately 9 folds) in the small cell line, with a dose-response effect ($P<0.05$, $P<0.01$ and $P<0.0001$, at 0.05, 0.1 and 1 µM AMG641, respectively). In both cell lines, the addion of NPS2390 reversed the effects of AMG641 on OPN mRNA levels, with significant reduction in large cells ($P<0.01$) and significant increase in small cells ($P<0.001$) whereas it had no effects on RUNX2 mRNA levels. In both cell lines, the CaSR relative abundance remained at comparable levels after agonist or antagonist/agonist treatments. Panels C, D: Quantitative Real Time RT-PCR analysis of CaSR, Nestin and GFAP transcripts in cells cultured in the conditions as described for Panels A,B. In both cell lines, AMG641 significantly increased Nestin mRNA level at the highest tested dose (1 µM, $P<0.05$; Panels C and D). The GFAP transcript was never detected in any examined condition (not shown). As well, in both cell lines, AMG641 significantly increased CaSR transcription level (up to six folds in the large cell line; $P<0.05$ and $P<0.001$ at 0.05 and 1 µM AMG641 respectively; Panel C and up to approximately 4 folds in the small cell line; $P<0.05$ an $P<0.001$ at 0.05 and 0.1 µM AMG641, respectively; Panel D). In both cell line types, no repeatable reverse effects were obtained upon NPS2390 addition (data not shown). For each sample, average Ct data (mean±SD of three independent experiments in duplicate) were normalized relatively to the abundance of HPRT1 mRNA (endogenous control) and normalized values were compared among groups. Student's t-Test: a,b $P<0.05$; c,d $P<0.01$; e,f $P<0.001$; * $P<0.01$; ** $P<0.001$.

to act reciprocally in mediating this process [63]. In ovine amniotic fluid MSCs, increasing $[Ca^{2+}]_o$ was reported to increase ALP activity [49]. Our data allow to confirm that Ca^{2+} is a potential osteo-inductive triggerer in UCM-MSCs, and that observed difference in the RUNX2 expression between the two cell lines tested in the present study could be related to differences in their developmental and functional stage (commitment level), as previously reported [12,13]. Similarly, Ca^{2+}-induced up-regulation of osteogenic biomarkers was associated with up-regulation of CaSR expression (significant increase in the large cell line and increasing trend in the small cell line), leading us to hypothesize that Ca^{2+}-induced stimulation of osteogenic differentiation could be mediated by CaSR.

The addition of AMG641 during osteogenic differentiation induced opposite effects in the two cell line types. In fact, in the large cell line, AMG641 promoted osteogenic differentiation as it significantly increased OPN transcription, ALP activity and cell mineralization level even if it had no effect on RUNX2 expression, as observed in the same cell line upon stimulation with high $[Ca^{2+}]_o$. Conversely, in the small cell line, AMG641 significantly down-regulated OPN and RUNX2 transcription even though it significantly increased ALP activity and calcium phosphate deposit formation. This apparent discrepancy may be explained considering that the formation of the organic glycoproteic and inorganic mineralized extracellular matrix are distinct events in the sequence leading to bone formation. Mineralization is regulated by a complex arrangement of stimulatory and inhibitory components [42] and AMG641-mediated CaSR stimulation may result in a balance between stimulatory and inhibitory factors involved in calcium phosphate crystal formation and prevention of eccessive mineralization. Our data on the effects of CaSR stimulation on osteogenic differentiation can be compared with those of the recently published study by Di Tomo et al., [49] who reported that the addition of the calcimimetic R-568, a selective CaSR agonist, in ovine amniotic fluid MSCs, increases cell mineralization (as expressed by ALP and Alizarin red S) and this effect is reversed by Calhex 231, a CaSR allosteric inhibitor. The same group confirmed these results in human amniotic fluid MSCs [53]. Our data allow us to confirm that CaSR is involved in the osteogenic differentiation of UCM-MSC because the research calcimimetic AMG641 used in the present study is a selective CaSR activator [59,60]. The different molecular cell responses observed in large and small cell lines, may be due to their different developmental and functional maturity (different commitment status, as discussed above), including possible differences in the CaSR gene structure, gene expression regulatory mechanisms or signal transduction pathways, as previously hypothesized by Martino et al, [13]. Interestingly, and unlike observed stimulation with high $[Ca^{2+}]_o$, the calcimimetic AMG641-induced regulation of osteogenic biomarkers expression was inversely related to that of CaSR transcript, which was significant down-regulated in the large cell line where osteogenic differentiation was promoted, but markedly up-regulated in the small cell line, where osteogenesis was inhibited. This finding is not in agreement with the R-568-induced significant increase of CaSR protein expression reported by Di Tomo et al., [49] in ovine amniotic fluid MSCs. These differences may be due to differences in the two calcimimetics action mechanisms, probably eliciting different signaling pathways, and/or to differences in the commitment status of analyzed cell lines. As a further confirmation to the observed CaSR-mediated effect on eUCM-MSC, we tried to revert the effect observed in the presence of AMG641 by using a CaSR antagonist, NPS2390. As previously observed, NPS2390 is a potent and selective non-competitive group I metabotropic glutamate receptor (mGluR) antagonist [64]. In relation to CaSR's reported high structural homology with mGluR1 [65], NPS2390 has been used as CaSR antagonist in previous studies [13,66–68]. Indeed, in the present study, NPS2390 reversed the effects of AMG641 on OPN mRNA transcription levels, which were down-regulated in the large cell line and up regulated in the small cell line. As well, in both cell lines it significantly reversed the AMG641-induced effect on ALP activity and calcium phosphate deposit formation. Taken together, our data allowed us to demonstrate that AMG641 significantly enhanced osteogenic differentiation efficiency in equine UCM-MSCs. All these findings suggest that Ca^{2+} and the calcimimetic AMG641 promote osteogenic differentiation via CaSR. However, differences in synergic (Ca^{2+}) or inverse (AMG641) regulation of CaSR and osteogenic markers mRNA levels, lead us to hypothesize that these two agonists may act through different pathways.

Concerning neurogenic differentiation, we also showed that keeping elevated $[Ca^{2+}]_o$, during differentiation culture resulted in the over-expression of a specific gene involved in neurogenesis. Indeed, in both cell lines (even with different significance levels in the two cell types), we found over-expression of the gene coding for Nestin, which is an intermediate filament protein associated with immaturity in the nervous system [69]. Nestin has been reported as a prerequisite for the acquisition of the capacity to progress towards the neural lineage [69] and also as a neuronal stem cells marker implied in neuronal differentiation of MSCs [70,71]. Moreover, expression of GFAP was never found in our trials, indicating that culture conditions examined in the present study are not useful to walk the differentiation road leading to the development of mature astrocytes [69]. These findings are in line with those of a previous study by Vizard et al., [45] in which it was reported that the effects of increased $[Ca^{2+}]_o$ in mouse late fetal sympathetic neurons in culture enhances axonal growth, thus showing that calcium is involved in the regulation of the growth of neural processes in the central and peripheral nervous system.

The addition of AMG641 during neurogenic differentiation increased CaSR and Nestin mRNA expression in both the large and the small cell line. Our observations of a synergic up-regulation of CaSR and the neurogenic biomarker Nestin mRNA levels, by both CaSR agonists ($Ca^{2+}$and AMG641) and in both cell lines, even associated with non quantitatively relevant effects on Nissl bodies formation and beta III tubulin immunopositivity, support our hypothesis that CaSR is involved in early-stage neurogenic differentiation of UCM-MSCs, as reported in previous studies in other cell systems [72]. The stimulatory effects of the CaSR agonist observed in our study are also in line with those reported by Vizard et al., [45] who showed that activating CaSR in perinatal sympathetic neurons with the calcimimetic NPS R-467 enhances axonal and dendritic growth in culture and this effect is reversed by the selective CaSR antagonist NPS89636 and cannot be obtained in CaSR deficient mice. Nevertheless, the study by Vizard et al. was performed on perinatal neurons [45]. Lack of reproducible reversion effects by NPS2390 on the analyzed neurogenic differentiation biomarkers (Nissl bodies formation and Nestin mRNA levels) was observed. However, the possibility that NPS2390 could reverse expression or activity of other CaSR-induced neurogenic differentiation biomarkers cannot be excluded.

In conclusion, this study demonstrates that CaSR stimulation, by means of the calcimimetic AMG641 in presence of high $[Ca^{2+}]_o$, increases cell proliferation and increases osteogenic differentiation efficiency and early-stage neurogenic differentiation in UCM-MSCs, a unique fetal adnexa-derived MSC family with components presenting various stemness degree, thus a unique versatile opportunity in future cell therapy strategies. Moreover, our findings showed that CaSR activation may play a fundamental role in selecting specific differentiation checkpoints of these two differentiation routes, as related to cell commitment status, including differences in CaSR gene and/or protein structure and/or function, and used agonists. This CaSR-mediated selection of specific differentiation checkpoints could be of considerable utility in future therapeutical applications. Lastly, our data open the way to the use of the calcimimetic AMG641 in bone and nervous system regenerative medicine.

Author Contributions

Conceived and designed the experiments: NAM SJR MED. Performed the experiments: NAM EC. Analyzed the data: EC NAM. Contributed reagents/materials/analysis tools: MED SJR. Wrote the paper: MED NAM EC SJR.

References

1. Kim DW, Staples M, Shinozuka K, Pantcheva P, Kang SD, et al. (2013) Wharton's jelly derived mesenchymal stem cells: phenotypic characterization and optimizing their therapeutical potential for clinical applications. Int J Mol Sci 14: 11692–11712.

2. Marcus AJ, Woodbury D (2008) Fetal stem cells from extra-embryonic tissues: do not discard. J Cell Mol Med 12: 730–742.
3. Pappa KI, Anagnou NP (2009) Novel sources of fetal stem cells: where do they fit on the developmental continuum? Regen Med 4: 423–433.
4. Hua J, Gong J, Meng H, Xu B, Yao L, et al. (2013) Comparison of different methods for the isolation of mesenchymal stem cells from umbilical cord matrix: proliferation and multilineage differentiation as compared to mesenchymal stem cells from umbilical cord blood and bone marrow. Cell Biol Int Oct 7. doi: 10.1002/cbin.10188.
5. Gatta V, D Aurora M, Lanuti P, Pierdomenico L, Sperduti S, et al. (2013) Gene expression modifications in Wharton's Jelly mesenchymal stem cells promoted by prolonged *in vitro* culturing. BMC Genomics 21: 635.
6. Liu S, Hou KD, Yuan M, Peng J, Zhang L, et al. (2013) Characteristics of mesenchymal stem cells derived from Wharton's jelly of human umbilical cord and for fabrication of non-scaffold tissue-engineered cartilage. J Biosci Bioeng Jul : 27.S1389-1723(13)00263-6.
7. Esposito M, Lucariello A, Costanzo C, Fiumarella A, Giannini A, et al. (2013) Differentiation of human umbilical cord-derived mesenchymal stem cells, WJ-MSCs, into chondrogenic cells in the presence of pulsed electromagnetic fields. In Vivo 27: 495–500.
8. Li TX, Yuan J, Chen Y, Pan LJ, Song C, et al. (2013) Differentiation of mesenchymal stem cells from human umbilical cord tissue into odontoblast-like cells using the conditioned medium of tooth germ cells *in vitro*. Biomed Res Int 2013:218543.
9. Hoynowski SM, Fry MM, Gardner BM, Leming MT, Tucker JR, et al. (2007) Characterization and differentiation of equine umbilical cord-derived matrix cells. Biochem and Biophys Res Commun 362: 347–353.
10. Cremonesi F, Violini S, Lange Consiglio A, Ramelli P, Ranzenigo G, et al. (2008) Isolation, *in vitro* culture and characterization of foal umbilical cord stem cells at birth. Vet Res Commun 32: 139–142.
11. Passeri S, Nocchi F, Lamanna R, Lapi S, Miragliotta V, et al. (2009) Isolation and expansion of equine umbilical cord-derived matrix cells (EUCMCs). Cell Biol Int 33: 100–105.
12. Corradetti B, Lange-Consiglio A, Barucca M, Cremonesi F, Bizzaro D (2011) Size-sieved subpopulations of mesenchymal stem cells from intervascular and perivascular equine umbilical cord matrix. Cell Prolif 44: 330–342.
13. Martino NA, Lange-Consiglio A, Cremonesi F, Valentini L, Caira M, et al. (2011) Functional expression of the extracellular calcium sensing receptor (CaSR) in equine umbilical cord matrix size-sieved stem cells. PLoS One 17: e17714.
14. Iacono E, Brunori L, Pirrone A, Pagliaro PP, Ricci F, et al. (2012) Isolation, characterization and differentiation of mesenchymal stem cells from amniotic fluid, umbilical cord blood and Wharton's jelly in the horse. Reproduction 143: 455–468.
15. Penny J, Harris P, Shakesheff KM, Mobasheri A (2012) The biology of equine mesenchymal stem cells: phenotypic characterization, cell surface markers and multilineage differentiation. Front Biosci (Landmark Ed) 1: 892–908.
16. Gittel C, Brehm W, Burk J, Juelke H, Staszyk C, et al. (2013) Isolation of equine multipotent mesenchymal stromal cells by enzymatic tissue digestion or explant technique: comparison of cellular properties. BMC Vet Res 29: 221.
17. Rho GJ, Kumar BM, Balasubramanian SS (2009) Porcine mesenchymal stem cells-current technological status and future perspective. Front Biosci 1: 3942–3961.
18. Wei F, Qu C, Song T, Ding G, Fan Z, et al. (2012) Vitamin C treatment promotes mesenchymal stem cell sheet formation and tissue regeneration by elevating telomerase activity. J Cell Physiol 227: 3216–3224.
19. Seo MS, Jeong YH, Park JR, Park SB, Rho KH, et al. (2009) Isolation and characterization of canine umbilical cord blood-derived mesenchymal stem cell. J Vet Sci 10: 181–187.
20. Byeon YE, Ryu HH, Park SS, Koyama Y, Kikuchi M, et al. (2010) Paracrine effect of canine allogenic umbilical cord blood-derived mesenchymal stromal cells mixed with beta-tricalcium phosphate on bone regeneration in ectopic implantations. Cytotherapy 12: 626–636.
21. Filioli Uranio M, Valentini L, Lange-Consiglio A, Caira M, Guaricci AC, et al. (2011) Isolation, proliferation, cytogenetic, and molecular characterization and *in vitro* differentiation potency of canine stem cells from foetal adnexa: a comparative study of amniotic fluid, amnion, and umbilical cord matrix. Mol Reprod Dev 78: 361–373.
22. Lee KS, Nah JJ, Lee BC, Lee HT, Lee HS, et al. (2013) Maintenance and characterization of multipotent mesenchymal stem cells isolated from canine umbilical cord matrix by collagenase digestion. Res Vet Sci 94: 144–151.
23. Borjesson DL, Peroni JF (2011) The regenerative medicine laboratory: facilitating stem cell therapy for equine disease. Clin Lab Med 31: 109–123.
24. Lange-Consiglio A, Tassan S, Corradetti B, Meucci A, Perego R, et al. (2013) Investigating the efficacy of amnion-derived compared with bone marrow-derived mesenchymal stromal cells in equine tendon and ligament injuries. Cytotherapy 15:1011–1020.
25. Hall MS, Vasey JR, Russell JW, Russell T (2013) Use of ultrasound-guided autologous bone marrow transfer for treatment of suspensory ligament desmitis in 30 race horses (2003–2010). Aust Vet J 91: 102–107.
26. Ricco S, Renzi S, Del Bue M, Conti V, Merli E, et al. (2013) Allogeneic adipose tissue-derived mesenchymal stem cells in combination with platelet rich plasma are safe and effective in the therapy of superficial digital flexor tendonitis in the horse. Int J Immunopathol Pharmacol 26: 61–68.
27. Reed SA, Leahy ER (2013) Growth and Development Symposium: Stem cell therapy in equine tendon injury. J Anim Sci 91: 59–65.
28. Uppalapati D, Ohta N, Zhang Y, Kawabata A, Pyle MM, et al. (2011) Identification and characterization of unique tumoricidal genes in rat umbilical cord matrix stem cells. Mol Pharm 3: 1549–1558.
29. Wu KH, Tsai C, Wu HP, Sieber M, Peng CT, et al. (2013) Human application of ex vivo expanded umbilical cord-derived mesenchymal stem cells: enhance hematopoiesis after cord blood transplantation. Cell Transplant 22: 2041–2051.
30. Brown EM, MacLeod RJ (2001) Extracellular Calcium Sensing and Extracellular Calcium Signaling. Physiol Rev 81: 239–297.
31. McNeil L, Hobson S, Nipper V, Rodland KD (1998) Functional calcium-sensing receptor expression in ovarian surface epithelial cells. Am J Obstet Gynecol 178: 305–313.
32. Brown EM, Vassilev PM, Hebert SC (1995) Calcium ions as extracellular messengers. Cell 83: 679–682.
33. Brown EM, Gamba G, Riccardi D, Lombardi M, Butters R, et al. (1993) Cloning and characterization of an Extracellular Ca2+-Sensing Receptor from bovine parathyroid. Nature 366: 575–580.
34. Huang S, Maher VM, McCormick JJ (1995) Extracellular Ca2+ stimulates the activation of mitogen-activated protein kinase and cell growth in human fibroblasts. Biochem J 310: 881–885.
35. Mailland M, Waelchli R, Ruat M, Boddeke HG, Seuwen K (1997) Stimulation of cell proliferation by calcium and a calcimimetic compound. Endocrinology 138: 3601–3605.
36. Yamaguchi T, Yamauchi M, Sugimoto T, Chauhan D, Anderson KC, et al. (2002) The extracellular calcium Ca2+o-sensing receptor is expressed in myeloma cells and modulates cell proliferation. Biochem Biophys Res Commun 13: 532–538.
37. Hobson SA, Wright J, Lee F, McNeil SE, Bilderback T, et al. (2003) Activation of the MAP kinase cascade by exogenous calcium-sensing receptor. Mol Cell Endocrinol 200: 189–198.
38. Tfelt-Hansen J, Chattopadhyay N, Yano S, Kanuparthi D, Rooney P, et al. (2004) Calcium-sensing receptor induces proliferation through p38 mitogenactivated protein kinase and phosphatidylinositol 3-kinase but not extracellularly regulated kinase in a model of humoral hypercalcemia of malignancy. Endocrinology 145: 1211–1217.
39. Riccardi D, Kemp PJ (2012) The Calcium-Sensing receptor beyond extracellular calcium homeostasis: conception, development, adult physiology, and disease. Annu Rev Physiol 74: 271–297.
40. Singh N, Promkan M, Liu G, Varani J, Chakrabarty S (2013) Role of Calcium sensing receptor (CaSR) in tumorigenesis. Best Pract Res Clin Endocrinol Metab 27: 455–463.
41. Brennan SC, Thiem U, Roth S, Aggarwal A, Fetahu ISh, et al. (2013) Calcium sensing receptor signalling in physiology and cancer. Biochim Biophys Acta 1833: 1732–1744.
42. Dvorak MM, Siddiqua A, Ward DT, Carter DH, Dallas SL, et al. (2004) Physiological changes in extracellular calcium concentration directly control osteoblast function in the absence of calciotropic hormones. Proc Natl Acad Sci 101: 5140–5145
43. Dvorak MM, Chen TH, Orwoll B, Garvey C, ChangW, et al. (2007) Constitutive activity of the osteoblast Ca2+−sensing receptor promotes loss of cancellous bone. Endocrinology 148: 3156–3163
44. Mentaverri R, Yano S, Chattopadhyay N, Petit L, Kifor O, et al. (2006) The calcium sensing receptor is directly involved in both osteoclast differentiation and apoptosis. FASEB J 20: 2562–2564
45. Vizard TN, O'Keeffe GW, Gutierrez H, Kos CH, Riccardi D, et al. (2008) Regulation of axonal and dendritic growth by the extracellular calcium-sensing receptor. Nat Neurosci 11: 285–291.
46. Arabzadeh A, Troy T-C, Turksen K (2009) Insights into the Role of the Calcium Sensing Receptor in Epidermal Differentiation *in Vivo*. Mol Biotechnol 43: 264–272
47. He YH, He Y, Liao XL, Niu YC, Wang G, et al. (2012) The Calcium-sensing receptor promotes adipocytes differentiation and adipogenesis through PPARg pathway. Mol Cell Biochem 361: 321–328.
48. Sun J, He W, Bai SZ, Peng X, Zhang N, et al. (2013) The expression of calcium-sensing receptor in mouse embryonic stem cells (mESCs) and its influence on differentiation of mESC into cardiomyocytes. Differentiation 85: 32–40.
49. Di Tomo P, Pipino C, Lanuti P, Morabito C, Pierdomenico L, et al. (2013) Calcium sensing receptor expression in ovine amniotic fluid mesenchymal stem cells and the potential role of R-568 during osteogenic differentiation. PLoS One 9:e73816.
50. Lange-Consiglio A, Corradetti B, Bizzaro D, Magatti M, Ressel L, et al. (2012) Characterization and potential applications of progenitor-like cells isolated from horse amniotic membrane. J Tissue Eng Regen Med 6: 622–635.
51. Mori G, Ballini A, Carbone C, Oranger A, Brunetti G, et al. (2012) Osteogenic Differentiation of Dental Follicle Stem Cells. Int. J. Med. Sci. 9: 480–487.
52. Hinrichs K, Choi YH, Walckenaer BE, Varner DD, Hartman DL (2007) *In vitro* produced equine embryos: production of foals after transfer assessment by differential staining and effect of medium concentration during culture. Theriogenology 68: 521–529.
53. Pipino C, Di Tomo P, Mandatori D, Cianci E, Lanuti P, et al. (2014) Calcium Sensing Receptor activation by calcimimetic R-568 in human amniotic fluid mesenchymal stem cells: correlation with osteogenic differentiation. Stem Cell Dev 2014 Aug 21 doi:10.1089/scd.2013.0627.

54. Lopez I, Mendoza FJ, Aguilera-Tejero E, Perez J, Guerrero F, et al. (2008) The effect of calcitriol, paricalcitol, and a calcimimetic on extraosseous calcifications in uremic rats. Kidney Int 73: 300–307.
55. Rodríguez M, Aguilera-Tejero E, Mendoza FJ, Guerrero F, López I (2008) Effects of calcimimetics on extraskeletal calcifications in chronic kidney disease. Kidney I 111: S50–54
56. Lopez I, Mendoza FJ, Guerrero F, Almaden Y, Henley C, et al. (2009) The calcimimetic AMG641 accelerates regression of extraosseous calcification in uremic rats. Am J Physiol Renal Physiol 296: F1376–1385.
57. Henley C, Davis J, Miller G, Shatzen E, Cattley R, et al. (2009) The calcimimetic AMG641 abrogates parathyroid hyperplasia, bone and vascular calcification abnormalities in uremic rats. Eur J Pharmacol 15: 306–313.
58. Mendoza FJ, Lopez I, Canalejo R, Almaden Y, Martin D, et al. (2009) Direct upregulation of parathyroid calcium-sensing receptor and vitamin D receptor by calcimimetics in uremic rats. Am J Physiol Renal Physiol 296: F605–613.
59. Mendoza FJ, Martinez-Moreno J, Almaden Y, Rodriguez-Ortiz ME, Lopez I, et al. (2011) Effect of calcium and the calcimimetic AMG 641 on matrix-Gla protein in vascular smooth muscle cells. Calcif Tissue Int 88: 169–178.
60. Mendoza FJ, Perez-Marin CC, Garcia-Marin L, Madueño JA, Henley C, et al. (2012) Localization, distribution, and function of the calcium-sensing receptor in sperm. J Androl 33: 96–104.
61. Henaut L, Boudot C, Massy ZA, Lopez-Fernandez I, Dupont S, et al. (2014) Calcimimetics increase CaSR expression and reduce mineralization in vascular smooth muscle cells: mechanisms of action. Cardiovasc Res. 101: 256–265.
62. Barradas AM, Fernandes HA, Groen N, Chai YC, Schrooten J, et al. (2012) A calcium-induced signaling cascade leading to osteogenic differentiation of human bone marrow-derived mesenchymal stromal cells. Biomaterials. 33: 3205–3215.
63. Koori K, Maeda H, Fujii S, Tomokiyo A, Kawaki G, et al. (2014) The roles of calcium-sensing receptor and calcium chanel in osteogenic differentiation of undifferentiated periodontal ligament cells. Cell Tissue Res 357: 707–718.
64. Lavreysen H, Janssen C, Bischoff F, Langlois X, Leysen JE, et al. (2003) [3H] R214127: a novel high-affinity radioligand for the mGlu1 receptor reveals a common binding site shared by multiple allosteric antagonists. Mol Pharm 63: 1082–1093.
65. Noeske T, Gutcaits A, Parsons CG, Weil T (2005) Allosteric modulation of family 3 GPCRs. QSAR Comb Sci 25: 134–146.
66. Jung SY, Kwak JO, Kim HW, Kim DS, Ryu SD, et al. (2005) Calcium sensing receptor forms complex with and is up regulated by caveolin-1 in cultured human osteosarcoma (Saos-2) cells. Exp Mol Med 37: 91–100.
67. Kwak JO, Kwak J, Kim HW, Oh KJ, Kim YT, et al. (2005) The extracellular calcium sensing receptor is expressed in mouse mesangial cells and modulates cell proliferation. Exp Mol Med 37: 457–465.
68. De Santis T, Casavola V, Reshkin SJ, Guerra L, Ambruosi B, et al. (2009) The extracellular calcium-sensing receptor is expressed in the cumulus-oocyte complex in mammalians and modulates oocyte meiotic maturation. Reproduction 138: 1–15.
69. Wislet-Gendebien S, Leprince P, Moonen G, Rogister B (2003) Regulation of neural markers nestin and GFAP expression by cultivated bone marrow stromal cells. J Cell Sci 116: 3295–3302.
70. Greco SJ, Zhou C, Ye J-H, Rameshwar P (2007) An interdisciplinary approach and characterization of neuronal cells transdifferentiated from human mesenchymal stem cells. Stem Cells Dev 16: 811–826.
71. Tondreau T, Dejeneffe M, Meuleman N, Stamatopoulos B, Delforge A, et al. (2008) Gene expression pattern of functional neuronal cells derived from human bone marrow mesenchymal stromal cells. BMC Genomics 11: 166.
72. de Torres C, Beleta H, Díaz R, Toran N, Rodríguez E, et al. (2009) The calcium-sensing receptor and parathyroid hormone-related protein are expressed in differentiated, favorable neuroblastic tumors. Cancer 115:2792–803.

Quantification of Heterogeneity as a Biomarker in Tumor Imaging

Lejla Alic[1,2]*, Wiro J. Niessen[1,3], Jifke F. Veenland[1]

1 Biomedical Imaging Group Rotterdam, Department of Radiology and Medical Informatics, Erasmus Medical Center Rotterdam, Rotterdam, The Netherlands, 2 Department of Intelligent Imaging, Netherlands Organization for Applied Scientific Research (TNO), The Hague, The Netherlands, 3 Imaging Physics, Faculty of Applied Sciences, Delft University of Technology, Delft, The Netherlands

Abstract

Background: Many techniques are proposed for the quantification of tumor heterogeneity as an imaging biomarker for differentiation between tumor types, tumor grading, response monitoring and outcome prediction. However, in clinical practice these methods are barely used. This study evaluates the reported performance of the described methods and identifies barriers to their implementation in clinical practice.

Methodology: The Ovid, Embase, and Cochrane Central databases were searched up to 20 September 2013. Heterogeneity analysis methods were classified into four categories, i.e., non-spatial methods (NSM), spatial grey level methods (SGLM), fractal analysis (FA) methods, and filters and transforms (F&T). The performance of the different methods was compared.

Principal Findings: Of the 7351 potentially relevant publications, 209 were included. Of these studies, 58% reported the use of NSM, 49% SGLM, 10% FA, and 28% F&T. Differentiation between tumor types, tumor grading and/or outcome prediction was the goal in 87% of the studies. Overall, the reported area under the curve (AUC) ranged from 0.5 to 1 (median 0.87). No relation was found between the performance and the quantification methods used, or between the performance and the imaging modality. A negative correlation was found between the tumor-feature ratio and the AUC, which is presumably caused by overfitting in small datasets. Cross-validation was reported in 63% of the classification studies. Retrospective analyses were conducted in 57% of the studies without a clear description.

Conclusions: In a research setting, heterogeneity quantification methods can differentiate between tumor types, grade tumors, and predict outcome and monitor treatment effects. To translate these methods to clinical practice, more prospective studies are required that use external datasets for validation: these datasets should be made available to the community to facilitate the development of new and improved methods.

Editor: Christos Hatzis, Yale University, United States of America

Funding: This study was supported by The Netherlands Organization for Scientific Research (NWO), grant number 017.002.019. The funders had no role in study design, data collection and analysis, decision to publish, or preparation of the manuscript.

Competing Interests: The authors have declared that no competing interests exist.

* Email: LejlaResearch@gmail.com

Introduction

Tumors are often inhomogeneous. Regional variations in cell death, metabolic activity, proliferation and vascular structure are observed. There is increasing evidence that solid tumors may consist of subpopulations of cells with different genotypes and phenotypes [1]. These distinct populations of cancer cells can interact in a competitive way [2] and may differ in sensitivity to treatments [3,4]. This heterogeneity can be detected using diagnostic imaging techniques at a genetic, molecular or cellular level [4,5], or at a cell population level. The advantage of diagnostic imaging techniques is their non-invasive nature and the fact that the whole tumor is taken into account, whereas cellular diagnostic techniques are invasive and limited to a discrete set of tumor samples. Various imaging techniques are available to visualize the heterogeneity in tissue characteristics, such as necrosis, metabolic activity, cell density and vascularity. Observed heterogeneity in an image is a reflection of the phenotypic variation of the tumor and is reported to be associated with underlying gene-expression patterns [6].

Image heterogeneity can be quantified using a variety of texture analysis methods. As such, image heterogeneity is potential biomarker for tumor characterization, for response prediction and monitoring. Parameters in hot spots, as quantified with dynamic contrast-enhanced magnetic resonance imaging (DCE-MRI), are more relevant for monitoring tumor response than parameters averaged over the whole tumor [7–9]. When a region of the tumor is not well vascularized or is hypoxic, chemotherapy and radiotherapy are more likely to fail. The existence of poorly vascularized or hypoxic areas within a tumor is an important component of tumor radiation resistance and correlates with treatment failure [10]. In radiotherapy, the heterogeneity can be used to guide treatment [11,12]: an ongoing trial is currently escalating the dose to the part of the tumor with high standardized uptake values [13]. Also for computed tomography (CT), image heterogeneity has prognostic value [6].

Several methods are available to quantify tumor heterogeneity from imaging data. Many studies have used histogram-derived features such as percentile values, standard deviation (SD) and enhancing fraction. However, these features do not take into account the spatial distribution of the intensity values. In contrast, texture methods take spatial information into account by quantifying the spatial variations in the images. Ideally, these methods are independent of the absolute signal intensities in the image. They provide additional and independent information (such as the average signal intensity) compared to histogram-derived measures. These methods result in features which can be considered to be imaging biomarkers providing information on the underlying tumor heterogeneity. Some of these features are related to image properties that are visually perceived by the radiologist, whereas others are more abstract [14].

By means of a systematic review, the aim of this study is to investigate the performance of different heterogeneity imaging biomarkers extracted from diagnostic tumor images for differentiation between tumor types, tumor grading, outcome prediction and treatment monitoring.

The following research questions were formulated:

- Which analysis methods are used to quantify heterogeneity or texture in tumor imaging, with the aim to differentiate between tumor types, tumor grading, outcome prediction and treatment monitoring?
- What are the reported performances of the different analysis methods? Is there a relation between performance and analysis method?

What is the potential clinical impact of the methods? Can the performance results be generalized? Is the performance evaluated in addition to established imaging biomarkers?

Methods

Data Sources and Search method

This review was performed in accordance with the PRISMA (Preferred Reporting Items for Systematic Review and Meta-Analyses) guidelines [15], with details summarized in Checklist S1. In January 2013 the study protocol was registered with the International Prospective Register of Systematic Reviews (Identification number: CRD42013003634) [16]. A systematic search was conducted in the databases of Medline, Embase, and Cochrane Central. The search was performed with the aid of an experienced librarian on September 20th 2013.

The following topics were used for the searches:

1. Neoplasms
2. Heterogeneity, texture
3. MRI, MRS, CT, PET, SPECT, ultrasonography
4. Differentiation between tumor types, tumor grading, classification, staging, treatment response, survival, and treatment outcome

Full details of the Embase search is included in Text S1. The results from all three searches were combined and verified to ensure exclusion of publications containing the same title, written by the same authors, and published in the same journal. The remaining publications were considered for study selection.

Study Selection

Two authors (L.A. and J.F.V.) independently reviewed the titles and abstracts. The selected publications then underwent full-text screening. During the title and abstract review, any discrepancies about study inclusion were resolved by full-text screening. Any discrepancies during the following stages were resolved by discussion. The bibliographies of seminal review papers [17–19] were reviewed to identify additional relevant articles.

Inclusion and exclusion criteria

We included only publications related to diagnostic imaging which reported quantification of tumor heterogeneity or tumor texture with the goal to differentiate between tumor types, tumor grading, outcome prediction and tumor response monitoring. No restrictions were made based on location, type, stage or grade of malignancy. Prior to review, a decision was made to exclude any study with too few participants, i.e., for patient studies ($n<10$) and for animal studies ($n<5$). Therefore, all case studies, and studies with no information on the number of subjects, were excluded. In addition, all the following types of studies were excluded:

- publications based on non-tumor images;
- publications not based on quantitative assessment of heterogeneity or texture in images
- publications without one of the following goals: differentiation between tumor types, tumor grading, or outcome prediction or treatment monitoring;
- publications not based on in vivo studies (histology, phantom, ex vivo, synthetic data);
- publications describing non-original research (editorial, letter to the editor, review, meta-analysis, opinion publications).

Data extraction

A data extraction form was designed. All selected publications were independently reviewed and data extraction was cross-checked. Disagreements between the reviewers were resolved by consensus. The following data were extracted from the full papers: year of publication, human or animal study, type of study (retrospective or prospective), number of subjects, number of tumors, location of tumor, imaging modality, tracer/contrast agent, goal of heterogeneity/texture analysis, and type of heterogeneity/texture quantification method used. For studies reporting on the same analysis method based on the identical dataset, only the latest publication was included. For publications reporting classification experiments, the following data were extracted: number of candidate heterogeneity features, dimensionally reduction technique used, number of selected features used in the best classification experiment, the results of the best classification experiment, i.e., accuracy, sensitivity, specificity, area under the receiver operator curve (AUC), type of cross-validation used, and use of an external validation set. For publications using statistical hypothesis testing the following data were extracted: the number of candidate features, and the number of features that showed a significant difference between outcome categories (before and after Holm-Bonferroni correction) [20]. All publications were divided into two categories:

- Publications reporting cross-sectional measurements with the aim to differentiate between tumor types, tumor grading, and treatment outcome prediction.
- Publications reporting longitudinal measurements for tumor treatment monitoring.

Data synthesis and analysis

The imaging modalities were summarized into four categories: i) magnetic resonance imaging (MRI), ii) computed tomography (CT), iii) positron emission tomography (PET), single photon emission computed tomography (SPECT), and iv) ultrasonography (US). No further subdivision was made regarding the type of imaging protocol or use of contrast agent.

Image analysis methods to estimate tumor heterogeneity were divided into four categories: non-spatial methods, local spatial distribution methods, fractal analysis, and a category consisting of filters and transforms.

Non-spatial methods (NSM). These methods characterize tumor heterogeneity by non-spatial descriptors, such as descriptors of the gray-level frequency distributions: standard deviation, skewness, maximum, minimum, range, peak height, peak position, and percentile values.

Spatial gray-level methods (SGLM). Methods included in the second category extract the local spatial image intensity distribution. This category includes grey-tone spatial-dependence matrix (GTSDM) [21], neighborhood gray-tone difference matrix (NGTDM) [22], run-length matrix (RLM), and Local Binary Pattern (LBP) [23]. The GTSDM, originally proposed by Haralick et al. [21], is often referred to as co-occurrence or the second-order histogram. When divided by the total number of neighboring pixels in the image, this matrix becomes the estimate of the joint probability of two pixels at a distance along a given direction having a particular gray value. The NGTDM, originally proposed by Amadasm and King [22], is based on spatial changes in gray values by inspecting the difference between gray levels of a specific pixel and the average gray level of their surrounding neighbors. The RLM, originally proposed by Galloway [24], is subsidiary to the observation that a coarse texture would have relatively longer gray level runs compared to a fine texture. This matrix provides information about runs of pixels with the same gray level values in a given direction. LBP, originally proposed by Ojala et al. [25] and later modified to a rotation and scale invariant approach [23], represents local texture. In its simplest form it labels the pixels of an image by thresholding the neighborhood of each pixel and considers the result as a binary number.

Fractal analysis (FA). The third category consists of FA methods that overcome the scale problem by providing a statistical measure reflecting pattern changes as a function scale. The two basic parameters in FA are fractal dimension (FD) and lacunarity [26]. An often used method to estimate FD is box counting [26]. This procedure systematically overlays an image with a series of grids with increasing/decreasing size. For each step, this procedure captures the predefined relevant features [27]. Another frequently used technique in FA is the blanket method [26], which is often used in its extended form, as described by Peleg et al. [28]. This method estimates the surface area by measuring the volume between an upper and lower blanket.

Filters and Transforms (F&T). The fourth category consists of a collection of image processing algorithms that extract texture features. Examples are methods that use techniques defined in the spatial domain such as filters (Gabor filters or Law's filters) or transformations to other domains (Fourier transform, Wavelet transform, S-transform, discrete cosine transform). Since the various methods have only been used in a limited number of publications included in the present review, these methods were grouped together.

Publications reporting classification experiments. Publications were considered classification studies if they reported a classification result such as accuracy, sensitivity, specificity or AUC values. Only publications in which the results of the classification experiments were solely based on texture parameters were further analyzed. These studies often utilize a high number of candidate features to describe a tumor. When the number of extracted features is too large to perform a statistically meaningful classification [29], the extracted features can be redundant in the information they retain. Because an increase of dimensionality in the feature space results in an increase of its volume, the feature space is sparsely filled. The use of an extensive number of features for classification purposes can result in over-fitting, which reduces the possibility of generalization; this paradox is generally referred to as the 'curse of dimensionality' [30].

To keep the system manageable, dimensionality reduction techniques were commonly applied to select a subset of features that were relevant for the classification problem. The ratio between the number of tumors classified and the dimensionality of the feature space (e.g., the number of selected features) should be chosen in a meaningful way. In pattern recognition applications, the rule of thumb is to use 5–10 datasets per feature per category [31]. Therefore, we evaluated the number of candidate features, the number of selected features, and the ratio between the number of tumors included in the study and the number of selected classification features. A one-way ANOVA was used to test for differences in classification results between the modalities and analysis methods.

Publications reporting on significance testing. A commonly used approach to test the validity of the selected features is significance testing. For heterogeneity analysis, many publications compute a large number of features. As multiple comparisons generally require a stronger level of evidence to be considered significant, the Holm-Bonferroni correction [20] can be applied. This correction allows for the significance levels for single and multiple comparisons to be directly comparable. In these publications, we evaluated whether a Holm-Bonferroni correction was applied and, if this was not the case, computed the number of significant features after correction using the available data. A one-way ANOVA was used to test for differences in the number of significant features, before and after Holm-Bonferroni correction, between the modalities and the analysis methods used.

Results

Figure 1 presents details on the literature search. In summary, of the 7351 potentially relevant articles, 480 (6.5%) were considered for inclusion after abstract review. After these latter papers had undergone full-text screening, an additional 249 publications were excluded. The remaining 231 original publications entered the data extraction phase. In this phase an additional 22 papers [32–53] were excluded as they reported results of a similar analysis method on the same dataset as that used in another paper; for these publications, the most recent one was included in the analysis. Finally, data from 209 studies [7,14,54–228] were extracted for further analysis.

General characteristics

Table 1 presents the characteristics of the included publications (after removing duplicate publications). A publication may include more than one imaging modality, analysis method, or goal. Two studies (1%) reported on two imaging modalities, and 66 studies (32%) reported on two or more analysis methods.

Since 2008, the number of imaging studies quantifying tumor heterogeneity has been steadily increasing, i.e. from 8 papers in 2006–2007 to 66 publications in 2012–2013 (figure 2-A). Prior to 2006, heterogeneity was mainly studied based on US data

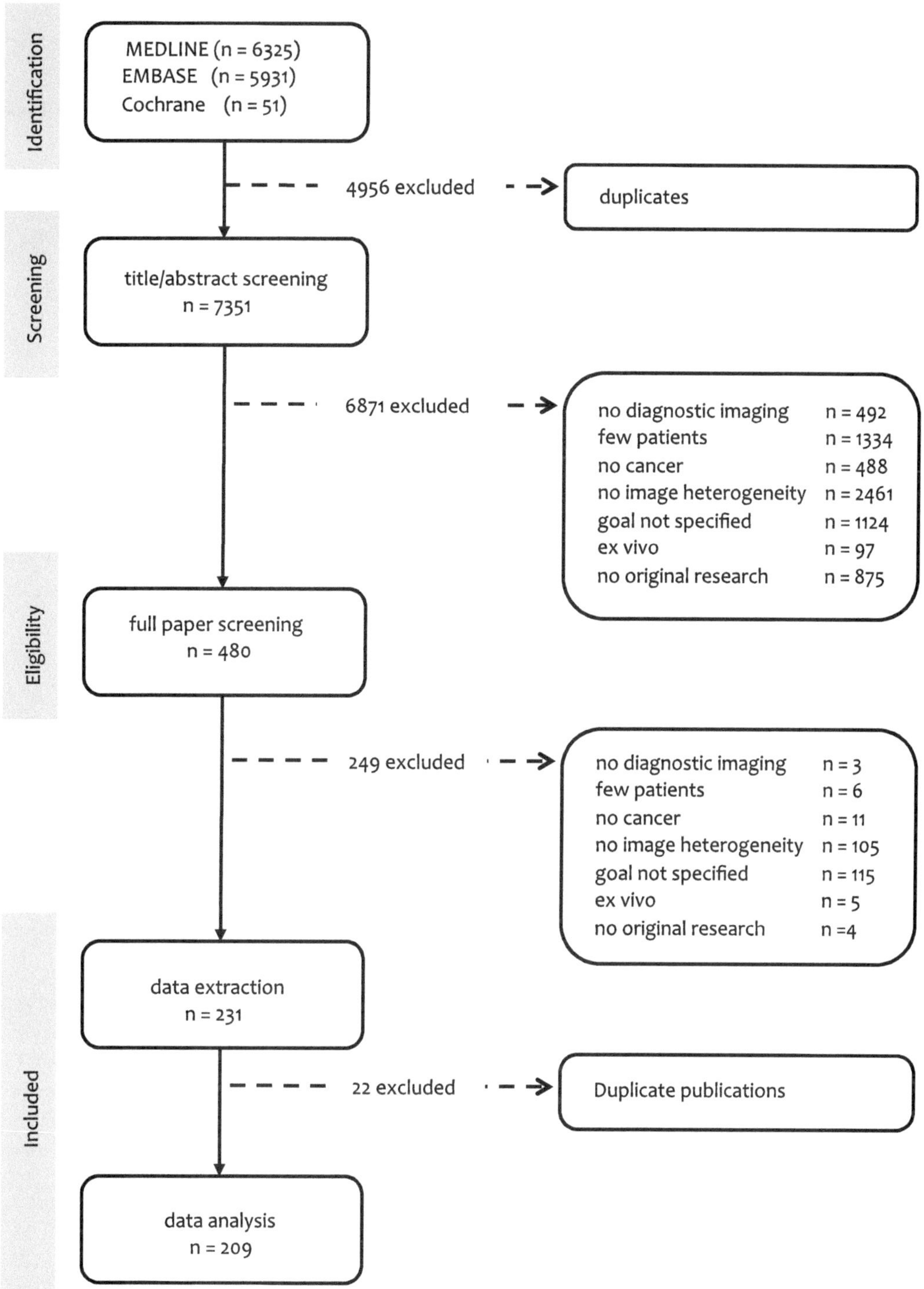

Figure 1. Results of the literature search. PRISMA flow diagram for study collection [15], showing the number of studies identified, screened, eligible, and included in the systematic review. This study is registered with the PROSPERO registry for systematic reviews (Identification number: CRD42013003634) [16].

(Figure 2-B). Since 2007, most studies quantifying tumor heterogeneity are based on MRI. Generally, the non-spatial method (NSM) and the spatial gray-level method (SGLM) are the most frequently used to analyze tumor heterogeneity (Figure 2-C). Although the number of publications using these methods has increased since 2007, their contribution to heterogeneity literature is relatively stable. The number of studies reporting tumor response monitoring has varied over the years, ranging from 0–20% (Figure 2-D).

Breast tumors were studied in 33% (n = 69) of the publications. Figure 3 shows the distribution of studies per tumor location. Figure 3-A shows the use of imaging modalities for quantification of tumor heterogeneity per primary tumor location. MRI is used primarily for brain and breast tumors, CT for lung and

Table 1. Characteristics of the included publications (n = 209).

Characteristic		n	%
Imaging method	MRI	75	36%
	CT	40	19%
	PET	14	7%
	US	81	39%
Analysis method	NSM	121	58%
	SGLM	103	49%
	FA	21	10%
	F&T	58	28%
Study goal	Diagnosis/grading/outcome pred.	182	87%
	Response monitoring	27	13%
Study type	Retrospective	118	56%
	Retrospective (with inclusion criteria)	63	30%
	Prospective	28	13%
Type of subjects	Human	197	94%
	Animal	12	6%
Type of experiment	Classification	139	67%
	Significance testing	64	30%
	Neither	6	3%

Imaging modalities: magnetic resonance imaging (MRI), computed tomography (CT), positron emission tomography (PET), ultrasonography (US).
Analysis methods: non-spatial methods (NSM), spatial grey level methods (SGLM), fractal analysis (FA) methods, and filters and transforms (F&T).

gastrointestinal tumors, PET for gastrointestinal, lung tumors and sarcoma, and US for breast tumors. Heterogeneity analysis of brain tumors was performed almost exclusively with MRI, while for breast tumors both MRI and US were used.

Figure 3-B presents the analysis methods used per primary tumor location. For almost all locations, all methods were used. For prostate, breast, and head and neck analysis, the SGLM was the most frequently used. For all other locations, the NSM was the favored modality. Heterogeneity analyses for longitudinal studies were mainly performed for gastrointestinal and breast tumors (Figure 3-C).

Figure S1 summarizes the publications included in the present review (n = 209) in a matrix form. The publications are divided into different imaging modalities and analysis methods, and are available for download for each cell separately. Each cell in the matrix links to the supplementary EndNote file containing the records for these publications.

Figure 4-A shows the relation between imaging modality and analysis methods for cross-sectional studies. In general, 74% of these studies used either MRI or US. The SGLM (37%) and NSM (36%) are most frequently used to grade and diagnose tumors. Figure 4-B shows the relation between imaging modality and analysis method for the longitudinal studies (n = 27). MRI was

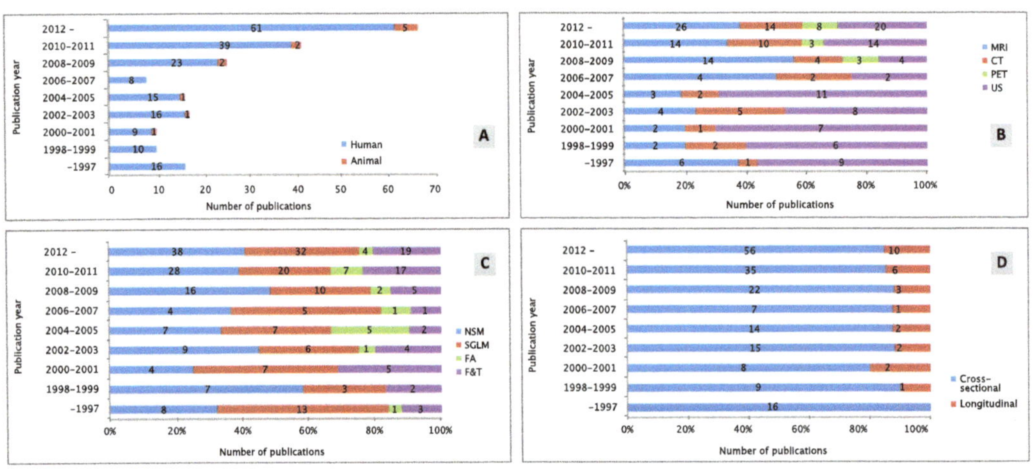

Figure 2. Number of publications reporting on tumor heterogeneity analysis for all publications bi-annually. Total number of publications (A), publications per imaging modality (B), publications per analysis method (C), and publications per goal (D).

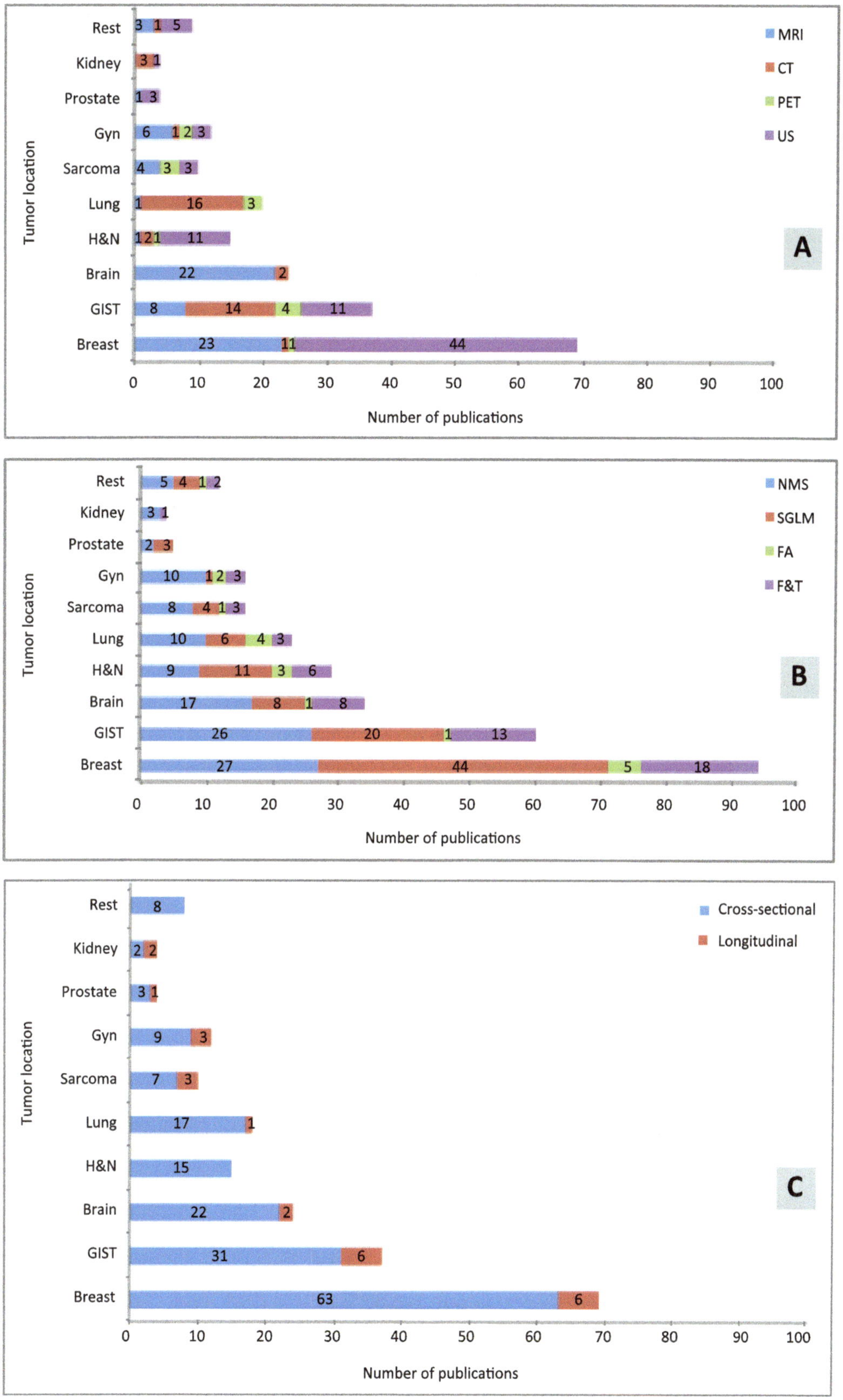

Figure 3. Publications reporting on quantification of tumor heterogeneity in cancer sites summarized for imaging modality (A), analysis method (B), and study aim (C). Publications can report on more than one analysis method. The acronyms used: Gyn – gynecological, H&N - head and neck, GIST – gastrointestinal.

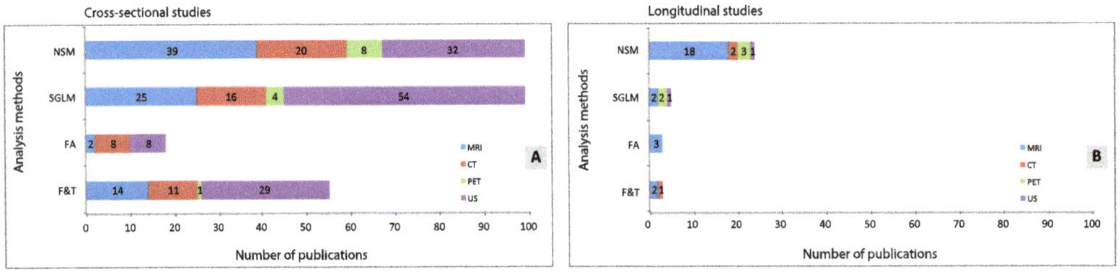

Figure 4. All included publications reporting cross-sectional (A) and longitudinal (B) studies. Several publications report more than one analysis method.

used in 70% of these studies and PET in 11%. In 7% of the studies, US-based heterogeneity quantification was used for tumor response monitoring. NSM is the most frequently used (69%) analysis method in longitudinal studies.

A relatively small number of all studies (13%) utilized a prospective study design. Figure 5-A shows the relation between imaging modality and analysis method used for cross-sectional studies (n = 12). US is the most frequently used modality, whereas NSM is the most frequently used analysis method. Figure 5-B shows the relation between imaging modality and analysis method for publications reporting longitudinal studies (n = 16). Again, most data were analyzed with NSM. In contrast to MRI, CT, US and PET are rarely used for heterogeneity quantification in prospective longitudinal studies.

Publications reporting classification experiments

Of all included studies, 67% (n = 139) reported classification experiments and 30% reported significance testing. The remaining 3% either did not report quantitative results or the experiments were not completely described. Also, 23 studies only reported results of classification experiments where the texture features were combined with non-texture features. For these latter publications, it was not possible to extract the performance of the texture features separately and, therefore, these results were excluded from further analysis. Additionally, 10 studies were excluded because the number of generated or selected features was lacking. Of the papers reporting classification experiments (n = 106), 45% used US, 37% used MRI, 13% used CT, and 5% used PET. In 42% of the classification papers, features originating from different texture analysis methods were combined. Some studies reporting classification experiments (n = 39) performed no feature reduction, and the median number of candidate features used in these studies (6) was significantly lower than that of candidate features in the studies using feature reduction techniques (38). The remaining 67 studies reporting classification experiments used one of the methods commonly applied in statistics, pattern recognition, or machine learning. These methods were summarized into three categories: filters, wrappers and embedded methods [229].

Figure 6 shows the relation between the number of candidate features and the number of selected features used in classification experiments for different imaging modalities (Figure 6-A) and different analysis methods (Figure 6-B). For the papers presented on the dotted line, no feature selection was performed. The number of candidate features ranged from 1–5280 (median 22) while the number of selected features ranged from 1–476 (median 3). The distribution of the numbers of selected features can be assessed as boxplots for imaging modality (Figure 6-C) and for analysis methods (Figure 6-D).

About 63% of the publications describing a classification experiment, reported cross- validation or training test sets as a technique to limit the effect of over-fitting on the available data. Figure 6-B shows that the combination of features from different methods generally leads to a higher number of candidate features. In general, in publications reporting the use of more than one analysis method more extensive feature reduction is applied compared to publications reporting on the use of the separate analysis methods.

In the classification experiments, one or more of the following performance measures were reported: sensitivity, specificity, accuracy, or AUC. Figure 7-A shows the AUC per imaging modality and Figure 7-B the AUC per analysis method. The differences in performance (as measured by AUC) are shown in Figure 7-C per imaging modality and in Figure 7-D per analysis method.

The supplementary material provides the figures for accuracy (Figure S2), sensitivity (Figure S3) and specificity (Figure S4) per imaging modality and per analysis method. In these figures, the reported performance is depicted as a function of the tumor-feature ratio (ratio between the number of tumors included and the number of selected features). In general, the tumor-feature

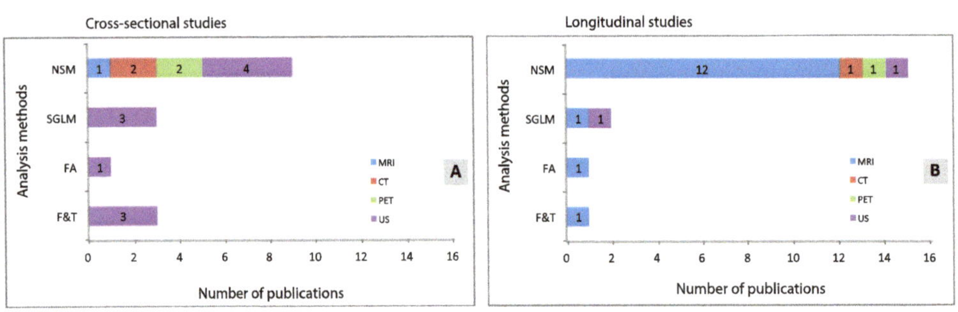

Figure 5. Publications reporting a prospective study design cross-sectional (At) and longitudinal (B) studies. Several publications report more than one analysis method.

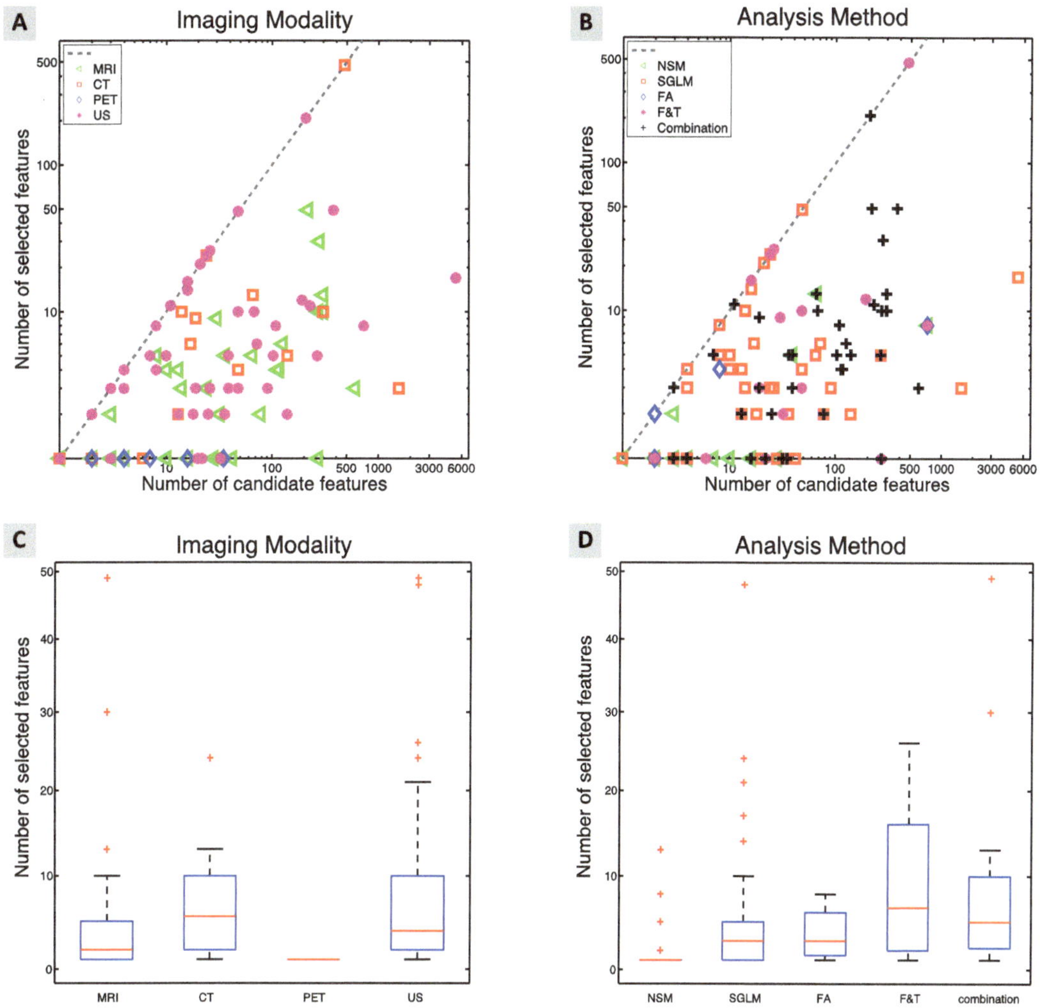

Figure 6. Number of features used in classification experiments for different imaging modalities (A) and for different analysis methods (B). Boxplot representing distribution in number selected features for imaging modality (C) and for analysis methods (D). To enhance visibility, we excluded for both boxplots two studies with large numbers of selected features.

ratio ranged from 0.46–502 (median 20) with (on average) 29% of the publications showing a tumor-feature ratio ≤10.

With respect to the analysis method, publications using the F&T, or a combination of methods, had the highest risk of a tumor-feature ratio ≤10, i.e. 53% and 42%, respectively. With regard to imaging modality, CT publications had the highest percentage (43%) with a tumor-feature ratio <10.

Using a one-way ANOVA, no significant differences were found in the performance measures between the modalities or between the analysis methods used. However, there was a negative correlation between the logarithm of the number of tumors per selected feature and the AUC ($r = -0.32$, $p<0.05$) and the specificity ($r = -0.48$, $p<0.05$).

Publications using statistical hypothesis testing

Of all included studies, 30% ($n = 64$) reported statistical hypothesis testing with the number of features ranging from 1–320 (median 4). Of these studies, 39% were based on MRI, 26%, on CT, 14% on PET, and 21% on US. Similarly, in 61% of the cases, data were analyzed using NSM, 12% using SGLM, 3% using FA, 6% using F&T, and 18% using a combination of these methods. The number of significant features, as reported by the authors, ranged from 0–76 (median 1). Since multiple comparisons generally require a stronger level of evidence to be considered significant, the Holm-Bonferroni correction [20] was applied by the original research authors, or by the authors of this review paper. This correction allows direct comparison to be made of the significance levels of single and multiple comparisons. For eight papers the correction could not be performed due to missing information. After the Holm-Bonferroni correction, the number of significant features ranged from 0–6 (median 1). Figure 8 shows the number of significant features before and after the Holm-Bonferroni correction per imaging modality (A) and per analysis method (B). In 45% of the papers the number of significant features decreased after correction. Using a one-way ANOVA, no significant differences were found in the number of significant features between the modalities. With respect to the analysis method used, a one-way ANOVA established a significant difference in the number of significant features ($p<0.018$). Publications using SGLM reported more significant features. However, after the Holm-Bonferroni correction, the numbers of significant features were similar between all analysis methods used.

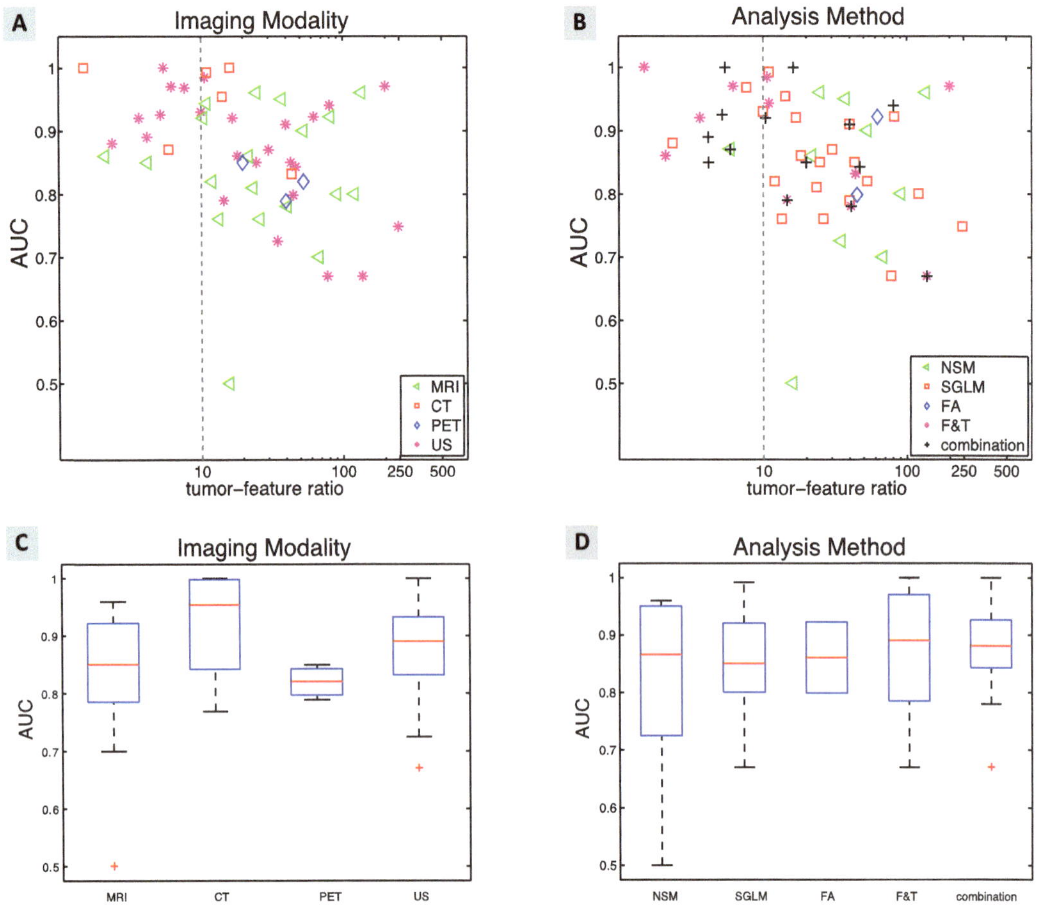

Figure 7. The AUC for different imaging modalities (A) and for different analysis methods (B) as a function of tumor-feature ratio in the classification experiments. The scatter plot shows each imaging modality and analysis method separately. Dotted line represents the ratio of 10 tumors per selected feature. Boxplot representing distribution in AUC for imaging modality (C) and for analysis methods (D).

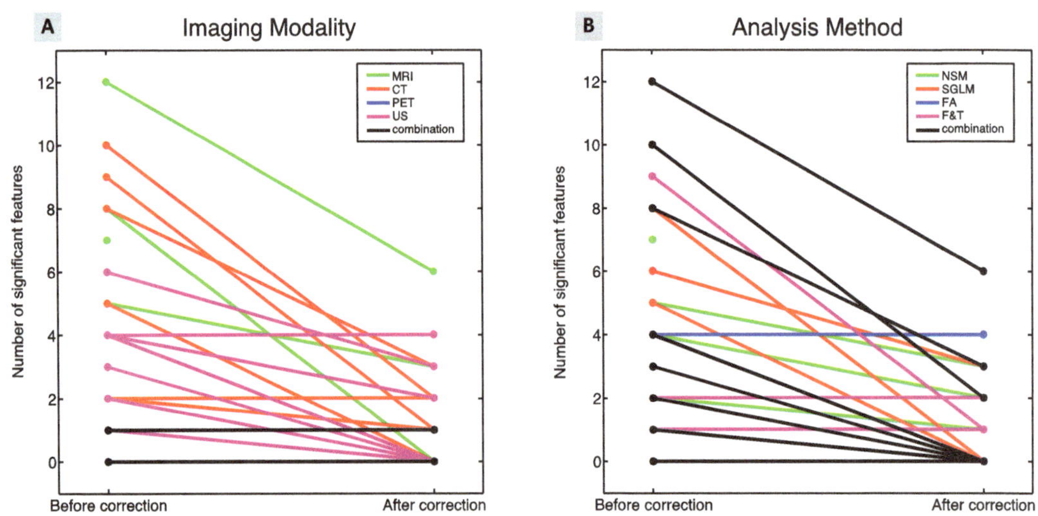

Figure 8. Number of significant features before and after Holm-Bonferroni correction in publications reporting on significance testing for all image modalities (A) and all analysis methods (B).

Discussion

This systematic review investigated the use and performance of heterogeneity or texture quantification methods in radiological images for differentiation between tumor types, tumor grading, outcome prediction and treatment response monitoring. After a systematic literature search yielding 7351, 209 unique studies reported on heterogeneity as an imaging biomarker in tumor imaging. Since 2008, an increasing number of publications have reported on quantification of tumor heterogeneity. Since the present review is based on the existing literature, it reflects the modalities, heterogeneity analysis methods, and location of tumors that were investigated by the authors of the included studies. Because almost all of the included publications presented positive results, it should be noted that this literature probably contains an over presentation of modalities, heterogeneity analysis methods and tumor locations for which heterogeneity analysis seems to work.

Until 2006 most heterogeneity papers were based on US, whereas after 2007 there was an increase in the number of studies using MRI. During the present study period, NSM and SGLM were the most frequently used methods. Most of the papers focus on heterogeneity quantification to differentiate between tumor types, tumor grading or outcome prediction; however, the number of papers with the goal of response monitoring has recently increased. In tumor heterogeneity quantification, US is the most frequently used imaging modality for differentiation between tumor types, tumor grading and outcome prediction, and MRI is the most frequently used modality for treatment response monitoring. For monitoring of treatment response, NSM is the most frequently used method. To differentiate between tumor types and tumor grading, all methods are evenly distributed over all the modalities.

The performance of the heterogeneity features was mostly (67%) evaluated by classification experiments reporting performance measures such as accuracy, sensitivity, specificity and AUC. Papers reporting only on the results of the combination of texture features with other features were excluded from the analysis. Some authors selectively report on sensitivity without mentioning the specificity. The AUC is the preferred measure to report performance as it is more comprehensive compared to a measure based on a single threshold, such as accuracy. Only one paper reported an AUC of 0.5, all other papers reported higher values. This is most likely caused by publication bias: only the positive performance of heterogeneity features tend to reach the journals. Only 63% of the publications reporting classification results described the use of the cross-validation technique to limit the effect of over-fitting on the available data. We found no relation between the performance measures and the modality, or with the analysis method used. However, a negative correlation was found between the tumor-feature ratio and the AUC. When more tumors were available per selected feature, the AUC was lower. This correlation may be the result of overfitting of the data when fewer tumors per feature are available.

Publications using statistical hypothesis testing often did not perform a correction of the significance levels for multiple comparisons. For eight papers, due to missing information, a retrospective Holm-Bonferroni correction could not be performed by the authors. For 45% of the papers, the number of significant features decreased after the Holm-Bonferroni correction. We found no relation between the number of significant features after the Holm-Bonferroni correction and the modality or the analysis method used.

The number of prospective studies is small, i.e. only 13% of all studies. These latter studies are mainly based on MRI and report NSM features. Although the use of retrospectively collected data is necessary to develop, test and evaluate heterogeneity as a biomarker for differentiation between tumor types, tumor grading, outcome prediction and treatment response monitoring, the real test is to evaluate the performance of the developed features in a prospective study design. When using a retrospective study design, the criteria for the inclusion of cases are often not (or not clearly) described, so that the performance of the heterogeneity feature can be overestimated. Using a prospective study design, with clear inclusion criteria, the actual performance of heterogeneity features can be more reliably assessed.

Moreover, in most included studies, performance of the heterogeneity feature is evaluated without taking into account currently accepted clinical features, such as mean signal intensity, tumor size, tumor grade, or border regularity of a tumor. Some studies report only the combined classification performance of heterogeneity and clinical features. A large number of publications even use the mean signal intensity as a feature to estimate tumor heterogeneity, even though this is clearly not a heterogeneity measure (i.e., mean signal intensity does not measure intra-tumor heterogeneity). Based on these types of studies, it is not possible to evaluate the added value of heterogeneity to currently accepted clinical features. Whereas researchers are interested in the performance of the feature itself, clinicians are interested in the additional value of the feature compared with the currently available clinical biomarkers. Since the quantification of heterogeneity is usually more complex and computationally more costly than computing the mean intensity, the benefit of the added effort to characterize heterogeneity needs sufficient motivation. To enable the translation of imaging biomarkers from the research stage to clinical practice, future research should focus on studies investigating the additional value of the proposed heterogeneity biomarker compared with the established clinical markers.

In this systematic review, comparison between the performance of different methods for a certain classification task was not possible due to the large variety in the datasets used and the classification tasks posed. The search for new and optimal (combinations of) heterogeneity features would benefit from developing reliable datasets (for different classification problems) that are available to the scientific community. Large well-defined datasets are a prerequisite for objective comparison of methods.

Future studies should have a design that takes the requirements from pattern recognition into account, i.e. a balanced number of subjects and features, cross-validation, independent test datasets, and a prospective study design. Satisfying these requirements will allow more reliable evaluation of the value of heterogeneity features.

Supporting Information

Figure S1 Numbers of publications for a specific imaging modality and analysis method. The supplementary EndNote files corresponding to the records for these publications (for each cell in the matrix separately) are publically available. To download separate files just click on a cell of interest in the figure.

Figure S2 The accuracy for different imaging modalities (A) and for different analysis methods (B) as a function of tumor-feature ratio in the classification experiments. The scatter plot shows each imaging modality and analysis method separately. Dotted line represents the ratio of 10 tumors per selected feature. Boxplot representing distribution in AUC for imaging modality (C) and for analysis methods (D).

Figure S3 The sensitivity for different imaging modalities (A) and for different analysis methods (B) as a function of tumor-feature ratio in the classification experiments. The scatter plot shows each imaging modality and analysis method separately. Dotted line represents the ratio of 10 tumors per selected feature. Boxplot representing distribution in AUC for imaging modality (C) and for analysis methods (D).

Figure S4 The specificity for different imaging modalities (A) and for different analysis methods (B) as a function of tumor-feature ratio in the classification experiments. The scatter plot shows each imaging modality and analysis method separately. Dotted line represents the ratio of 10 tumors per selected feature. Boxplot representing distribution in AUC for imaging modality (C) and for analysis methods (D).

Text S1 Comprehensive EMBASE search strategy used in the systematic review.

Checklist S1 PRISMA checklist for the systematic review: Quantification of heterogeneity as a biomarker in tumor imaging.

Author Contributions

Conceived and designed the experiments: LA JFV WJN. Performed the experiments: LA JFV. Analyzed the data: LA JFV. Contributed reagents/materials/analysis tools: LA JFV. Wrote the paper: LA JFV WJN.

References

1. Fisher R, Pusztai L, Swanton C (2013) Cancer heterogeneity: implications for targeted therapeutics. Br J Cancer 108: 479–485.
2. Ng CK, Pemberton HN, Reis-Filho JS (2012) Breast cancer intratumor genetic heterogeneity: causes and implications. Expert Rev Anticancer Ther 12: 1021–1032.
3. Brown JR, DiGiovanna MP, Killelea B, Lannin DR, Rimm DL (2014) Quantitative assessment Ki-67 score for prediction of response to neoadjuvant chemotherapy in breast cancer. Lab Invest 94: 98–106.
4. Fasching PA, Heusinger K, Haeberle L, Niklos M, Hein A, et al. (2011) Ki67, chemotherapy response, and prognosis in breast cancer patients receiving neoadjuvant treatment. BMC Cancer 11: 486–498.
5. Szerlip NJ, Pedraza A, Chakravarty D, Azim M, McGuire J, et al. (2012) Intratumoral heterogeneity of receptor tyrosine kinases EGFR and PDGFRA amplification in glioblastoma defines subpopulations with distinct growth factor response. Proc Natl Acad Sci USA 109: 3041–3046.
6. Aerts HJ, Velazquez ER, Leijenaar RT, Parmar C, Grossmann P, et al. (2014) Decoding tumour phenotype by noninvasive imaging using a quantitative radiomics approach. Nat Commun 5: 1–8.
7. Hayes C, Padhani AR, Leach MO (2002) Assessing changes in tumour vascular function using dynamic contrast-enhanced magnetic resonance imaging. NMR Biomed 15: 154–163.
8. van Rijswijk CS, Geirnaerdt MJ, Hogendoorn PC, Peterse JL, van Coevorden F, et al. (2003) Dynamic contrast-enhanced MR imaging in monitoring response to isolated limb perfusion in high-grade soft tissue sarcoma: initial results. Eur Radiol 13: 1849–1858.
9. Pickles MD, Manton DJ, Lowry M, Turnbull LW (2009) Prognostic value of pre-treatment DCE-MRI parameters in predicting disease free and overall survival for breast cancer patients undergoing neoadjuvant chemotherapy. Eur J Radiol 71: 498–505.
10. Brizel DM, Sibley GS, Prosnitz LR, Scher RL, Dewhirst MW (1997) Tumor hypoxia adversely affects the prognosis of carcinoma of the head and neck. Int J Radiat Oncol Biol Phys 38: 285–289.
11. Aerts HJ, Bussink J, Oyen WJ, van Elmpt W, Folgering AM, et al. (2012) Identification of residual metabolic-active areas within NSCLC tumours using a pre-radiotherapy FDG-PET-CT scan: a prospective validation. Lung Cancer 75: 73–76.
12. Lambin P, Petit SF, Aerts HJ, van Elmpt WJ, Oberije CJ, et al. (2010) The ESTRO Breur Lecture 2009. From population to voxel-based radiotherapy: exploiting intra-tumour and intra-organ heterogeneity for advanced treatment of non-small cell lung cancer. Radiother Oncol 96: 145–152.
13. PET Boost trial. Dose escalation by boosting radiation dose within the primary tumor on the basis of a pre-treatment FDG-PET-CT scan in stage IB, II and III NSCLC: a randomized Phase II trial. Available: www.clinicaltrials.gov.
14. Sinha S, Lucas-Quesada FA, DeBruhl ND, Sayre J, Farria D, et al. (1997) Multifeature analysis of Gd-enhanced MR images of breast lesions. J Magn Reson Imaging 7: 1016–1026.
15. Moher D, Liberati A, Tetzlaff J, Altman DG, Group P (2009) Preferred reporting items for systematic reviews and meta-analyses: the PRISMA statement. PLoS Med 6: e1000097.
16. Alic L, Veenland JV, Niessen WJ (2011) Quantification of heterogeneity as a biomarker in tumour imaging: a systematic review. Available: http://wwwmetaxiscom/prospero/full_docasp?RecordID=3634 2013: 732848.
17. Yang X, Knopp MV (2011) Quantifying tumor vascular heterogeneity with dynamic contrast-enhanced magnetic resonance imaging: a review. J Biomed Biotechnol 2011: 732848.
18. Asselin MC, O'Connor JP, Boellaard R, Thacker NA, Jackson A (2012) Quantifying heterogeneity in human tumours using MRI and PET. Eur J Cancer 48: 447–455.
19. Davnall F, Yip CS, Ljungqvist G, Selmi M, Ng F, et al. (2012) Assessment of tumor heterogeneity: an emerging imaging tool for clinical practice? Insights Imaging 3: 573–589.
20. Holm S (1979) A simple sequentially rejective multiple test procedure. Scand J Statistics 6: 65–70.
21. Haralick RM, Shanmugam K, Dinstein J (1973) Textural features for image classification. IEEE Trans Syst Man Cybern 6: 610–621.
22. Amadasun M, King R (1989) Textural features corresponding to textural properties. IEEE Trans Syst, Man Cybernet 19: 1264–1273.
23. Ojala T, Pietikäinen M, Mäenpää T (2002) Multiresolution gray-scale and rotation invariant texture classification with local binary patterns. IEEE Trans Pattern Analy Mach Intell 24: 971–987.
24. Galloway MM (1975) Texture analysis using gray level run lengths. Comp Graphics Image Processing 4: 172–179.
25. Ojala T, Pietikäinen M, Harwood D (1996) A comparative study of texture measures with classification based on feature distributions. Pattern Recognition 29: 51–59.
26. Mandelbrot BB (1983) The fractal geometry of nature. New York: W.H. Freeman. 468 p.
27. Smith TG Jr, Lange GD, Marks WB (1996) Fractal methods and results in cellular morphology–dimensions, lacunarity and multifractals. J Neurosci Methods 69: 123–136.
28. Peleg S, Naor J, Hartley R, Avnir D (1984) Multiple resolution texture analysis and classification. IEEE Trans Pattern Anal Mach Intell 6: 518–523.
29. Tabachnick BG, Fidell LS (2013) Using multivariate statistics. Boston: Pearson Education. xxxi, 983 p.
30. Pekalska E, Duin RPW (2005) The dissimilarity representation for pattern recognition: foundations and applications. Hackensack, N.J.: World Scientific. xxvi, 607 p.
31. Young TY, Calvert TW (1974) Classification, estimation, and pattern recognition: American Elsevier Pub. Co. 366 p.
32. Acharya UR, Faust O, Sree SV, Molinari F, Garberoglio R, et al. (2011) Cost-effective and non-invasive automated benign and malignant thyroid lesion classification in 3D contrast-enhanced ultrasound using combination of wavelets and textures: a class of ThyroScan algorithms. Technol Cancer Res Treat 10: 371–380.
33. Acharya UR, Faust O, Sree SV, Molinari F, Suri JS (2012) ThyroScreen system: high resolution ultrasound thyroid image characterization into benign and malignant classes using novel combination of texture and discrete wavelet transform. Comput Meth Progr Biomed 107: 233–241.
34. Chang RF, Wu WJ, Moon WK, Chen DR (2003) Improvement in breast tumor discrimination by support vector machines and speckle-emphasis texture analysis. Ultrasound Med Biol 29: 679–686.
35. Chang RF, Wu WJ, Moon WK, Chou YH, Chen DR (2003) Support vector machines for diagnosis of breast tumors on US images. Acad Radiol 10: 189–197.
36. Chen D, Chang RF, Huang YL (2000) Breast cancer diagnosis using self-organizing map for sonography. Ultrasound Med Biol 26: 405–411.
37. Chen DR, Chang RF, Huang YL (1999) Computer-aided diagnosis applied to US of solid breast nodules by using neural networks. Radiology 213: 407–412.
38. Chen DR, Kuo WJ, Chang RF, Moon WK, Lee CC (2002) Use of the bootstrap technique with small training sets for computer-aided diagnosis in breast ultrasound. Ultrasound Med Biol 28: 897–902.
39. Chen SJ, Cheng KS, Dai YC, Sun YN, Chen YT, et al. (2005) Quantitatively characterizing the textural features of sonographic images for breast cancer with histopathologic correlation. J Ultrasound Med 24: 651–661.

40. Chen W, Giger ML, Bick U, Newstead GM (2006) Automatic identification and classification of characteristic kinetic curves of breast lesions on DCE-MRI. Med Phys 33: 2878–2887.
41. Ganeshan B, Abaleke S, Young RC, Chatwin CR, Miles KA (2010) Texture analysis of non-small cell lung cancer on unenhanced computed tomography: initial evidence for a relationship with tumour glucose metabolism and stage. Cancer Imaging 10: 137–143.
42. Georgiadis P, Cavouras D, Kalatzis I, Daskalakis A, Kagadis GC, et al. (2008) Improving brain tumor characterization on MRI by probabilistic neural networks and non-linear transformation of textural features. Comput Meth Programs Biomed 89: 24–32.
43. Georgiadis P, Kostopoulos S, Cavouras D, Glotsos D, Kalatzis I, et al. (2011) Quantitative combination of volumetric MR imaging and MR spectroscopy data for the discrimination of meningiomas from metastatic brain tumors by means of pattern recognition. Magn Reson Imaging 29: 525–535.
44. Harrison L, Dastidar P, Eskola H, Jarvenpaa R, Pertovaara H, et al. (2008) Texture analysis on MRI images of non-Hodgkin lymphoma. Comput Biol Med 38: 519–524.
45. Kido S, Kuriyama K, Higashiyama M, Kasugai T, Kuroda C (2002) Fractal analysis of small peripheral pulmonary nodules in thin-section CT: evaluation of the lung-nodule interfaces. J Comput Assist Tomogr 26: 573–578.
46. Klein HM, Klose KC, Eisele T, Brenner M, Ameling W, et al. (1993) [The diagnosis of focal liver lesions by the texture analysis of dynamic computed tomograms]. Rofo 159: 10–15.
47. McNitt-Gray MF, Hart EM, Wyckoff N, Sayre JW, Goldin JG, et al. (1999) A pattern classification approach to characterizing solitary pulmonary nodules imaged on high resolution CT: preliminary results. Med Phys 26: 880–888.
48. Ng F, Kozarski R, Ganeshan B, Goh V (2013) Assessment of tumor heterogeneity by CT texture analysis: can the largest cross-sectional area be used as an alternative to whole tumor analysis? Eur J Radiol 82: 342–348.
49. O'Sullivan F, Roy S, Eary J (2003) A statistical measure of tissue heterogeneity with application to 3D PET sarcoma data. Biostatistics 4: 433–448.
50. Sun T, Wang J, Li X, Lv P, Liu F, et al. (2013) Comparative evaluation of support vector machines for computer aided diagnosis of lung cancer in CT based on a multi-dimensional data set. Comput Meth Programs Biomed 111: 519–524.
51. Thijssen JM, Verbeek AM, Romijn RL, de Wolff-Rouendaal D, Oosterhuis JA (1991) Echographic differentiation of histological types of intraocular melanoma. Ultrasound Med Biol 17: 127–138.
52. Way TW, Hadjiiski LM, Sahiner B, Chan HP, Cascade PN, et al. (2006) Computer-aided diagnosis of pulmonary nodules on CT scans: segmentation and classification using 3D active contours. Med Phys 33: 2323–2337.
53. Wu WJ, Moon WK (2008) Ultrasound breast tumor image computer-aided diagnosis with texture and morphological features. Acad Radiol 15: 873–880.
54. Chen DR, Chang RF, Huang YL, Chou YH, Tiu CM, et al. (2000) Texture analysis of breast tumors on sonograms. Semin Ultrasound CT MR 21: 308–316.
55. Chen DR, Chang RF, Kuo WJ, Chen MC, Huang YL (2002) Diagnosis of breast tumors with sonographic texture analysis using wavelet transform and neural networks. Ultrasound Med Biol 28: 1301–1310.
56. Chen DR, Huang YL, Lin SH (2011) Computer-aided diagnosis with textural features for breast lesions in sonograms. Comput Med Imaging Graph 35: 220–226.
57. Chen DR, Liang WM, Kuo HW, Chang RF (1999) Computerized quantitative assessment of sonomammographic homogeneity of fibroadenoma and breast carcinoma. J of Med Ultrasound 7: 157–162.
58. Chen EL, Chung YN, Chung PC, Tsai HM, Huang YS (2001) Using a fuzzy engine and complete set of features for hepatic diseases diagnosis: Integrating contrast and non-contrast CT images. Biomed Eng - Applications, Basis and Communications 13: 159–167.
59. Chen SJ, Chang CY, Chang KY, Tzeng JE, Chen YT, et al. (2010) Classification of the thyroid nodules based on characteristic sonographic textural feature and correlated histopathology using hierarchical support vector machines. Ultrasound Med Biol 36: 2018–2026.
60. Chen SJ, Cheng KS, Dai YC, Sun YN, Chen YT, et al. (2005) The representations of sonographic image texture for breast cancer using co-occurrence matrix. J Med and Biol Eng 25: 193–199.
61. Chen SJ, Lin CH, Chang CY, Chang KY, Ho HC, et al. (2012) Characterizing the major sonographic textural difference between metastatic and common benign lymph nodes using support vector machine with histopathologic correlation. Clin Imaging 36: 353–359 e352.
62. Chen SJ, Yu SN, Tzeng JE, Chen YT, Chang KY, et al. (2009) Characterization of the major histopathological components of thyroid nodules using sonographic textural features for clinical diagnosis and management. Ultrasound Med Biol 35: 201–208.
63. Chen W, Giger ML, Li H, Bick U, Newstead GM (2007) Volumetric texture analysis of breast lesions on contrast-enhanced magnetic resonance images. Magn Reson Med 58: 562–571.
64. Chen WM, Chang RF, Kuo SJ, Chang CS, Moon WK, et al. (2005) 3-D ultrasound texture classification using run difference matrix. Ultrasound Med Biol 31: 763–770.
65. Chikui T, Tokumori K, Yoshiura K, Oobu K, Nakamura S, et al. (2005) Sonographic texture characterization of salivary gland tumors by fractal analyses. Ultrasound Med Biol 31: 1297–1304.
66. Cook GJR, Yip C, Siddique M, Goh V, Chicklore S, et al. (2013) Are pretreatment 18F-FDG PET tumor textural features in non-small cell lung cancer associated with response and survival after chemoradiotherapy? J Nuc Med 54: 19–26.
67. Cui C, Cai H, Liu L, Li L, Tian H, et al. (2011) Quantitative analysis and prediction of regional lymph node status in rectal cancer based on computed tomography imaging. Eur Radiol 21: 2318–2325.
68. Cui J, Sahiner B, Chan HP, Nees A, Paramagul C, et al. (2009) A new automated method for the segmentation and characterization of breast masses on ultrasound images. Med Phys 36: 1553–1565.
69. de Langen AJ, van den Boogaart V, Lubberink M, Backes WH, Marcus JT, et al. (2011) Monitoring response to antiangiogenic therapy in non-small cell lung cancer using imaging markers derived from PET and dynamic contrast-enhanced MRI. J Nucl Med 52: 48–55.
70. de Lussanet QG, Backes WH, Griffioen AW, Padhani AR, Baeten CI, et al. (2005) Dynamic contrast-enhanced magnetic resonance imaging of radiation therapy-induced microcirculation changes in rectal cancer. Int J Radiat Oncol Biol Phys 63: 1309–1315.
71. Ding J, Cheng H, Ning C, Huang J, Zhang Y (2011) Quantitative measurement for thyroid cancer characterization based on elastography. J Ultrasound Med 30: 1259–1266.
72. Dominietto M, Lehmann S, Keist R, Rudin M (2012) Pattern analysis accounts for heterogeneity observed in MRI studies of tumor angiogenesis. Magn Reson Med 70: 1481–1490.
73. Dong X, Xing L, Wu P, Fu Z, Wan H, et al. (2013) Three-dimensional positron emission tomography image texture analysis of esophageal squamous cell carcinoma: relationship between tumor 18F-fluorodeoxyglucose uptake heterogeneity, maximum standardized uptake value, and tumor stage. Nucl Med Commun 34: 40–46.
74. Donohue KD, Forsberg F, Piccoli CV, Goldberg BB (1999) Analysis and classification of tissue with scatterer structure templates. IEEE Trans Ultrason Ferroelectr Freq Control 46: 300–310.
75. Donohue KD, Huang L, Burks T, Forsberg F, Piccoli CW (2001) Tissue classification with generalized spectrum parameters. Ultrasound Med Biol 27: 1505–1514.
76. Downey K, Riches SF, Morgan VA, Giles SL, Attygalle AD, et al. (2013) Relationship between imaging biomarkers of stage I cervical cancer and poor-prognosis histologic features: quantitative histogram analysis of diffusion-weighted MR images. Am J Roentgenol 200: 314–320.
77. Drabycz S, Roldan G, de Robles P, Adler D, McIntyre JB, et al. (2010) An analysis of image texture, tumor location, and MGMT promoter methylation in glioblastoma using magnetic resonance imaging. Neuroimage 49: 1398–1405.
78. Dumrongpisutikul N, Intrapiromkul J, Yousem DM (2012) Distinguishing between germinomas and pineal cell tumors on MR imaging. AJNR Am J Neuroradiol 33: 550–555.
79. Eary JF, O'Sullivan F, O'Sullivan J, Conrad EU (2008) Spatial heterogeneity in sarcoma 18F-FDG uptake as a predictor of patient outcome. J Nucl Med 49: 1973–1979.
80. Eliat PA, Lechaux D, Gervais A, Rioux-Leclerc N, Franconi F, et al. (2001) Is magnetic resonance imaging texture analysis a useful tool for cell therapy in vivo monitoring? Anticancer Res 21: 3857–3860.
81. Eliat PA, Olivie D, Saikali S, Carsin B, Saint-Jalmes H, et al. (2012) Can dynamic contrast-enhanced magnetic resonance imaging combined with texture analysis differentiate malignant glioneuronal tumors from other glioblastoma? Neurol Res Int 2012: 1–7.
82. Emblem KE, Nedregaard B, Nome T, Due-Tonnessen P, Hald JK, et al. (2008) Glioma grading by using histogram analysis of blood volume heterogeneity from MR-derived cerebral blood volume maps. Radiology 247: 808–817.
83. Engelbrecht MR, Hitge-Boetes C, Coolen J, Thijssen JM, Makkus AC, et al. (1998) Follow-up of Wilms' tumour during pre-operative chemotherapy by qualitative and quantitative sonography. Eur J Ultrasound 8: 157–165.
84. Farace P, Galie M, Merigo F, Daducci A, Calderan L, et al. (2009) Inhibition of tyrosine kinase receptors by SU6668 promotes abnormal stromal development at the periphery of carcinomas. Br J Cancer 100: 1575–1580.
85. Faschingbauer F, Beckmann MW, Weyert Goecke T, Renner S, Haberle L, et al. (2013) Automatic texture-based analysis in ultrasound imaging of ovarian masses. Ultraschall Med 34: 145–150.
86. Fetit AE, Novak J, Rodriguez D, Auer DP, Clark CA, et al. (2013) MRI texture analysis in paediatric oncology: a preliminary study. Stud Health Technol Inform 190: 169–171.
87. Fruehwald-Pallamar J, Czerny C, Holzer-Fruehwald L, Nemec SF, Mueller-Mang C, et al. (2013) Texture-based and diffusion-weighted discrimination of parotid gland lesions on MR images at 3.0 Tesla. NMR Biomed 26: 1372–1379.
88. Ganeshan B, Panayiotou E, Burnand K, Dizdarevic S, Miles K (2012) Tumour heterogeneity in non-small cell lung carcinoma assessed by CT texture analysis: a potential marker of survival. Eur Radiol 22: 796–802.
89. Ganeshan B, Skogen K, Pressney I, Coutroubis D, Miles K (2012) Tumour heterogeneity in oesophageal cancer assessed by CT texture analysis: preliminary evidence of an association with tumour metabolism, stage, and survival. Clin Radiol 67: 157–164.

90. Garra BS, Krasner BH, Horii SC, Ascher S, Mun SK, et al. (1993) Improving the distinction between benign and malignant breast lesions: the value of sonographic texture analysis. Ultrason Imaging 15: 267–285.
91. Gensure RH, Foran DJ, Lee VM, Gendel VM, Jabbour SK, et al. (2012) Evaluation of hepatic tumor response to yttrium-90 radioembolization therapy using texture signatures generated from contrast-enhanced CT images. Acad Radiol 19: 1201–1207.
92. Georgiadis P, Cavouras D, Kalatzis I, Glotsos D, Athanasiadis E, et al. (2009) Enhancing the discrimination accuracy between metastases, gliomas and meningiomas on brain MRI by volumetric textural features and ensemble pattern recognition methods. Magn Reson Imaging 27: 120–130.
93. Gibbs P, Turnbull LW (2003) Textural analysis of contrast-enhanced MR images of the breast. Magn Reson Med 50: 92–98.
94. Giger ML, Al-Hallaq H, Huo Z, Moran C, Wolverton DE, et al. (1999) Computerized analysis of lesions in US images of the breast. Acad Radiol 6: 665–674.
95. Gletsos M, Mougiakakou SG, Matsopoulos GK, Nikita KS, Nikita AS, et al. (2003) A computer-aided diagnostic system to characterize CT focal liver lesions: design and optimization of a neural network classifier. IEEE Trans Inf Technol Biomed 7: 153–162.
96. Glotsos D, Kalatzis I, Theocharakis P, Georgiadis P, Daskalakis A, et al. (2010) A multi-classifier system for the characterization of normal, infectious, and cancerous prostate tissues employing transrectal ultrasound images. Comput Meth Programs Biomed 97: 53–61.
97. Goh V, Ganeshan B, Nathan P, Juttla JK, Vinayan A, et al. (2011) Assessment of response to tyrosine kinase inhibitors in metastatic renal cell cancer: CT texture as a predictive biomarker. Radiology 261: 165–171.
98. Goldberg V, Manduca A, Ewert DL, Gisvold JJ, Greenleaf JF (1992) Improvement in specificity of ultrasonography for diagnosis of breast tumors by means of artificial intelligence. Med Phys 19: 1475–1481.
99. Gomez W, Pereira WC, Infantosi AF (2012) Analysis of co-occurrence texture statistics as a function of gray-level quantization for classifying breast ultrasound. IEEE Trans Med Imaging 31: 1889–1899.
100. Haney CR, Fan X, Markiewicz E, Mustafi D, Karczmar GS, et al. (2013) Monitoring anti-angiogenic therapy in colorectal cancer murine model using dynamic contrast-enhanced MRI: comparing pixel-by-pixel with region of interest analysis. Technol Cancer Res Treat 12: 71–78.
101. Hatt M, Tixier F, Cheze Le Rest C, Pradier O, Visvikis D (2013) Robustness of intratumour (18)F-FDG PET uptake heterogeneity quantification for therapy response prediction in oesophageal carcinoma. Eur J Nucl Med Mol Imaging 40: 1662–1671.
102. Herts BR, Coll DM, Novick AC, Obuchowski N, Linnell G, et al. (2002) Enhancement characteristics of papillary renal neoplasms revealed on triphasic helical CT of the kidneys. AJR Am J Roentgenol 178: 367–372.
103. Hirano M, Satake H, Ishigaki S, Ikeda M, Kawai H, et al. (2012) Diffusion-weighted imaging of breast masses: comparison of diagnostic performance using various apparent diffusion coefficient parameters. AJR Am J Roentgenol 198: 717–722.
104. Hirning T, Zuna I, Schlaps D, Lorenz D, Meybier H, et al. (1989) Quantification and classification of echographic findings in the thyroid gland by computerized B-mode texture analysis. Eur J Radiol 9: 244–247.
105. Holli K, Laaperi AL, Harrison L, Luukkaala T, Toivonen T, et al. (2010) Characterization of breast cancer types by texture analysis of magnetic resonance images. Acad Radiol 17: 135–141.
106. Horsch K, Giger ML, Venta LA, Vyborny CJ (2002) Computerized diagnosis of breast lesions on ultrasound. Med Phys 29: 157–164.
107. Huang B, Chan T, Kwong DL, Chan WK, Khong PL (2012) Nasopharyngeal carcinoma: investigation of intratumoral heterogeneity with FDG PET/CT. AJR Am J Roentgenol 199: 169–174.
108. Huang YL, Chen JH, Shen WC (2006) Diagnosis of hepatic tumors with texture analysis in nonenhanced computed tomography images. Acad Radiol 13: 713–720.
109. Huang YL, Kuo SJ, Chang CS, Liu YK, Moon WK, et al. (2005) Image retrieval with principal component analysis for breast cancer diagnosis on various ultrasonic systems. Ultrasound Obstet Gynecol 26: 558–566.
110. Huang Z, Mayr NA, Lo SS, Grecula JC, Wang JZ, et al. (2012) Characterizing at-risk voxels by using perfusion magnetic resonance imaging for cervical cancer during radiotherapy. J Cancer Sci Ther 4: 254–259.
111. Huber S, Danes J, Zuna I, Teubner J, Medl M, et al. (2000) Relevance of sonographic B-mode criteria and computer-aided ultrasonic tissue characterization in differential/diagnosis of solid breast masses. Ultrasound Med Biol 26: 1243–1252.
112. Iakovidis DK, Keramidas EG, Maroulis D (2010) Fusion of fuzzy statistical distributions for classification of thyroid ultrasound patterns. Artif Intell Med 50: 33–41.
113. Issa B, Buckley DL, Turnbull LW (1999) Heterogeneity analysis of Gd-DTPA uptake: improvement in breast lesion differentiation. J Comput Assist Tomogr 23: 615–621.
114. Jansen JF, Schoder H, Lee NY, Stambuk HE, Wang Y, et al. (2012) Tumor metabolism and perfusion in head and neck squamous cell carcinoma: pretreatment multimodality imaging with 1H magnetic resonance spectroscopy, dynamic contrast-enhanced MRI, and [18F]FDG-PET. Int J Radiat Oncol Biol Phys 82: 299–307.
115. Jung SC, Cho JY, Kim SH (2012) Subtype differentiation of small renal cell carcinomas on three-phase MDCT: usefulness of the measurement of degree and heterogeneity of enhancement. Acta Radiol 53: 112–118.
116. Juntu J, Sijbers J, De Backer S, Rajan J, Van Dyck D (2010) Machine learning study of several classifiers trained with texture analysis features to differentiate benign from malignant soft-tissue tumors in T1-MRI images. J Magn Reson Imaging 31: 680–689.
117. Karahaliou A, Vassiou K, Arikidis NS, Skiadopoulos S, Kanavou T, et al. (2010) Assessing heterogeneity of lesion enhancement kinetics in dynamic contrast-enhanced MRI for breast cancer diagnosis. Br J Radiol 83: 296–309.
118. Kidd EA, Grigsby PW (2008) Intratumoral metabolic heterogeneity of cervical cancer. Clin Cancer Res 14: 5236–5241.
119. Kido S, Kuriyama K, Higashiyama M, Kasugai T, Kuroda C (2003) Fractal analysis of internal and peripheral textures of small peripheral bronchogenic carcinomas in thin-section computed tomography: comparison of bronchioloalveolar cell carcinomas with nonbronchioloalveolar cell carcinomas. J Comput Assist Tomogr 27: 56–61.
120. Kim DY, Kim JH, Noh SM, Park JW (2003) Pulmonary nodule detection using chest CT images. Acta Radiol 44: 252–257.
121. Kim KG, Cho SW, Min SJ, Kim JH, Min BG, et al. (2005) Computerized scheme for assessing ultrasonographic features of breast masses. Acad Radiol 12: 58–66.
122. Kim KG, Kim JH, Min BG (2001) Comparative analysis of texture characteristics of malignant and benign tumors in breast ultrasonograms. J Digit Imaging 14: 208–210.
123. Kjaer L, Ring P, Thomsen C, Henriksen O (1995) Texture analysis in quantitative MR imaging. Tissue characterisation of normal brain and intracranial tumours at 1.5 T. Acta Radiol 36: 127–135.
124. Klein HM, Eisele T, Klose KC, Stauss I, Brenner M, et al. (1996) Pattern recognition system for focal liver lesions using "crisp" and "fuzzy" classifiers. Invest Radiol 31: 6–10.
125. Kratzik C, Schuster E, Hainz A, Kuber W, Lunglmayr G (1988) Texture analysis–a new method of differentiating prostatic carcinoma from prostatic hypertrophy. Urol Res 16: 395–397.
126. Kuntz C, Glaser F, Zuna I, Buhr HJ, Herfarth C (1994) Endorectal ultrasound and computerized B-scan texture analysis to assess sessile adenoma and small rectal carcinoma. Endoskopie Heute 7: 173–178.
127. Kuo WJ, Chang RF, Lee CC, Moon WK, Chen DR (2002) Retrieval technique for the diagnosis of solid breast tumors on sonogram. Ultrasound Med Biol 28: 903–909.
128. Kuo WJ, Chang RF, Moon WK, Lee CC, Chen DR (2002) Computer-aided diagnosis of breast tumors with different US systems. Acad Radiol 9: 793–799.
129. Kurki T, Lundbom N, Kalimo H, Valtonen S (1995) MR classification of brain gliomas: value of magnetization transfer and conventional imaging. Magn Reson Imaging 13: 501–511.
130. Lai YC, Huang YS, Wang DW, Tiu CM, Chou YH, et al. (2013) Computer-aided diagnosis for 3-d power Doppler breast ultrasound. Ultrasound Med Biol 39: 555–567.
131. Larkin TJ, Canuto HC, Kettunen MI, Booth TC, Hu DE, et al. (2013) Analysis of image heterogeneity using 2D Minkowski functionals detects tumor responses to treatment. Magn Reson Med 7.
132. Lee CC, Shih CY (2010) Learning patterns of liver masses using improved RBF networks. Biomedical Engineering - Applications, Basis and Communications 22: 137–147.
133. Lefebvre F, Meunier M, Thibault F, Laugier P, Berger G (2000) Computerized ultrasound B-scan characterization of breast nodules. Ultrasound Med Biol 26: 1421–1428.
134. Li X, Lu Y, Pirzkall A, McKnight T, Nelson SJ (2002) Analysis of the spatial characteristics of metabolic abnormalities in newly diagnosed glioma patients. J Magn Reson Imaging 16: 229–237.
135. Liao YY, Tsui PH, Li CH, Chang KJ, Kuo WH, et al. (2011) Classification of scattering media within benign and malignant breast tumors based on ultrasound texture-feature-based and Nakagami-parameter images. Med Phys 38: 2198–2207.
136. Liu F, Kornecki A, Shmuilovich O, Gelman N (2011) Optimization of time-to-peak analysis for differentiating malignant and benign breast lesions with dynamic contrast-enhanced MRI. Acad Radiol 18: 694–704.
137. Liu Y, Cheng HD, Huang JH, Zhang YT, Tang XL, et al. (2012) Computer aided diagnosis system for breast cancer based on color Doppler flow imaging. J Med Syst 36: 3975–3982.
138. Liu YH, Muftah M, Das T, Bai L, Robson K, et al. (2012) Classification of MR tumor images based on Gabor wavelet analysis. J Med Biol Eng 32: 22–28.
139. Loren DE, Seghal CM, Ginsberg GG, Kochman ML (2002) Computer-assisted analysis of lymph nodes detected by EUS in patients with esophageal carcinoma. Gastrointest Endosc 56: 742–746.
140. Ma JH, Kim HS, Rim NJ, Kim SH, Cho KG (2010) Differentiation among glioblastoma multiforme, solitary metastatic tumor, and lymphoma using whole-tumor histogram analysis of the normalized cerebral blood volume in enhancing and perienhancing lesions. Am J Neuroradiol 31: 1699–1706.
141. Maruyama H, Takahashi M, Sekimoto T, Kamesaki H, Shimada T, et al. (2012) Heterogeneity of microbubble accumulation: a novel approach to discriminate between well-differentiated hepatocellular carcinomas and regenerative nodules. Ultrasound Med Biol 38: 383–388.

142. Mattonen SA, Palma DA, Haasbeek CJ, Senan S, Ward AD (2013) Distinguishing radiation fibrosis from tumour recurrence after stereotactic ablative radiotherapy (SABR) for lung cancer: a quantitative analysis of CT density changes. Acta Oncol 52: 910–918.
143. Mayerhoefer ME, Breitenseher M, Amann G, Dominkus M (2008) Are signal intensity and homogeneity useful parameters for distinguishing between benign and malignant soft tissue masses on MR images? Objective evaluation by means of texture analysis. Magn Reson Imaging 26: 1316–1322.
144. Mayerhoefer ME, Schima W, Trattnig S, Pinker K, Berger-Kulemann V, et al. (2010) Texture-based classification of focal liver lesions on MRI at 3.0 Tesla: a feasibility study in cysts and hemangiomas. J Magn Reson Imaging 32: 352–359.
145. Mayr NA, Yuh WT, Arnholt JC, Ehrhardt JC, Sorosky JI, et al. (2000) Pixel analysis of MR perfusion imaging in predicting radiation therapy outcome in cervical cancer. J Magn Reson Imaging 12: 1027–1033.
146. McLaren CE, Chen WP, Nie K, Su MY (2009) Prediction of malignant breast lesions from MRI features: a comparison of artificial neural network and logistic regression techniques. Acad Radiol 16: 842–851.
147. McNitt-Gray MF, Wyckoff N, Sayre JW, Goldin JG, Aberle DR (1999) The effects of co-occurrence matrix based texture parameters on the classification of solitary pulmonary nodules imaged on computed tomography. Comput Med Imaging Graph 23: 339–348.
148. Meinel LA, Stolpen AH, Berbaum KS, Fajardo LL, Reinhardt JM (2007) Breast MRI lesion classification: improved performance of human readers with a backpropagation neural network computer-aided diagnosis (CAD) system. J Magn Reson Imaging 25: 89–95.
149. Miles KA, Ganeshan B, Griffiths MR, Young RC, Chatwin CR (2009) Colorectal cancer: texture analysis of portal phase hepatic CT images as a potential marker of survival. Radiology 250: 444–452.
150. Mitrea D, Mitrea P, Nedevschi S, Badea R, Lupsor M, et al. (2012) Abdominal tumor characterization and recognition using superior-order cooccurrence matrices, based on ultrasound images. Comput Math Methods Med 2012: 348135.
151. Mittal D, Kumar V, Saxena SC, Khandelwal N, Kalra N (2011) Neural network based focal liver lesion diagnosis using ultrasound images. Comput Med Imaging Graph 35: 315–323.
152. Moon WK, Shen YW, Huang CS, Chiang LR, Chang RF (2011) Computer-aided diagnosis for the classification of breast masses in automated whole breast ultrasound images. Ultrasound Med Biol 37: 539–548.
153. Mougiakakou SG, Valavanis IK, Nikita A, Nikita KS (2007) Differential diagnosis of CT focal liver lesions using texture features, feature selection and ensemble driven classifiers. Artif Intell Med 41: 25–37.
154. Mouthuy N, Cosnard G, Abarca-Quinones J, Michoux N (2012) Multi-parametric magnetic resonance imaging to differentiate high-grade gliomas and brain metastases. J Neuroradiol 39: 301–307.
155. Mussurakis S, Gibbs P, Horsman A (1998) Peripheral enhancement and spatial contrast uptake heterogeneity of primary breast tumours: quantitative assessment with dynamic MRI. J Comput Assist Tomogr 22: 35–46.
156. Nagarajan MB, Huber MB, Schlossbauer T, Leinsinger G, Krol A, et al. (2013) Classification of Small Lesions in Breast MRI: Evaluating The Role of Dynamically Extracted Texture Features Through Feature Selection. J Med Biol Eng 33: 59–68.
157. Negendank WG, al-Katib AM, Karanes C, Smith MR (1990) Lymphomas: MR imaging contrast characteristics with clinical-pathologic correlations. Radiology 177: 209–216.
158. Newell D, Nie K, Chen JH, Hsu CC, Yu HJ, et al. (2010) Selection of diagnostic features on breast MRI to differentiate between malignant and benign lesions using computer-aided diagnosis: differences in lesions presenting as mass and non-mass-like enhancement. Eur Radiol 20: 771–781.
159. Ng F, Ganeshan B, Kozarski R, Miles KA, Goh V (2013) Assessment of primary colorectal cancer heterogeneity by using whole-tumor texture analysis: contrast-enhanced CT texture as a biomarker of 5-year survival. Radiology 266: 177–184.
160. Nguyen P, Bashirzadeh F, Hundloe J, Salvado O, Dowson N, et al. (2012) Optical differentiation between malignant and benign lymphadenopathy by grey scale texture analysis of endobronchial ultrasound convex probe images. Chest 141: 709–715.
161. Nguyen VX, Nguyen CC, Li B, Das A (2010) Digital image analysis is a useful adjunct to endoscopic ultrasonographic diagnosis of subepithelial lesions of the gastrointestinal tract. J Ultrasound Med 29: 1345–1351.
162. Nie K, Chen JH, Yu HJ, Chu Y, Nalcioglu O, et al. (2008) Quantitative analysis of lesion morphology and texture features for diagnostic prediction in breast MRI. Acad Radiol 15: 1513–1525.
163. O'Connor JP, Rose CJ, Jackson A, Watson Y, Cheung S, et al. (2011) DCE-MRI biomarkers of tumour heterogeneity predict CRC liver metastasis shrinkage following bevacizumab and FOLFOX-6. Br J Cancer 105: 139–145.
164. O'Sullivan F, Wolsztynski E, O'Sullivan J, Richards T, Conrad EU, et al. (2011) A statistical modeling approach to the analysis of spatial patterns of FDG-PET uptake in human sarcoma. IEEE Trans Med Imaging 30: 2059–2071.
165. Padma A, Sukanesh R (2013) Combined texture feature analysis of segmentation and classification of benign and malignant tumour CT slices. J Med Eng Technol 37: 1–9.
166. Pang Y, Li L, Hu W, Peng Y, Liu L, et al. (2012) Computerized segmentation and characterization of breast lesions in dynamic contrast-enhanced MR images using fuzzy c-means clustering and snake algorithm. Comput Math Methods Med 2012: 634907.
167. Peeters F, Rommel D, Abarca-Quinones J, Gregoire V, Duprez T (2012) Early (72-hour) detection of radiotherapy-induced changes in an experimental tumor model using diffusion-weighted imaging, diffusion tensor imaging, and Q-space imaging parameters: a comparative study. J Magn Reson Imaging 35: 409–417.
168. Peng SL, Chen CF, Liu HL, Lui CC, Huang YJ, et al. (2012) Analysis of parametric histogram from dynamic contrast-enhanced MRI: application in evaluating brain tumor response to radiotherapy. NMR Biomed 26: 443–451.
169. Piliouras N, Kalatzis I, Dimitropoulos N, Cavouras D (2004) Development of the cubic least squares mapping linear-kernel support vector machine classifier for improving the characterization of breast lesions on ultrasound. Comput Med Imaging Graph 28: 247–255.
170. Plant RL (1998) Image analysis of benign and malignant neck masses. Ann Otol Rhinol Laryngol 107: 689–696.
171. Preim U, Glasser S, Preim B, Fischbach F, Ricke J (2012) Computer-aided diagnosis in breast DCE-MRI–quantification of the heterogeneity of breast lesions. Eur J Radiol 81: 1532–1538.
172. Prescott JW, Zhang D, Wang JZ, Mayr NA, Yuh WT, et al. (2010) Temporal analysis of tumor heterogeneity and volume for cervical cancer treatment outcome prediction: preliminary evaluation. J Digit Imaging 23: 342–357.
173. Raja JV, Khan M, Ramachandra VK, Al-Kadi O (2012) Texture analysis of CT images in the characterization of oral cancers involving buccal mucosa. Dentomaxillofac Radiol 41: 475–480.
174. Rakoczy M, McGaughey D, Korenberg MJ, Levman J, Martel AL (2013) Feature selection in computer-aided breast cancer diagnosis via dynamic contrast-enhanced magnetic resonance images. J Digit Imaging 26: 198–208.
175. Ravanelli M, Farina D, Morassi M, Roca E, Cavalleri G, et al. (2013) Texture analysis of advanced non-small cell lung cancer (NSCLC) on contrast-enhanced computed tomography: prediction of the response to the first-line chemotherapy. Eur Radiol 23: 3450–3454.
176. Rehn S, Sperber GO, Nyman R, Glimelius B, Hagberg H, et al. (1993) Quantification of inhomogeneities in malignancy grading of non-Hodgkin lymphoma with MR imaging. Acta Radiol 34: 3–9.
177. Rehn SM, Rodriguez M, Bergstrom SR, Nyman RS, Glimelius BL (1997) Tumour inhomogeneities on magnetic resonance imaging, a new factor with prognostic information in non-Hodgkin's lymphomas. Leuk Lymphoma 24: 501–511.
178. Retico A, Fantacci ME, Gori I, Kasae P, Golosio B, et al. (2009) Pleural nodule identification in low-dose and thin-slice lung computed tomography. Comput Biol Med 39: 1137–1144.
179. Revert Ventura AJ, Sanz Requena R, Marti-Bonmati L, Pallardo Y, Jornet J, et al. (2012) The heterogeneity of blood flow on magnetic resonance imaging: a biomarker for grading cerebral astrocytomas. Radiologia 56.
180. Rokita E, Taton G, Sierzega M, Kulig J, Urbanik A (2009) Quantitative analysis of 3D US images in the relationship with liver lesion diagnosis. Polish J Radiol 74: 28–34.
181. Rose CJ, Mills SJ, O'Connor JP, Buonaccorsi GA, Roberts C, et al. (2009) Quantifying spatial heterogeneity in dynamic contrast-enhanced MRI parameter maps. Magn Reson Med 62: 488–499.
182. Sachdeva J, Kumar V, Gupta I, Khandelwal N, Ahuja CK (2012) A dual neural network ensemble approach for multiclass brain tumor classification. Int J Numer Method Biomed Eng 28: 1107–1120.
183. Sadeghi-Naini A, Falou O, Tadayyon H, Al-Mahrouki A, Tran W, et al. (2013) Conventional frequency ultrasonic biomarkers of cancer treatment response in vivo. Transl Oncol 6: 234–243.
184. Sahiner B, Chan HP, Roubidoux MA, Helvie MA, Hadjiiski LM, et al. (2004) Computerized characterization of breast masses on three-dimensional ultrasound volumes. Med Phys 31: 744–754.
185. Sarty GE, Kendall EJ, Loewy J, Dhir A, Olatunbosun OA, et al. (2004) Magnetic resonance diffusion imaging of ovarian masses: a first experience with 12 cases. MAGMA 16: 182–193.
186. Sasikala M, Kumaravel N (2008) A wavelet-based optimal texture feature set for classification of brain tumours. J Med Eng Technol 32: 198–205.
187. Scheipers U, Siebers S, Gottwald F, Ashfaq M, Bozzato A, et al. (2005) Sonohistology for the computerized differentiation of parotid gland tumors. Ultrasound Med Biol 31: 1287–1296.
188. Schulte M, von Baer A, Schultheiss M, Scheil-Bertram S (2010) [Classification of solid soft tissue tumours by ultrasonography]. Ultraschall Med 31: 182–190.
189. Selvan S, Kavitha M, Devi SS, Suresh S (2012) Fuzzy-based classification of breast lesions using ultrasound echography and elastography. Ultrasound Q 28: 159–167.
190. Shah SK, McNitt-Gray MF, Rogers SR, Goldin JG, Suh RD, et al. (2005) Computer-aided diagnosis of the solitary pulmonary nodule. Acad Radiol 12: 570–575.
191. Sidiropoulos KP, Kostopoulos SA, Glotsos DT, Athanasiadis EI, Dimitropoulos ND, et al. (2013) Multimodality GPU-based computer-assisted diagnosis of breast cancer using ultrasound and digital mammography images. Int J Comput Assist Radiol Surg 8: 547–560.

192. Siebers S, Zenk J, Bozzato A, Klintworth N, Iro H, et al. (2010) Computer aided diagnosis of parotid gland lesions using ultrasonic multi-feature tissue characterization. Ultrasound Med Biol 36: 1525–1534.
193. Sivaramakrishna R, Powell KA, Lieber ML, Chilcote WA, Shekhar R (2002) Texture analysis of lesions in breast ultrasound images. Comput Med Imaging Graph 26: 303–307.
194. Skogen K, Ganeshan B, Good C, Critchley G, Miles K (2013) Measurements of heterogeneity in gliomas on computed tomography relationship to tumour grade. J Neurooncol 111: 213–219.
195. Spector DI, Fischetti AJ, Kovak-McClaran JR (2011) Computed tomographic characteristics of intrapelvic masses in dogs. Vet Radiol Ultrasound 52: 71–74.
196. Spira D, Sokler M, Vogel W, Loffler S, Spira SM, et al. (2011) Volume and attenuation computed tomography measurements for interim evaluation of Hodgkin and follicular lymphoma as an additional surrogate parameter for more confident response monitoring: a pilot study. Cancer Imaging 11: 155–162.
197. Spira D, Wecker M, Spira SM, Hetzel J, Spengler W, et al. (2013) Does volume perfusion computed tomography enable differentiation of metastatic and non-metastatic mediastinal lymph nodes in lung cancer patients? A feasibility study. Cancer Imaging 13: 323–331.
198. Stantz KM, Cao M, Cao N, Liang Y, Miller KD (2011) Monitoring the longitudinal intra-tumor physiological impulse response to VEGFR2 blockade in breast tumors using DCE-CT. Mol Imaging Biol 13: 1183–1195.
199. Strzelecki M, Materka A, Drozdz J, Krzeminska-Pakula M, Kasprzak JD (2006) Classification and segmentation of intracardiac masses in cardiac tumor echocardiograms. Comput Med Imaging Graph 30: 95–107.
200. Su Y, Wang Y, Jiao J, Guo Y (2011) Automatic detection and classification of breast tumors in ultrasonic images using texture and morphological features. Open Med Inform J 5: 26–37.
201. Sujana H, Swarnamani S, Suresh S (1996) Application of artificial neural networks for the classification of liver lesions by image texture parameters. Ultrasound Med Biol 22: 1177–1181.
202. Sun T, Zhang R, Wang J, Li X, Guo X (2013) Computer-aided diagnosis for early-stage lung cancer based on longitudinal and balanced data. PLoS One 8: 1–6.
203. Tan S, Kligerman S, Chen W, Lu M, Kim G, et al. (2013) Spatial-temporal [(1)(8)F]FDG-PET features for predicting pathologic response of esophageal cancer to neoadjuvant chemoradiation therapy. Int J Radiat Oncol Biol Phys 85: 1375–1382.
204. Thijssen JM, Verbeek AM, Romijn RL, de Wolf-Rouendaal D, Oosterhuis JA (1992) Echographic differentiation of intraocular melanomas by computer analysis. Acta Ophthalmol Suppl 204: 26–34.
205. Tixier F, Le Rest CC, Hatt M, Albarghach N, Pradier O, et al. (2011) Intratumor heterogeneity characterized by textural features on baseline 18F-FDG PET images predicts response to concomitant radiochemotherapy in esophageal cancer. J Nucl Med 52: 369–378.
206. Tozer DJ, Jager HR, Danchaivijitr N, Benton CE, Tofts PS, et al. (2007) Apparent diffusion coefficient histograms may predict low-grade glioma subtype. NMR Biomed 20: 49–57.
207. Tsantis S, Cavouras D, Kalatzis I, Piliouras N, Dimitropoulos N, et al. (2005) Development of a support vector machine-based image analysis system for assessing the thyroid nodule malignancy risk on ultrasound. Ultrasound Med Biol 31: 1451–1459.
208. Tse DM, Joshi N, Anderson EM, Brady M, Gleeson FV (2012) A computer-aided algorithm to quantitatively predict lymph node status on MRI in rectal cancer. Br J Radiol 85: 1272–1278.
209. Tuma J, Novakova B, Schwarzenbach HR, Jungius KP, Hollerweger A, et al. (2011) [Image analysis in the differential diagnosis of renal parenchyma lesions]. Ultraschall Med 32: 286–292.
210. Vaidya M, Creach KM, Frye J, Dehdashti F, Bradley JD, et al. (2012) Combined PET/CT image characteristics for radiotherapy tumor response in lung cancer. Radiother Oncol 102: 239–245.
211. Virmani J, Kumar V, Kalra N, Khandelwal N (2013) A comparative study of computer-aided classification systems for focal hepatic lesions from B-mode ultrasound. J Med Eng Technol 37: 292–306.
212. Virmani J, Kumar V, Kalra N, Khandelwal N (2013) SVM-based characterization of liver ultrasound images using wavelet packet texture descriptors. J Digit Imaging 26: 530–543.
213. Wang H, Guo XH, Jia ZW, Li HK, Liang ZG, et al. (2010) Multilevel binomial logistic prediction model for malignant pulmonary nodules based on texture features of CT image. Eur J Radiol 74: 124–129.
214. Way TW, Sahiner B, Chan HP, Hadjiiski L, Cascade PN, et al. (2009) Computer-aided diagnosis of pulmonary nodules on CT scans: improvement of classification performance with nodule surface features. Med Phys 36: 3086–3098.
215. Willaime JM, Turkheimer FE, Kenny LM, Aboagye EO (2013) Quantification of intra-tumour cell proliferation heterogeneity using imaging descriptors of 18F fluorothymidine-positron emission tomography. Phys Med Biol 58: 187–203.
216. Win T, Miles KA, Janes SM, Ganeshan B, Shastry M, et al. (2013) Tumor heterogeneity and permeability as measured on the CT component of PET/CT predict survival in patients with non-small cell lung cancer. Clin Cancer Res 19: 3591–3599.
217. Wu H, Sun T, Wang J, Li X, Wang W, et al. (2013) Combination of radiological and gray level co-occurrence matrix textural features used to distinguish solitary pulmonary nodules by computed tomography. J Digit Imaging 26: 797–802.
218. Wu WJ, Lin SW, Moon WK (2012) Combining support vector machine with genetic algorithm to classify ultrasound breast tumor images. Comput Med Imaging Graph 36: 627–633.
219. Yan K, Yu Y, Tinney E, Baraldi R, Liao L (2012) Clinical study of a noninvasive multimodal sono-contrast induced spectroscopy system for breast cancer diagnosis. Med Phys 39: 1571–1578.
220. Yang X, Mrozek E, Lustberg M, Jia G, Sammet S, et al. (2012) Microcirculatory fraction (MCF(I)) as a potential imaging marker for tumor heterogeneity in breast cancer. Magn Reson Imaging 30: 1059–1067.
221. Yoshida H, Casalino DD, Keserci B, Coskun A, Ozturk O, et al. (2003) Wavelet-packet-based texture analysis for differentiation between benign and malignant liver tumours in ultrasound images. Phys Med Biol 48: 3735–3753.
222. Yoshida H, Nappi J, MacEneaney P, Rubin DT, Dachman AH (2002) Computer-aided diagnosis scheme for detection of polyps at CT colonography. Radiographics 22: 963–979.
223. Yoshiura K, Miwa K, Yuasa K, Tokumori K, Kanda S, et al. (1997) Ultrasonographic texture characterization of salivary and neck masses using two-dimensional gray-scale clustering. Dentomaxillofac Radiol 26: 332–336.
224. Zacharaki EI, Wang S, Chawla S, Soo Yoo D, Wolf R, et al. (2009) Classification of brain tumor type and grade using MRI texture and shape in a machine learning scheme. Magn Reson Med 62: 1609–1618.
225. Zhang X, Kanematsu M, Fujita H, Zhou X, Hara T, et al. (2009) Application of an artificial neural network to the computer-aided differentiation of focal liver disease in MR imaging. Radiol Phys Technol 2: 175–182.
226. Zheng Y, Englander S, Baloch S, Zacharaki EI, Fan Y, et al. (2009) STEP: spatiotemporal enhancement pattern for MR-based breast tumor diagnosis. Med Phys 36: 3192–3204.
227. Zhou S, Shi J, Zhu J, Cai Y, Wang R (2013) Shearlet-based texture feature extraction for classification of breast tumor in ultrasound image. Biomed Signal Process Control 8: 688–696.
228. Zhu Y, Tan Y, Hua Y, Wang M, Zhang G, et al. (2010) Feature selection and performance evaluation of support vector machine (SVM)-based classifier for differentiating benign and malignant pulmonary nodules by computed tomography. J Digit Imaging 23: 51–65.
229. Liu H, Motoda H (2008) Computational methods of feature selection; Liu H, Motoda H, editors. Boca Raton: Chapman & Hall/CRC.

17

Circulating MicroRNAs as a Novel Class of Diagnostic Biomarkers in Gastrointestinal Tumors Detection

Ran Wang[1,2], Hong Wen[2], Yongcheng Xu[3], Qiulan Chen[2], Yi Luo[2], Yiqin Lin[2], Yu Luo[2], Angao Xu[1,3]*

1 Department of Gastroenterology, Nanfang Hospital, Southern Medical University, Guangzhou, China, **2** Department of Ultrasound, HuiZhou Municipal Central Hospital, Huizhou, China, **3** Department of Gastroenterology, HuiZhou Municipal Central Hospital, Huizhou, China

Abstract

Objective: MicroRNAs (miRNAs) have become the focus of most recent efforts in cancer research. However, there have been inconsistencies in the literature regarding the suitability of circulating miRNAs for early detection of gastrointestinal cancers. This study aims to assess the diagnostic performance of circulating miRNAs in detection of gastrointestinal cancer through a meta-analysis.

Methods: Eligible studies were selected by conducting a systematic literature search of public databases. The sensitivity and specificity were used to plot the summary receiver operator characteristic (SROC) curve and calculate the area under the SROC curve (AUC). The between-study heterogeneity was evaluated by *Q* test and I^2 statistics. Subgroup analyses and meta-regression were further performed to explore the potential sources of heterogeneity. All analyses were performed using the STATA 12.0 software.

Results: A total of 107 studies from 42 articles were included for the meta-analysis according to the inclusion criteria. The overall analysis of all gastrointestinal cancers showed that circulating miRNAs have a relatively good diagnostic performance in gastrointestinal cancers, with a sensitivity of 0.75, a specificity of 0.81 and an AUC of 0.85. In addition, subgroup analyses based on different type of miRNA assay suggested that single-miRNA assay displayed a relatively low diagnostic performance with the AUC values of 0.84 for gastric cancer (GC) and 0.79 for colorectal cancer (CRC), while multiple-miRNAs assay significantly improved the diagnosing accuracy with AUC rising to 0.92 for GC and 0.89 for CRC. Another interesting finding was that plasma-based miRNA assay reach a higher accuracy compared with serum-based one for GC, while opposite conclusion was drawn for CRC.

Conclusions: In conclusion, circulating miRNAs, particularly the combination of multiple miRNAs, may present as promising biomarkers for the diagnosis of gastrointestinal cancers. Further large-scale prospective studies are necessary to validate their potential applicability in human cancer diagnosis.

Editor: Olga Y. Gorlova, Geisel School of Medicine at Dartmouth College, United States of America

Funding: The authors have no support or funding to support.

Competing Interests: The authors have declared that no competing interests exist.

* Email: angao_xu@163.com

Introduction

Gastrointestinal tract cancers, especially gastric, colorectal, and esophageal cancers, are one of the most common causes of cancer-related deaths [1]. It was estimated that tumors in esophagus, stomach, and colorectum account for approximately 11% of all newly diagnosed cancers and 14% of cancer related deaths in the United States in 2013, which make it an epidemiological health concern [2]. Currently, one of the biggest challenges in cancer treatment is the lack of specific and sensitive biomarker for early cancer diagnosis, which hinders the patients from receiving the timely treatment. The 5-year survival rate after surgical resection reaches 90% for gastric cancer (GC) patients at stage I, but this rate dramatically drops to 5% in cases at stage IV [3]. For colorectal cancer (CRC) patients, the 5-year survival rate of stage II cases is over 80% after surgical resection, but less than 10% at advanced [4]. In addition, the locoregional recurrence and/or distant metastasis can be frequently observed in the late-stage cancer patients even if they have already received the resection and multimodality therapy [5]. Therefore, the low survival rate of cancer patients at advanced stages highlights the importance of early cancer diagnosis. Unfortunately, most human cancers show no symptom in at early stages, which makes it hard for early diagnosis, and the cost-effectiveness of available diagnostic techniques is unsatisfactory.

Currently, the wide range of conventional diagnostic methods, including gastroscopy, random biopsies, colonoscopy, double contrast barium enema (DCBE), and computed tomographic colonography (CTC), are applied to diagnose and monitor gastrointestinal cancers. Although gastroscopy/colonoscopy is currently considered to be the most reliable screening tool with reportedly high accuracy, its invasive nature and expensive cost have hindered its widespread application in cancer diagnosis as a screening tool [6,7]. DCBE and CTC can detect some intestinal cancers at an early stage, but the complicated diagnostic procedures as well as the associated radiation hazards also limit their clinical applications [8]. In addition, fecal-based analyses, such as occult blood and stool DNA tests, are currently most common non-invasive procedure for early cancer diagnosis [9,10]. However, the lack of sufficient sensitivity and specificity hampers their utility in the detection of premalignant lesions.

It is generally believed that cancer-related biomarkers in blood would be quite helpful in early cancer diagnosis and tumor progression monitoring. Several currently available circulating biomarkers, such as carbohydrate antigen 19-9 (CA 19-9), carcinoembryonic antigen (CEA), pepsinogen (PG) I/II ratio, estrogen receptor (ER), and progesterone receptor (PR), are being used as non-invasive methods for cancer diagnosis without involving a biopsy or a surgical procedure [11–13]; Unfortunately, they also suffer from the limitation of low sensitivities and specificities. Therefore, there is a pressing need for novel and more sensitive non-invasive biomarkers to improve the diagnostic accuracy for gastrointestinal cancers.

Recently, circulating miRNAs have attracted considerable attention in its diagnostic value for human cancers. MiRNAs are a family of small non-coding functional RNAs with 19–24 nucleotides modulating the expression of messenger RNA (mRNA) [14]. In recent years, miRNAs have been found to be dysregulated in a variety of diseases, particularly in human cancers [15,16]. It has been observed that miRNAs could present extensively in the cell-free body fluids and excretions, including serum, plasma, urine, tears, saliva, bronchial lavage, and feces, etc [17]. Furthermore, biochemical analyses indicate that circulating miRNAs have a remarkable stability and are tolerant to RNase activity and extreme physiological environment [18], making it plausible to use circulating miRNAs as novel non-invasive biomarkers in diagnosing and monitoring human cancers.

The role of miRNAs as novel biomarkers in cancer was first recognized in a study considering miR-15 and miR-16, which were found to be down-regulated in B-cell chronic lymphocytic leukemia (B-CLL) [19]. Subsequent evidence has indicated that unique miRNA expression profiles in circulation may contribute to the diagnosis of cancers, such as colorectal cancer [20], gastric cancer [21], esophageal cancer [22], breast cancer [23], lung cancer [24], hepatocellular carcinoma [25], prostate cancer [26], and pancreatic cancer [27]. However, there have been inconsistencies or discrepancies in the literature reviews regarding the reliability of circulating miRNAs for early detection of gastro-

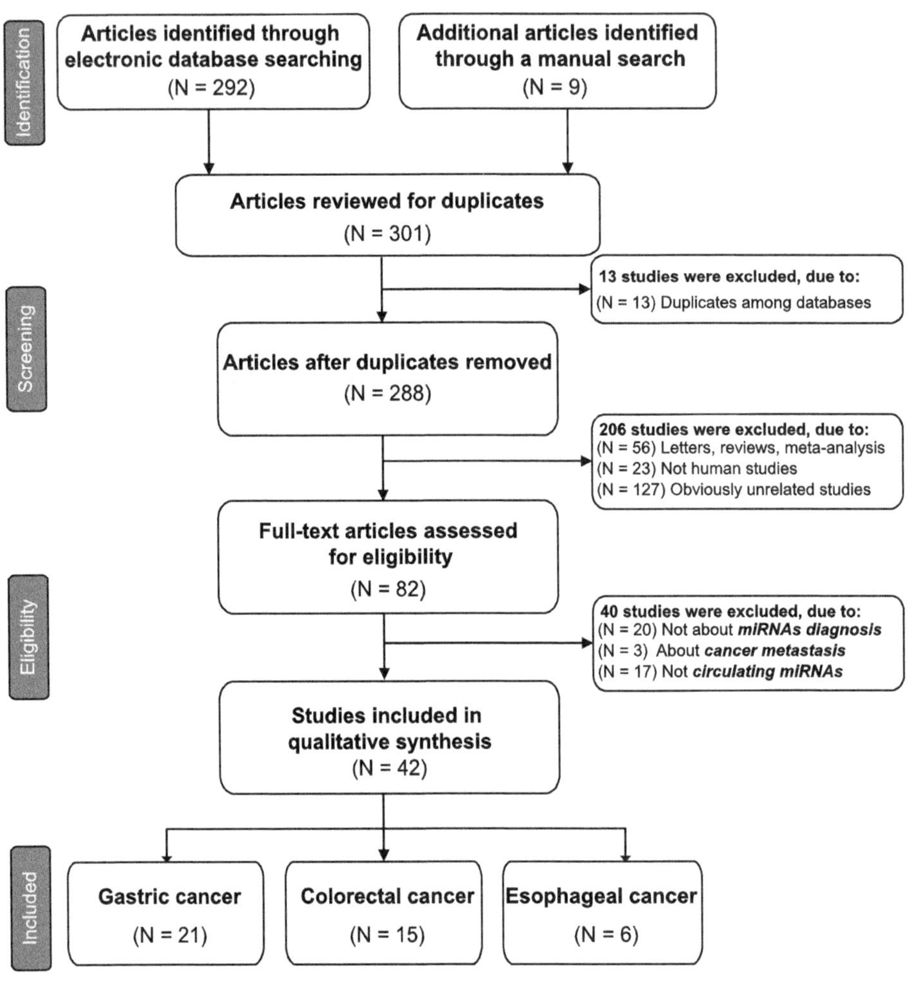

Figure 1. Flow diagram of study selection process.

Table 1. Main characteristics of 42 studies included in meta-analysis.

Included studies	Cancer type	Location	Ethnicity	Study design	Case/Control			miRNA profiling	Specimen	QUADAS
					Number	Mean age	Male ratio			
Cai H, 2013	GC	China	Asian	Case-control	90/90	46.2/46.1	0.81/0.81	miR-106b, -20a, -221	Plasma	5
Chen Q, 2014	GC	China	Asian	Case-control	36/36	56/59	0.78/0.78	miR-122, -192	Plasma	6
Konishi H, 2012	GC	Japan	Asian	Case-control	56/30	66/NA	0.55/NA	miR-451, -486	Plasma	7
Li BS, 2012	GC	China	Asian	Case-control	60/60	54/51	0.70/0.63	miR-223, -21, -218	Plasma	4
Li C, 2013	GC	China	Asian	Case-control	180/80	58.1/58.9	0.31/0.35	miR-199a-3p, -151-5p	Plasma	5
Li ZQ, 2012	GC	China	Asian	Case-control	46/21	58.8/57	0.65/0.67	miR-27a, -181b	Plasma	5
Liu H, 2012	GC	China	Asian	Case-control	40/41	56/58	0.66/0.66	miR-371-5p, -187, -378	Serum	3
Liu R, 2011	GC	China	Asian	Case-control	164/127	60.2/60	0.84/0.8	miR-1, -20a, -27a, -34, -423-5p	Serum	4
Peng WZ, 2014	GC	China	Asian	Case-control	57/58	NA/43	NA/0.48	miR-191, -425	Serum	5
Sheinerman KS, 2013	GC	America	Caucasian	Case-control	10/30	55.8/51.9	0.10/0.30	miR-203, -146b-5p, -192	Plasma	6
Shiotani A, 2013	GC	Japan	Asian	Case-control	64/64	67.9/68.4	0.70/0.64	miR-106b, let-7	Serum	5
Song MY, 2012	GC	China	Asian	Retrospective	68/68	60.4/60.4	0.71/0.71	7 miRNAs[a]	Serum	4
Tsujiura M, 2010	GC	Japan	Asian	Case-control	69/30	NA/NA	NA/NA	miR-106b	Plasma	5
Valladares M, 2012	GC	Spain	Caucasian	Case-control	52/15	65.9/65.3	0.81/0.81	miR-200c	Plasma	7
Wang B, 2012	GC	China	Asian	Case-control	30/39	58/46	0.73/0.77	miR-21	Serum	3
Xu Q, 2013	GC	China	Asian	Case-control	94/103	60.2/59.1	0.63/0.63	miR-320a	Serum	4
Zheng Y, 2011	GC	China	Asian	Case-control	53/20	60/60	0.66/0.66	miR-21	Serum	4
Zhou H, 2010	GC	China	Asian	Case-control	90/27	62.3/NA	0.70/NA	miR-106a, -17	Serum	4
Zhou H, 2012	GC	China	Asian	Case-control	40/17	64.6/64.6	0.73/0.73	miR-421	Serum	4
Zhu C, 2014	GC	China	Asian	Case-control	40/40	53.8/53.5	0.73/0.73	miR-16, -25, -92a, -451, -468-5p	Plasma	3
Zhu CJ, 2011	GC	China	Asian	Case-control	48/27	61.2/55.4	0.83/0.74	miR-191, -27a	Plasma	6
Feng L, 2013	CRC	China	Asian	Case-control	98/50	54.3/52.7	0.53/0.52	miR-92a	Serum	7
Giraldez MD, 2013	CRC	Spain	Caucasian	Cohort	42/53	62.8/62.1	0.51/0.49	miR-19a, -19b, -15b	Plasma	4
Huang Z, 2010	CRC	China	Asian	Case-control	100/59	61/58	0.51/0.53	miR-29a, -92a	Plasma	3
Liu et al, 2013	CRC	China	Asian	Cohort	200/80	57.9/57.5	0.63/0.52	miR-21, 92a	Serum	6
Liu HS, 2012	CRC	China	Asian	Case-control	47/28	58.6/56.2	0.66/0.68	miR-129-3p, -767-3p, -877	Serum	4
Luo X, 2013	CRC	Germany	Caucasian	Case-control	80/144	68/62.5	0.56/0.42	12 miRNAs[b]	Plasma	5
Ng EK, 2009	CRC	China	Asian	Case-control	90/50	71/69	0.52/0.52	miR-17-3p, -92	Plasma	5
Pu XX, 2010	CRC	China	Asian	Cohort	103/37	58/32	0.64/0.51	miR-221	Plasma	7
Sheinerman KS, 2013	CRC	America	Caucasian	Case-control	10/30	57.8/57.3	0.80/0.30	miR-203, -146b-5p, -192, -215, -303-3p	Plasma	3
Toiyama Y, 2013	CRC	Japan	Asian	Cohort	186/53	67.5/64	0.57/0.51	miR-21	Serum	3

Table 1. Cont.

Included studies	Cancer type	Location	Ethnicity	Study design	Case/Control			miRNA profiling	Specimen	QUADAS
					Number	Mean age	Male ratio			
Wang Q, 2012	CRC	China	Asian	Case-control	90/58	62/58	0.50/0.52	miR-601, -760, -29a, -92a	Plasma	6
Wang S, 2013	CRC	China	Asian	Cohort	77/84	64/44	0.42/0.60	miR-409-3p, -7, -93	Plasma	4
Yong FL, 2013	CRC	Malaysia	Asian	Case-control	70/32	64.4/61.5	0.60/0.48	miR-193a-3p, -23a, -338-5p	Serum	5
Zanutto S, 2014	CRC	Italy	Caucasian	Cohort	29/29	NA/NA	NA/NA	miR-378, -21	Plasma	5
Zhang GJ, 2013	CRC	China	Asian	Case-control	78/86	61.4/60.3	0.55/0.62	miR-200c, 18a	Plasma	4
Hirajima S, 2013	EC	Japan	Asian	Case-control	106/54	65/NA	0.82/NA	miR-18a	Plasma	5
Komatsu S, 2011	EC	Japan	Asian	Case-control	50/20	65/NA	0.88/NA	miR-21/-375	Plasma	7
Takeshita N, 2013	EC	Japan	Asian	Case-control	101/46	NA/NA	0.89/NA	miR-1246	Serum	3
Zhang C, 2010	EC	China	Asian	Cohort	149/100	62/50	0.78/0.74	7 miRNAs[c]	Serum	4
Zhang T, 2011	EC	China	Asian	Cohort	201/202	NA/NA	0.66/0.63	miR-31	Serum	3
Zhang T, 2013	EC	China	Asian	Case-control	201/201	NA/NA	0.66/0.62	miR-1322	Serum	6

[a]miR-221, -744, -376c, -27a, -27b, -222, -191.
[b]miR-18a, -20a, -21, -29a, -92a, -106b, -133a, -143, -145, -181b, -342-3p, -532-3p.
[c]miR-10a, -22, -100, -148b, -223, -133a, -127-3p.
NA, not available; GC, gastric cancer; CRC, colorectal cancer; EC, esophageal cancer; QUADAS-2, the revised Quality Assessment of Diagnostic Accuracy Studies.

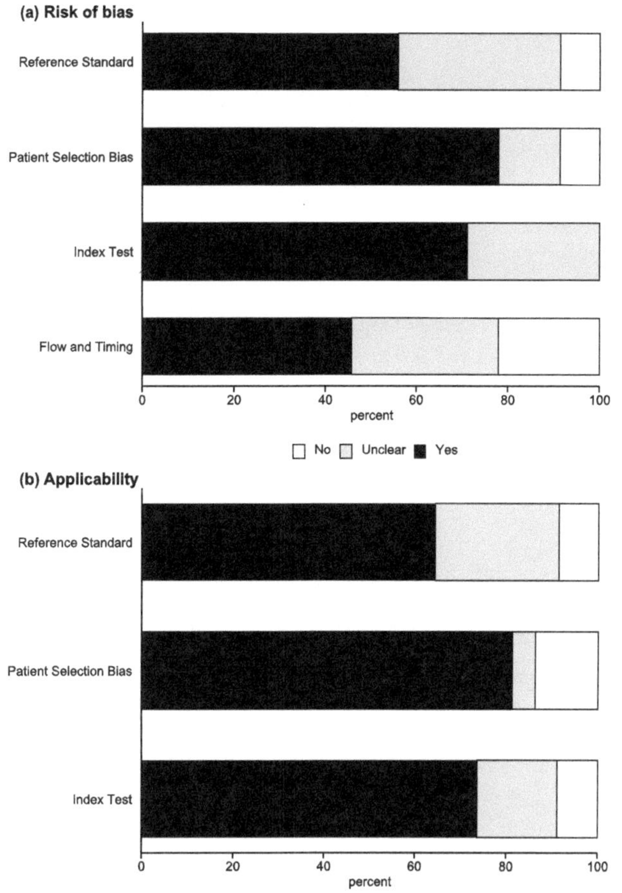

Figure 2. Overall quality assessment of included studies using the QUADAS-2 criteria (a: risk of bias; b: applicability).

intestinal cancers. In this meta-analysis, we summarize an overview of circulating miRNAs present in blood circulation to further elucidate their diagnostic performance and provide information for the early detection of gastrointestinal cancers.

Materials and Methods

This meta-analysis was conducted according to the Preferred Reporting Items for Systematic Reviews and Meta-analyses (PRISMA) guidance (Supplement S1).

Literature search

This meta-analysis was conducted according to guidelines for diagnostic meta-analysis [28]. Eligible studies published up to 1 April 2014 were selected for meta-analysis by conducting a systematic literature search of public databases including PubMed, Embase, Chinese National Knowledge Infrastructure (CNKI), and Chinese Biology Medicine (CBM) databases, without language limitation. The following retrieval strategy was used: ('gastro-intestinal tumor' OR 'gastric tumor' OR 'gastric cancer' OR 'colorectal tumor' OR 'colorectal cancer' OR 'esophageal tumor' OR 'esophageal cancer') AND ('microRNA' OR 'miRNA' OR 'miR') AND ('blood' OR 'serum' OR 'plasma' or 'circulating') AND ('diagnosis' OR 'sensitivity and specificity' OR 'ROC curve'). In addition, reference lists of eligible articles were independently searched manually to obtain additional sources.

Inclusion and exclusion criteria

Eligible studies included in this meta-analysis have to fulfill the following criteria: (1) studies regarding the diagnostic potential of circulating miRNAs for gastrointestinal cancers; (2) studies with a gold reference standard for the gastrointestinal cancers diagnosis; (3) studies with sufficient data for construction of two-by-two tables [i.e., true positive (TP), false positive (FP), true negative (TN) and false negative (FN)]. Exclusion criteria were: (1) publications unrelated to the diagnostic values of circulating miRNAs for gastrointestinal cancers; (2) studies with duplicate data reported in other studies; (3) letters, editorials, case reports or reviews.

Data extraction

Two reviewers independently extracted data from all the eligible studies: (1) basic characteristics of studies, including name of the first author, year of publication, country of origin, ethnicity, study design, sample size, mean age, male ratio, cancer type, type of miRNA assay, methods of miRNAs detection, type of specimens; and (2) diagnostic performance, including sensitivity, specificity, TP, FP, FN, and TN.

Quality assessment

The qualities of included studies were scored independently by two reviewers using the revised Quality Assessment of Diagnostic Accuracy Studies (QUADAS-2) criteria [29]. The QUADAS-2 tool is comprised of 4 key domains: patient selection, index test, reference standard and flow and timing, and uses seven questions to evaluate the quality of included studies (Supplements S2). Each question is answered with "yes", "no", or "unclear". An answer of "yes" means that the risk of bias can be judged low, while an answer of "no" or "unclear" means that the risk of bias can be judged high. In case of conflict, a third reviewer was consulted, and disagreement was settled through multilateral discussion.

Statistical analysis

All analyses were performed using the STATA 12.0 software. The bivariate meta-analysis model was employed to summarize the sensitivity (SEN), specificity (SPE), positive likelihood ratio (PLR), negative likelihood ratio (NLR) and diagnostic odds ratio (DOR) [30,31]. The sensitivity and specificity of each included study were used to plot the summary receiver operator characteristic (SROC) curve and calculate the area under the SROC curve (AUC). The AUC can be statistically interpreted as the probability to correctly distinguish patients from normal controls. The between-study heterogeneity was evaluated by Q test and I^2 statistics. A P value less than 0.10 for Q test or I^2 values $\geq 50\%$ indicates substantial heterogeneity, and then the random-effects model was applied [32,33]. To further explore the potential sources of heterogeneity, subgroup analyses and meta-regression were performed according to the characteristics of the included studies. As publication bias is a concern for meta-analyses, Deeks' funnel plot asymmetry test was used, with $P<0.10$ indicating statistically significant [34].

Results

Procedure of literature retrieval

The procedure of the literature retrieval was presented in Figure 1. The initial search returned a total of 301 articles, of which 13 duplicate publications among databases were removed. After the review of titles and abstracts, 206 articles were excluded: 56 were reviews or letters, 23 were not human studies, and 127 were not related to our research topic, leaving 82 articles available for further full-text review. After careful reading, 40 articles were

Table 2. Summary estimates of diagnostic criteria and their 95% confidence intervals (95% CI).

Analysis	No. of studies	SEN (95%CI)	SPE (95%CI)	PLR (95%CI)	NLR (95%CI)	DOR (95%CI)	AUC (95%CI)
Gastric cancer	47	0.77 (0.72–0.80)	0.81 (0.77–0.84)	4.0 (3.2–4.9)	0.29 (0.24–0.36)	14 (9–20)	0.86 (0.82–0.88)
MiRNA profiling							
Single-miRNA	39	0.75 (0.70–0.79)	0.80 (0.75–0.84)	3.7 (2.9–4.6)	0.32 (0.26–0.39)	11 (8–17)	0.84 (0.80–0.87)
Multiple-miRNAs	8	0.87 (0.75–0.94)	0.84 (0.75–0.91)	5.6 (3.1–10)	0.15 (0.07–0.33)	37 (10–134)	0.92 (0.89–0.94)
Source material							
Plasma-based	26	0.82 (0.78–0.86)	0.85 (0.80–0.89)	5.6 (4.0–7.8)	0.21 (0.16–0.27)	27 (16–47)	0.90 (0.88–0.93)
Serum-based	21	0.67 (0.61–0.73)	0.74 (0.69–0.78)	2.5 (2.1–3.1)	0.44 (0.37–0.53)	6 (4–8)	0.77 (0.73–0.80)
Colorectal cancer	47	0.73 (0.69–0.77)	0.80 (0.76–0.83)	3.6 (3.0–4.2)	0.34 (0.29–0.39)	11 (8–14)	0.83 (0.80–0.86)
MiRNA profiling							
Single-miRNA	29	0.68 (0.62–0.73)	0.77 (0.72–0.81)	2.9 (2.4–3.5)	0.42 (0.36–0.50)	7 (5–10)	0.79 (0.75–0.82)
Multiple-miRNAs	18	0.81 (0.77–0.84)	0.83 (0.79–0.87)	4.9 (3.8–6.2)	0.23 (0.19–0.27)	22 (15–30)	0.89 (0.86–0.91)
Source material							
Plasma-based	33	0.72 (0.65–0.77)	0.77 (0.73–0.80)	3.1 (2.5–3.7)	0.37 (0.30–0.46)	8 (6–12)	0.81 (0.77–0.84)
Serum-based	14	0.77 (0.72–0.81)	0.85 (0.80–0.89)	5.1 (3.9–6.7)	0.28 (0.23–0.33)	18 (13–26)	0.88 (0.85–0.90)
Esophageal cancer	13	0.79 (0.74–0.84)	0.85 (0.81–0.89)	5.4 (4.1–7.1)	0.24 (0.19–0.31)	22 (14–35)	0.89 (0.86–0.92)
All studies	107	0.75 (0.73–0.78)	0.81 (0.79–0.83)	4.0 (3.5–4.5)	0.30 (0.27–0.34)	13 (10–16)	0.85 (0.82–0.88)

CI, confidence interval; SEN, sensitivity; SPE, specificity; PLR, positive likelihood ratio; NLR, negative likelihood ratio; DOR, diagnostic odds ratio; AUC, area under the curve.

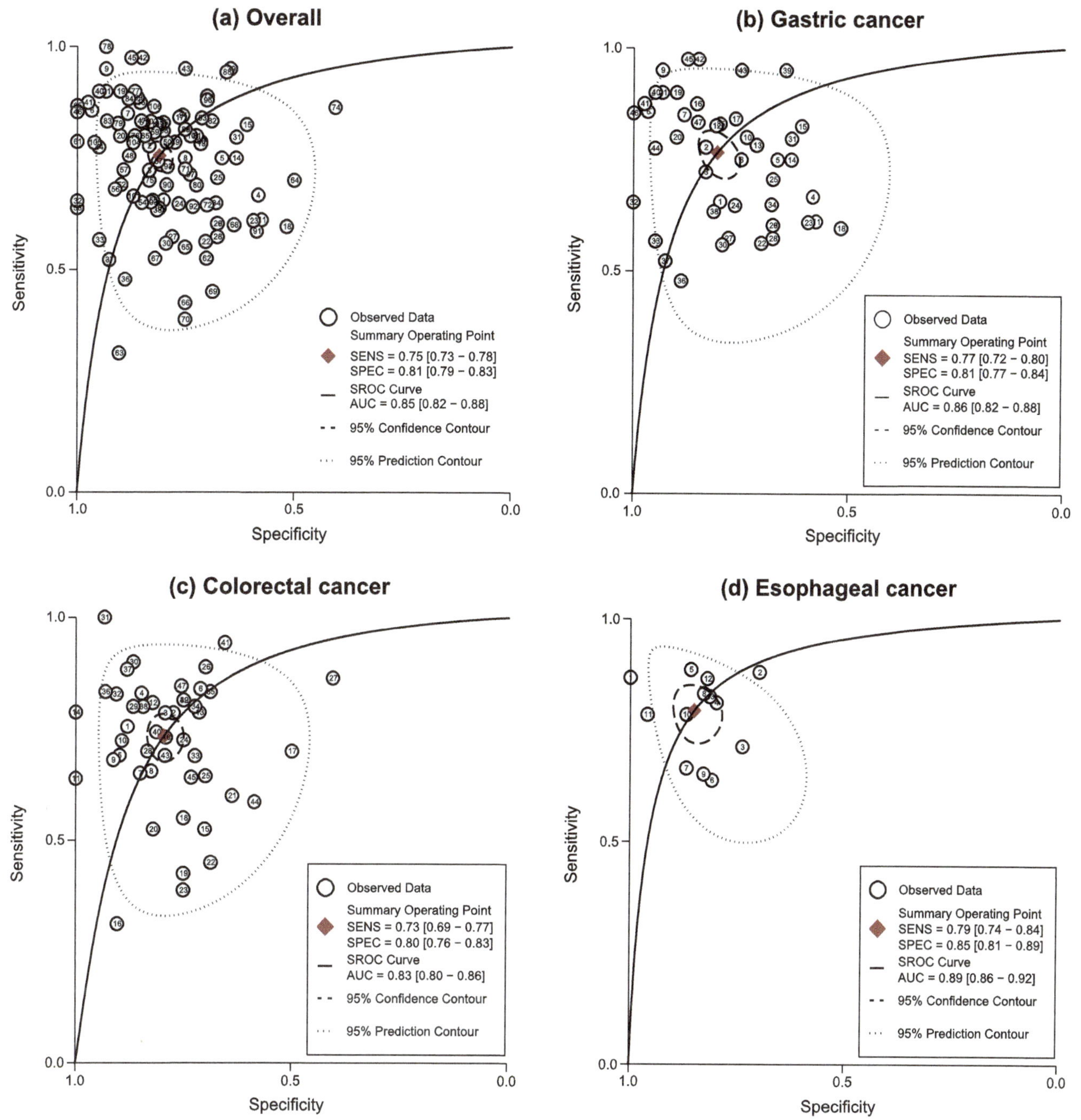

Figure 3. SROC curve with pooled estimates of sensitivity, specificity and AUC (a: overall studies on gastrointestinal cancers; b: GC; c: CRC; d: EC).

further excluded: 20 were not about gastrointestinal cancers diagnosis, 3 were relevant to metastasis in cancers, and 17 were not circulating miRNAs. Finally, 42 articles were included according to the inclusion criteria, 21 of which focused on GC [21,35–54], 15 on CRC [20,49,55–67], and the other 6 on EC [22,68–72].

Baseline characteristics of included studies

The main characteristics of 42 articles were shown in Table 1. In total, 107 studies from these 42 articles were involved in the current meta-analysis. As for GC, 47 studies from 21 articles were available for analysis. 38 of these 47 studies investigated the diagnostic value of single-miRNA assay in GC detection, while only 8 focused on multiple-miRNAs assay. 26 studies used plasma as specimen, and the other 21 based on serum. Similarly, for 47 studies from the 15 articles focusing on CRC, 29 of them assessed the performance of single-miRNA assay in CRC detection, whereas 18 focused on multiple-miRNAs assay. 33 studies used plasma as specimen, while serum was applied in the other 14 studies. For EC diagnosis, 13 studies from 6 articles were available. The publication years of the included articles range from 2010 to 2014. All studies used the quantitative real-time reverse transcrip-

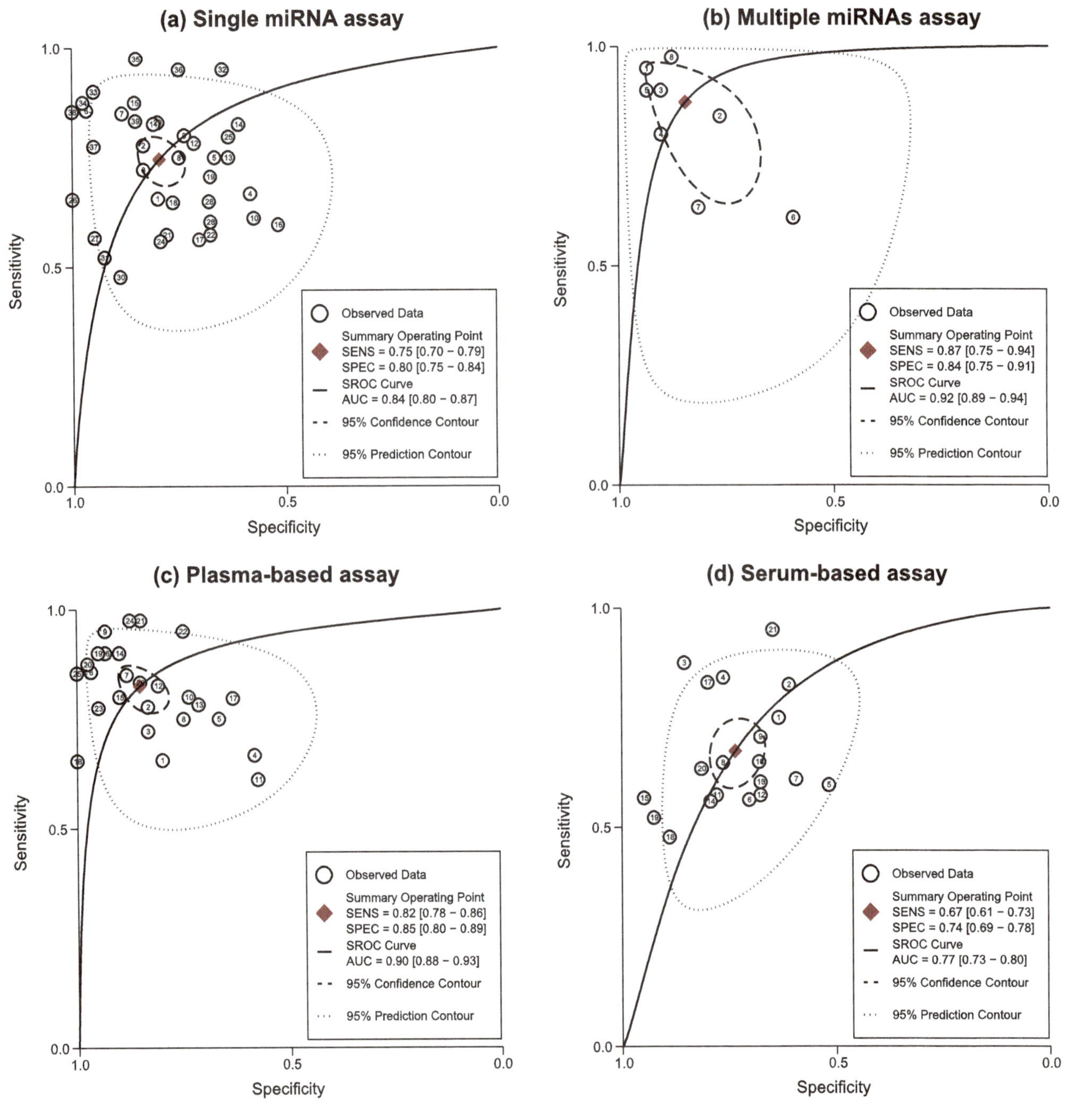

Figure 4. SROC curve with pooled estimates of sensitivity, specificity and AUC on the diagnostic value of circulating miRNAs in GC detection (a: single-miRNA assay; b: multiple-miRNAs assay; c: plasma-based assay; d: serum-based assay).

tion-PCR (qRT-PCR) method to measure the expression of circulating miRNAs. Quality assessment for the overall studies was shown with a bar graph according to the QUADAS-2 tool in Figure 2. The majority of all included studies in this meta-analysis fulfilled 4 or more of the 7 items in QUADAS-2, indicating that the overall quality of included studies is generally good.

Diagnostic accuracy of miRNAs in gastrointestinal cancers

The pooled estimates of gastrointestinal cancers (GC/CRC/EC) for the diagnostic accuracy of circulating miRNAs were presented in Table 2. The overall analysis of all types gastrointestinal cancers showed that circulating miRNAs have a relatively good diagnostic performance in gastrointestinal cancers, with SEN of 0.75 (95% CI: 0.73–0.78), SPE of 0.81 (95% CI: 0.79–0.83) and AUC of 0.85 (95% CI: 0.82–0.88) (Figure 3A). Since only 13 studies from 6 publications were involved in EC, subgroup analyses were conducted for GC and CRC. For EC, the diagnostic accuracy of circulating miRNAs was even better than the overall results, with SEN of 0.79 (95% CI: 0.74–0.84), SPE of 0.85 (95% CI: 0.81–0.89) and AUC of 0.89 (95% CI: 0.86–0.92) (Figure 3D).

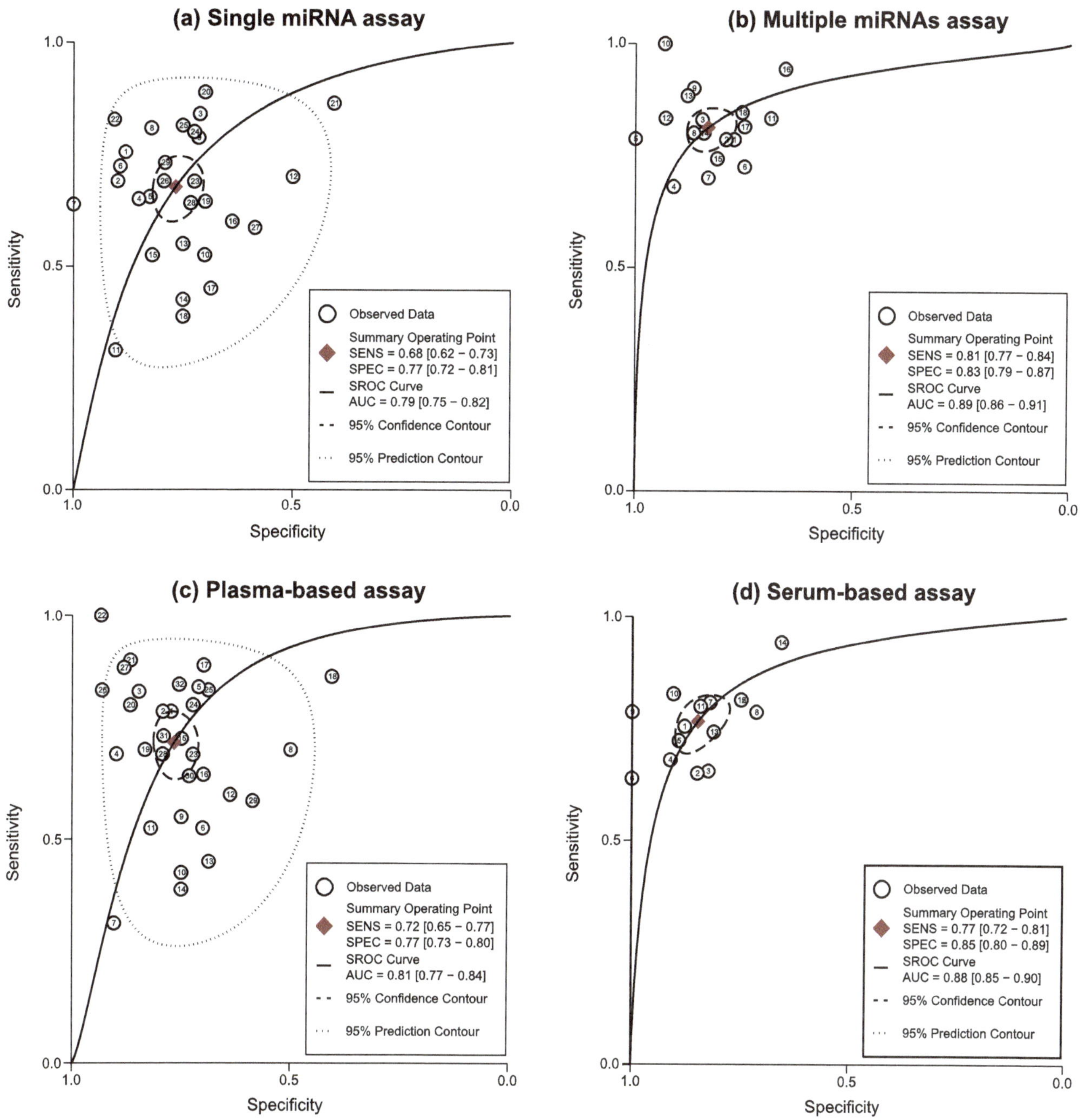

Figure 5. SROC curve with pooled estimates of sensitivity, specificity and AUC on the diagnostic value of circulating miRNAs in CRC detection (a: single-miRNA assay; b: multiple-miRNAs assay; c: plasma-based assay; d: serum-based assay).

As for GC, since significant heterogeneity between studies was observed in sensitivity and specificity data ($I^2 = 84.53\%$ and $I^2 = 78.98\%$, respectively), the random-effects model was used. The pooled parameters calculated from all 47 studies on GC were as follows: SEN, 0.77 (95% CI: 0.72–0.80); SPE, 0.81 (95% CI: 0.77–0.84); PLR, 4.0 (95% CI: 3.2–4.9); NLR, 0.29 (95% CI: 0.24–0.36); and DOR, 14 (95% CI: 9–20). Figure 3B shows the corresponding SROC curve with the AUC of 0.86 (95%CI: 0.82–0.88), indicating that circulating miRNAs may be able to differentiate GC patients from controls with a relatively high accuracy. Subgroup analysis based on different type of miRNA assay suggested that multiple-miRNAs assay showed superior diagnostic properties (Figure 4B) than single one (Figure 4A), with SEN of 0.87 versus 0.75, SPE of 0.84 versus 0.80, and AUC of 0.92 versus 0.84 (Table 2). Notably, we found that plasma-based assay (Figure 4C) has a higher accuracy compared with serum-based assay (Figure 4D), suggesting that plasma is a better matrix for miRNA detection.

Similarly, the random-effects model was used for meta-analysis of studies on CRC since significant heterogeneity existed ($I^2 = 87.18\%$ and $I^2 = 83.27\%$, respectively). The pooled estimates all 47 studies on CRC are as follows: SEN of 0.73 (95% CI: 0.69–

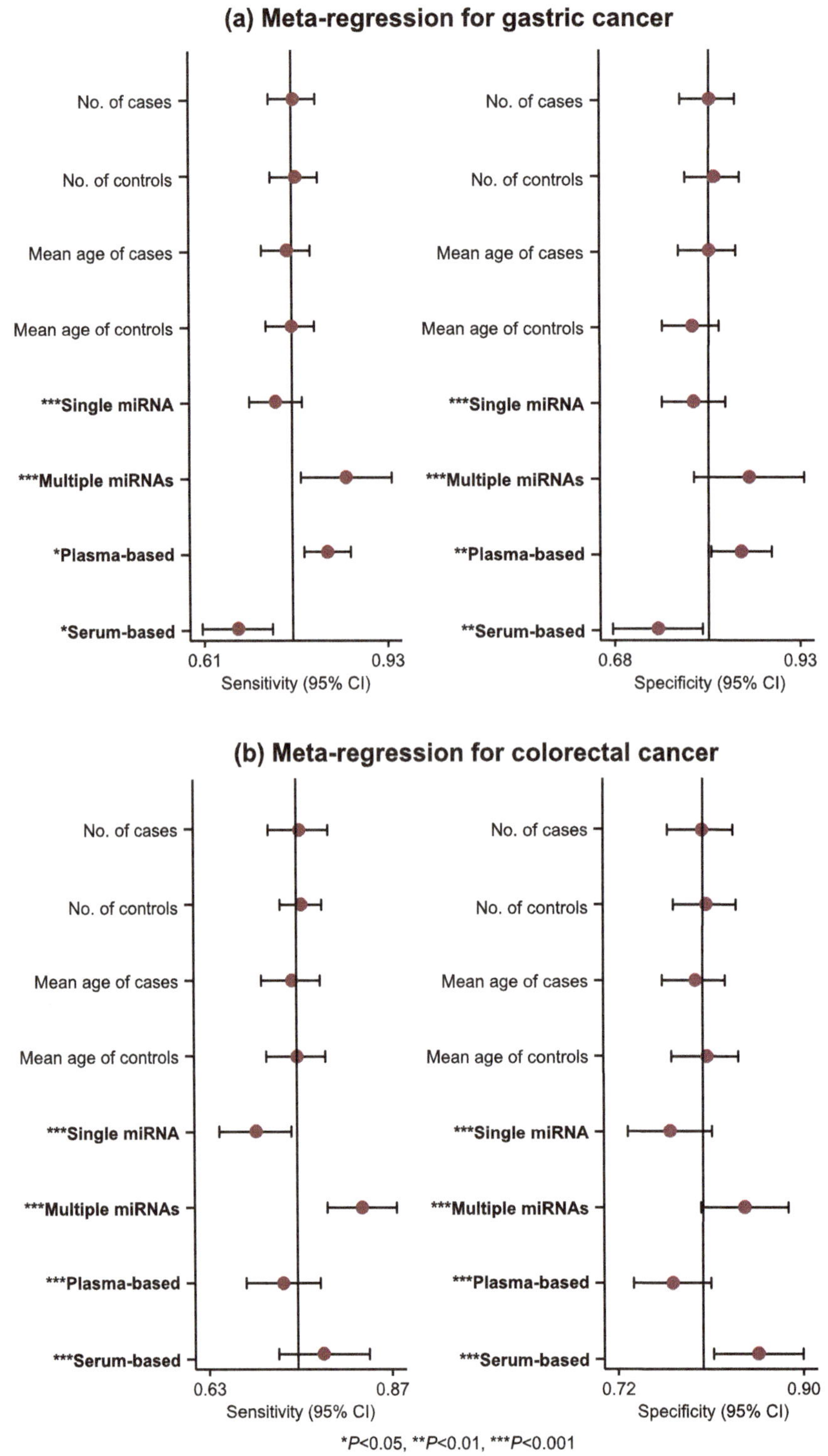

Figure 6. Forest plots of multivariable meta-regression analyses for sensitivity and specificity (a: single-miRNA assay; b: multiple-miRNAs assay).

0.77), SPE of 0.80 (95% CI: 0.76–0.83), PLR of 3.6 (95% CI: 3.0–4.2), NLR of 0.34 (95% CI: 0.29–0.39), and DOR of 11 (95% CI: 8–14) (Table 2). Figure 3C shows the corresponding SROC curve with the AUC of 0.83 (95%CI: 0.80–0.86), indicating that the diagnostic accuracy of miRNAs in CRC detection is slightly worse than the overall diagnostic performance of miRNAs in gastrointestinal cancers detection. Similar to miRNAs in GC detection, we found that multiple-miRNAs assay (Figure 5B) in differentiating CRC patients from controls achieve a better diagnostic performance than single-miRNA assay (Figure 5A). However,

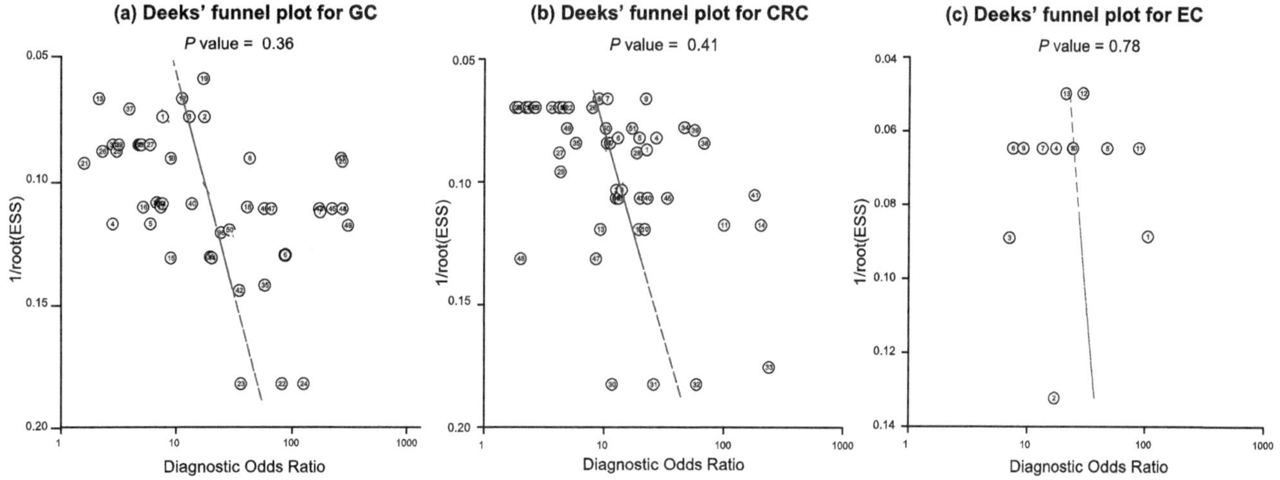

Figure 7. The Deeks' test of the diagnostic meta-analysis (a: Deeks' funnel for GC; b: Deeks' funnel for CRC; c: Deeks' funnel for EC. The dotted line indicates the regression line. No publication bias was detected for this meta-analysis (GC: $P = 0.38$; CRC: $P = 0.41$; EC: $P = 0.78$).

contrast to the results of GC, serum-based miRNAs assay (Figure 5D) has a higher accuracy compared with plasma-based assay (Figure 5C) in CRC detection.

Meta-regression and publication bias

The meta-regression analyses for both GC (Figure 6A) and CRC (Figure 6B) were performed to analyze the potential sources of inter-study heterogeneity. Overall, miRNA profiling and sample types may be the major sources of heterogeneity for miRNAs assay either in GC or CRC detection. To assess publication bias of included studies, the Deeks' funnel plot asymmetry test was conducted (Figure 7). As shown in Figure 7, the slope coefficient was associated with a P-value of 0.38 for GC, 0.41 for CRC, 0.78 for EC, suggesting a low likelihood of publication bias in our meta-analysis.

Discussion

Gastrointestinal cancers, including esophageal, gastric, and colorectal cancer, together with breast and lung tumors, are responsible for the most cancer-related mortality [1]. Although endoscopic examinations and random biopsies are currently the most reliable screening tool for gastrointestinal cancers, their invasive, unpleasant, and inconvenient nature as well as potential sampling errors have hampered the wide clinic application. Conventional cancer-specific biomarkers are sufficiently simple and fast; unfortunately, their diagnostic performances have mostly been insufficient for application as a primary tool in population-based screening. Therefore, large number of studies on the search for ideal candidate biomarkers of tumors is still ongoing. During the past few years, miRNAs have become the focus of most recent efforts in cancer research. Since their discovery, emerging evidences suggest that the miRNAs may play important role in tumor suppressing, since the aberrant expression of miRNA was discovered between cancer patients and healthy controls [73,74]. Subsequently, miRNAs as molecular markers have attracted much attention in cancer diagnosis [20,21,44,54,67].

Circulating miRNAs, also known as cell-free miRNAs, have a promising future as a novel class of reliable minimally invasive biomarkers for early cancer diagnosis due to their remarkable stability, relatively easy detection, and convenience to measure its sensitivity and specificity [73]. Since circulating miRNAs in serum was first reported [75], a tremendous growth of interest is attracted to the feasibility of circulating miRNAs as potential biomarkers in gastrointestinal malignancies diagnosis. However, inconsistencies are still existed in the literature reviews regarding the reliability of circulating miRNAs for early detection of gastrointestinal cancers. The variations and discrepancies in individual studies are possibly due to their small sample sizes, variations in miRNA assay, and different type of cancers. In this meta-analysis, we summarize the recent findings focusing on the potential of circulating miRNAs as diagnostic biomarkers in gastrointestinal tumors, including esophageal, gastric, and colorectal cancer.

To the best of our knowledge, this is the first evidence-based meta-analysis to evaluate the diagnostic value of circulating miRNA on gastrointestinal malignancies. The pooled results based on all included studies showed circulating miRNAs yielding an AUC of 0.85 with 75% sensitivity and 81% specificity in discriminating gastrointestinal cancer patients from controls. Although the origin and function of circulating miRNAs in cancer diagnosis have not been systematically elucidated, they have displayed a superior diagnostic performance compared with conventional blood biomarkers like CEA (AUC of 0.549) for EC and CA19-9 for GC (AUC of 0.60). Accordingly, further studies are required to elucidate the mechanism and target of miRNAs and their roles in cellular and molecular pathways. Interestingly, our results suggest that plasma-based miRNA assay reaches a higher accuracy than serum-based one for GC; the conclusion is, however, opposite for CRC. The origin of source-related difference is still unclear and might be explained by unknown mechanism. Thus, large scale investigations are needed in the following study to determine whether the source-related differences truly exist.

Another interesting finding of our study is that single-miRNA assay displayed a relatively low diagnostic performance with the AUC values of 0.84 for gastric cancer (GC) and 0.79 for colorectal cancer (CRC), while multiple-miRNAs assay significantly improved the diagnosing accuracy with AUC rising to 0.92 for GC and 0.89 for CRC, implying that the advantage of using combination of miRNAs to obtain a complete picture. It is widely accepted that using single tumor-related miRNA as disease fingerprints is much simpler and more straightforward than comprehensively detecting panels of miRNAs, but the specificity of biomarkers based on single miRNA is relatively poor. The molecular basis for the limitation of single miRNA as a tumor biomarker is that aberrant levels of single miRNA might be associated with several different types of cancers [76]. Furthermore, cancer develops can be regarded as a result of complex multi-stage process of epigenetic and genomic abnormalities, and thus, should be targeted by multiple miRNAs [77]. Accordingly, employing panels of miRNAs instead of an individual miRNA as biomarkers represents a rational option to circumvent the limitations in utilizing miRNAs as a non-invasive blood-based biomarker in cancer detection, especially for the localized pathological conditions, where regular biopsies are hard to get.

Although circulating miRNAs have a promising potential as relevant novel non-invasive cancer biomarkers in future as shown in the current study, several limitations need to be addressed. First, methodologies for an accurate absolute quantification of miRNAs suffer from a lack of convention, which limits the cross-comparison between studies performed by different laboratories. Standardized protocol, which should be preferably followed across all studies, needs to be established aiming to minimize protocol-based bias. In addition, some researchers have showed correlations of grade and stage of cancers with specific circulating miRNAs. Therefore, further studies addressing the relationships between miRNAs expression and clinical/pathological parameters are very important and desirable. Third, most included studies in this meta-analysis only distinguished the cancer patients from healthy controls. It is vital to identify and develop panels of miRNAs that can distinguish cancer from other diseases, especially from those with similar symptom diseases. Last but not least, as shown in Table 1, most of included studies were on Asian and little bit on Caucasian/African populations. Therefore, further studies on Caucasian/African populations may be needed.

Based on recent observations in gastrointestinal cancer, we conclude that circulating miRNAs, particularly the combination of multiple-miRNAs, may present as promising minimally invasive approach for the diagnosis and monitoring of gastrointestinal tumors. Further large-scale prospective studies are necessary to validate their potential applicability in human cancer diagnosis.

Supporting Information

Supplement S1 PRISMA Checklist.

Supplement S2 QUADAS-2 Checklist.

Author Contributions

Conceived and designed the experiments: AX. Performed the experiments: RW HW. Analyzed the data: YCX QLC. Contributed reagents/materials/analysis tools: Yi Luo Yiqin Lin Yu Luo. Wrote the paper: RW HW YCX.

References

1. Jemal A, Bray F, Center MM, Ferlay J, Ward E, et al. (2011) Global cancer statistics. CA Cancer J Clin 61: 69–90.
2. Siegel R, Naishadham D, Jemal A (2013) Cancer statistics, 2013. CA Cancer J Clin 63: 11–30.
3. Suzuki H, Gotoda T, Sasako M, Saito D (2006) Detection of early gastric cancer: misunderstanding the role of mass screening. Gastric Cancer 9: 315–319.
4. McFarland EG, Levin B, Lieberman DA, Pickhardt PJ, Johnson CD, et al. (2008) Revised colorectal screening guidelines: joint effort of the American Cancer Society, U.S. Multisociety Task Force on Colorectal Cancer, and American College of Radiology. Radiology 248: 717–720.
5. Hartgrink HH, Jansen EP, van Grieken NC, van de Velde CJ (2009) Gastric cancer. Lancet 374: 477–490.
6. Takahashi S, Hirayama M, Kuroiwa G, Kawano Y, Takada K, et al. (2013) Diagnostic validity of CT gastrography versus gastroscopy for primary lesions in gastric cancer: evaluating the response to chemotherapy, a retrospective analysis. Gastric Cancer 16: 543–548.
7. Brenner H, Chang-Claude J, Jansen L, Knebel P, Stock C, et al. (2014) Reduced risk of colorectal cancer up to 10 years after screening, surveillance, or diagnostic colonoscopy. Gastroenterology 146: 709–717.
8. Neri E, Faggioni L, Cerri F, Turini F, Angeli S, et al. (2010) CT colonography versus double-contrast barium enema for screening of colorectal cancer: comparison of radiation burden. Abdom Imaging 35: 596–601.
9. Duffy MJ (2007) Role of tumor markers in patients with solid cancers: A critical review. Eur J Intern Med 18: 175–184.
10. Choong MK, Tsafnat G (2012) Genetic and epigenetic biomarkers of colorectal cancer. Clin Gastroenterol Hepatol 10: 9–15.
11. Tarro G, Perna A, Esposito C (2005) Early diagnosis of lung cancer by detection of tumor liberated protein. J Cell Physiol 203: 1–5.
12. Sorio C, Mauri P, Pederzoli P, Scarpa A (2006) Non-invasive cancer detection: strategies for the identification of novel cancer markers. IUBMB Life 58: 193–198.
13. Dbouk HA, Tawil A, Nasr F, Kandakarjian L, Abou-Merhi R (2007) Significance of CEA and VEGF as Diagnostic Markers of Colorectal Cancer in Lebanese Patients. Open Clin Cancer J 1: 1–5.
14. Lee RC, Feinbaum RL, Ambros V (1993) The C. elegans heterochronic gene lin-4 encodes small RNAs with antisense complementarity to lin-14. Cell 75: 843–854.
15. Bartel DP (2004) MicroRNAs: genomics, biogenesis, mechanism, and function. Cell 116: 281–297.
16. Davis BN, Hata A (2009) Regulation of MicroRNA Biogenesis: A miRiad of mechanisms. Cell Commun Signal 7: 18.
17. Weber JA, Baxter DH, Zhang S, Huang DY, Huang KH, et al. (2010) The microRNA spectrum in 12 body fluids. Clin Chem 56: 1733–1741.
18. Chen X, Ba Y, Ma L, Cai X, Yin Y, et al. (2008) Characterization of microRNAs in serum: a novel class of biomarkers for diagnosis of cancer and other diseases. Cell Res 18: 997–1006.
19. Calin GA, Dumitru CD, Shimizu M, Bichi R, Zupo S, et al. (2002) Frequent deletions and down-regulation of micro- RNA genes miR15 and miR16 at 13q14 in chronic lymphocytic leukemia. Proc Natl Acad Sci U S A 99: 15524–15529.
20. Ng EK, Chong WW, Jin H, Lam EK, Shin VY, et al. (2009) Differential expression of microRNAs in plasma of patients with colorectal cancer: a potential marker for colorectal cancer screening. Gut 58: 1375–1381.
21. Tsujiura M, Ichikawa D, Komatsu S, Shiozaki A, Takeshita H, et al. (2010) Circulating microRNAs in plasma of patients with gastric cancers. Br J Cancer 102: 1174–1179.
22. Zhang C, Wang C, Chen X, Yang C, Li K, et al. (2010) Expression profile of microRNAs in serum: a fingerprint for esophageal squamous cell carcinoma. Clin Chem 56: 1871–1879.
23. Heneghan HM, Miller N, Kelly R, Newell J, Kerin MJ (2010) Systemic miRNA-195 differentiates breast cancer from other malignancies and is a potential biomarker for detecting noninvasive and early stage disease. Oncologist 15: 673–682.
24. Keller A, Leidinger P, Borries A, Wendschlag A, Wucherpfennig F, et al. (2009) miRNAs in lung cancer - studying complex fingerprints in patient's blood cells by microarray experiments. BMC Cancer 9: 353.
25. Li LM, Hu ZB, Zhou ZX, Chen X, Liu FY, et al. (2010) Serum microRNA profiles serve as novel biomarkers for HBV infection and diagnosis of HBV-positive hepatocarcinoma. Cancer Res 70: 9798–9807.
26. Mitchell PS, Parkin RK, Kroh EM, Fritz BR, Wyman SK, et al. (2008) Circulating microRNAs as stable blood-based markers for cancer detection. Proc Natl Acad Sci U S A 105: 10513–10518.
27. Dillhoff M, Liu J, Frankel W, Croce C, Bloomston M (2008) MicroRNA-21 is overexpressed in pancreatic cancer and a potential predictor of survival. J Gastrointest Surg 12: 2171–2176.
28. Leeflang MM, Deeks JJ, Gatsonis C, Bossuyt PM (2008) Systematic reviews of diagnostic test accuracy. Ann Intern Med 149: 889–897.
29. Whiting PF, Rutjes AW, Westwood ME, Mallett S, Deeks JJ, et al. (2011) QUADAS-2: a revised tool for the quality assessment of diagnostic accuracy studies. Ann Intern Med 155: 529–536.
30. Deeks JJ (2001) Systematic reviews in health care: Systematic reviews of evaluations of diagnostic and screening tests. BMJ 323: 157–162.
31. Glas AS, Lijmer JG, Prins MH, Bonsel GJ, Bossuyt PM (2003) The diagnostic odds ratio: a single indicator of test performance. J Clin Epidemiol 56: 1129–1135.
32. Higgins JP, Thompson SG, Deeks JJ, Altman DG (2003) Measuring inconsistency in meta-analyses. BMJ 327: 557–560.
33. Jackson D, White IR, Thompson SG (2010) Extending DerSimonian and Laird's methodology to perform multivariate random effects meta-analyses. Stat Med 29: 1282–1297.

34. Deeks JJ, Macaskill P, Irwig L (2005) The performance of tests of publication bias and other sample size effects in systematic reviews of diagnostic test accuracy was assessed. J Clin Epidemiol 58: 882–893.
35. Zhou H, Guo JM, Lou YR, Zhang XJ, Zhong FD, et al. (2010) Detection of circulating tumor cells in peripheral blood from patients with gastric cancer using microRNA as a marker. J Mol Med (Berl) 88: 709–717.
36. Liu R, Zhang C, Hu Z, Li G, Wang C, et al. (2011) A five-microRNA signature identified from genome-wide serum microRNA expression profiling serves as a fingerprint for gastric cancer diagnosis. Eur J Cancer 47: 784–791.
37. Zheng Y, Cui L, Sun W, Zhou H, Yuan X, et al. (2011) MicroRNA-21 is a new marker of circulating tumor cells in gastric cancer patients. Cancer Biomark 10: 71–77.
38. Zhu CJ, Zhang JY, Wei J, Liu YQ, Shu YQ (2011) [MiR-191 and miR-29a in plasma are promising novel biomakers for detection of gastric cancer]. Acta Universitatis Medicinalis Nanjing(Natural Science) 31: 1173–1178.
39. Konishi H, Ichikawa D, Komatsu S, Shiozaki A, Tsujiura M, et al. (2012) Detection of gastric cancer-associated microRNAs on microRNA microarray comparing pre- and post-operative plasma. Br J Cancer 106: 740–747.
40. Li BS, Zhao YL, Guo G, Li W, Zhu ED, et al. (2012) Plasma microRNAs, miR-223, miR-21 and miR-218, as novel potential biomarkers for gastric cancer detection. PLoS One 7: e41629.
41. Li ZQ, Huang PW, Zhu CJ, Chen CP, Cheng T, et al. (2012) [Diagnostic value of expressions of miR-27a and miR-181b for early detection of gastric cancer]. Jiangsu Med J 38: 1665–1667.
42. Liu H, Zhu L, Liu B, Yang L, Meng X, et al. (2012) Genome-wide microRNA profiles identify miR-378 as a serum biomarker for early detection of gastric cancer. Cancer Lett 316: 196–203.
43. Song MY, Pan KF, Su HJ, Zhang L, Ma JL, et al. (2012) Identification of serum microRNAs as novel non-invasive biomarkers for early detection of gastric cancer. PLoS One 7: e33608.
44. Valladares-Ayerbes M, Reboredo M, Medina-Villaamil V, Iglesias-Diaz P, Lorenzo-Patino MJ, et al. (2012) Circulating miR-200c as a diagnostic and prognostic biomarker for gastric cancer. J Transl Med 10: 186.
45. Wang B, Zhang Q (2012) The expression and clinical significance of circulating microRNA-21 in serum of five solid tumors. J Cancer Res Clin Oncol 138: 1659–1666.
46. Zhou H, Xiao B, Zhou F, Deng H, Zhang X, et al. (2012) MiR-421 is a functional marker of circulating tumor cells in gastric cancer patients. Biomarkers 17: 104–110.
47. Cai H, Yuan Y, Hao YF, Guo TK, Wei X, et al. (2013) Plasma microRNAs serve as novel potential biomarkers for early detection of gastric cancer. Med Oncol 30: 452.
48. Li C, Li JF, Cai Q, Qiu QQ, Yan M, et al. (2013) miRNA-199a-3p in plasma as a potential diagnostic biomarker for gastric cancer. Ann Surg Oncol 20 Suppl 3: S397–405.
49. Sheinerman KS, Tsivinsky VG, Umansky SR (2013) Analysis of organ-enriched microRNAs in plasma as an approach to development of Universal Screening Test: feasibility study. J Transl Med 11: 304.
50. Shiotani A, Murao T, Kimura Y, Matsumoto H, Kamada T, et al. (2013) Identification of serum miRNAs as novel non-invasive biomarkers for detection of high risk for early gastric cancer. Br J Cancer 109: 2323–2330.
51. Xu Q, Dong QG, Sun LP, He CY, Yuan Y (2013) Expression of serum miR-20a-5p, let-7a, and miR-320a and their correlations with pepsinogen in atrophic gastritis and gastric cancer: a case-control study. BMC Clin Pathol 13: 11.
52. Chen Q, Ge X, Zhang Y, Xia H, Yuan D, et al. (2014) Plasma miR-122 and miR-192 as potential novel biomarkers for the early detection of distant metastasis of gastric cancer. Oncol Rep 31: 1863–1870.
53. Peng WZ, Ma R, Wang F, Yu J, Liu ZB (2014) Role of miR-191/425 Cluster in Tumorigenesis and Diagnosis of Gastric Cancer. Int J Mol Sci 15: 4031–4048.
54. Zhu C, Ren C, Han J, Ding Y, Du J, et al. (2014) A five-microRNA panel in plasma was identified as potential biomarker for early detection of gastric cancer. Br J Cancer.
55. Huang Z, Huang D, Ni S, Peng Z, Sheng W, et al. (2010) Plasma microRNAs are promising novel biomarkers for early detection of colorectal cancer. International Journal of Cancer 127: 118–126.
56. Pu XX, Huang GL, Guo HQ, Guo CC, Li H, et al. (2010) Circulating miR-221 directly amplified from plasma is a potential diagnostic and prognostic marker of colorectal cancer and is correlated with p53 expression. J Gastroenterol Hepatol 25: 1674–1680.
57. Liu HS, Ma YY, Xiao HS (2012) [The diagnostic value of serum microRNAs including miR-129-3p, miR-767-3p and miR-877* for colorectal cancer]. Tumor 32: 42–48.
58. Wang Q, Huang Z, Ni S, Xiao X, Xu Q, et al. (2012) Plasma miR-601 and miR-760 are novel biomarkers for the early detection of colorectal cancer. PLoS ONE 7: e44398.
59. Feng L, Pang Z, Sha S, Wu B, Xu F, et al. (2013) [The value of diagnosis and prognosis prediction of serum miR-29a and miR-92a for colorectal cancer]. Chin J Clin Oncol Rehabil: 1313–1315.
60. Giraldez MD, Lozano JJ, Ramirez G, Hijona E, Bujanda L, et al. (2013) Circulating MicroRNAs as biomarkers of colorectal cancer: Results from a genome-wide profiling and validation study. Clinical Gastroenterology and Hepatology 11: 681–688.e683.
61. Liu GH, Zhou ZG, Chen R, Wang MJ, Zhou B, et al. (2013) Serum miR-21 and miR-92a as biomarkers in the diagnosis and prognosis of colorectal cancer. Tumour Biol 34: 2175–2181.
62. Luo X, Stock C, Burwinkel B, Brenner H (2013) Identification and evaluation of plasma microRNAs for early detection of colorectal cancer. PLoS ONE 8: e62880.
63. Toiyama Y, Takahashi M, Hur K, Nagasaka T, Tanaka K, et al. (2013) Serum miR-21 as a diagnostic and prognostic biomarker in colorectal cancer. Journal of the National Cancer Institute 105: 849–859.
64. Wang S, Xiang J, Li Z, Lu S, Hu J, et al. (2013) A plasma microRNA panel for early detection of colorectal cancer. Int J Cancer.
65. Yong FL, Law CW, Wang CW (2013) Potentiality of a triple microRNA classifier: MiR-193a-3p, miR-23a and miR-338-5p for early detection of colorectal cancer. BMC Cancer 13.
66. Zhang GJ, Zhou T, Liu ZL, Tian HP, Xia SS (2013) Plasma miR-200c and miR-18a as potential biomarkers for the detection of colorectal carcinoma. Molecular and Clinical Oncology 1: 379–384.
67. Zanutto S, Pizzamiglio S, Ghilotti M, Bertan C, Ravagnani F, et al. (2014) Circulating miR-378 in plasma: a reliable, haemolysis-independent biomarker for colorectal cancer. Br J Cancer 110: 1001–1007.
68. Komatsu S, Ichikawa D, Takeshita H, Tsujiura M, Morimura R, et al. (2011) Circulating microRNAs in plasma of patients with oesophageal squamous cell carcinoma. Br J Cancer 105: 104–111.
69. Zhang T, Wang Q, Zhao D, Cui Y, Cao B, et al. (2011) The oncogenetic role of microRNA-31 as a potential biomarker in oesophageal squamous cell carcinoma. Clin Sci (Lond) 121: 437–447.
70. Hirajima S, Komatsu S, Ichikawa D, Takeshita H, Konishi H, et al. (2013) Clinical impact of circulating miR-18a in plasma of patients with oesophageal squamous cell carcinoma. Br J Cancer 108: 1822–1829.
71. Takeshita N, Hoshino I, Mori M, Akutsu Y, Hanari N, et al. (2013) Serum microRNA expression profile: miR-1246 as a novel diagnostic and prognostic biomarker for oesophageal squamous cell carcinoma. Br J Cancer 108: 644–652.
72. Zhang T, Zhao D, Wang Q, Yu X, Cui Y, et al. (2013) MicroRNA-1322 regulates ECRG2 allele specifically and acts as a potential biomarker in patients with esophageal squamous cell carcinoma. Mol Carcinog 52: 581–590.
73. Redova M, Sana J, Slaby O (2013) Circulating miRNAs as new blood-based biomarkers for solid cancers. Future Oncol 9: 387–402.
74. Shen J, Stass SA, Jiang F (2013) MicroRNAs as potential biomarkers in human solid tumors. Cancer Lett 329: 125–136.
75. Lawrie CH, Gal S, Dunlop HM, Pushkaran B, Liggins AP, et al. (2008) Detection of elevated levels of tumour-associated microRNAs in serum of patients with diffuse large B-cell lymphoma. Br J Haematol 141: 672–675.
76. Sita-Lumsden A, Dart DA, Waxman J, Bevan CL (2013) Circulating microRNAs as potential new biomarkers for prostate cancer. Br J Cancer 108: 1925–1930.
77. Zen K, Zhang CY (2012) Circulating MicroRNAs: A novel class of biomarkers to diagnose and monitor human cancers. Medicinal Research Reviews 32: 326–348.

Permissions

All chapters in this book were first published in PLOS ONE, by The Public Library of Science; hereby published with permission under the Creative Commons Attribution License or equivalent. Every chapter published in this book has been scrutinized by our experts. Their significance has been extensively debated. The topics covered herein carry significant findings which will fuel the growth of the discipline. They may even be implemented as practical applications or may be referred to as a beginning point for another development.

The contributors of this book come from diverse backgrounds, making this book a truly international effort. This book will bring forth new frontiers with its revolutionizing research information and detailed analysis of the nascent developments around the world.

We would like to thank all the contributing authors for lending their expertise to make the book truly unique. They have played a crucial role in the development of this book. Without their invaluable contributions this book wouldn't have been possible. They have made vital efforts to compile up to date information on the varied aspects of this subject to make this book a valuable addition to the collection of many professionals and students.

This book was conceptualized with the vision of imparting up-to-date information and advanced data in this field. To ensure the same, a matchless editorial board was set up. Every individual on the board went through rigorous rounds of assessment to prove their worth. After which they invested a large part of their time researching and compiling the most relevant data for our readers.

The editorial board has been involved in producing this book since its inception. They have spent rigorous hours researching and exploring the diverse topics which have resulted in the successful publishing of this book. They have passed on their knowledge of decades through this book. To expedite this challenging task, the publisher supported the team at every step. A small team of assistant editors was also appointed to further simplify the editing procedure and attain best results for the readers.

Apart from the editorial board, the designing team has also invested a significant amount of their time in understanding the subject and creating the most relevant covers. They scrutinized every image to scout for the most suitable representation of the subject and create an appropriate cover for the book.

The publishing team has been an ardent support to the editorial, designing and production team. Their endless efforts to recruit the best for this project, has resulted in the accomplishment of this book. They are a veteran in the field of academics and their pool of knowledge is as vast as their experience in printing. Their expertise and guidance has proved useful at every step. Their uncompromising quality standards have made this book an exceptional effort. Their encouragement from time to time has been an inspiration for everyone.

The publisher and the editorial board hope that this book will prove to be a valuable piece of knowledge for researchers, students, practitioners and scholars across the globe.

List of Contributors

Mengling Tang, Kun Chen, Fangxing Yang and Weiping Liu
MOE Key Laboratory of Environmental Remediation and Ecosystem Health, College of Environmental and Resource Sciences, Zhejiang University, Hangzhou, China
Department of Epidemiology & Health Statistics, School of Public Health, Zhejiang University, Hangzhou, China

Thomas Boillot
Clinique Vétérinaire Vetea, Saintes, France

Serge G. Rosolen
INSERM, U968, Institut de la Vision, Paris, France
Sorbonne Universite´ s, UPMC Univ Paris 06, UMR_S 968, Institut de la Vision, Paris, France
CNRS, UMR 7210, Institut de la Vision, Paris, France
Clinique Veterinaire Voltaire, Asnie`res sur Seine, France

Thomas Dulauren and Pierre-François Isard
Centre Hospitalier Veterinaire Saint-Martin, Saint-Martin de Bellevue, France

Frédéric Goulle
Clinique Veterinaire Aquivet, Eysines, France

Philippe Thomas
Clinique Veterinaire Saint-Pierre, Saint-Chamond, France

Thierry Azoulay
Clinique Veterinaire des Halles, Strasbourg, France

Stéphanie Lafarge-Beurlet
Vébio, Arcueil, France

Mike Woods
Pimrose Hill Veterinary Clinic, Dun Laoghaire, Co. Dublin, Ireland

Sylvie Lavillegrand
Clinique Veterinaire Voltaire, Asniéres sur Seine, France

Ivana Ivkovic and Nicolas Froger
INSERM, U968, Institut de la Vision, Paris, France
Sorbonne Universités, UPMC Univ Paris 06, UMR_S 968, Institut de la Vision, Paris, France
CNRS, UMR 7210, Institut de la Vision, Paris, France

Nathalie Neveux
Department of Nutrition, Faculty of Pharmacy, Paris Descartes University, Paris, France
Clinical Chemistry, Hôtel-Dieu-Cochin Hospitals, AP-HP, Paris, France

José -Alain Sahel
INSERM, U968, Institut de la Vision, Paris, France
Sorbonne Universite´ s, UPMC Univ Paris 06, UMR_S 968, Institut de la Vision, Paris, France
CNRS, UMR 7210, Institut de la Vision, Paris, France
Fondation Ophtalmologique Adolphe de Rothschild, Paris, France
Centre hospitalier d9ophtalmologie des Quize-Vingts, Paris, France
University College London, London, United Kingdom

Serge Picaud
INSERM, U968, Institut de la Vision, Paris, France
Sorbonne Universités, UPMC Univ Paris 06, UMR_S 968, Institut de la Vision, Paris, France
CNRS, UMR 7210, Institut de la Vision, Paris, France

Hyunsoo Kim and Jiyoung Park
Department of Biomedical Sciences, Seoul National University College of Medicine, Seoul, Republic of Korea

Kyunggon Kim and Jonghwa Jin
Department of Biomedical Engineering, Seoul National University College of Medicine, Seoul, Republic of Korea

Jung-Hwan Yoon and Su Jong Yu
Department of Internal Medicine, Seoul National University College of Medicine, Seoul, Republic of Korea

Youngsoo Kim
Department of Biomedical Sciences, Seoul National University College of Medicine, Seoul, Republic of Korea

Department of Biomedical Engineering, Seoul National University College of Medicine, Seoul, Republic of Korea

Sigrid Hatse, Barbara Brouwers, Patrick Schöffski and Hans Wildiers
Laboratory of Experimental Oncology (LEO), Department of Oncology, KU Leuven, and Department of General Medical Oncology, University Hospitals Leuven, Leuven Cancer Institute, Leuven, Belgium

Bruna Dalmasso
Laboratory of Experimental Oncology (LEO), Department of Oncology, KU Leuven, and Department of General Medical Oncology, University Hospitals Leuven, Leuven Cancer Institute, Leuven, Belgium
Department of Internal Medicine, Istituto di Ricerca a Carattere Clinico e Scientifico (IRCCS), Azienda Ospedaliera Universitaria (AOU) San Martino Istituto Nazionale Tumori (IST), Genoa, Italy

Annouschka Laenen
Interuniversity Centre for Biostatistics and Statistical Bioinformatics, Leuven, Belgium

Cindy Kenis
Laboratory of Experimental Oncology (LEO), Department of Oncology, KU Leuven, and Department of General Medical Oncology, University Hospitals Leuven, Leuven Cancer Institute, Leuven, Belgium
Department of Geriatric Medicine, University Hospitals Leuven, Leuven, Belgium

Joo Myung Lee, Jonghanne Park, Ki-Hyun Jeon, Ji-hyun Jung, Sang Eun Lee, Jung-Kyu Han, Han-Mo Yang, Kyung Woo Park, Hyun-Jae Kang and Bon-Kwon Koo
Department of Internal Medicine and Cardiovascular Center, Seoul National University Hospital, Seoul, Korea

Hyo-Soo Kim
Department of Internal Medicine and Cardiovascular Center, Seoul National University Hospital, Seoul, Korea
Department of Molecular Medicine and Biopharmaceutical Sciences, Graduate School of Convergence
Science and Technology, Seoul National University, Seoul, Korea

Sang-Ho Jo
Division of Cardiology, Department of Internal Medicine, Hallym University Sacred Heart Hospital, Anyang-si, Gyeonggi-do, Korea

Hack-Lyoung Kim
Cardiovascular Center, Seoul National University, Boramae Medical Center, Seoul, Korea

Tomoko Yamazaki, Mayumi Mori, Satoko Arai, Akemi Nishijima, Toshihiro Kai and Kayo Aoyama
Laboratory of Molecular Biomedicine for Pathogenesis, Center for Disease Biology and Integrative
Medicine, Faculty of Medicine, The University of Tokyo, Tokyo, Japan

Ryosuke Tateishi and azuhiko Koike
Department of Gastroenterology, Graduate School of Medicine, The University of Tokyo, Tokyo, Japan

Masanori Abe and Yoichi Hiasa
Department of Gastroenterology and Metabology, Ehime University Graduate School of Medicine, Ehime, Japan

Mihoko Ban, Maki Maeda, Shinji Seto, Kiyohiro Izumino, Jun Takahashi and Ken-ichiro Inoue
Shunkaikai, Inoue Hospital, Nagasaki, Japan

Takeharu Asano and Yukio Yoshida
Department of Gastroenterology, Jichi Medical University, Saitama Medical Center, Omiya, Japan

Sei Harada and Toru Takebayashi
Department of Preventive Medicine and Public Health, School of Medicine, Keio University, Tokyo, Japan

Toshiaki Gunji
Center for Preventive Medicine, NTT Medical Center Tokyo, Tokyo, Japan

Shin Ohnishi
National Center for Global Health and Medicine, Tokyo, Japan

Ken-ichi Yamamura
Center for Animal Resources and Development, Kumamoto University, Kumamoto, Japan

Toru Miyazaki
Laboratory of Molecular Biomedicine for Pathogenesis, Center for Disease Biology and Integrative

Medicine, Faculty of Medicine, The University of Tokyo, Tokyo, Japan
Max Planck-The University of Tokyo Center for Integrative Inflammology, Tokyo, Japan
CREST, Japan Science and Technology Agency, Tokyo, Japan

Irina Gromova and Pavel Gromov
Danish Cancer Society Research Center, Genome Integrity Unit, Copenhagen, Denmark

Jaime A. Espinoza
Department of Pathology, Center for Investigation in Translational Oncology (CITO), School of Medicine, Pontificia Universidad Católica de Chile, Santiago, Chile

Maj-Lis Talman and Vera Timmermans Wielenga
Department of Pathology, the Centre of Diagnostic Investigations, Copenhagen University Hospital, Copenhagen, Denmark

Naoko Honma
Research Team for Geriatric Pathology, Tokyo Metropolitan Institute of Gerontology, Tokyo, Japan

Niels Kroman
Department of Breast Surgery, Copenhagen University Hospital, Copenhagen, Denmark

José M. A. Moreira
Section of Molecular Disease Biology and Sino-Danish Breast Cancer Research Centre, Department of Veterinary Disease Biology, Faculty of Health and Medical Sciences, University of Copenhagen, Copenhagen, Denmark

Daniel M. Pearlman
Neuroinflammation Research Group, Epilepsy Center Division, Department of Neurology, NYU School of Medicine, New York, New York, United States of America
The Dartmouth Institute for Health Policy and Clinical Practice, Audrey and Theodor Geisel School of Medicine at Dartmouth, Hanover, New Hampshire, United States of America

Jeremiah R. Brown and Todd A. MacKenzie
The Dartmouth Institute for Health Policy and Clinical Practice, Audrey and Theodor Geisel School of Medicine at Dartmouth, Hanover, New Hampshire, United States of America
Section of Epidemiology and Biostatistics, Department of Community and Family Medicine, Audrey and Theodor Geisel School of Medicine at Dartmouth, Hanover, New Hampshire, United States of America
Section of Cardiology, Department of Medicine, Audrey and Theodor Geisel School of Medicine at Dartmouth, Hanover, New Hampshire, United States of America

Felix Hernandez Jr.
Cardiothoracic Surgery, Eastern Maine Medical Center, Bangor, Maine, United States of America

Souhel Najjar
Neuroinflammation Research Group, Epilepsy Center Division, Department of Neurology, NYU School of Medicine, New York, New York, United States of America

Mohamed Diwan M. AbdulHameed, Gregory J. Tawa, Kamal Kumar and Anders Wallqvist
Department of Defense Biotechnology High Performance Computing Software Applications Institute, Telemedicine and Advanced Technology Research Center, U.S. Army Medical Research and Materiel Command, Fort Detrick, Maryland, United States of America

Danielle L. Ippolito, John A. Lewis and Jonathan D. Stallings
U.S. Army Center for Environmental Health Research, Fort Detrick, MD, United States of America

Annette M. Hormann, Frederick S. vom Saal, Richard W. Stahlhut, Carol L. Moyer and Julia A. Taylor
Division of Biological Sciences, University of Missouri, Columbia, Missouri, United States of America

Susan C. Nagel
Department of Obstetrics, Gynecology and Women's Health,nUniversity of Missouri, Columbia, Missouri, United States of America

Mark R. Ellersieck
Department of Statistics, University of Missouri, Columbia, Missouri, United States of America

Wade V. Welshons
Department of Biomedical Sciences, University of Missouri, Columbia, Missouri, United States of America

Pierre-Louis Toutain
Universitè de Toulouse, INPT, ENVT, UPS, UMR1331, F- 31062 Toulouse, France
INRA, UMR1331, Toxalim, Research Centre in Food Toxicology, F-31027 Toulouse, France

Wouter Wegdam, Marrije R. Buist, Gemma G. Kenter and Danielle Meijer
Department of Gynecology, Academic Medical Center, University of Amsterdam, Amsterdam, the Netherlands

Carmen A. Argmann
Department of Genetics and Genomic Sciences, Icahn Institute for Genomics and Multiscale Biology, Icahn School of Medicine at Mount Sinai, New York, New York, United States of America

Gertjan Kramer, Johannes M. F. G. Aerts
Clinical Proteomics Group, Department of Medical Biochemistry, Academic Medical Center, University of Amsterdam, Amsterdam, the Netherlands

Johannes P. Vissers
Waters Corporation MS Technologies Center, Manchester, United Kingdom

Perry D. Moerland
Bioinformatics Laboratory, Department of Clinical Epidemiology, Biostatistics and Bioinformatics, Academic Medical Center, University of Amsterdam, Amsterdam, the Netherlands

Paul R. West, Alan M. Smith, Laura A. Egnash, Mark E. Ross, Jessica A. Palmer, Burr R. Fontaine, Kevin R. Conard, Gabriela G. Cezar, Elizabeth L. R. Donley and Robert E. Burrier
Stemina Biomarker Discovery, Madison, Wisconsin, United States of America

David G. Amaral
The M.I.N.D. Institute and Department of Psychiatry and Behavioral Sciences, University of California Davis, Davis, California, United States of America

Preeti Bais
The Jackson Laboratory for Genomic medicine, University of Connecticut Health Center, Farmington, Connecticut, United States of America

Blythe A. Corbett
Department of Psychiatry, Psychology and Kennedy Center, Vanderbilt University, Nashville, Tennessee, United States of America

Bo Yang
Department of Preventive Medicine, Wenzhou Medical University, Wenzhou, China

Duo Li and Feng-Lei Wang
Department of Food Science and Nutrition, Zhejiang University, Hangzhou, China

Xiao-Li Ren
Medical Laboratory Animal Center, Wenzhou Medical University, Wenzhou, China

Mohammad Azhar Aziz, Ibrahim AlAbdulkarim, Majed Al Otaibi, Abdulaziz Alfahed and Glowi Alasiri
Medical Genomics, King Abdullah International Medical Research Center, Riyadh, Saudi Arabia

Sathish Periyasamy
Bioinformatics, King Abdullah International Medical Research Center, Riyadh, Saudi Arabia

Zeyad Al Yousef
Surgery, National Guard Health Affairs, Riyadh, Saudi Arabia

Nicola Antonio Martino and Maria Elena Dell'Aquila
Department of Emergency and Organ Transplantation (DETO) - Section of Veterinary Clinics and Animal Productions, University of Bari Aldo Moro, Valenzano, Bari, Italy

Stephan Joel Reshkin and Elena Ciani
Department of Biosciences, Biotechnologies and Biopharmaceutics (DBBB), University Campus "Ernesto Quagliariello" University of Bari Aldo Moro, Bari, Italy

Lejla Alic
Biomedical Imaging Group Rotterdam, Department of Radiology and Medical Informatics, Erasmus Medical Center Rotterdam, Rotterdam, The Netherlands
Department of Intelligent Imaging, Netherlands Organization for Applied Scientific Research (TNO), The Hague, The Netherlands

Wiro J. Niessen
Biomedical Imaging Group Rotterdam, Department of Radiology and Medical Informatics, Erasmus Medical Center Rotterdam, Rotterdam, The Netherlands

Imaging Physics, Faculty of Applied Sciences, Delft University of Technology, Delft, The Netherlands

Jifke F. Veenland
Biomedical Imaging Group Rotterdam, Department of Radiology and Medical Informatics, Erasmus Medical Center Rotterdam, Rotterdam, The Netherlands

Ran Wang
Department of Gastroenterology, Nanfang Hospital, Southern Medical University, Guangzhou, China
Department of Ultrasound, HuiZhou Municipal Central Hospital, Huizhou, China

Hong Wen, Qiulan Chen, Yi Luo, Yiqin Lin and Yu Luo
Department of Ultrasound, HuiZhou Municipal Central Hospital, Huizhou, China

Yongcheng Xu
Department of Gastroenterology, HuiZhou Municipal Central Hospital, Huizhou, China

Angao Xu
Department of Gastroenterology, Nanfang Hospital, Southern Medical University, Guangzhou, China
Department of Gastroenterology, HuiZhou Municipal Central Hospital, Huizhou, China

Index